Resources for Nursing Research

An Annotated Bibliography

Fourth Edition

CYNTHIA G L CLAMP
STEPHEN GOUGH
and
LUCY LAND

Sage Publications
London • Thousand Oaks • New Delhi

SAGE Publications Ltd
1 Oliver's Yard
55 City Road
London EC1Y 1SP

SAGE Publications Inc.
2455 Teller Road
Thousand Oaks, California 91320

SAGE Publications India Pvt Ltd
B-42, Panchsheel Enclave
Post Box 4109
New Delhi 110 017

British Library Cataloguing in Publication data

A catalogue record for this book is available from the British
Library

ISBN 0 7619 4991 7

Library of Congress Control Number available: 2003115353

Typeset by C&M Digitals (P) Ltd., Chennai, India
Printed in India at Gopsons Papers Ltd, Noida

This book is dedicated to the memory of Lisbeth Hockey – an outstanding nurse, researcher and a very special friend.

Contents

Foreword

At the time of writing , I regret that Lisbeth Hockey is unable to share this virtual podium with me. She has been an indispensable source of inspiration and support for many a nurse researcher and, I believe, for this extraordinary reference work. Just as Lisbeth's career maps in microcosm many elements of the history of nursing research in the UK, so this book reflects the expansion and shifting boundaries of research in nursing. The volume is unique in the sense of providing a historical record and reference point for analysing 'growth areas', through the development of research resources and categories over time. Each edition brings with it an even more encyclopaedic reach and range of material.

The beauty of this book is not a blinding blizzard of detail but a well tried and tested taxonomy. Within the information-rich era in which we live, skills in accessing and the utilization of information come to the fore. To have assembled and synthesized the myriad entries within this single volume reflects an achievement of significant magnitude and commitment. One may wonder whether this accelerated age justifies the publication of a resource in paper form? Such doubts will be dispelled since this 'route map' through the disciplinary highways and by-ways of research still has much to offer the would-be and seasoned researcher. Not surprisingly, the section on electronic sources has been expanded and others updated. New material from a range of countries, including China, poised to become an increasingly important player in international health care, has been added.

The signpost approach adopted helps to take the 'sting' out of searching for those new to the field as well as leading the reader on an investigative trail that points the path from 'novice to expert'. The result of a creative collaboration between a librarian and two nurse researchers, an attempt is made to address different audiences' needs in the text. The international dimension provides a further index of the topical and methodological interests and investments in nursing research over time. Many useful pointers are provided on policy and funding opportunities, frameworks, career structures and contexts that can make or break research. This book helps the researcher access information and take the first steps towards turning it into useful knowledge. I commend this text to you.

Anne Marie Rafferty DPhil (Oxon) RGN DN

Acknowledgements

Many relatives, friends and colleagues have assisted in the development of this resource book and we would like to record our sincere thanks to them all. I would like to express gratitude to my two co-authors, and especially to Stephen, whose patience, thoughtfulness and support in times of difficulty have made this new edition possible.

Anne Marie Rafferty, an outstanding British researcher, has kindly written the foreword and we appreciate this very much. To have her endorsement is praise indeed.

Thanks also go to Raymond Poland, and David and Stuart Land, Phillipa Jordan and Fiona Bantock. Stephen Gough sends a particular thank you and much love to Tricia O'Connor and Kyle for all their help, and to Calum. We are also grateful to the many librarians who have assisted us.

The staff at Sage Publications have been very supportive and we wish to thank Rachel Burrows, Sarah Bury, Alison Poyner and Louise Wise.

Introduction

The fourth edition of this annotated bibliography provides a guide to sources of literature, papers, books and Internet resources on research methodology and the background to research in nursing. It is designed to complement existing texts on research methods and to act as a 'signpost' to available literature, mainly from the disciplines of nursing, medicine and the social sciences. It is intended for all those with an interest in nursing research – students, teachers, librarians, practitioners and researchers.

The Internet and many databases have been used to find the literature included here, but the authors believe that there is value in having available in one place, in book form, references to literature covering the whole span of research methodology and its use, particularly for the novice researcher and those in clinical practice.

The book includes just under 3,000 entries, 70 per cent of which are new, and these cite literature published since 1998. Many websites are included throughout the text for nurses to continue their own searching. The criteria for inclusion are current usage, focus and relevance.

The book is divided into: Part 1: Sources of literature, Part 2: Methods of inquiry, and Part 3: The background to research in nursing, with author and subject indexes at the end of the book. Details of the book's structure, format and numbering system are explained on the following page in 'How to use this book'.

The entries have been extensively cross-referenced, and in addition examples are given in most sections where a particular element of the research process has been used. Definitions relating to each element are also included from published sources (Appendix D).

All books have been checked for the latest editions but not all remain in print. Material on research methods can date slowly and in some instances has not been superseded. The number of entries varies considerably between sections and this largely reflects the state of the literature. Because of the increasing amount of literature on research methods now available, the authors have tried to select a broad spread from which readers may then pursue their own areas of interest.

The varying amount of literature included from around the world largely reflects the length of time in which nurses have been learning about research in their educational programmes. An almost equal proportion of the citations are from Britain and the United States. Literature from Australia, Canada, China, Europe, India, New Zealand, South Africa and South America is also included.

Based on comments from users of previous editions, it is clear that the book can be used in a variety of ways, e.g. as a conventional bibliography and as a dictionary. It also provides an overview of research processes that teachers may like to use as part of a course, and suggests possible collection development strategies for librarians.

The authors hope that use of this book will save time during the literature searching process by giving pointers to existing material. It will also assist nurses to develop skills in evaluating and perhaps undertaking research studies for the benefit of their patients.

How to Use this Book

INDEXES

There are two indexes in this book, author and subject, which will be found at the end. At the beginning an expanded contents list will enable readers to see its structure and quickly find the relevant sections.

STRUCTURE OF THE BOOK

The book is divided into three major parts:

Part 1   Sources of literature
Part 2   Methods of inquiry
Part 3   The background to research in nursing

FORMAT OF SECTIONS

The format of each section follows a similar pattern, although not all sections include each item. Entries are listed in alphabetical order.

Title
Introductory statement
Definition(s)
Example

Major text/article [specific to sub-section]

Annotations

NUMBERING SYSTEM

The numbering system used in the book should enable items to be found easily.

Part 1   items are numbered   1.1 to 1.7
Part 2   items are numbered   2.1 to 2.102
Part 3   items are numbered   3.1 to 3.22

Within each section entries have individual numbers, e.g. 1.1.1, 2.1.2 or 3.1.3 and this number is also used in the cross-referencing system.

CROSS-REFERENCING SYSTEM

Many books and articles contain information that comes under several headings in the book. Where this occurs other item reference number(s) are given at the end of the annotation so that further relevant entries can be found. The number may indicate a whole section, e.g. CR 2.15, or a particular annotation, e.g. CR 2.15.6. In general cross-referencing has not been done within sections as so many items relate to each other.

NOTES

Every effort has been made to ensure the accuracy of entries, but the authors would be pleased to know of any errors.

British English has been used throughout the text, except in book and journal titles, in order to achieve consistency.

The authors' policy has been to see most of the books and articles and these have been annotated. In a few instances this has not been possible, but the bibliographical data is included so that readers can still follow up the reference.

Where website addresses (URLs or Uniform Resource Locators) have been included, they were correct at the time of going to press.

PART 1: SOURCES OF LITERATURE

Literature Searching and Libraries

1.1 LIBRARIES

The purpose of this section is to highlight major health care or nursing library resources as well as materials which describe particular collections and the use of libraries in general. It is not an exhaustive list.

Annotations

1.1.1 Akinsanya, J. (1984) Learning about nursing research. *Nursing Times* 80 (16) 59–61 Occasional Paper 10 References

Describes a small-scale survey of theses and dissertations in the Steinberg Collection at the Royal College of Nursing, London. The study, carried out by Diploma in Nursing students, aimed to show the range and scope of nursing literature in this collection.

1.1.2 Coffman, S. (1999) Nursing bites and bytes: the Virginia Henderson International Nursing Library. *Australian Journal of Advanced Nursing* 16 (3) 30

1.1.3 Dale, P. (ed.) (2000) *Guide to libraries and information sources in medicine and health care* (3rd edition). London: British Library. ISBN 0712308563

Provides basic information on individual libraries plus the major literature-searching services and sources.

1.1.4 eLSC (electronic Library for Social Care) www.elsc.org.uk

The eLSC enables access to research, training in the skills needed to understand and critically appraise research and the tools required to use the research in practice. It hosts the Caredata database.

1.1.5 NeLH (National electronic Library for Health) www.nelh.nhs.uk

The role of the NeLH is to provide health care professionals and the public with a focal resource in the decision-making process. As well as original material, it also links to such resources as the Cochrane Library.

1.1.6 NLM (United States National Library of Medicine) www.nlm.nih.gov

The United States National Library of Medicine is a comprehensive collection of health care-related materials and services and should be seen as an international resource. Services include a range of databases, including Medline, and the PubMed and NLM Gateway search interfaces.

1.1.7 NN/LM (United States National Network of Libraries of Medicine) nnlm.gov/

A web-based directory that lists United States libraries with health care collections. It is fully searchable.

1.1.8 Osborne, H. (2001) In other words … Finding the information you need at a medical library. *On-Call* 4 (9) 30–1

Discusses the services provided by medical libraries.

1.1.9 Phillips, R. (2001) How to … make the most of your library. *MIDIRS Midwifery Digest* 11(2) 288

A brief guide to library services.

1.1.10 Root, J.A. (2001) Virginia Henderson International Nursing Library. Finding nursing research: it just got easier. *Reflections on Nursing Leadership* 27 (2) 48

A brief overview of the services provided by the Virginia Henderson International Nursing Library.

1.1.11 Shepherd, T. (1996) The RCN Library at your service. *Paediatric Nursing* 8 (8) 11

An overview guide to the services of the Royal College of Nursing. This is a subscription service based on membership of the Royal College of Nursing.

1.1.12 Strauch, K.P. (ed.) (1992) *Library Research Guide to Nursing.* Ann Arbor, MI: Pierian Press. ISBN 0876502532

This book is designed to identify a variety of current materials in nursing, how to locate and evaluate them easily and quickly. Features include: comprehensive listing of general reference sources, annotated lists of nursing literature organized by subject, separate listings of periodicals related to nursing, a list of audio-visual material and names and addresses of publishers.

1.1.13 Thomas, J. (2000) Library resources and getting the best out of them. *British Journal of Perioperative Nursing* 10 (2) 90–3   5 References

Discusses the use of libraries as gateways to information and how to get the most from them.

1.1.14 Virginia Henderson International Nursing Library www.stti.iupui.edu/library/

The Virginia Henderson International Nursing Library is a major collection of nursing resources and includes the *Online Journal of Knowledge Synthesis for Nursing and Registry of Nursing Research.* With the exception of the Registry of Nursing Research, it is a subscription service.

1.2 LITERATURE SEARCHING

This section includes material which describes the process of literature searching as well as documents on particular services, strategies and techniques.

Annotations

1.2.1 Allen, M. & Levy, J. (2002) Evidence-based searching for nursing and allied health. *Bibliotheca Medica Canadiana* 23 (3) 90–5   27 References

Reviews literature searching, looking at a wide range of sources and techniques.

1.2.2 Anonymous (1996) Literature searches: part 3. *Practice Nurse* 11 (1) 35–7   1 Reference

Describes how to organize a search of the literature.

1.2.3 Anonymous (2000) For the enquiring mind. Guidelines for conducting a literature search. *Cannt Journal* 10 (3) 57

General guidelines for conducting a search of the literature.

1.2.4 Anonymous (2001) HealthWeb – evidence-based health care. *Library of the Health Sciences at Chicago, University of Illinois at Chicago*

Description of the HealthWeb Gateway in relation to evidence-based practice.

1.2.5 Anonymous (2001) Internet basics. Does Medline give you much too much information? These tips will keep you from drowning in data. *Internet Medicine* 6 (11) 1, 6

Medline is a vast database which, for the inexperienced searcher, can be overwhelming. This article describes the use of filters and other devices to limit the search results to those of direct use.

1.2.6 Anonymous (2001) Search solutions. Cited reference searches in Dialog: how to find articles that cite a given author. *Chronolog* 10

Citation searching can be an important tool in gathering information. This article describes using the Dialog database search interface to identify cited authors.

1.2.7 Avenell, A., Handoll, H.H.G. & Grant, A.M. (2001) Lessons for search strategies from a systematic review, in the Cochrane Library, of nutritional supplementation trials in patients after hip fracture. *American Journal of Clinical Nutrition* 73 (3) 505–10   29 References

Using the example of a systematic review for the Cochrane Library, this article analyses the search strategy and concludes that a reliance on a narrow focus of database sources is inadequate.

1.2.8 Bachmann, L.M., Coray, R., Estermann, P. & ter Riet, G. (2002) Identifying diagnostic studies in MEDLINE: reducing the number needed to read. *Journal of the American Informatics Association* 9 (6) 653–8   11 References

An analysis of the use of the diagnostic studies filter in PubMed. It also proposes an alternative.

1.2.9 Barnsteiner, J.H. (1994) The Online Journal of Knowledge Synthesis for Nursing. *Reflections* 20 (2) 10–11

A description of the journal, one of the first in nursing to be exclusively available on the Internet.

1.2.10 Barroso, J., Gollop, C.J., Sandelowski, M., Meynell, J., Pearce, P.F. & Collins, L.J. (2003) The challenges of searching for and retrieving qualitative studies. *Western Journal of Nursing Research* 25 (2) 153–78   29 References

Although aimed specifically at developing literature searches for conducting qualitative meta-synthesis studies, the strategies used demonstrate clearly the need for cross-database and format investigation to produce a near comprehensive result. The article includes a very useful table covering several of the major databases and gives some indication of their coverage.

1.2.11 Bechtel, G.A. & Cosey, E.J. (2000) Technology. Using electronic resources for a thorough nursing literature search. *Nurse Author & Editor* 10 (4) 4, 7–8

Looks at the use of CINAHL, Medline and other health care databases and the World Wide Web for conducting literature searches.

1.2.12 Behm, K. & Baier, M. (1998) News, notes & tips. Evaluating online literature searches. *Nurse Educator* 23 (2) 9–10

Looks at the techniques researchers can use to ensure that their literature search using electronic resources such as CINAHL and Medline has been comprehensive.

1.2.13 Benner, J. (1997) Nursing the Net. Researching health care topics on the Internet. *Nursing* 27 (9) 28–9

A brief guide to searching for specific topics on the Internet.

1.2.14 Benton, N. (2002) Health Services and Science Research Resources (HSRR) Database. *NLM Technical Bulletin* (329) www.nlm.nih.gov/pubs/techbull/tb.html

Provides a brief introduction to the HSRR and a description of the type and content of the different records that can be found there.

1.2.15 Bereczki, D. & Gesztelyi, G. (2000) A Hungarian example for hand searching specialized national health care journals of small countries for controlled trials. Is it worth the trouble? *Health Libraries Review* 17 (3) 144–7   24 References

The authors objective was to determine whether any clinical trials were reported that were not also indexed by Medline or reported on in Medline-indexed publications. Their conclusion was that to obtain a comprehensive controlled trials register, specialized health care journals with low print runs, from smaller countries should be included.

1.2.16 Booth, A. (1991) The place of CINAHL within the British context. *Health Libraries Review* 8 (4) 220–3

Highlights the differences in terminology and organizational practice which affect search strategies in Britain when executed on a database from North America. Many of the points made highlight the evolutionary nature of technical language and variations in practice (some cultural) and are equally applicable in the wider international health care community.

1.2.17 Brown, C.M. (1998) The benefits of searching EMBASE versus MEDLINE for pharmaceutical information. *Online & Cdrom Review* 22 (1) 3–8

Demonstrates the difference in search results from using the same strategy on two apparently similar databases.

1.2.18 Burnard, P. (1993) Facilities for searching the literature and storing references. *Nurse Researcher* 1 (1) 56–63   4 References

Discusses the use of computers to search for references and store bibliographical information.

1.2.19 Burr, B. & Kautzmann, A.M. (1998) Web versus CD-ROM: format follows function. *Searcher: The Magazine for Database Professionals* 6 (1) 59–63   11 References

The choice between CD-ROM and Internet-based services is becoming less easy to make. This article highlights the differences based on their functions.

1.2.20 Canese, K. (2003) New Entrez Database: MeSH. *NLM Technical Bulletin* (331) www.nlm.nih.gov/pubs/techbull/tb.html

MeSH subject searches can be considerably eased if MeSH is used effectively. This article explains how to use the Entrez MeSH database to find the best subject terms to use in a search.

1.2.21 Coma, I., Campmany, I., Montcusi, I. & Puig, C. (1997) Reference sources for journal articles: CINAHL database (Spanish). *Enfermeria Clinica* 7 (1) 39–41   2 References

An explanation of the CINAHL database and how it may be accessed.

1.2.22 Coma, I., Campmany, I., Sanchez, R.D. & Puig, C.M. (1999) Sources of information for nursing: comparison between CINAHL and MEDLINE databases (Spanish). *Metas de Enfermeria* 2 (14) 21–7   4 References

A direct comparison of the two databases, indicating their strengths and weaknesses.

1.2.23 Davies, R. (2001) Sources of information for nurses on the Internet. *Nursing & Residential Care* 3 (1) 21–4, 40–1   2 References

A discussion of some of the issues which need to be considered when searching the Internet and suggests some strategies for searching.

1.2.24 Demsey, A. (2001) Hands on: sending NLM Gateway results via email. *NLM. Technical Bulletin* (323) www.nlm.nih.gov/pubs/techbull/tb.html

Although not strictly a feature of searching the literature, this Bulletin does point to one feature which can make searching a little easier. Several database services now offer an email option.

1.2.25 Demsey, A. & Shoosan, S. (2003) Access to ClinicalTrials.gov in the NLM Gateway. *NLM Technical Bulletin* (330) www.nlm.nih.gov/pubs/ techbull/tb.html

An overview of how to search ClinicalTrials.gov using the NLM Gateway.

1.2.26 DeZelar-Tiedman, C. (1997) Known item searching on the World Wide Web. *Internet Reference Services Quarterly* 2 (1) 5–14

A comparison of search engine effectiveness using a known item as the test.

1.2.27 Dollar, D.M. (2001) Using the National Library of Medicine's PubMed to improve clinical practice. *Clinical Excellence for Nurse Practitioners* 5 (2) 119–24   1 Reference

Strategies and tips for searching PubMed.

1.2.28 Drabenstott, K.M. (2001) Web search strategy development. *Online* 25 (4) 18–20, 22–4, 26–7   11 References

Searching the World Wide Web can be a confusing and intricate process. This article seeks to show how to develop strategies for effective searching.

1.2.29 Fain, J.A. (2001) Using the Internet to support evidence-based practice. *Diabetes Educator* 27 (2) 150, 152

An exploration of the Internet resources available in support of evidence-based practice.

1.2.30 Filler, R. (1998) Bits and bytes. Cybernurse…useful library sites for researchers and nurses. *Australian Journal of Advanced Nursing* 15 (4) 21

1.2.31 Forward, L. & Hobby, L. (2002) A practical guide to conducting a systematic review. *Nursing Times* 98 (2) 36–7   2 References

A practical explanation of the literature search in the context of a systematic review.

1.2.32 Gash, S. (2000) *Effective literature searching for research* (2nd edition). Aldershot: Gower. ISBN 0566082772

A comprehensive general guide to literature searching when conducting research.

1.2.33 Glover, J. (2002) Informatics education: searching for the evidence using PubMed. *Medical Reference Services Quarterly* 21 (4) 57–65   3 References

Outlines the use of four searching techniques – Simple Limit, Preview/Index, Clinical Queries and MeSH Browser – for identifying material on PubMed.

1.2.34 Grandage, K.K., Slawson, D.C. & Shaughnessy, A.F. (2002) When less is more: a practical approach to searching for evidence-based answers. *Journal of the Medical Library Association* 90 (3) 298–304   35 References

Description of a pyramidal strategy for identifying the evidence-based literature.

1.2.35 Hart, C. (2001) *Doing a literature search: a comprehensive guide for the social sciences.* London: Sage. ISBN 0761968105

Aimed primarily at the social sciences, this guide covers such areas as the purpose of the literature search, planning, management, quick reference materials, finding books, journal articles, grey literature, official publications, statistics and citations. It also has a chapter on using the Internet and goes on to outline advanced searching techniques. There are useful appendices giving information on how to cite sources and a list of Internet file types.

1.2.36 Hassig, R.A. & Gluck, J.C. (2001) First hand: how to find evidence-based information that matters for your clinical care decisions and improvements. *National Network* 25 (4) 14–6

A general overview of the resources and services available for finding evidence-based information.

1.2.37 Hek, G., Langton, H. & Blunden, G. (2000) Systematically searching and reviewing literature. *Nurse Researcher* 7 (3) 40–57   37 References

Starting with cancer nursing education, this paper discusses the principles of a systematic review and the processes involved in identifying the literature.

1.2.38 Helmer, D., Savoie, I., Green, C. & Kazanijan, A. (2001) Evidence-based practice: extending the search to find material for the systematic review. *Bulletin of the Medical Library Association* 89 (4) 346–52   27 References

This small-scale study looked at methods for uncovering material for the systematic review. It particularly addresses material which is not included in specialized databases.

1.2.39 Hock, R.E. (1998) Precision searching with Web search engines. *Cyberskeptic's Guide to Internet Research* 3 (1) 4

Looks at getting the best from using search engines to find information on the World Wide Web.

1.2.40 Hood, W.W. & Wilson, C.S. (2001) The scatter of documents over databases in different subject domains: how many databases are needed? *Journal of the American Society for Information Science & Technology* 52 (14) 1242–54   23 References

The proliferation of databases and areas of nursing research interest has meant that it is no longer possible to perform a systematic literature search using only one or two services. This article discusses this situation.

1.2.41   Hsu, P.P. (1993) ClinPSYC, PsycLIT, and MEDLINE for health professionals. *Medical Reference Services Quarterly* 12 (4) 7–22   12 References

A comparison of the three databases.

1.2.42   Hutcherson, M. (1999) Principles for effective PubMed searching. *Health Care on the Internet* 3 (4) 59–69

A detailed exploration of the basic principles for searching Medline using the PubMed search interface. It includes descriptions of the advanced search options illustrated with a sample search as well as explanations of Medline syntax.

1.2.43   Hutchinson, D. (1997) A nurse's guide to the Internet. *RN* 60 (1) 46–52   6 References

A general guide to the Internet.

1.2.44   Hutchinson, D. (1997) The Internet for healthcare professionals. *ORL-Head & Neck Nursing* 15 (3) 9–14   28 References

Provides a summary of different types of Internet resource and suggests a basic strategy for its use. The emphasis is on Otolaryngology and several sites are listed and described.

1.2.45   Katcher, B.S. (1999) *Medline: a guide to effective searching.* San Francisco: Ashbury. ISBN 096734459X

Though the pace of development has meant that there are many features in Medline and the Medline search interfaces not covered in this text, it is still a sound introduction to the principles of searching and the search strategies that can be used to search the database effectively.

1.2.46   Kiley, R. (ed.) (2001) *A guide to health care resources on the Internet.* London: Royal Society of Medicine. ISBN 1853154733 References

Contains information on a wide range of medical resources on the Internet. Topics covered include evidence-based health care, cancer, mental health, women's health, nursing information and finding health information on the Internet (CR 2.85).

1.2.47   Kinniburgh, J. (2001) Using the Internet to support evidence-based practice. *Journal of Community Nursing* 15 (8) 4, 6, 8   14 References

Focusing on community nursing, this article gives an overview of searching the Internet.

1.2.48   Kleyman, P. (1998) Media currents. Using the Net for good health…assessing websites. *Aging Today* 19 (1) 18–19

Based around consumer health information, this article gives advice on the assessment of the efficacy of websites.

1.2.49   Knecht, L., Canese, K. & Port, T. (1998) PubMed: truncation, automatic explosion, mapping and MeSH headings. *NLM Technical Bulletin* (302) www.nlm.nih.gov/pubs/techbull/tb.html

An explanation of how to conduct an effective search in PubMed using some of the main features of MeSH.

1.2.50   Korn, K. (1998) Pharmacology resources on the Internet. *Journal of the American Academy of Nurse Practitioners* 10 (1) 29–30

1.2.51   Kuster, J.M. (2000) Subject guides: cyberspace launch pads. *ASHA Leader* 5 (15) 7

A description of how to use web-based subject guides as the starting point to a search.

1.2.52   LaBruzza, A.L. (1997) *The essential Internet: a guide for psychotherapists and other Mental Health Professionals.* Northvale, NJ: Jason Aronson. ISBN 0765701057

A very useful guide for those working in the field of mental health.

1.2.53   Levy, J. (2001) Searching the CINAHL database. *CINAHLnews* 20 (1, 2) 6–7

Describes the basic search tools available on the CINAHL database.

1.2.54   Levy, J.R. (2002) Searching the CINAHL database. Part 1: Evidence-based practice. *CINAHLnews* 21 (1) 10, 12, 15

Related to the CINAHL database, this article gives an overview of evidence-based practice and practical tips for identifying material using CINAHL subject headings and filters.

1.2.55   Levy, J.R. (2002) Searching the CINAHL database. Part 2: abstracts, cited references and full text. *CINAHLnews* 21 (2) 4, 6, 11

Second in the series, this article again gives practical advice on the use of subject heading and filters.

1.2.56 Lindell, C. (2001) Four steps to better search results on the Internet. *Nursing Spectrum (New England Edition)* 5 (9) 32–3

A straightforward guide to improving search strategies on the Internet.

1.2.57 Lingle, V.A. (1997) Journal searching in non-MEDLINE resources on Internet websites. *Medical Reference Services Quarterly* 16 (3) 27–43   10 References

Provides a review of a selection of non-Medline-based searches and sources on the Internet.

1.2.58 LoBinondo-Wood, G. (2002) Evaluating the validity of Internet resources. *Inside Case Management* 8 (11) 1, 3–4, 11   3 References

Discusses methods for evaluating resources identified on the Internet.

1.2.59 Logan, M. (2001) Academic education: fostering use of the Internet for research of clinical issues. *Critical Care Nurse* 21 (6) 30–2, 34   14 References

As well as looking at Medline and CINAHL this article also looks at finding research information on the Internet.

1.2.60 Makulowich, J.S. & Bates, M.E. (1995) 10 tips on managing your Internet searching. *Online* 19 (4) 32–4, 36–7   2 References

The resources available via the Internet are vast and it is very easy to become overwhelmed and lose track. This article gives advice on how to control a search so that key resources are identified and can be tracked.

1.2.61 Mason, C. (1993) Doing a literature review. *Nurse Researcher* 1 (1) 43–55   15 References

Provides a step-by-step guide to searching and reviewing the literature.

1.2.62 Matthews, E.J., Edwards, A.G.K., Barker, M., Bloor, M., Covey, J., Hood, K., Pill, R., Russell, I., Stott, N. & Wilkinson, C. (1999) Efficient literature searching in diffuse topics: lessons from a systematic review of research on communicating risk to patients in primary care *Health Libraries Review* 16 (2) 112–20   7 References

This study shows how to conduct an effective literature search on a diffuse subject. It also clearly identifies the problem of cross-database searching

and effective recall when a subject can be approached from a number of different conceptual starting points.

1.2.63 McEntyre, J. & Lipman, D. (2001) PubMed: bridging the information gap. *CMAJ: Canadian Medical Association Journal* 164 (9) 1317–9   2 References

An introduction to using PubMed.

1.2.64 McGhee, M. (2000) Hands on – using Limits in a PubMed search. *NLM Technical Bulletin* (315) www.nlm.nih.gov/pubs/techbull/tb.html

By using the Limits option in PubMed it is possible to refine a search. A brief explanation of their use is given in this article.

1.2.65 McGuire, T.J. (1997) Medlineing: why and how to conduct a literature search. *JEMS: Journal of Emergency Medical Services* 22 (4) 56–7, 59–60   7 References

Discusses in some detail the reasons for doing a literature review and some of the strategies that can be employed with particular reference to the Medline database.

1.2.66 McKenzie, B.C. (1996) *Medicine and the Internet: introducing online resources and terminology.* Oxford: Oxford University Press. ISBN 0192627058

With the progress made in developing database resources and interfaces in recent years this book has dated. However, much of the basic information about the resources is still current and there is a very good exploration of the terminology.

1.2.67 McKibbon, K.A. & Marks, S. (1998) EBN Notebook. Searching for the best evidence. Part 1: where to look. *Evidence-Based Nursing* 1 (3) 68–70   5 References

First in a two-part series, this article gives a general overview of literature searching in evidence-based nursing.

1.2.68 McKibbon, K.A. & Marks, S. (1998) Searching for the best evidence. Part 2: searching CINAHL and Medline. *Evidence-Based Nursing* 1 (4) 105–7   5 References

Second in the series, this article looks specifically at strategies for searching CINAHL and Medline for evidence-based nursing material.

1.2.69 McLellan, F. (2001) 1966 and all that – when is a literature search done? *Lancet* 358 (9282) 646

Discusses some of the objective limits that can be applied to a literature search.

1.2.70 Mendelsohn, S. (1996) First person: CDROM, online or the Internet? *Information World Review* 114 30–1

A useful comparison of three electronic services.

1.2.71 Monash University: Monash University Library (2000) How to use CINAHL via OVID www.lib.monash.edu.au/vl/cinahl/cinprfl.htm (Accessed 21/02/2003)

A step-by-step tutorial which takes the user through a search using the OVID web interface. Though occasionally referring to services provided by Monash University, it can be applied to any access point for OVID CINAHL.

1.2.72 Morrisey, L.J. & DeBourgh, G.A. (2001) Finding evidence: refining literature searching skills for the advanced practice nurse. *AACN Clinical Issues: Advanced Practice in Acute & Critical Care* 12 (4) 560–77 35 References

Starting from the premise of the diversity of sources, this article identifies databases, reviews search terminology and gives practical strategies.

1.2.73 Munoz, M.B., Sanchez, A.G. & Sanchez, M.M. (1997) How to make a bibliographic search in rehabilitation. *Rehabilitation* 31 (2) 108–17 32 References

Provides a thorough comparison of many of the main databases and sources with particular emphasis on Spanish sources such as Indice Medico Espanol.

1.2.74 Nahin, A.M. (2002) New PubMed filter: systematic reviews. *NLM Technical Bulletin* (324) www.nlm.nih.gov/pubs/techbull/tb.html 2 References

Describes the filter available on PubMed which enables searches to be limited to only systematic reviews.

1.2.75 Notess, G.R. (1997) On the Net. Internet search techniques and strategies. *Online* 21 (4) 63–6

Sound advice on developing effective search techniques and applying strategies.

1.2.76 Pierce, L.R. & Ball, J. (2000) How to conduct a literature search on the topic of interdisciplinary health care research. *National Academies of Practice Forum: Issues in Interdisciplinary Care* 2 (1) 55–7 3 References

1.2.77 Playle, J. (2000) Developing research questions and searching the literature. *Journal of Community Nursing* 14 (2) 20, 22, 24 14 References

Discusses the development of a research question and establishing, through the literature search, current knowledge.

1.2.78 Potter, L.A. (1995) A systematic approach to finding answers over the Internet. *Bulletin of the Medical Library Association* 83 (3) 280–5 6 References

Applied specifically to health care, this article discusses the application of systematic methodology to finding answers to specific questions via the Internet.

1.2.79 Poynder, R. (1998) Patient information on the Internet. *Online and CDROM Review* 22 (1) 9–17

Suggests strategies for searching for patient information on the Internet as well as some of the services available.

1.2.80 Reiswig, J. (2001) MEDLINEplus: better than ever for consumer health information. *Health Care on the Internet* 5 (2) 61–8 2 References

Aimed at the general public MEDLINEplus is a good example of an Internet portal site. It combines a mixture of articles relevant to public health and health concerns with links to other Internet services such as Medline.

1.2.81 Shojania, K.G. & Olmsted, R.N. (2002) Current methodological concepts. Searching the health care literature efficiently: from clinical decision-making to continuing education. *AJIC: American Journal of Infection Control* 30 (3) 187–95 68 References

Using examples from infection control, this article demonstrates the efficient use of Medline for identifying the answers to specific clinical questions. It refers in particular to selecting appropriate MeSH headings and targeting systematic reviews and meta-analyses.

1.2.82 Shoosan, S. (2000) NLM Gateway: your entrance to the knowledge resources of the National Library of Medicine. *NLM Technical Bulletin* (317) www.nlm.nih.gov/pubs/techbull/tb.html

Because of the speed of developments in the organization of the databases provided through the US National Library of Medicine this overview of the NLM Gateway is now slightly dated. However, it does give clear information on the scope of coverage, training and searching techniques.

1.2.83 Shooshan, S. (2001) How to search OLDMEDLINE using the NLM Gateway. *NLM Technical Bulletin* (320) www.nlm.nih.gov/pubs/techbull/tb.html

A practical article showing how to search OldMedline, browse and download the results to a file.

1.2.84　Smart, N. Welcome to the Internet for allied health. www.vts.rdn.ac.uk/tutorial/allied/ (Accessed 04/05/2003)

A tutorial aimed at increasing the knowledge and skill levels of allied health professionals in using the Internet effectively. A BIOME service.

1.2.85　Subirana, M., Sola, I., Garcia, J.M., Guillamet, A., Paz, E., Gich, I. & Urrutia, G. (2002) Importance of the database in the literature search: the first step in a systematic review. *Enfermeria Clinica* 12 (6) 296–300　7 References

A comparison of CINAHL and Medline in retrieving references relevant to nursing which comes to the conclusion that both databases should be used to produce a comprehensive search.

1.2.86　Tse, T. (2000) Searching ClinicalTrials.gov. *NLM Technical Bulletin* (316) www.nlm.nih.gov/pubs/techbull/tb.html

A brief overview of how to perform a search of ClinicalTrials.gov.

1.2.87　United States National Library of Medicine (2002) Fact Sheet: Medical Subject Headings (MeSH) www.nlm.nih.gov/pubs/factsheets/mesh.html (Accessed 27/04/2003)

A fact sheet designed to describe the MeSH. Useful for anyone unsure of what MeSH is.

1.2.88　United States National Library of Medicine (2002) Fact Sheet: PubMed: MEDLINE retrieval on the World Wide Web www.nlm.nih.gov/pubs/factsheets/pubmed.html (Accessed 27/04/ 2003)

Describes the PubMed search interface.

1.2.89　United States National Library of Medicine (2002) Fact Sheet: What's the difference between Medline and PubMed? www.nlm.nih.gov/pubs/factsheets/dif_med_pub.html (Accessed 27/04/2003)

One of a number of fact sheets produced by the US National Library of Medicine. It gives a brief description of the Medline database and the additional features available through the PubMed search interface.

1.2.90　United States National Library of Medicine (2002) PubMed tutorial www.nlm.nih.gov/bsd/pubmed_tutorial/m1001.html (Accessed 04/05/2003)

A web-based tutorial for the PubMed search interface.

1.2.91　United States National Library of Medicine (2003) NLM Gateway www.nlm.nih.gov/pubs/manuals/gateway.pdf (Accessed 01/05/2003)

The training manual for the NLM Gateway, a search interface which allows the users to search across several NLM databases.

1.2.92　United States National Library of Medicine (2003) MeSH vocabulary and Boolean logic www.nlm.nih.gov/pubs/manuals/mesh.pdf (Accessed 04/05/2003)

This training manual deals with the MeSH vocabulary and Boolean operators, key areas to understand for a successful search of Medline. The explanation of Boolean operators (AND, NOT, OR etc.) and their uses can be used with any database.

1.2.93　United States National Library of Medicine (2003) PubMed www.nlm.nih.gov/pubs/manuals/pubmed.pdf (Accessed 01/05/2003)

The training manual for the PubMed search interface available from the US National Library of Medicine. It is a detailed document which is invaluable in learning to exploit this resource effectively. It follows directly from the training manual for the MeSH vocabulary and Boolean operators.

1.2.94　University of Alberta (2003) Medline Glossary www.med.ualberta.ca/ebm/medglos.htm (Accessed 30/04/2003)

Searching databases has its own language which can be confusing for the novice. This glossary seeks to unravel some of the common terms used on the Medline database. Many of the terms are equally applicable in other databases such as CINAHL.

1.2.95　University of Rochester Medical Center (2000) Evidence-based filters for OVID Medline *www.urmc.rochester.edu/Miner/Educ/Expertsearch. html* (Accessed 30/04/2003)

Explains how to save searches and then reuse the search strategy within the OVID Medline interface to develop evidence-based filters. A number of examples are given.

1.2.96　University of Rochester Medical Center (2003) Evidence-based filters for OVID CINAHL www.urmc.rochester.edu/Miner/Educ/ebnfilt.htm (Accessed 30/04/2003)

Explains how to save searches and then reuse the search strategy within the OVID CINAHL interface to develop evidence-based filters. A number of examples are given.

1.2.97　University of York: NHS Centre for Reviews and Dissemination (2002) Search strategies to identify reviews and meta-analyses in

MEDLINE and CINAHL www.york.ac.uk/inst/crd/search.htm (Accessed 30/04/2003)

Gives example strategies with their degree of precision for identifying systematic reviews and meta-analyses in the Medline and CINAHL databases.

1.2.98 Ward, R. Welcome to the Internet for nursing, midwifery and health visiting. www.vts.rdn.ac.uk/tutorial/nurse (Accessed 22/04/2003)

A tutorial aimed at increasing the knowledge and skill levels of nurses in using the Internet effectively. A BIOME service.

1.2.99 Williams, M. (2001) Question of the month. Need to locate research in a hurry? Try PubMed. *Journal of the American Dietetic Association* 101 (5) 571

A guide to finding research quickly on Medline using the US National Library of Medicine PubMed search interface.

1.2.100 Williams, R.M., Baker, L.M. & Marshall, J.G. (1992) *Information Searching in Health Care*. Thorofare, NJ: Slack Inc. ISBN 1556420935

Designed for health professionals, this book provides a foundation in information searching skills. It also includes guidance on the critical appraisal of research evidence. Chapters include the process (knowing where to start), the resources (putting them to work), and the analysis of information. An appendix gives advice on reading clinical journals (CR 2.95).

1.2.101 Yensen, J. (1998) Connecting points: electronic nursing resources. Systematic, fast, comprehensive search strategis in nursing. *Computers in Nursing* 16 (1) 23–9   23 References

A very useful article describing in detail some of the possible strategies to adopt to get the best from searching the Internet.

1.3 BIBLIOGRAPHIES/CATALOGUES

Bibliographies are listings of books and other materials which can be grouped by a common factor. Library catalogues are also included in this section. Both of these can be effective means of identifying relevant, usually book-based, material in a literature search.

Annotations

1.3.1 *Bibliography of nursing literature 1859–1960: with an historical introduction* (1968) Edited by Thompson, A.M.C. London: Library Association.   ISBN 0853654700

and

1.3.2 *Bibliography of nursing literature 1961–1970* (1974) Edited by Thompson, A.M.C. London: Library Association.   ISBN 085365316X

and

1.3.3 *Bibliography of nursing literature 1971–1975* (1985) Edited by Walsh, F. London: Library Association.   ISBN 0853656231

and

1.3.4 *Bibliography of nursing literature 1976–1980* (1986) Edited by Walsh, F. London: Library Association.   ISBN 0853657467

These bibliographies are of value to anyone researching the history of nursing. The entries include journal articles as well as books. However, The listings are not comprehensive.

1.3.5 British Library Catalogue blpc.bl.uk

All materials received by the Copyright Receipt Office of the British Library can be found on the catalogue. It is a useful tool for checking whether a book has been published in the United Kingdom.

1.3.6 Library of Congress Catalog catalog.loc.gov/

The Library of Congress Catalog serves a similar purpose to the British Library Catalogue. It is searchable by subject and therefore particularly useful for identifying material without first knowing author or title.

1.3.7 The University of Queensland Cybrary: National Library Catalogues Worldwide www.library.uq.edu.au/ssah/jeast

A useful site for locating the catalogues of National Libraries.

1.3.8 United States National Library of Medicine Catalog locatorplus.gov

An internationally significant resource in determining what has been published in the field of health care.

1.3.9 University of Central England Library Catalogue talis.uce.ac.uk:8001/www-bin/www_talis32

Included as an example of a typical university library catalogue.

1.4 CURRENT AWARENESS SERVICES

Current awareness services are produced to provide up-to-date listings, sometimes annotated, of items usually of interest to a specific group. Some of the bibliographic databases, such as CINAHL, also include different forms of current awareness service.

Annotations

1.4.1 Midwives Information and Resource Service (MIDIRS) www.midirs.org/
Publisher: MIDIRS
Frequency: Three times a year

A service that includes original source material. Useful to teachers of midwifery, midwives, health visitors and students.

1.4.2 Royal College of Midwives Current Awareness Service
Publisher: Royal College of Midwives
Frequency: Quarterly

Gives lists of journals and available bibliographies. Also included are book reviews of items in current awareness service, information on books, reports, press releases, useful addresses and journal holdings of the library.

1.5   INDEXING SERVICES/DATABASES

Indexing services/databases are the principal tools for identifying journals and other material. This is not intended as a comprehensive listing but reflects the breadth of services available and gives some indication of their content. Where the database is only available via a subscription service (vendor), then it is indicated by (Information page) following the URL.

Annotations

1.5.1   AMED (Allied and Complementary Medicine Database) www.bl.uk/services/information/amed.html (Information page)

AMED is a British Library bibliographic database available through a number of vendor organizations. It covers complementary medicine, physiotherapy, occupational therapy, rehabilitation, podiatry, palliative care and speech and language therapy from 1995.

1.5.2   ASSIAnet (Applied Social Sciences Index and Abstracts) www.csa.com/csa/index.html (Information page)

An indexing and abstracting tool covering health, social services, psychology, sociology, economics, politics, race relations and education, including over 650 journals from 16 countries.

1.5.3   BEI (British Education Index) www.leeds.ac.uk/bei/bei.htm (Information page)

BEI covers all aspects of education from the UK literature, including nursing.

1.5.4   BNI (British Nursing Index) www.bni-plus.co.uk (Information page)

BNI is the leading UK-generated bibliographic database for nurses. It indexes over 220 English language journals based on the collections of Bournemouth University, the Royal College of Nursing, Poole Hospital NHS Trust and Salisbury Health Care NHS Trust. It uses subject headings which reflect UK terminology, practice and definitions.

1.5.5   Campbell Collaboration www.campbell-collaboration.org/

The Campbell Collaboration is a non-profit organization that aims to aid informed decision-making about the effects of interventions in the social, behavioural and educational arenas. It provides access to information about trials of interventions.

1.5.6   Caredata www.elsc.org.uk/caredata.htm

Caredata supports management and practice through extensive abstracting of relevant social work and social care literature. It contains over 50,000 abstracts of books, UK government reports, research papers, publications of voluntary organizations and articles from journals.

1.5.7   CINAHL (Cumulative Index of Nursing and Allied Health Literature) www.cinahl.com/mainentry.htm (Information page)

The leading specialist database for nurses and allied health disciplines, the CINAHL subject headings reflect the needs of the target professions and use an extensive thesaurus to ensure searches are not language dependent. The coverage of the professional literature is extensive. There are several companies providing CINAHL web access.

1.5.8   ClinicalTrials clinicaltrials.gov

A database of information about clinical research studies provided by the US National Institutes of Health.

1.5.9   ClinPSYCH   www.apa.org/psychinfo/products/clinpsyc.html (Information page)

ClinPSYC is a subset of PSYCHInfo covering clinical applications in the behavioural sciences and mental health.

1.5.10   Cochrane Library www.nelh.nhs.uk/cochrane.asp

www.areas.it/index.asp?IDL=ITA
www.centrocochranedobrasil.org/
www.chinacochrane.org/
www.cochrane.ch
www.cochrane.de
www.cochrane.dk
www.cochrane.es/Castellano
cochrane.mcmaster.ca
www.med.monash.edu.au/healthservices/cochrane/
library/library.htm
www.cochrane.nl
www.cochrane.ru/
www.cochrane.us
www.mrc.ac.za/cochrane/cochrane.htm
www.spc.univ-lyon1.fr/citccf/

The Cochrane Library consists of the Cochrane
Database of Systematic Reviews (full text reviews
of evidence that include a conclusion of effective-
ness), the Database of Abstracts of Reviews of
Effectiveness (including critical appraisal), the
Cochrane Controlled Trials Register and Health
Technology Assessment reports. For the researcher
this is a crucial element in any literature search.

1.5.11 EMBASE www.elsevier.nl/homepage/
sah/spd/site/embase/embase_main.html (Information
page)

EMBASE coverage is very similar to Medline but
should not be seen as a true alternative. The main
strength of EMBASE is drug-related literature.

1.5.12 Fitzpatrick, R.B. (2000) The Cochrane
Library and Cochrane Collaboration. *Medical
Reference Services Quarterly* 19 (4) 73–8

A general overview of the Cochrane service.

1.5.13 Health Service Abstracts
Publisher: UK Department of Health
Frequency: Monthly

Covers a broad range of subjects of interest in the
health services.

1.5.14 HerbMed www.herbmed.org/

HerbMed provides hyperlinked access to the scientific data underlying the use of herbs for health.

**1.5.15 HSRR (Health Services and Sciences
Research Resources)** wwwcf.nlm.nih.gov/hsrr_
search/home_search.cfm

The HSRR is a database of descriptions of research
datasets, instruments/indexes and software applications, frequently used in health services research
and in the behavioural and social sciences. It is
maintained by the US National Information Center
on Health Services Research & Health Care
Technology (NICHSR).

1.5.16 Index to Theses www.theses.com
(Information page)

A comprehensive index to theses (including abstracts)
accepted for higher degrees by UK universities.

1.5.17 Medline www.ncbi.nlm.nih.gov/entrez/
query.fcgi?CMD=Limits&DB=PubMed

This is the US National Library of Medicine
PubMed interface for the Medline database.
Medline is also available from other suppliers.
Medline is the most comprehensive of the medical
databases covering the international literature
(mainly journals) on medicine. It uses the MeSH
(Medical Subject Headings) controlled vocabulary.
PubMed has a number of useful features, including
links to full-text journal articles. There are also
added features such as tutorial support – www.nlm.
nih.gov/bsd/pubmed_tutorial/m2016.html

1.5.18 MeSH Browser www.nlm.nih.gov/mesh/
Mbrowser.html

The MeSH Browser is not in itself a bibliographic
database but allows the user to identify the MeSH
terms that can be used in a search of any of the bibliographic databases which use Medical Subject
Headings.

1.5.19 OldMedline gateway.nlm.nih.gov/gw/Cmd

Available via the NLM Gateway, OldMedline
covers the period 1957 to 1965.

**1.5.20 ProQuest Digital Dissertations
(Dissertation Abstracts)** wwwlib.umi.com/
dissertations/

Covering doctoral dissertations and masters theses
from over 1,000 graduate schools and universities
this is the web version of Dissertation Abstracts. The
most recent two years are fully searchable without a
subscription.

1.5.21 PsychINFO www.apa.org/psycinfo/products/
psychinfo.html (Information page)

PsychINFO is a bibliographic database of citations
and abstracts for the behavioural sciences and
mental health. It is the major resource in these
subject areas and is provided by the American
Psychological Association.

**1.5.22 ReFeR (Research Findings electronic
Register)** tap.ukwebhost.eds.com/doh/refr_web.
nsf/basicsearch?OpenForm

The ReFeR database covers completed projects
from the UK National Health Service R&D
Programme and the UK Department of Health
Policy Research Programme.

1.5.23 Registry of Nursing Research (RNR) www.stti.iupui.edu

Organized by Sigma Theta Tau who are also responsible for the Virginia Henderson International Nursing Library, the RNR contains information and abstracts from over 17,000 studies. It can be searched by researcher, study details, findings and keywords.

1.5.24 Rndex www.rndex.com

A database covering nursing, case management and managed care literature in the English language.

1.5.25 Royal College of Midwives (1987) *Midwifery Index: A Source of Journal References on Midwifery and Related Topics 1980–1986* (with selective coverage of 1976–79). Edited and compiled by Ayres, J. London: Royal College of Midwives. ISBN 1870822005

A cumulation of the main sections of the Royal College of Midwives' Library's Current Awareness Service. A list of subject headings and an author index are given. Journals only are covered and these are not listed.

1.5.26 Saba, V.K., Pravikoff, D.S. & Pletzke, C.J. (2000) Electronic access to military/uniformed services nursing research. *Military Medicine* 165 (11) 835–8   8 References

A description of the Electronic Military/Uniformed Services Nursing Research (EMUSNR) database.

1.5.27 Social Sciences Citation Index www.isinet. com/isi/products/citation/ssci/ (Information page)

Comprises a citation index, source index, permuterm subject index and a corporate index. Citation services rely on the citations given by authors and are of particular use in establishing a body of literature on a subject and identifying key authors, studies or seminal works. Nursing journals are covered by this service.

1.5.28 Sociological Abstracts www.csa.com/ detailsV5/socioabs.html (Information page)

Covers research in the areas of sociology and related disciplines in the social and behavioural sciences. International in its coverage, it includes over 2,500 journals, conference papers, books and dissertations. It is updated monthly with a backfile to 1963.

1.5.29 SRM Database www.niwi.knaw.nl/ srmonline/index.htm

Unique in its coverage, this database indexes the literature on social and behavioural research methodology, statistical analysis and computer software. The indexing language is the Thesaurus of Social Research Methodology (SRM-Thesaurus). Documents for inclusion are from the English, French, German and Dutch literature.

1.5.30 Tsalapatani, I. (2001) Greek electronic information resources for nursing. *Icus & Nursing Web Journal* (7) 1–8   16 References

An evaluative article on the databases available to Greek nurses.

1.5.31 United States National Library of Medicine (2003) ClinicalTrials.gov www.nlm. nih.gov/pubs/manuals/clinicaltrials.pdf (Accessed 01/05/2003)

This is the second part of the training manual for the NLM Gateway and ClinicalTrials.gov. It gives clear details of potential search strategies, how to read search results and ways to develop a search.

1.5.32 United States National Library of Medicine (2002) Fact Sheet: Medline www.nlm. nih.gov/pubs/factsheets/medline.html (Accessed 27/04/2003)

A description of the Medline database.

1.5.33 United States National Library of Medicine (2003) Fact Sheet: The NLM Gateway www.nlm.nih.gov/pubs/factsheets/gateway.html (Accessed 27/03/2003)

The NLM Gateway is a recent development to allow searching across several of the US National Library of Medicine database services. Databases include Medline, OldMedline, ClinicalTrials.gov and HSRProj – a database of health services research projects.

1.5.34 United States National Library of Medicine (2003) NLM Technical Bulletin Home Page   www.nlm.nih.gov/pubs/techbull/tb.html (Accessed 30/04/2003)

Individual bulletins have been listed elsewhere in this section but the catalogue is worth exploring because it is regularly updated with information explaining particular features of the databases (Medline) and services (PubMed) provided by the US National Library of Medicine.

1.5.35 United States National Library of Medicine (2003) NLM Training Manuals: PubMed, NLM Gateway, ClinicalTrials.gov, and TOXNET   www.nlm.gov/pubs/web_based.html (Accessed 04/05/2003)

The parent site for the US National Library of Medicine Training Manuals.

1.5.36 Zetoc zetoc.mimas.ac.uk/about.html (Information page)

Zetoc is the British Library's Electronic Table of Contents database. The database contains approximately 20 million conference and journal records across all disciplines from 1993. All material is available from the British Library's Document Supply Centre.

1.6 INTERNET/WORLD WIDE WEB PORTALS

Portals are services which provide links to other web-based services. They usually provide a structure through a subject index/contents and some will also have a search engine. These are thematic links pages.

Annotations

1.6.1 American Nurses Association Nursing World www.nursingworld.org/index.htm

Largely centred on the activities of the American Nurses' Association, this website includes links to the *Online Journal of Issues in Nursing*, nursing-related resources and State Nursing Associations.

1.6.2 Anonymous (1998) Resources. websites of interest to RNs. *Chart* 95 (1) 4

A brief but very useful article which lists and describes a number of websites.

1.6.3 BIOME biome.ac.uk

Host to a series of web links searchable databases, such as NMAP and OMNI, in the health and life sciences.

1.6.4 BUBL (Bulletin Board for Libraries) www.bubl.ac.uk/nursing/

Provides links to other Internet services for nurses. UK focused.

1.6.5 Hardin Meta Directory of Health Internet Sites www.lib.uiowa.edu/hardin/md/ index.html

This website is structured as an index and is designed to provide easy access to leading websites that act as 'directories' in the health sciences. It has general and subject-specific listings.

1.6.6 Healthfinder www.healthfinder.gov

Sponsored by the Office of Disease Prevention and Health Promotion of the US Department of Health and Human Services, this portal provides links to a range of web-based resources including a specific section for research.

1.6.7 HealthWeb healthweb.org

This portal is organized by broad condition and profession categories.

1.6.8 HON (Health on the Net Foundation) www.hon.ch/MedProf/med_prof.html

The Health on the Net Foundation, based in Switzerland, provides access to quality assessed web-based information. It is now a United Nations-recognized NGO.

1.6.9 Horan, T. (2002) Research has never been easier. *World of Irish Nursing* 10 (3) 16–17

A description of the nurse2nurse website of the Irish Nurses' Organization.

1.6.10 Mental Health Network www.opd.state. md.us/mhnet.htm

Self-help mental health resources and links to related websites are provided. There is clear subject distinction in the structure of the site but with overlapping links between categories.

1.6.11 Netting the Evidence www.sheffield.ac. uk/~scharr/ir/netting/first.html

An Internet portal which provides links to resources organizations, learning resources, an evidence-based virtual library, databases and some journals.

1.6.12 NMAP nmap.ac.uk

A fully searchable database of web links aimed at nurses and the allied health professions. A BIOME service.

1.6.13 NursingCenter www.nursingcenter.com/ library/index.asp (Accessed 01/05/2003)

A web portal which includes a library of web accessible journals.

1.6.14 NursingNet www.nursingnet.org/allied.htm

A subject directory to nursing on the World Wide Web, it includes subject categorization of links.

1.6.15 OMNI – Organizing Medical Networked Information omni.ac.uk

With emphasis on the United Kingdom but also with international coverage, it provides a comprehensive catalogue of networked biomedical and health-related resources. The database is fully browsable, using alphabetical listings, National Library of Medicine Classification and Medical Subject Headings (MeSH). It includes an invaluable section on evaluating Internet resources.

1.6.16 Resources for Nurses and Families
pegasus.cc.ucf.edu/~wink/home.html

Aimed at family health services nurses and families, this website provides links to sites based around these two groups needs.

1.6.17 Royal College of Nursing, Research & Development Co-ordinating Centre: Dissemination & Utilization Databases www.man.ac.uk/rcn/d&udatabase.html

Lists databases used to disseminate information about research and development within the field of nursing, midwifery and health visiting. Bias is towards British-based services.

1.6.18 SOSIG (Social Science Information Gateway) www.sosig.ac.uk

Aims to provide a source of quality assessed Internet information for students, academics, researchers and practitioners in the social sciences, business and law.

1.6.19 University of Bristol: Institute for Learning and Research (2002) Making sense of the Internet for social scientists: the Social Science Information Gateway www.sosig.ac.uk/about_us/docs/workbook.pdf (Accessed 03/05/2003)

A workbook and guide to the Social Science Information Gateway, it covers finding resources through the SOSIG Gateway, other specialist services and Internet search engines.

1.6.20 University of Central England in Birmingham: Library Services library.uce.ac.uk/

This website is included as an example of a typical academic institution's set of pages which provide links to resources on the Internet. The structured links give access to general search engines, health care and nursing-specific sites, government departments and agencies, databases, library catalogues and source material. Most institutions now have home pages with this type of structure which can serve as a good starting point for any search of the Internet.

1.7   DIRECTORIES

Directories are useful and often essential for identifying sources of information, people and possible assistance. However, not all are comprehensive as questionnaire returns are often the method used for compilation. The entries here are not intended to be a complete listing. ISBN numbers and editions have been excluded for titles where the frequency of publication is regular.

Annotations

1.7.1 Associations Unlimited. Detroit: Gale

Available both on CD-ROM and the Internet via GaleNet, this suite of databases is based on the Gale series *The Encyclopedia of Associations*. The three main elements are (1) National, (2) International, and (3) Regional, State and Local. There are over 400,000 organizations listed. Updates are three times a year on GaleNet and annually for the CD-ROM.

1.7.2 Centres, Bureaux and Research Institutes (2000) 14th edition. Beckenham: CBD Research. ISBN 0900246855

Lists over 2,000 establishments indexed by subject.

1.7.3 Councils, Committees and Boards (2001) 12th edition. Beckenham: CBD Research. ISBN 0900246871

Arranged alphabetically, each entry gives details of structure and purpose.

1.7.4 Current British Directories (2000) 13th edition. Beckenham: CBD Research. ISBN 0900246758

A directory of directories, yearbooks, guides and registers with nearly 2,500 entries. Includes subject and publishers indexes.

1.7.5 Current Research in Britain, Social Sciences. London: Longman

A national register of current research being carried out in universities, colleges and other institutions in the UK. The series is divided into four areas: physical sciences (annual – 2 parts); biological sciences (annual – 2 parts); social sciences (annual); humanities (biennial). Contains a department index, lists research in progress and has name, study area and keyword indexes. Social sciences covers nursing and medicine.

1.7.6 Directory of British Associations and Associations in Ireland (2002) 16th edition. Beckenham: CBD Research. ISBN 0900246928

Arranged alphabetically, each entry includes a statement or purpose, publication, whether there is a library and gives website and email addresses. A subject index is also included.

1.7.7 Directory of Libraries in Canada (2002) 17th edition. Toronto: Micromedia. ISBN 1895021898

Includes over 7,000 listings of libraries and branches, information and resource centres, archive and learning centres. Health science libraries are included.

1.7.8 Directory of Health Library and Information Services in the United Kingdom and Republic of Ireland 2002–3. (2001) 11th edition. London: Library Association. ISBN 1856043789

Each entry includes the name, address, telephone number, URLs, email addresses, type of library, opening hours, stock policy, holdings classification system, publications and network membership.

1.7.9 DIRLINE (Directory of Health Organizations Online) dirline.nlm.nih.gov

DIRLINE is provided by the US National Library of Medicine. It is fully searchable and covers information resources in subject areas such as federal, state and local government agencies, professional societies, academic and research institutions and their programmes, information systems and research facilities. Specific topics include most diseases, health services research and technology assessment.

1.7.10 Encyclopedia of Associations: Regional, State and Local Organizations (1998) 8th edition. Gale. Detroit: ISBN 078761386X

    Volume 1: Great Lakes States. ISBN 0787613908
    Volume 2: Northeastern States. ISBN 0787613878
    Volume 3: Southern and Middle Atlantic States. ISBN 0787613886
    Volume 4: South Central and Great Plains States. ISBN 0787613916
    Volume 5: Western States. ISBN 0787613894

Includes professional and social welfare non-profit membership organizations giving detailed information for each entry.

1.7.11 Gale Directory of Databases. Detroit: Gale (CD-ROM and paper)

Over 13,000 databases available online, on CD-ROM, diskette or magnetic tape are listed. It is possible to search by subject and is updated twice yearly.

1.7.12 Government Research Directory (2003) 17th edition. Detroit: Gale. ISBN 0787659266

Over 4,800 federal research programmes and facilities of the US and Canadian governments are listed. Indexes include keywords, subject and geographic.

1.7.13 International Directories in Print Edited by Towell, J.E. & Montney, C.B. Detroit: Gale

1.7.14 International Research Centers Directory (2003) 17th edition. Detroit: Gale. ISBN 0787669075

Covers government, university, independent, non-profit and commercial research activities. Full contact details, staff, research programme descriptions and publications are listed.

1.7.15 Library Services for Nurses www.nursing-libraries.org

This web-based service offers digital maps for the United Kingdom, service information and a searchable database of contact information.

1.7.16 Medical and Health Information Directory (2002) 15th edition. Detroit: Gale

    Volume 1: Organizations, Agencies and Institutions. ISBN 0787664510
    Volume 2: Publications, Libraries and Other Information. ISBN 0787664529
    Volume 3: Health Services. ISBN 0787664537

A comprehensive guide to organizations, agencies, institutions, services and information sources in medicine and health-related fields.

1.7.17 New Research Centers Directory (2004) 31st edition. Detroit: Gale. ISBN 0787669490

An inter-edition supplement to the Research Centers Directory and the International Research Centers Directory.

1.7.18 Ready Reference Shelf. Detroit: Gale

Available on CD-ROM and the Internet via GaleNet, entries are drawn from the *Encyclopedia of Associations, Publishers Directory, Directories in Print, Gale Directory of Databases, Directory of Special Libraries and Information Centers, Research Centers Directory, International Research Centers Directory* and *Government Research Centers Directory.*

1.7.19 Research Centers Directory (2002) 30th edition. Detroit: Gale. ISBN 078764288

A directory listing of the programmes, facilities, publications and educational services of North American non-profit research institutes.

1.7.20 Subject Directory of Special Libraries and Information Centers (2002) 28th edition. Detroit: Gale

    Volume 1. ISBN 0787661937
    Volume 2. ISBN 0787661945
    Volume 3. ISBN 0787661953

This directory is arranged by subject over three volumes and includes web and Internet addresses as well as many online services.

1.7.21   The CenterWatch Directory of Drugs in Clinical Trials (2001) 2nd edition. Detroit: Gale

Covers approximately 1,900 drugs currently in clinical development.

1.7.22   World Guide to Special Libraries (2001) 5th edition. Detroit: Gale.   ISBN 3598222572

Includes information on over 37,000 special libraries and is divided by subject.

PART 2: METHODS OF INQUIRY

An Introduction to Research

2.1 RESEARCH TEXTS

Two major categories of research methodology texts are included in this section, those written for and by nurses and general texts suitable for any discipline. Others may be found in sections 2.9, 2.29 and 2.36.

Annotations

2.1.1 Abbott, P. & Sapsford, R. (1998) *Research methods for nursing and the caring professions* (2nd edition). Buckingham: Open University Press ISBN 0335196977 References

This text will assist those undertaking or evaluating research for the first time. Small-scale social research papers are discussed and exercises are included (CR 2.14, 2.95).

2.1.2 Armstrong, D. & Grace, J. (2000) *Research methods and audit for general practice* (3rd edition). Oxford: Oxford University Press ISBN 0192631918 References

Book for general practitioners which shows how research may be conducted in their own practice. It includes study design, data collection and analysis, statistics and writing up results.

2.1.3 Balnaves, M., Caputi, P. & McHoul, A. (2001) *Introduction to quantitative research methods: an investigative approach.* London: Sage ISBN 0761968040

Book is an innovative and accessible introduction to quantitative research methods and basic statistics. A detective theme is used throughout the text and in multimedia tutorials to show how quantitative methods have been used to solve real-life problems. Examples and illustrations are drawn from historical and contemporary research in the social sciences (CR 2.29).

2.1.4 Beanland, C., Schneider, Z., LoBiondo-Wood, G. & Haber, J. (1999) *Nursing research:*

methods, critical appraisal and utilization. St Louis, MO: Mosby ISBN 1875897623 References

Nursing Research, the first Australasian edition, provides the latest information and research methods from US nurse researchers integrated with Australasian cases, examples and methodologies pertinent to the local curriculum. The adaptation will maintain and build upon the features that have led to the US edition of the text being adopted for use at all academic levels.

2.1.5 Blaxter, L., Hughes, C. & Tight, M. (2001) *How to research* (2nd edition). Buckingham: Open University Press ISBN 0335209033 References

Book is intended for less experienced researchers undertaking small-scale projects. It gives an overview of the research process and addresses both theoretical and practical considerations. It also addresses issues ignored by many texts, for example, gaining access, time management, project management and choosing supervisors. Novices would need to use this book in conjunction with a more in-depth research text. It contains exercises, helpful hints, health warnings, key points and further reading.

2.1.6 Bowling, A. (2002) *Research methods in health: investigating health and health services* (2nd edition). Buckingham: Open University Press ISBN 0335206433 References

Book is not a manual of how to do research, but rather it provides rationales and explanations for the methods discussed. Case studies and review questions are included (CR 2.2).

2.1.7 Breakwell, G.M., Hammond, S. & Fife-Schaw, C. (eds) (2000) *Research methods in psychology* (2nd edition). London: Sage ISBN 0761965912 References

Book introduces the key research methods used in psychology. Each part covers a discrete area of the research process and the text is illustrated with examples from current research. Step-by-step advice is given together with exercises and lists for further reading. New to this edition are chapters on research with special groups, cross-cultural research, content analysis and structural equation modelling (CR 2.34, 2.35, 2.53, 2.67, 2.88, 2.89, 2.92).

2.1.8 Brewerton, P.M. & Millward, L.J. (2001) *Organizational research methods: a practical guide for students and researchers.* London: Sage ISBN 0761971017 References

Book guides readers with clear pointers for conducting organizational research. Each aspect of the research process is discussed and related to this field of study.

2.1.9 Brockopp, Y. & Hastings-Tolsma, M.T. (2003) *Fundamentals of nursing research* (3rd edition). Sudbury, MA: Jones & Bartlett ISBN 0763715670 References

Book is intended for students and practitioners and covers qualitative and quantitative methods. The text's framework is solidly grounded in contemporary nursing science and theory (CR 2.9, 2.29, 2.36).

2.1.10 Brown, A. & Dowling, P. (1998) *Doing research/reading research: a mode of interrogation for education.* London: Falmer Press ISBN 0750707194 References

This is not a research methods 'cookbook', but authors have developed a systematic procedure that can be applied to both reading and conducting research in education and the social sciences. This mode of interrogation enables the researcher/professional to evaluate the research they are reading and to bring insight and rigour into the planning and implementation of their own projects (CR 2.95).

2.1.11 Bryman, A. (2001) *Social research methods.* Oxford: Oxford University Press ISBN 0198742045 References

Book is a comprehensive introduction to the study and implementation of social research methods for undergraduates. All major methods and designs are covered and illustrated by practical examples. Powerpoint slides are available for each chapter and links to appropriate web resources are included (CR 2.2).

2.1.12 Burns, N. & Grove, S.K. (1999) *Understanding nursing research* (2nd edition). Philadelphia, PA: W.B. Saunders ISBN 0721681069 References

Book introduces each step of the research process and shows how to read, summarize, critique and use findings in clinical practice. Highlights from published studies and critique questions will help in the learning process. An Instructor's Manual (on CD-ROM) [ISBN 0721681077] and Study Guide with

Study Disk [ISBN 0721681085] are also available (CR 2.102).

2.1.13 Burns, N. & Grove, S.K. (2001) *The practice of nursing research: conduct, critique and utilization,* (4th edition). Philadelphia, PA: W.B. Saunders ISBN 0721691773 References

Text expands coverage of previous editions, using real examples, and relevant websites are also included. Comprehensive coverage of qualitative research methods is given. Book emphasizes critical thinking and readers are guided through discussions about evidence-based practice. Also available is an Instructor's Electronic Resource that includes Instructor's Manual, PowerPoint Lecture Slides and a Computerized Test Bank (CR 2.36, 2.43).

2.1.14 Burns, R.B. (2000) *Introduction to research methods* (4th edition). London: Sage ISBN 0761965939 References

Book provides students with an understanding of the concepts and techniques of qualitative and quantitative research. Examples and exercises are given to demystify complex theories and methodologies (CR 2.9, 2.29, 2.36).

2.1.15 Burton, D. (ed.) (2000) *Research training for social scientists: a handbook for postgraduate researchers.* London: Sage ISBN 0761963510 References

Provides the beginning researcher with the conceptual and practical skills to undertake successful research. Both qualitative and quantitative methods are included (CR 2.5, 2.9, 2.10, 2.17, 2.29, 2.36).

2.1.16 Carter, Y. & Thomas, C. (eds) (1997) *Research methods in primary care.* Oxford: Radcliffe Medical Press ISBN 1857751981 References

Book introduces readers to the basic range of research skills in primary care. Reasons for doing research and a brief history of that undertaken in general practice are given. The role of qualitative methods is emphasized (CR 2.9, 2.36).

2.1.17 *Central Archive for Empirical Social Research* Cologne: University of Cologne www.gesis.org/en/methods_consultation/index.htm (Accessed 12/01/03)

Provides an advisory service on methodological questions in empirical social research and includes most aspects of a study. Scientists in higher education and research institutes in Germany and other countries can use these services. Further advice on types of research is also available.

2.1.18 Cherulnik, P.D. (2001) *Methods for behavioural research: a systematic approach.*

Thousand Oaks, CA: Sage ISBN 0761921990
References

Providing both a theoretical understanding of research issues and a nuts-and-bolts guide, this book presents the critical issues in psychological research.

2.1.19 Cluett, E.R. & Bluff, R. (eds) (2000) *Principles and practice of research in midwifery.* Edinburgh: Ballière Tindall ISBN 0702024252 References

Book provides an introduction to all aspects of research from a midwifery perspective. Equal weight is given to qualitative and quantitative methods and the principles underlying these approaches are described. Examples from midwifery and neonatal care are included (CR 2.9, 2.29, 2.36).

2.1.20 Cohen, L., Manion, L. & Morrison, K. (eds) (2000) *Research methods in education.* (5th edition). London: Routledge/Falmer ISBN 0415195411 References

Completely rewritten and updated, this classic text covers the whole range of methods currently used by novices and experienced researchers. The theory that underpins research methodology and detailed practical guidelines are given and much new material is included (CR 2.10, 2.14, 2.51, 2.77, 2.85).

2.1.21 Coleman, M. & Briggs, A.R.J. (eds) (2002) *Research methods in educational leadership and management.* London: Paul Chapman Publishing ISBN 0761971858 References

Text examines the concept of research and its philosophical bases, fundamental issues like ethics, reliability and validity, survey, case study and action research, and some major tools for collecting data. Advice is also given on analysing and presenting data.

2.1.22 Coombes, H. (2001) *Research using IT.* Basingstoke: Palgrave ISBN 0333914503 References

Book introduces students to research methods and shows how to use the computer to aid the process (CR 2.2, 2.85).

2.1.23 Cormack, D.F.S. (ed.) (2000) *The research process in nursing* (4th edition). Oxford: Blackwell Science ISBN 0632051582 References

This new edition continues to provide a comprehensive and practical guide to the stages in research. It has been extensively revised and updated and contains new chapters on reliability, validity, single-case and longitudinal studies (CR 2.24, 2.25, 2.34, 2.48).

2.1.24 Curran, J. & Blackburn, R. (2000) *Researching the small enterprise.* London: Sage ISBN 0761952950 References

Book discusses the need for small business research and takes readers through the necessary steps to conduct their project.

2.1.25 de Vaus, D. (2001) *Research design in social research.* London: Sage ISBN 0761953477 References

Book argues that the core of research methods is the structure and design of the research. It includes sections on research design, experimental, longitudinal, cross-sectional and case study designs (CR 2.29, 2.39, 2.48, 2.86, 2.87).

2.1.26 Denscombe, M. (1998) *The good research guide for small scale social research projects.* Buckingham: Open University Press ISBN 0335198058 References

Provides practical guidance and a vision of key issues involved in social research. Checklists are included which will enable elementary errors to be avoided.

2.1.27 Downs, F.S. (1999) *Readings in research methodology* (2nd edition). Philadelphia, PA: Lippincott ISBN 0781719240 References

Book comprises a series of articles derived from the methodology corner of *Nursing Research*. Parts cover samples and sampling issues, qualitative techniques, measuring differences and change, correlational techniques, measurement and measurement issues, and special analytic techniques (CR 2.22, 2.36, 2.40, 2.54).

2.1.28 Easterby-Smith, M., Thorpe, R. & Lowe, A. (2001) *Management research: an introduction.* (2nd edition). London: Sage ISBN 0761972854 References

Intended for graduate researchers at masters and doctoral level, this book considers not only methods but also the nature of management research, its philosophy and politics.

2.1.29 Edwards, A. & Talbot, R. (1999) *The hard-pressed researcher: a research handbook for the caring professions (*2nd edition). Longman: London ISBN 058236972X References

This introductory text is for students and practitioners undertaking research for the first time. Readers are taken through the research process and examples are given throughout.

2.1.30 Field, D., Davis, C., Corner, J. & Clark, D. (eds) (2001) *Researching palliative care.* Buckingham:

Open University Press ISBN 0335204368
References

Book on research methods has been specifically designed for those involved in the study and delivery of palliative care, but would also be of value to other health care professionals. The strengths and weaknesses of appropriate research methods are explored and examples given.

2.1.31 Fitzpatrick, J.J. (ed.) (1998) *Encyclopedia of nursing research.* New York: Springer Publishing Company ISBN 082611170X

This encyclopedia contains over 300 articles by the world's leading authorities in nursing research and will be of value to all who have an interest in improving patient care through research. Key terms and concepts are comprehensively explained and an extensive cross-referenced index is included. Entries include applied and clinical nursing research, concept analysis, data management, ethics of research, the Internet, journals in nursing research, measurement and scales, qualitative and qualitative research, statistical techniques and research utilization (CR 2.2, 2.5, 2.17, 2.29, 2.36, 2.79, 2.80, 2.85, 2.102, Appendix B).

2.1.32 Gilbert, N. (ed.) (2001) *Researching social life* (2nd edition). London: Sage ISBN 0761972455 References

This fully revised and updated text includes an even broader range of methods that are emerging as a result of the adoption of new technologies and media, such as the Internet, the analysis of multimedia and especially visual materials, and the secondary analysis of longitudinal datasets (CR 2.36, 2.48, 2.86, 2.91).

2.1.33 Gill, J. & Johnson, P. (1997) *Research methods for managers,* (2nd edition). London: Paul Chapman Publishing ISBN 185396350X References

This introductory text will assist students when undertaking management research at all levels of study.

2.1.34 Gillis, A. & Jackson, W. (2002) *Research for nurses: methods and interpretation.* Philadelphia, PA: F.A. Davis Co. ISBN 0803608969 References

Text aims to take the mystery out of research and illustrates the synergy and importance of research in nursing practice. Both qualitative and quantitative approaches are included. Case studies, sample projects, a statistics primer, an overview of NUD*IST, a series of laboratory assignments, studies in the use of SPSS and numerous website addresses are included (CR 2.9, 2.29, 2.36, Appendix A).

2.1.35 Glicken, M.D. (2003) *Social research: a simple guide.* Boston, MA: Allyn & Bacon/ Longman ISBN 0205334288 References

Book aims to make research fun and interesting by using concrete examples, funny vignettes and worked-out problems.

2.1.36 Green, S. (2000) *Research methods in health, social and early years care.* Cheltenham: Stanley Thornes ISBN 0748754628 References

Book covers key issues of research methodology and provides guidance on planning, conducting and presenting a project. It is intended for first-time researchers and those taking Advanced NVQ in Health and Social Care (CR 2.14).

2.1.37 Greenfield, T. (ed.) (2002) *Research methods for postgraduates.* London: Edward Arnold ISBN 0340806567 References

A book for masters level students covering a variety of topics in addition to research methods.

2.1.38 Hansen, A., Cottle, S., Negrine, R. & Newbold, C. (1998) *Mass communication research methods.* Basingstoke: Palgrave ISBN 033361710X References

Book provides an introduction to research methods in the study of media and mass communication processes. Chapters include asking the right questions, selected data collection methods and analysing various types of data (CR 2.20, 2.52, 2.72, 2.84, 2.88).

2.1.39 Hayes, N. (2000) *Doing psychological research: gathering and analysing data.* Buckingham: Open University Press ISBN 0335203795 References

Book is a comprehensive introductory account of both qualitative and quantitative research methods. Parts discuss the different ways of gathering and analysing data (CR 2.9, 2.29, 2.36, 2.39, 2.42, 2.64, 2.68, 2.72, 2.75, 2.81, 2.86, 2.87).

2.1.40 Hek, G., Judd, M. & Moule, P. (2002) *Making sense of research: an introduction for health and social care practitioners* (2nd edition). London: Continuum ISBN 0826455565 References

Book aims to 'demystify' and explain research by introducing its central elements. It emphasizes the development of critical skills and gives advice on implementing research findings (CR 2.98, 2.102).

2.1.41 Hopkins, D. (2002) *A teacher's guide to classroom research* (3rd edition). Buckingham: Open University Press ISBN 033521004X References

This guide is for teachers wishing to undertake research in their classrooms with a view to improving practice. The book emphasizes the contribution teacher research can make to creating a discourse around teaching and learning, whole school development and creating learning communities within schools. Examples are included together with case studies, discussions and a description of methods for collecting and analysing data. Ways in which classroom research can be reported, published and linked to the curriculum, teaching and staff development are also described.

2.1.42 Hott, J.R. & Budin, W.C. (1999) *Notter's essentials of nursing research* (6th edition). New York: Springer ISBN 0826115993 References

Book provides a contemporary explanation of basic knowledge and skills that form the foundation of nursing research in clinical practice. New features include a comprehensive list of websites for research activities, a glossary of terms, information about funding, references on presenting research and how to write a research abstract (CR 2.2, 2.97, 2.99, 3.13).

2.1.43 Kumar, R. (1999) *Research methodology: a step-by-step guide for beginners*. London: Sage ISBN 076196214X

Provides information about the research process in a systematic way from the simple to the complex, using flow chart diagrams and examples to communicate the concepts described. No knowledge is assumed and each chapter contains a summary and exercises.

2.1.44 Laws, S., Harper, C. & Marcus, R. (2002) *Research for development: a practical guide*. London: Sage ISBN 0761973273 Published in Association with Save the Children Fund References

Book is designed as a quick reference manual and a learning tool for all those engaged in development work.

2.1.45 Leary, M.R. (2001) *Introduction to behavioral research methods* (3rd edition). Boston, MA: Allyn & Bacon ISBN 0205322042

Book is written to help students who are afraid/less interested in studying research methods. It contains many examples, questions for review and discussion, and exercises to interest and help to consolidate learning. It mainly covers experimental approaches and statistical concepts are included (CR 2.2).

2.1.46 LoBiondo-Wood, G. & Haber, J. (2001) *Nursing research methods: critical appraisal and utilization* (5th edition). St Louis, MO: Mosby ISBN 0323012876 References

Text examines the roles of research in nursing, quantitative and qualitative research, application and analysis of research and evidence-based practice. This new edition highlights critiquing elements in each chapter and interactive features include articles, critical thinking challenges and critiquing criteria. It also includes an Electronic Instructor's Resource Online and an Outline Workbook (CR 2.1.47).

2.1.47 LoBiondo-Wood, G. & Haber, J. (2001) *Online workbook for nursing research methods: critical appraisal and utilization* (5th edition). St Louis, MO: Mosby ISBN 0323014666

Designed to accompany the 5th edition of *Nursing research methods*, this interactive learning feature reinforces concepts presented in the text, including the roles of research in nursing, the processes of qualitative and quantitative research, application and analysis of research and evidence-based practice (CR 2.1.46, 2.9, 2.36).

2.1.48 Marks, D.F. & Yardley, L. (eds) (2003) *Research methods for clinical and health psychology*. London: Sage ISBN 0761971912 References

This single volume research methods text has been geared specifically to the needs of both clinical and health psychologists, and both quantitative and qualitative approaches are discussed (CR 2.9, 2.29, 2.36).

2.1.49 May, T. (2001) *Social research: issues, methods and process* (3rd edition). Buckingham: Open University Press ISBN 0335206123 References

Book is designed as a complete course of study for social policy students and aims to bridge the gap between theory and methods. The latest developments in the interdisciplinary field in social research are included.

2.1.50 McTavish, D.G. & Loether, H.J. (2002) *Social research: an evolving process* (2nd edition). Boston, MA: Allyn & Bacon/Longman ISBN 02053374449 References

This text covers both qualitative and quantitative approaches and issues relating to the research process. It emphasizes the social aspects of serious research, the flaws that can result, and ways to detect and correct those flaws (CR 2.29, 2.36).

2.1.51 Miell, D. & Wetherell, M. (eds) (1998) *Doing social psychology*. London: Sage ISBN 0761960503 References

Textbook gives step-by-step guidance through every stage of the research process and challenges the reader to tackle the key methodological and theoretical issues in conducting research (CR 2.67, 2.77).

2.1.52   Miller, D.C. & Salkind, N.J. (2002) *Handbook of research design and social measurement* (6th edition). Thousand Oaks, CA: Sage ISBN 0761920463   References

Handbook covers many aspects of research design, applied and evaluation research and expanded coverage of qualitative methods. Data collection techniques, data libraries and guides to statistical analysis and the use of computers are all included.

2.1.53   Miller, R.L. & Brewer, J. (eds) (2003) *The a–z of social research: a dictionary of key social science research.* London: Sage   ISBN 0761971335   References

This A–Z is a collection of 94 entries ranging from qualitative research techniques to statistical testing, and the practicalities of using the Internet as a research tool. The book provides a practical, fast and concise introduction to the key concepts and methods in social research, and helps demystify a field that students often find daunting (CR 2.29, 2.36, 2.85).

2.1.54   Neutens, J.J. & Rubinson, L. (2001) *Research techniques for the health sciences.* Reading, MA: Benjamin Cummings ISBN 0205340962   References

Book focuses on pragmatic aspects of health science research. Underlying concepts and theory are explored and illustrated by case studies. New to this edition are online research and an evidence-based approach to literature reviews (CR 2.12, 2.85).

2.1.55   Nieswiadomy, R.M. (2002) *Foundations of nursing research* (4th edition). Upper Saddle River, NJ: Prentice-Hall ISBN 0130339911 References

Book provides a comprehensive, step-by-step approach to the research process. Additional features include concepts of evidence-based practice, nursing research on the World Wide Web, excerpts from published studies, get-involved activities, self-tests and critiquing guidelines. It also includes information on online course management systems. Appendix A (338–40) contains a list of sources of research instruments (CR 2.2, 2.56, 2.57, 2.58, 2.60, 2.61, 2.63, 2.85, 2.95).

2.1.56   Norwood, S.L. (2000) *Research strategies for advanced practice nurses.* London: Prentice Hall ISBN 0838584063   References

Guide offers presentation and utilization strategies that help make the nursing research process more 'do-able' and exciting. More emphasis is placed on implementing research in a variety of settings than

on undertaking original research. It incorporates current research and guidelines for writing and conveying research results throughout (CR 2.95, 2.97, 2.98, 2.100, 2.102).

2.1.57   Parahoo, K. (1997) *Nursing research: principles, process and issues.* Basingstoke: Macmillan Press   ISBN 0333699181   References

Written for students with little or no previous knowledge of research, this book aims to equip readers with a comprehensive understanding of the concepts and principles of research so that it may be read critically and utilized where appropriate (CR 2.2, 2.95).

2.1.58   Partington, D. (ed.) (2002) *Essential skills for management research.* London: Sage   ISBN 0761970088   References

Text will guide management researchers and students at postgraduate and MBA levels. It covers philosophy and research, research processes, approaches and techniques (CR 2.5, 2.6, 2.7, 2.9, 2.17, 2.39, 2.42, 2.45, 2.77, 2.97, 3.16).

2.1.59   Polgar, S. & Thomas, S.A. (2000) *Introduction to research in the health sciences* (4th edition). Melbourne: Churchill Livingstone ISBN 044306265X   References

Assuming no prior knowledge of statistics, this book introduces quantitative research techniques and shows how to plan, implement and evaluate a project. It includes self-quizzes, questions and answers and a glossary (CR 2.2, 2.29, 2.95).

2.1.60   Polit, D.F. & Hungler, B.P. (1999) *Nursing research: principles and methods* (6th edition). Philadelphia, PA: Lippincott ISBN 0781715628   References

Book retains all the features of previous editions and includes a balanced presentation of both qualitative and quantitative methods. A new chapter on qualitative research design and approaches is included, together with expanded discussion of multi-method research. A study guide, instructor's manual and test-bank are available to complement the text (CR 2.1.61, 2.2, 2.9, 2.36, 2.84).

2.1.61   Polit, D.F. & Hungler, B.P. (1999) *Study guide to accompany nursing research: principles and methods* (6th edition). Philadelphia, PA: Lippincott Williams & Wilkins   ISBN 0781715636

Book gives opportunities to reinforce the acquisition of basic research skills through systematic learning exercises. It will also help to bridge the gap between passive readings of complex abstract materials and active development of these skills (CR 2.1.60).

2.1.62 Remenyi, D., Williams, B., Money, A. & Swartz, E. (1998) *Doing research in business and management: an introduction to process and method.* London: Sage ISBN 0761959505 References

Book provides a comprehensive overview of management research and research methodology.

2.1.63 Robson, C. (2002) *Real world research: a resource for social scientists and practitioner-researchers* (2nd edition). Oxford: Blackwell ISBN 0631213058 References

Book covers quantitative and qualitative methods, which may be used when undertaking research in applied settings (CR 2.2, 2.9, 2.29, 2.36).

2.1.64 Salkind, N.J. (2002) *Exploring research* (5th edition). New York: Prentice-Hall ISBN 0130983527 References

Book is for advanced level students and it introduces all aspects of the research process. A chapter on qualitative research has been added and the section on the Internet has been revised and updated. There is also an accompanying website (CR 2.2).

2.1.65 Schutt, R.K. (2001) *Investigating the social world: the process and practice of research* (3rd edition). Thousand Oaks, CA: Pine Forge Press ISBN 0761987274 References

This textbook on research strategy retains its earlier features but now includes separate sections on qualitative methods in each chapter. Also in each chapter is a section on developing a research proposal. Many new web exercises and SPSS exercises, updated to GSS.98 data sets are included (CR 2.29, 2.36, 2.85, 2.90, 2.96, Appendix A).

2.1.66 Schneider, Z. & Elliott, D. (2002) *Nursing research: methods, critical appraisal and utilization* (2nd edition). St Louis, MO: Mosby ISBN 0729536653 References

Book examines the role of research in nursing practice and introduces students to the processes and methods used to conduct nursing research and how to use findings in clinical practice. There is free access to a website that contains student activities, lecturer support materials, additional research papers and relevant nursing research web links (CR 2.3, 2.29, 2.36).

2.1.67 Sumser, J. (2001) *A guide to empirical research in communication: rules for looking.* Thousand Oaks, CA: Sage ISBN 0761922229 References

Book explains difficult scientific and statistical concepts in simple terms and examines how the rules of looking are applied in four different areas of study: field research, experimentation, survey research and content analysis (CR 2.29, 2.36, 2.52, 2.88).

2.1.68 Thietart, R.-A. (2001) *Doing management research: a comprehensive guide.* London: Sage ISBN 0761965173 References

Book provides answers to questions and problems which researchers invariably encounter. The research process is described from beginning to end (CR 2.16).

2.1.69 Trochim, W.M. *Bill Trochim's center for social research methods* trochim.human.cornell.edu/ (Accessed 12/01/03)

This website is for those involved in applied social research and evaluation. It includes: the *Knowledge Base* – an online hypertext textbook on applied social research methods; the *Research Pointers Page* – references to other useful websites on social research and methods; *Selecting Statistics* – an online statistical advisor; the *Simulation Book* – a book of manual and computer simulation exercises of common research designs; *Research Papers* – published and unpublished; and the *World Wide Web Resource Center* – resources to assist in using the World Wide Web as a research tool (CR 2.1.70, 2.51, 2.83, 2.85).

2.1.70 Trochim, W.M. *Research methods knowledge base.* trochim.human.cornell.edu/kb (Accessed 12/01/03)

Comprises a comprehensive web-based textbook suitable for introductory or graduate courses in social research methods. It covers the entire research process and also discusses the theoretical and philosophical underpinnings of research. It was designed to be different from many other texts and uses an informal, conversational style to engage novices and more experienced students. Workbooks, study guides, online testing, test item data banks and other features are also included. It is a fully hyper-linked text that can be integrated into existing courses. A printed copy is also available.

2.1.71 University of Miami Libraries *Research methods in the social sciences: an Internet resource list.* www.miami.edu/netguides/psymeth.html (Accessed 20/01/03)

Provides an example of an Internet resource list that includes general information, tests and measures, survey method, quantitative research primers/dictionaries/datasets/other sources, qualitative research, research and writing and software (CR 2.2, 2.29, 2.36, 2.52, 2.54, Appendix A).

2.1.72 Walliman, N. & Baiche, B. (2001) *Your research project: a step-by-step guide for the*

first-time researcher. London: Sage ISBN 0761965394 References

The aim of this book is to guide novice researchers towards an understanding of the theory and approaches to research, and assist in the development of the necessary skills. Exercises are given throughout the text (CR 2.14).

2.1.73 Wilkinson, D. (ed.) (2000) *The researcher's toolkit: the complete guide to practitioner research.* London: Routledge/Falmer ISBN 0415215668 References

Book provides a short guide for novice researchers in the social sciences but it would need to be supplemented by other methods texts.

2.1.74 Wood, N. (2000) *The health project book: a handbook for new researchers in the field of health.* London: Routledge ISBN 1415243211 References

Book is an introduction to research and a 'dip-in' resource. Information is given on databases, data analysis packages and use of the Internet. A resource section provides additional material, including references to more advanced texts (CR 2.12, Appendix A).

2.2 LANGUAGE OF RESEARCH AND STATISTICS

Research, as with any other discipline, has its own terminology, and this section makes reference to dictionaries, chapters and articles where words or phrases are defined. Because no one source contains all the words to be found in this bibliography, definitions, taken from the literature, are given in each section where appropriate. Their original sources may be found in Appendix D. Definitions of statistical terms may be found in dictionaries in this section or methods textbook glossaries.

Annotations

2.2.1 *The a–z of social research: a dictionary of key social science research* (2003) Edited by Miller, R.L. & Brewer, J.D. London: Sage ISBN 0761971327

Provides critical guidance to the whole expanse of social science research methods and is a collection of 94 entries ranging from qualitative research techniques to statistical testing and the practicalities of using the Internet as a research tool. Entries are accessible, reader-friendly and vary in length from 800 to 3,000 words. Most are supported by suggestions for further reading.

2.2.2 *Cambridge dictionary of statistics in the medical sciences* (1995) Edited by Everitt, B.S.

Cambridge: Cambridge University Press ISBN 0521479282

Provides simple definitions and explanations of statistical concepts, especially those used in biomedicine.

2.2.3 Carnwell, R. (2000) Essential differences between research and evidence-based practice. *Nurse Researcher: The International Journal of Research Methodology in Nursing and Health Care* 8 (2) 55–68   12 References

There is considerable uncertainty in nursing about the differences between evidence-based practice and research. The author reviews a range of definitions of research and evidence-based practice, and delineates their defining features (CR 2.43, 2.102).

2.2.4 Clarke, M. & Oxman, A. (2001) *The Cochrane reviewers' handbook glossary.* Version 4.1.4 [Updated March 2001] (32pp). In: The Cochrane Library Issue 2 (2002). Oxford: Update Software   Updated quarterly www.update-software.com/ccweb/ (Accessed 14/02/03)

This glossary accompanies the *Cochrane Reviewers' Handbook* and defines words used in their published reviews (CR 2.12.5).

2.2.5 *Dictionary of clinical research* (2002) 3rd edition. Revised by Hutchinson, D.R. Richmond, Surrey: Brookwood Medical Publishers ISBN 1874409145

Contains glossaries of abbreviations and terms commonly encountered in clinical research.

2.2.6 *Dictionary of evidence-based medicine* (1998) Edited by Po, A.L.W. Oxford: Radcliffe Medical Press   ISBN 1857753054

An extensive guide to terms, ideas and concepts associated with evidence-based medicine. It is more than a simple dictionary and complements brief glossaries found in competing texts and in 'evidence-based' journals.

2.2.7 *Dictionary of nursing theory and research* (1995) 2nd edition. Edited by Powers, B.A. & Knapp, T.R. Thousand Oaks, CA: Sage ISBN 0803956266

Book contains a compilation of definitions, and discussion of both research and statistical terms, likely to be encountered in the nursing scientific literature. Also included are examples of where terms are used and citations to books and articles where they are more fully explained.

2.2.8 *Dictionary of social and market research* (1997) Edited by Koschnick, W.J. New York: John Wiley   ISBN 0470237333

Provides an exhaustive source of definitions, explanations of terms, techniques and concepts pertaining to the theory and practice of social and market research.

2.2.9 *Dictionary of social science methods* (1990) Edited by Miller, P.McC. & Wilson, M.J. New York: John Wiley ISBN 0471900362

Collects in one source accounts of current methods of inquiry that the empirical social sciences share in common. Definitions and explanations are also given, and a cross-referencing system leads to other relevant items. Many statistical terms are also included.

2.2.10 *Dictionary of statistics* (1998) Edited by Porkes, R. London: Collins ISBN 0004343549

Book is intended for the student and layperson, and is encyclopedic in nature. The text contains definitions, graphs, diagrams and worked examples of more advanced topics. Appendices include lists of symbols, formulae and statistical tables.

2.2.11 *Dictionary of statistics and methodology: a non-technical guide for the social sciences* (1999) 2nd edition. Edited by Vogt, W.P. Thousand Oaks, CA: Sage ISBN 0761912738

Book gives non-technical definitions of terms used in the social and behavioural sciences. The emphasis is on concepts rather than calculations. Items are cross-referenced.

2.2.12 Doordan, A.M. (1998) *Research survival guide*. Philadelphia, PA: Lippincott ISBN 0781710405

Book is designed to serve as a reference to research and research terminology for novices and experienced researchers. It contains an overview of research, a glossary of over 1,000 terms and a compendium of supplementary resources (CR 2.14).

2.2.13 Earl-Slater, A. (2002) *The handbook of clinical trials and other research*. Oxford: Radcliffe Medical Press ISBN 1857754859 References

A comprehensive book itemizing an A–Z of terms used in clinical research. Provides definitions of a wide range of clinical and research terms and uses worked examples to illustrate meaning. The book also gives references that can provide further explanations (CR 2.9, 2.29).

2.2.14 Gay, J.M. *Clinical epidemiology and evidence-based medicine glossary* www.vetmed.wsu.edu/courses-imgay/GlossClinEpiEBM.htm (Accessed 08/02/03)

Paper lists words, synonyms, common abbreviations and complete definitions for the most important

concepts unique or useful to epidemiology and evidence-based medicine. To assist understanding, the terms are classified into groups according to their usage, context and related words rather than being listed strictly alphabetically. A list of similar online dictionaries is also included (CR 2.41, 2.43).

2.2.15 Gubrium, J.F. & Holstein, J.A. (1997) *The new language of qualitative method*. New York: Oxford University Press ISBN 019709994X

Considering research methodologies as a set of idioms, this book examines alternate vocabularies for conveying social reality. It offers a new theoretical view that reintegrates the traditional emphasis on the *whats* of social life with a contemporary understanding of the *hows* and *whys* (CR 2.36).

2.2.16 Jary, D. & Jary, J. (2000) *Collins dictionary of sociology* (3rd edition). Glasgow: Harper Collins ISBN 0004708040

Covers terms and concepts used in sociology and related language in psychology, economics, political science and anthropology.

2.2.17 Lawson, T. & Garrod, J. (2000) *The complete a–z sociology handbook* (2nd edition). London: Hodder & Stoughton ISBN 0340772204

An alphabetical glossary designed for ease of use. Major concepts in the discipline of sociology have been included – each entry beginning with a one-sentence definition. The length of entry usually depends on the relative importance of the concept and often on the degree of controversy it arouses. Entries therefore provide illustrative examples or introduce the major points in support or criticism.

2.2.18 Munhall, P.L. (2001) Language of nursing research. In Author *Nursing research: a qualitative perspective* (3rd edition). Sudbury, MA: Jones & Bartlett and National League for Nursing ISBN 0763711357 Chapter 1 3–35 64 References

Chapter explores the qualitative/quantitative dichotomy to clearly reveal the possible differences between these two traditions. Nursing research and the quest for theory development are discussed from the point of view of language development and usage (CR 2.7, 2.9, 2.36.98).

2.2.19 *New Fontana dictionary of modern thought* (1999) 3rd edition. Edited by Bullock, A. & Trombley, S. London: Harper Collins ISBN 0006863833

Dictionary is a classic work of reference and companion to all fields of modern thought.

2.2.20 Schwandt, T.A. (2001) *Dictionary of qualitative inquiry* (2nd edition). Thousand Oaks, CA: Sage   ISBN 0761921664

Book considers the key concepts and issues that help to shape the field of qualitative research. The definitions acknowledge the multiple and often contested points of view that characterize these approaches. It focuses primarily on philosophical and methodological concepts rather than on the technical aspects of methods and procedures (CR 2.36).

2.3   NATURE AND PURPOSE OF RESEARCH IN NURSING

'As nurses we want to be able to give the very best care to our patients and clients. In order to do this we need to know what is the best and how to give it. Research findings and evidence can give us some of the knowledge to help us decide what is best and therefore to deliver the highest standards of care possible.' (Hek, Judd & Moule, 1996: 9)

Definitions [See Appendix D for sources]

Applied research – research without emphasis on theory, explanation or prediction but rather on application and development of research-based knowledge

Basic research – ... primarily concerned with developing the knowledge base and extending the theory in academic and/or practice disciplines ... findings cannot always be applied directly to practice

Clinical research – ... investigating questions emerging from clinical experience, paying attention to and revealing any underlying values and assumptions ... and directing the results towards clinical participants

Community health nursing research – research which attempts to prevent potential patients from becoming actual patients and to promote the health and well-being of both groups outside an institutional setting

Comparative research – research that creates empirical or explanatory knowledge about health, health services or health systems, by making comparisons using scientific methods that are appropriate for the subject studied and for the purpose of research

Empirical research – ... data-based investigations in which researchers systematically study some aspect of human behaviour

Fixed-design research – ... a research strategy where the research design is fixed (i.e. highly pre-specified) prior to the main phase of collection. Almost always involves collection of quantitative data and use of statistical analysis. The experiment is a prime example of fixed-design research

Flexible-design research – a research strategy when the research design develops (emerges, unfolds) during the process of data collection and analysis. Almost always involves the collection of qualitative data but can also involve the collection of quantitative data

Methodological research – is research into research. It is the ancient from of inquiry, with roots in philosophy, which tries to understand not what is true, but how we may know the truth

Nursing research – research into those aspects of health care which are the appropriate and predominant responsibility of nurses

Research – an attempt to extend the available knowledge by means of a systematically and scientifically defensible process of inquiry

Research methodology – ... the methods for collecting, processing and analysing research data

Research-mindedness – ... implies a critical, questioning approach to one's work, the desire and ability to find out about the latest research in that area, and the ability to assess its value to the situation and apply it as appropriate. It also implies recognition of the importance of research to the profession and to patient care, and a willingness to support nurse researchers in their work

---

Annotations

2.3.1   Chapman, J. (1991) Research: what it is and what it is not. In Perry, A. & Jolley, M. (eds) *Nursing: a knowledge base for practice.* London: Edward Arnold   ISBN 0340514922   Chapter 2   28–51   25 References

Provides an overview of research in nursing and outlines ways in which researchers explore problems to generate knowledge (CR 2.6, 2.14, 2.95, 3.7).

2.3.2   Gage, N.L. (1993) The obviousness of social and educational research results. In Hammersley, M. (ed.) *Social research: philosophy, politics and practice.* London: Sage   ISBN 0803988052   Chapter 17 226–37   11 References

Chapter discusses the obviousness of research and therefore whether it should be undertaken.

Critiques, positions and studies by several researchers are cited to illustrate the points made.

2.3.3   Hockey, L. (1981) Knowledge is a precious possession. *Nursing Mirror* 152 (13) 23 September 46–9   1 Reference

Examines what nursing research is and what it is not. The scepticism and enthusiasm of some nurses for research is contrasted, as well as the value of and necessity for research as a basis for practice.

2.3.4   Hockey, L. (2000) The nature and purpose of research. In Cormack, D.F.S. (ed.) *The research process in nursing* (4th edition). Oxford: Blackwell Science   ISBN 063204019X   Chapter 1   1–15 29 References

Chapter explores the nature, purpose and urgency of nursing research. Nurses' research involvement is discussed and the author speculates about the future (CR 2.1.23).

2.3.5   Holden, J.E. (1996) Physiological research is nursing research. *Nursing Research* 45 (5) 312–13   1 Reference

Author believes that what should drive nursing research is the question asked, not the bodily category in which it falls. Some of the confusion may have come from the struggle of nursing to gain autonomy as a separate profession from medicine. Nurses should take a holistic view so physical, psychosocial, spiritual and environmental factors are all important.

2.3.6   Hutchins, S.A. & Eckes, R. (1996) Clinical research: considerations for prospective participants. *Nursing Clinics of North America* 31 (1) 125–35   17 References

Article describes the purpose and process of clinical research, the patient perspective, ethical considerations and the role of the nurse in biomedical research (CR 2.17, 2.22, 3.16).

2.3.7   Martin, P.A. (1995) Is it research? *Applied Nursing Research* 8 (4) 199–201   11 References

Discusses some of the differences between research and organization improvement processes that can sometimes cause confusion. The pitfalls are highlighted when there is no clarity about which process is being used and the terminology is different. The implications of these problems are discussed.

2.3.8   Muir Gray, J.A. (2001) Appraising the quality of research. In Muir Gray, J.A. (ed.) *Evidence-based health care: how to make health policy and management decisions* (2nd edition). Edinburgh:

Churchill Livingstone   ISBN 0443062889   Chapter 5 117–67 5 References

Chapter asks what is research, choosing the right method, systematic reviews, randomized clinical trials, case-control studies, cohort studies and surveys. Decision analysis, qualitative research and hallmarks for knowledge are also discussed (CR 2.6, 2.12, 2.14, 2.29, 2.36, 2.41, 2.43, 2.48, 2.52).

2.3.9   Nolan, M. & Behi, R. (1995) What is research? Some definitions and dilemmas. *British Journal of Nursing* 4 (2) 111–15   24 References

Issues are addressed concerning the meaning and purpose of research and some of the principal differences between the major approaches are described (CR 2.2).

2.3.10   O'Brien, M. (1993) Social research and sociology. In Gilbert, N. (ed.) *Researching social life.* London: Sage   ISBN 0803986823   Chapter 1 1–17   References

Chapter outlines some of the key features of sociology as an approach to understanding social life. The role of theory in social research is discussed and two examples of research are given for illustration (CR 2.7).

2.3.11   Playle, J. (2000) The nature of research. *Journal of Community Nursing* 14 (1) 14, 16, 19, 20 16 References

Defines the nature of research as the basis for nursing practice.

2.3.12   Walliman, N.S.R. & Baiche, B. (2001) More about the nature of research. In Authors *Your research project: a step-by-step guide for the first-time researcher.* London: Sage   ISBN 0761965394 Chapter 5 151–88

Explores some aspects of the philosophy of research and the debate about the nature of knowledge. The forms and characteristics of the scientific method, alternative approaches, the nature of hypotheses and their roles in research are all discussed (CR 2.1.72, 2.5, 2.6, 2.8, 2.20).

2.4   RESEARCH PROCESSES

Although the phrase research process is frequently used, the practice of research often involves a series of processes. Science does not occur in stages or follow a linear path, but instead consists of overlapping processes in all parts of the investigation. The literature in this section provides brief overviews of these processes.

Definitions [See Appendix D for sources]

Research approaches – a set of methods and techniques for designing a study and collecting and analysing data: quantitative data for quantitative research, and qualitative data in qualitative research

Research processes – the use of quantitative and qualitative methods to collect and analyse data for the purposes of prediction and explanation [adapted]

Annotations

2.4.1   Arber, S. (1993) The research process. In Gilbert, N. (ed.) *Researching social life*. London: Sage   ISBN 0803986823   Chapter 3 32–50 References

Gives a personal account of a survey as an example of planning the research process. It also discusses the realities of research that are not always in accord with the ideas set out in manuals on methods (CR 2.14, 2.16, 2.52).

2.4.2   Barzun, J. (1998) *The modern researcher* (6th edition). San Diego, CA: Harcourt Brace College Publishers   ISBN 0155055291 References

Contains detailed information for researchers with particular reference to historical research. Advice is given on all aspects of writing reports (CR 2.46, 2.97).

2.4.3   Bush, C.T. (2001) What is nursing research? In Chitty, K.K. (ed.) *Professional nursing: concepts and challenges* (3rd edition). Philadelphia, PA: W.B. Saunders   ISBN 0721687113   Chapter 12 282–91   References

Chapter outlines the research process, how it may contribute to practice and its relationship to nursing theory and practice. Sources of support are identified and the roles of nurses in research discussed (CR 2.7, 3.16).

2.4.4   Carnwell, R. (2000) Essential differences between research and evidence-based practice. *Nurse Researcher* 8 (2) 55–68   12 References

Provides a step-by-step comparison of the differences between the processes and methodology involved in research and evidence-based practice (CR 2.43).

2.4.5   Fitch, M.I. (1995) Introduction to the process of research: a focus on oncology nursing research. *Canadian Oncology Nursing Journal* 5 (4) 130–5   41 References

Article offers a user-friendly approach for oncology nurses to instil confidence about some of the terminology and concepts used in research (CR 2.2).

2.4.6   Hockey, L. (2000) Research. In Lawton, S., Cantrell, J. & Harris, J. (eds) *District nursing: providing care in a supportive context*. Edinburgh: Churchill Livingstone   ISBN 0443062501 Chapter 6 101–12   References

Chapter brings research as a concept and as an activity right into the domain of district nursing. A definition of research is given together with a broad description of some basic research approaches. The involvement of district nurses is discussed together with issues of financing research. The author concludes with a glimpse into the future (CR 2.2, 2.14, 2.29, 2.36, 2.43, 2.52, 2.69, 2.102, 3.16).

2.4.7   Kirk, K. (1996) Embarking on the research process: a guide. *Health Visitor* 69 (9) 370–2   11 References

Readers are taken through the research process from inspiration to dissemination. Useful sources to support each stage are described.

2.4.8   Rees, C. (1994) A step-by-step guide to the research process. *British Journal of Midwifery* 2 (10) 479–84   4 References

Outlines the stages involved in the research process.

2.4.9   Rothwell, H. (1999) A beginner's picture of research (III) the end of the beginning. *The Practising Midwife* 2 (1) 35–7   3 References

Summarizes the research process (CR 2.14).

Conceptualizing Nursing Research

2.5 PHILOSOPHICAL BASES FOR RESEARCH

'[A] plurality of philosophies may be necessary to reflect the many facets of nursing science, that is, no one view may be sufficient to embrace or drive nursing knowledge in its totality.' (Omery, Kasper & Page, 1995: x)

Definitions [See Appendix D for sources]

Cartesianism – the philosophy of Descartes

Concept – a word picture or mental idea of a phenomenon

Conceptual framework – a background or foundation for a study, a less well-developed structure than a theoretical framework [… concepts are related in a logical manner by the researcher]

Conceptual model – symbolic presentation of concepts and the relationships between these concepts

Constructivism – … a philosophical perspective interested in the ways in which human beings individually and collectively interpret or construct the social and psychological world in specific linguistic, social and historical contexts

Critical realism – … while we have no option but to assume the existence of an objective reality, our knowledge of it is destined to be forever 'fallible'

Hermeneutics – the science or art of interpretation

Modernism – a particular view of the possibilities and direction of human social life, rooted in the Enlightenment and grounded in faith in rational thought. [From a modernist perspective, truth, beauty and morality exist as objective realities that can be discovered, known, and understood, through rational and scientific means]

Ontology – a sub-field of philosophy that focuses on the question of what actually exists and what does not

Operationalization – the process of figuring out how to measure concepts using empirical evidence

Paradigm – [*theoretical perspective*] … a set of assumptions about the nature of things that underlies the questions we ask and the kind of answers we arrive at as a result

Philosophy – love and pursuit of wisdom by intellectual means

Positivism – a way of thinking based on the assumption that it is possible to observe social life and establish reliable, valid knowledge about how it works

Positivist – an adherent or supporter of positivism

Post-modern thought – while diverse, there are clearly important points of connection between different (post) modern theorists in their discussions of the decentring of the subject, the rejection of 'grand narratives', the espousal of 'local narratives' … the dread of totalising discourses leading to totalitarianism … political pluralism and recovery of the 'other'

Post-modernism – … represents a reaction to, critique of, or departure from 'modernism' … an attitude toward the social world, more of a diagnosis than a theory

Post-positivism – … an attitude toward knowledge evident after the demise of epistemologies of science associated with logical positivism and logical empiricism – philosophies that sought to establish the foundation for all knowledge in sense experience

Post-structuralism – … a body of diverse theories

Realism – a philosophical approach to understanding reality that emphasizes the importance of taking into account not only what can be observed with the senses but [also] what cannot

Relativism – the theory that truths are relative and may vary according to the individual, group, place or time

Spatial ability – the ability to produce and manipulate or modify figural images

Structuralism – ... a way of thinking about the world and a methodology for investigating the world that is concerned with identifying and describing its underlying structures that cannot be observed but must be inferred

[The working distinction between post-modern and post-structural theoretical perspectives, posited by Agger (1991: 112): 'for my purposes here, post-structuralism ... is a theory of knowledge and language, whereas post-modernism ... is a theory of society, culture and history.']

Annotations

2.5.1 Alvesson, M. (2002) *Postmodernism and social research.* Buckingham: Open University Press   ISBN 033520631X   References

Book integrates philosophical and theoretical ideas with fieldwork and supports the development of research methods with a sharper interpretative and self-critical edge. It provides an overview of post-modern themes, evaluates the possibilities and dangers of post-modernist thinking and develops ideas on how a selective, sceptical incorporation of post-modernism can make social research more aware of pitfalls and more creative in working with data (CR 2.7).

2.5.2 Appleton, J.V. & King, L. (2002) Journeying from the philosophical contemplation of constructivism to the methodological pragmatics of health services research. *Journal of Advanced Nursing* 40 (6) 641–8   40 References

Paper describes a journey through the philosophical background of constructivism and the five principles underlying this paradigm. The philosophical roots of constructivism are then compared with post-positivism, critical realism and participatory inquiry. These methodologies are contrasted and their common features described. Such commonalities have resulted in the emergence of a generic research strategy that is gaining increased popularity in health services research and recent studies are used for illustration. The role of philosophy and the extent to which it should or does underpin or influence qualitative strategies are discussed.

2.5.3 DiBartolo, M.C. (1998) Philosophy of science in doctoral nursing education revisited. *Journal of Professional Nursing* 14 (6) November–December 350–60   49 References

Nurse scientists have been challenged recently to examine the discipline's philosophical underpinnings in order to understand the evolutionary process of nursing science. There is some disagreement as to whether the study of the philosophy of science should be included in the doctoral nursing curriculum, but it does provide a useful frame of reference in which to appreciate the unfolding of nursing as a discipline. Doctoral programmes are the most logical place in which to educate future scholars regarding the unique philosophical foundations of nursing, their implications for scientific inquiry and continued knowledge development (CR 2.7, 3.17).

2.5.4 Edwards, S.D. (2001) *Philosophy of nursing: an introduction.* Basingstoke: Palgrave   ISBN 033374991X   References

Book describes the nature of the philosophy of nursing and focuses on three areas of inquiry central to nursing theory and practice: knowledge, persons and care. The work of leading nurse writers is discussed and illuminating answers are supplied to issues in nursing upon which the very nature of nursing theory and practice depends (CR 2.6, 2.7, 2.8).

2.5.5 Francis, B. (2000) Poststructuralism and nursing: uncomfortable bedfellows? *Nursing Inquiry* 7 (1) 20–8   60 References

Debates the nature of post-structuralism and feminist research in relation to nursing. Argues that the former is useful for deconstructing existing discourse and practice, but incompatible and inadequate in changing or improving practice (CR 2.7, 2.10).

2.5.6 Fry, S.T. (1999) The philosophy of nursing. *Scholarly Inquiry for Nursing Practice* 13 (1) 5–15   39 References

Article provides an overview of the philosophy of nursing. The ontological, epistemological and ethical issues that comprise the field of inquiry are identified, and an examination is made of how some of these issues are being addressed in this particular issue of *Scholarly Inquiry for Nursing Practice.* Suggestions are made for further development of the philosophy of nursing in the twenty-first century (CR 2.6, 2.17).

2.5.7 Gartrell, C.D. & Gartrell, J.W. (2002) Positivism in sociological research: USA and UK (1966–1990). *British Journal of Sociology* 53 (4) 639–57   59 References

The results of a content analysis of sociological journal articles are discussed. They reveal that logical positivism remained a significant influence on sociological theory and this raises questions about sociologists' philosophy of science.

2.5.8 Geanellos, R. (1998a) Hermeneutic philosophy. Part 1: implications of its use as a methodology in interpretive nursing research. *Nursing Inquiry* 5 (3) September 154–63   64 References

AND

2.5.9 Geanellos, R. (1998b) Hermeneutic philosophy. Part 2: a nursing research example of the hermeneutic imperative to address forestructures/pre-understandings. *Nursing Inquiry* 5 (4) December 238–47 38 References

This two-part article reviews hermeneutically informed nursing research and methodological implications regarding the use of hermeneutic philosophy. This was in relation to: the need to address forestructures and pre-understandings; checking interpretations with research participants; seeking objectivity, consensus and accuracy in textual interpretation; evaluating interpretations and gaining entry into the hermeneutic circle. The author's research involved explicating the practice knowledge of nursing on residential adolescent mental health units where she had worked. The processes undertaken are described and this work was used to consider the presence of pre-understandings during textual interpretation in an attempt to prevent premature interpretative closure. The forestructures/pre-understandings were brought to consciousness and were reflected upon, their origins, adequacy and legitimacy questioned and their influence on the research taken into account (CR 2.68).

2.5.10 Goding, L. & Edwards, K. (2002) Evidence-based practice. *Nurse Researcher: The International Journal of Research Methodology in Nursing and Health Care* 9 (4) 45–57 29 References

Article provides an insight into the philosophical assumptions underpinning evidence-based practice. The authors believe that it has often been adopted within nursing, midwifery and health visiting without careful consideration of the nature of such evidence. The issues surrounding different research methodologies and methods, in particular the dichotomous relationships between positivism, constructivism and post-modernism are explored. Authors believe that nursing involves complex, intangible human behaviour that demands an interpretative, holistic approach investigating perceptions rather than a reductionist approach (CR 2.9, 2.29).

2.5.11 Jacox, A., Suppe, F., Campbell, J. & Stashinko, E. (1999) Diversity in philosophical approaches. In Hinshaw, A.S., Feetham, S.L. & Shaver, J.L.F. (eds) *Handbook of clinical nursing research*. Thousand Oaks, CA: Sage ISBN 080393784X Part 1 3–17 70 References

Chapter discusses the historical context for development of nursing theory and research, characterizes three philosophical approaches and the relationship of middle-range theory to the three philosophical approaches and illustrations of these in nursing.

Socio-political influences on contemporary nursing science, highlighting implications for clinical research are also discussed (CR 2.7, 3.5, 3.6.4).

2.5.12 Lines, K. (2001) A philosophical analysis of evidence-based practice in mental health nursing. *Australian & New Zealand Journal of Mental Health Nursing* 10 (3) 167–75 31 References

Paper examines some of the major philosophical problems in the debate over the use of evidence-based practice in mental health nursing, using both Foucault's formulation of discourse analysis and Derrida's construal of deconstruction. Author believes that post-modern philosophy offers a way to rid nursing of incessant attacks on either quantitative or qualitative research methods that underpin the debate over evidence-based practice in mental health nursing (CR 2.9, 2.43, 2.89).

2.5.13 Marinoff, L. (2001) *Philosophical practice.* New York: Academic Press ISBN 012475559 References

Book aims to familiarize readers with the developmental, theoretical, methodological and professional aspects of philosophical practice. It explains what philosophical practice is 'from the inside out', where and how it works, and how to establish a professional practice.

2.5.14 McVey, M.D. (2001) Understanding concepts in research methodology: the role of spatial ability. *Research in Education* 65 May 100–2 8 References

Students often experience difficulty learning the abstract concepts of research design. A brief report examined whether there is a link between spatial and research concepts. Further work is now being undertaken.

2.5.15 Pring, R. (2000) *Philosophy of educational research.* London: Continuum ISBN 0826448135 References

Three issues feature as central themes in this book: the nature of social science in general; the nature of educational inquiry in particular; and the links between the language and concepts of research, on the one hand, and those of practice and policy on the other.

2.5.16 Procter, S. (1998) Linking philosophy and method in the research process: the case for realism. *Nurse Researcher* 5 (4) 73–90 33 References

Paper discusses philosophical and methodological decision-making during the research process. Also considered are the links between philosophy, methodology and chosen method, and the importance of consistency between the aims of the study, research question, chosen methods and personal philosophy of the researcher. The discussion is based on reflections and decisions made during the early stages of a study that explored the issue of service quality in maternity care (CR 2.6, 2.14, 2.16, 2.26, 2.29, 2.49).

2.5.17   Radwin, L. & Fawcett, J. (2002) A conceptual model-based programme of nursing research: retrospective and prospective applications. *Journal of Advanced Nursing* 40 (3) 355–60 20 References

Article explains how one nurse researcher, working with a theoretician, formed a conceptual model that has provided a frame of reference for her past, present and future studies. This has allowed a view of her disparate studies as a more coherent programme of research. New possibilities were discovered and unanticipated areas for future study identified (CR 2.16).

2.5.18   Rodgers, B.L. & Knafl, K.A. (2000) *Concept development in nursing: foundations, techniques and applications* (2nd edition). Philadelphia, PA: W.B. Saunders ISBN 0443052018 References

This text presents state-of-the-art methods for developing concepts appropriate for nursing. It offers a wide array of approaches to concept development, ranging from the classic to the cutting-edge in a manner that balances philosophical foundations with techniques and practical examples.

2.5.19   Rolfe, G. (ed.) (2000) *Research, truth, authority: postmodern perspective on nursing.* Basingstoke: Macmillan ISBN 0333776372 References

Book traces the history of modernist and post-modernist thought from Galileo to the present day. Editor shows how post-modernism can offer new insights into the relationship between truth and power, and how these may be applied to nursing research and practice (CR 2.10, 2.78).

2.5.20   Rolfe, G. (2001) Postmodernism for health care workers in 13 easy steps. *Nurse Education Today* 21 (1) 38–47   42 References

Despite a growing literature on post-modernism in nursing and other health care disciplines, it continues to be dogged by mistrust, misunderstanding and outright hostility. This introduction to post-modernism attempts to straddle the discourses of modernism and post-modernism in both form and content, and offers a mixture of argument, example and speculation.

2.5.21   Smith, M.J. (1998) *Social science in question: towards a post-disciplinary framework.* London: Sage/Open University   ISBN 0761960414 References

Book makes the key ideas of philosophy of social science accessible to students, teachers and the community of social and cultural researchers.

2.5.22   Smith, M.J. (ed.) (2003) *Philosophy and methodology of the social sciences.* London: Sage   ISBN 076194737X   3 volumes

The source materials selected are drawn from debates within the natural sciences as well as social scientific practice. The set covers the traditional literature on the philosophy of the social sciences, and the contemporary philosophical and methodological debates developing at the heart of the disciplinary and interdisciplinary groups in the social sciences (CR 2.36).

2.5.23   Stevenson, C. & Beech, I. (2001) Paradigms lost, paradigms regained: defending nursing against a single reading of post-modernism. *Nursing Philosophy* 2 (2) 143–50   42 References

Iterates the post-modern position and recalls arguments for and against its application in nursing.

2.5.24   Tappan, M.B. (1997) Interpretive psychology: stories, circles and understanding lived experience. *Journal of Social Issues* 53 (4) Winter 645–56   34 References   (Accessed 24/07/01)

Essay provides an overview of an 'interpretative' or 'hermeneutic' approach to psychological research. It draws primarily on the work of Wilhelm Dilthey (1833–1911), a philosopher and literary historian, who is generally recognized as the 'father' of modern hermeneutic enterprise in the social and human sciences (CR 2.17).

2.5.25   Watson, M.J. (1999) *Postmodern nursing and beyond.* Edinburgh: Churchill Livingstone ISBN   0443057443

The author re-establishes the critical balance between caring and curing. It blends the technical aspects of modern medicine with the holistic focus traditionally associated with nursing, and serves as a model for nursing practice. The sections cover transpersonal nursing as ontological archetype, ontological artist and ontological architect.

2.5.26   Weiss, S. & Wesley, K. *Postmodernism and its critics* www.as.ua.edu/ant/Faculty/murphy/436/pomo.htm (Accessed 06/05/03)

Paper discusses the basic premises of post-modernism, points of reaction, leading figures, key works, principal concepts, methodologies, criticisms, comments and sources.

2.5.27   Yegdich, T. (2000) In the name of Husserl: nursing in pursuit of things-in-themselves. *Nursing Inquiry* 7 (1) 29–40   71 References

Explores the notion that nurse phenomenologists' pursuit of humanistic inquiry has led them to combine humanism and Husserlian phenomenology. Through an examination of Husserl and Kant's philosophies it is argued that there are inconsistencies between Husserl's thinking and nursing interpretations of his thought.

2.6   EPISTEMOLOGY

'Knowledge progresses not by absolute establishment of conclusions, but by the conjectures or hypotheses to criticism, and to the possibility of refutation. However not even this process yields certainty, for a position that is soundly criticizable today might undergo resuscitation tomorrow. Progress follows a tentative and meandering course.' (Phillips, D.C., 1987: 116)

Definitions [See Appendix D for sources]

Empiricism – the theory that all knowledge is derived from experience, or more specifically from sense-experience, scientific observation and experiment

Epistemology – a concept in philosophy that relates to the theories of knowledge or how people come to have knowledge of the world

Human Becoming Theory – a school of thought within the discipline of nursing

Praxis – practical application or exercise of a branch of learning

Science of Unitary Human Beings – ... an irreducible, indivisible, pan-dimensional energy field identified by pattern and manifesting characteristics that are specific to the whole and that cannot be predicted from knowledge of the parts

Example

Fisher, M.A. & Mitchell, G.J. (1998) Patients' views of quality of life: transforming the knowledge base of nursing. *Clinical Nurse Specialist* 12 (3) 99–105   28 References

Nurses in advanced practice roles are leaders in changing nurses' knowledge base. Findings from a qualitative research study, guided by the nursing theory of human becoming, are presented. The study aimed to enhance understanding of quality of life for patients receiving acute psychiatric care. Findings show directions for practice and further research.

Annotations

2.6.1   Alligood, M.R. & Fawcett, J. (1999) Acceptance of the invitation to dialogue: examination of an interpretive approach for the Science of Unitary Human Beings. *Visions: The Journal of Rogerian Nursing Science* 7 (1) 5–13   30 References

Paper argues that rational interpretative hermeneutics is compatible with the Science of Unitary Human Beings (SUHB). Following an invitation to discuss issues of (in)compatibility between the world view and research rules of the SUHB, the authors offer an interactive dialogue building on the questions raised and an examination of the compatibility of rational interpretative hermeneutics for this theory (CR 2.8).

2.6.2   Björnsdottir, K. (2001) Language, research and nursing practice. *Journal of Advanced Nursing* 33 (2) 159–66   46 References

Paper highlights the centrality of language in constructing knowledge. It aims at making us sensitive to the political nature of knowledge and the complex power relationships that may emerge as a result of our efforts to create new knowledge.

2.6.3   Benner, P. (2002) Uncovering the knowledge embedded in clinical nursing practice. In Rafferty, A.M. & Traynor, M. (eds) *Exemplary research for nursing and midwifery.* London: Routledge   ISBN 0415241634   Chapter 7 145–52

Examines the differences between practical and theoretical knowledge, and provides examples of competencies identified from the study of nursing practice. Aspects of practical knowledge are described, together with strategies for preserving and extending knowledge (CR 3.21.5).

2.6.4   Ceci, C. (2000) Not innocent: relationships between knowers and knowledge. *Canadian Journal of Nursing Research* 32 (2) 57–73   16 References

Discussions about nursing knowledge have tended to focus on determining what kinds of knowledge are the most appropriate or most useful for nursing. Should our methods be primarily empirical? What is the place of interpretative work? What kind of knowledge should have ascendancy in nursing? Framed in this way these questions seem unanswerable. However, if the terms of discussion are shifted from appropriate kinds of knowledge and the relationship between knowledge and knowers, we can reflect, as knowers, on what we think we know.

2.6.5   Chinn, P.L. & Kramer, M.K. (1999) *Knowledge and nursing: an integrated approach* (5th edition). St Louis, MO: Mosby   ISBN 0323003176   References

Book will help students develop a solid foundation by providing a comprehensive review of the fundamental patterns of knowing in nursing. It contains a thorough explanation of nursing theory, critical evaluation, knowledge development and evolution, and its contribution to the profession. Knowledge development content is expanded in this edition to include aesthetic, ethical, personal and empirical knowledge (CR 2.7).

2.6.6 Cooper, C. (2001) *The art of nursing: a practical introduction.* Philadelphia, PA: W.B. Saunders ISBN 0721682162 References

Using rich nursing narratives from practising nurses as well as scholarly conceptual sources, this book paints a vivid picture of the diversity and richness embodied in the artful practice of nursing. These stories illustrate the forms of knowledge used by nurses and demonstrate essential nursing concepts, such as care, spirituality, presence, compassion, self-care and advocacy (CR 2.78).

2.6.7 Coyle, J. & Williams, B. (2000) An exploration of the epistemological intricacies of using qualitative data to develop a quantitative measure of user views of health care. *Journal of Advanced Nursing* 31 (5) 1235–43 53 References

Paper highlights the epistemological and methodological complexities involved in combining qualitative and quantitative methods when developing an instrument to examine person-centredness in health care from a qualitative study of dissatisfaction. The intricacies of the project relate to epistemological continuity and inconsistency, research roles, reflexivity, confirmation and completeness. Authors believe that conceptually sound quantitative measures could be developed by extending the concept of reflexivity to the quantitative components of mixed method studies (CR 2.9, 2.29, 2.36, 2.58).

2.6.8 Cutcliffe, J.R. & McKenna, H.P. (2001) When do we know that we know? Considering the truth of research findings and the craft of qualitative research. *International Journal of Nursing Studies* 39 (6) 611–18 References

It can be argued that nurse researchers and theoreticians have paid insufficient attention to answering the fundamental question – when do we know what we know? This paper critically examines some of the key epistemological, philosophical and methodological issues and challenges some widely accepted, yet seldom confronted, myths. It examines and discusses 'knowing' in both quantitative and qualitative paradigms (CR 2.5, 2.7, 2.29, 2.36, 2.93).

2.6.9 Dancy, J. & Sosa, E. (eds) (1993) *A companion to epistemology.* Oxford: Blackwell ISBN 0631192581 References

This volume, in the Blackwell *Companion to Philosophy* series, is organized as a standard reference book with 250 alphabetically arranged entries. It contains contributions from leading epistemologists and includes summaries of technical terms and extended essays on major topics (CR 2.2).

2.6.10 Dixon, J.K. & Dixon, J.P. (2002) An integrative model for environmental health research. *Advances in Nursing Science* 24 (3) 43–57 50 References

Examines four domains that determine the health of individuals and populations and proposes an integrative model as a rational means of advancing knowledge in environmental health.

2.6.11 Freshwater, D. & Rolfe, G. (2001) Critical reflexivity: a politically and ethically engaged research method for nursing … including commentary by Pryce, A. *NT Research* 6 (1) 526–38 52 References

Paper proposes a research method that legitimizes practice as a source of knowledge. Beginning with an analysis of knowledge and power, the contribution of reflexivity to the development of a politically and ethically engaged research process in nursing is explored. In discussing critical reflexivity as a research method the role of reflexive research and reflexive researcher are discussed. Arguing against the superiority of theoretical over practitioner research, the authors present a challenge to technical rationality, suggesting not only a new approach to research but also a new approach to practice.

2.6.12 Gunter, B. (1999) *Media research methods: measuring audiences, reactions and impact.* London: Sage ISBN 076195659X References

By tracing the epistemological and theoretical roots of the major methodological perspectives, the author identifies the various schools of social scientific research that have determined the major perspectives in the area. The relative advantages and disadvantages of each approach are discussed and recent trends signal a convergence of methods (CR 2.5, 2.36).

2.6.13 Harvey, J., Pettigrew, A. & Ferlie, E. (2002) The determinants of research group performance: towards mode 2. *Journal of Management Studies* 39 (6) September 747–74 78 References

Paper explores the determinants of performance of research groups in the context of the emergence of knowledge as a key, intangible asset. It focuses on how best to configure knowledge produced for optimal effectiveness in the current research environment. It examines the under-researched area of organization and management of groups located in and around the interface of university research, focusing on medical and medical-related groups.

2.6.14 Hicks, F.D. (2001) Critical thinking: toward a nursing science perspective. *Nursing Science Quarterly* 14 (1) 14–21   57 References

Explores the nature of critical thinking in nursing, examining the foundations and current research approaches regarding critical thinking knowledge. The paper provides a discussion regarding the future of a nursing science perspective.

2.6.15 Hinshaw, A.S. (1998) Methodological innovations in knowledge development. In: *Knowledge development: clinicians and researchers in partnership.* Helsinki: The Finnish Federation of Nurses ISSN 0251–4753 Proceedings of the Workgroup of European Nurse Researchers (9th Biennial Conference 5–8 July 1998 Helsinki, Finland) Volume 1 29–46   23 References

Paper examines several of the innovative and challenging issues involved with the research methods and measures being used by the nursing scientific community (CR 2.5, 2.9, 2.28).

2.6.16 Johnson, P. & Duberley, J. (2000) *Understanding management research: an introduction to epistemology.* London: Sage ISBN 0761952950 References

Book provides an overview of the principal epistemological debates in social science. It examines how they are expressed and may lead to different ways of conceiving and undertaking organizational research. Topics include how to frame questions, assess the relevance and value of different research methodologies and evaluate the outputs of research (CR 2.14, 2.20, 2.95).

2.6.17 Kim, H.S. (1998) Structuring the nursing knowledge system: a typology of four domains … including commentary by Hinshaw, A.S. and Kim, H.S. *Scholarly Inquiry for Nursing Practice* 12 (4) 367–88   46 References

In order to develop a typology that can be used to systematize research and the ever-accumulating knowledge in nursing, a classification of four domains is proposed as a conceptual 'map' of nursing and as a 'sensitizing' scheme for further research. These are: client, environment, client–nurse and the practice domains.

2.6.18 Lawler, J. (2002) Knowing the body and embodiment – methodologies, discourses and nursing. In Rafferty, A.M. & Traynor, M. (eds) *Exemplary research for nursing and midwifery.* London: Routledge ISBN 0415241634 Chapter 9 166–87   36 References

The question explored in this chapter is how are we, as nurses, to know and understand the body and abstract concepts as researchable topics of importance to the discipline? The author argues that our knowledge and discourse(s) should both reflect and affect the manner of our practice as nurses. However, our recorded discourses and formalized knowledge are more reflective on influences external to nursing than the practice of nursing as it might emerge from clinical practice settings (CR 2.9, 2.16, 2.18, 3.21.5).

2.6.19 Manias, E. & Street, A. (2000) Legitimation of nurses' knowledge through policies and protocols in clinical practice. *Journal of Advanced Nursing* 32 (6) 1467–75   33 References

Paper examines the power relations at play between doctors and nurses, and among nurses, and the ways in which nurses used policies and protocols as a means of mediating communication in a small study. While policies and protocols provided nurses with legitimacy of their knowledge, doctors tended to rely on their past experience and background to inform their knowledge and activities. These differing views are discussed as complex power relations that can create tensions in clinical practice (CR 2.15, 2.42).

2.6.20 Meleis, A.I. & Im, E.-O. (1999). Transcending marginalization in knowledge development. *Nursing Inquiry* 6 (2) 94–102 50 References

Quality care requires a body of knowledge that reflects the experiences and responses of marginalized populations in both health and illness. It also requires the demarginalization of nursing knowledge. The authors discuss the development of knowledge that is not marginalizing, developing knowledge about marginalized populations, integrating nursing knowledge and making it visible, and the future of research enterprise.

2.6.21 Peters, M. (2000) Does constructivist epistemology have a place in nurse education? *Journal of Nursing Education* 39 (4) April 166–72 56 References

Constructivist epistemology offers an alternative to traditional pedagogy in that it is student-focused and considers previous learning as a foundation on which to modify, build and expand new knowledge. It also appears to be congruent with adult education theory and therefore offers great potential for the enhancement of self-directed learning. Learning within a constructivist framework benefits nurses in the practice setting, helping them to make the transition from inexperienced to experienced practitioners. Students are also provided with learning skills that enhance knowledge acquisition with understanding (CR 3.17).

2.6.22   Platt, J. (1996) *A history of sociological research methods in America 1920–1960.* Cambridge: Cambridge University Press ISBN 0521441730 References

Book provides systematic archival, documentary and interview data that question many conventional views, and it raises wider issues of method in the history of ideas. It discusses the production of methodological writing, showing that neither it nor theoretical work adequately describes research practice. The dominance and meaning of scientism is discussed, together with the impact of research funding on the development and practice of research (CR 2.7, 2.8, 2.46, 3.13).

2.6.23   Playle, J. (2000) The nature of research. *Journal of Community Nursing* 14 (1) 14, 16, 19–20   16 References

Identifies different forms of knowledge, and the process and purposes of research as a basis for nursing practice (CR 2.3, 2.4).

2.6.24   Ramprogus, V. (2002) Eliciting nursing knowledge from practice: the dualism of nursing. *Nurse Researcher: The International Journal of Research Methodology in Nursing and Health Care* 19 (1) 52–64   19 References

Challenges the traditional approach to how nursing knowledge is defined and the common understanding of the purpose of nursing research. It is argued that adhering to empirical vigour while investigating or measuring nursing practice interferes with the very act and experience of nursing. It becomes an either/or situation. It is also argued that nursing is not an empirical subject, and therefore the purpose of researching nursing is not about seeking the truth but about improving practice to achieve better patient care. The author hopes these ideas will provoke discussion and debate among researchers.

2.6.25   Rancourt, R., Guimond-Papai, P. & Prud'homme-Brisson, D. (2000) Faculty ways of knowing: the crux of nursing curricula. *Nurse Educator* 25 (3) 117–20   18 References

The director and three staff members from a fictitious nursing school portray three epistemological structures found in nursing curricula. These fundamentally different ways of knowledge acquisition are discussed and the authors believe they should be blended together when developing curricula.

2.6.26   Rolfe, G. (1998) *Expanding nursing knowledge: understanding and researching your own practice.* Oxford: Butterworth-Heinemann ISBN 0750630132 References

Book explores ways in which nurses and other health care practitioners can carry out personal research studies into their own practice. A new paradigm of nursing is advocated, the types of knowledge and theory needed are discussed, and suggestions are made as to how this can be acquired (CR 2.13, 2.34, 2.37, 2.39).

2.6.27   Schmidt, V.H. (2001) Over-socialized epistemology: a critical appraisal of constructivism. *Sociology* 35 (1) 135–57   75 References

Explores the strengths and weaknesses in attempting to socialize the concepts of knowledge and cites flaws in the constructivist literature concerning epistemology (CR 2.5).

2.6.28   Scott, D. (2000) *Realism and educational research: new perspectives and possibilities.* London: Routledge/Falmer ISBN 0750709189 References

Book critiques traditional perspectives on knowledge and educational research, and develops a realistic framework as an alternative. It explores a series of controversial debates that have taken place in the field of education, including biography and autobiography, race and ethnicity and post-modernism (CR 2.71, 3.11). •

2.6.29   Thorne, S.E. & Hayes, V.E. (eds) (1997) *Nursing praxis: knowledge and action.* London: Sage ISBN 076190011X References

As nursing theory and knowledge evolve, relationships between ideas and actions become blurred. Contributors to this book present some of the ways in which nursing scholars are confronting this problem by reflecting on the nature of nursing knowledge and the application of theory in practice.

2.6.30   Vinson, J.A. (2000) Nursing's epistemology revisited in relation to professional education competencies. *Journal of Professional Nursing* 16 (1) 39–46   40 References

A discussion of the epistemology of the nursing profession, needed competencies and the goals of higher education are presented in this article. Patterns of knowing distinguish disciplines from one another. Nursing patterns of knowing and subsequent clinical, conceptual and empirical knowledge need to be taught in institutions of higher learning that promote both professional competencies and attitudes.

2.7   DEVELOPMENT OF THEORY

The nature of nursing as a science and an art requires a strong theoretical basis that needs translating into practice. Nurse researchers are increasingly developing this base, which will inform all future studies and ultimately patient care.

Definitions [See Appendix D for sources]

Chaos theory – ... explains how complex systems behave

Critical theory – a sociological theory that aims to dig beneath the surface of social life and uncover the assumptions and masks that keep us from a full and true understanding of how the world works

Facet theory – a meta-theoretical approach to scientific research

Functionalism – ... theories or models [that] aim to explain human behaviour (e.g. rituals, customs, ceremonies) and social-cultural institutions (e.g. family, church, state) in terms of the functions they perform in a particular group, society, culture or community

Grand theories – theories that are concerned with a broad range of phenomena in the environment or in the experience of humans

Middle-range theories – theories that have a narrow focus, are concerned with only a small area of the environment or of human experience

Reductionism – the attempt to explain everything in terms of a single hypothesis or to reduce all theories to one basic theory

Taxonomy – the science, laws or principles of classification

Theoretical frameworks – a set of integrated hypotheses designed to explain particular classes of events

Theoretical substruction – a powerful tool for conceptualizing and assessing congruence between the theoretical and operational components of research

Theory – a set of statements that tentatively describes, explains or predicts relationships between concepts that have been systematically selected and organized as an abstract representation of some phenomena

Example

Forbes, M.A. (1999) Hope in the older adult with chronic illness: a comparison of two research methods in theory building. *Advances in Nursing Science* 22 (2) 74–87   26 References

When current theory about a concept of interest is insufficient, the researcher may desire to build or expand theory. Two research methods for building

nursing theory were compared by asking the same question using each method. Phenomenology was used to analyse the interviews of six older adults with chronic illness regarding their experience of hope. Eight categories emerged, and using concept mapping, statements about hope were generated. The procedures were compared and the outcome and results are reported.

Annotations

2.7.1 Alderson, P. (1998) The importance of theories in health care. *British Medical Journal* 317 (7164) 10 October 1007–10   13 References

States that theories are integral to health care practice, promotion and research and the choice of theory, although often unacknowledged, shapes the way practitioners and researchers collect and interpret evidence. Positivism, functionalism, social construction, post-modernism and critical theory are all discussed.

2.7.2 Alligood, M.R. & Marriner-Tomey, A. (2002) *Nursing theory: utilization and application.* St Louis, MO: Mosby   ISBN 0323011942   References

This new edition demonstrates how theory-based nursing guides critical thinking for decision-making in practice. The work of some nursing theorists is explored and areas for further development and directions for theory-based practice are discussed.

2.7.3 Barnum, B.S. (1998) Theory, research and knowledge. In Author *Nursing theory: analysis, application, evaluation* (5th edition). Philadelphia, PA: Lippincott   ISBN 0781711045   Chapter 20 263–77   16 References

Chapter discusses realism versus conceptualism, research and the nature of reality, theory and research, phenomenology, hermeneutics, critical social theory and recapitulation (CR 2.5, 2.49).

2.7.4 Cheek, J. (2000) *Postmodern and poststructural approaches to nursing research.* Thousand Oaks, CA: Sage   ISBN 0761906754   References

Book examines definitions of post-modern and post-structural approaches and ways in which they can be used to influence and inform about health care. The practical aspects of proposing and carrying out projects using these approaches are described, and by reviewing the 'intellectual journey' required in coming to grips with their meaning and application, the author suggests ways in which the reader can continue to 'grow'.

2.7.5 Chinn, P.L. & Kramer, M.K. (1995) *Theory and nursing: a systematic approach (*4th edition). St Louis, MO: Mosby   ISBN 0801679478   References

Book examines the relationships between theory and nursing and discusses ways in which nursing research studies can be theoretically sound.

2.7.6   Clift, J. & Barrett, E. (1998) Testing nursing theory cross-culturally. *International Nursing Review* 45 (4) July-August 123–26   8 References

For nursing science to be recognized globally, nursing theory must be tested in various cultural settings to prove its universality. This study provides an overview of cross-cultural theory development in three German-speaking countries of Europe and its implications for practice (CR 2.53, 3.3).

2.7.7   Dudley-Brown, S.L. (1997) The evaluation of nursing theory: a method for our madness. *International Journal of Nursing Studies* 34 (1) 76–83   21 References

Paper attempts to define theory, including nursing theory, and then analyses criteria for its evaluation. A more comprehensive set of criteria is proposed which may stimulate more informed decision-making regarding the choice of nursing theory for use in practice, education and research, and from which new ones may emerge.

2.7.8   Eisenhardt, K.M. (2002) Building theories from case study research. In Huberman, A.M. & Miles, M.B. (eds) *The qualitative researcher's companion.* Thousand Oaks, CA: Sage   ISBN 076191191X   Chapter 1 5–35   41 References

Chapter describes the process of theory-building from case studies (CR 2.36.62, 2.39).

2.7.9   Fawcett, J. (1999) *The relationship of theory and research* (3rd edition). Philadelphia, PA: F.A. Davis Co.   ISBN 0803604068   References

Book fills a major gap in the literature and presents a detailed discussion of the relationship between theory and research. Emphasis is placed on information needed by novices and scholars for analysing and evaluating research reports and creating proposals for new studies. This edition has been extensively revised and new examples are included. Appendices contain analyses and evaluation of descriptive, correlational and experimental studies. A comprehensive bibliography related to nursing theory and theorizing in nursing is also included (CR 2.29, 2.36, 2.40, 2.95, 2.96, 2.99).

2.7.10   Fawcett, J. & Gigliotti, E. (2001) Using conceptual models of nursing to guide nursing research: the case of the Neuman Systems Model. *Nursing Science Quarterly* 14 (4) October. 339–45 20 References

Conceptual models of nursing inform thinking and give meaning and direction to nursing research. The Neuman Systems Model is used to exemplify five steps, which provide direction for conceptual model-based research. These are to develop a comprehensive understanding of the substantive content and research rules of the model; review existing research guided by the model; construct a conceptual-theoretical-empirical structure; clearly communicate this structure, and evaluate the empirical adequacy of the middle-range theory and credibility of the conceptual model (CR 2.5, 2.6).

2.7.11   Fawcett, J., Watson, J., Neuman, B., Walker, P.H. & Fitzpatrick, J.J. (2001) On nursing theories and evidence. *Journal of Nursing Scholarship* 33 (2) 2nd Quarter 115–19   21 References

Article expands the understanding of what constitutes evidence for theory-guided, evidence-based nursing practice from a narrow focus on empirics to a more comprehensive focus on diverse patterns of knowing (CR 2.6, 2.43).

2.7.12   Gastaldo, D. & Holmes, D. (1999) Foucault and nursing: a history of the present. *Nursing Inquiry* 6 (4) 231–40   49 References

Paper identifies publications by nurses that employ a Foucauldian perspective, and provides a summative review of 27 works between 1987 and 1998 in English, Portuguese and German. The most frequent concepts in the literature reviewed were power/knowledge, surveillance, discourse, discipline, resistance, docile bodies, clinical gaze and panoptican. A Foucauldian reading of nursing enables nurses to move into a broader interdisciplinary and critical scholarship.

2.7.13   Hartrick, G. (1998) A critical pedagogy for family nursing. *Journal of Nursing Education* 37 (2) February 80–4   12 References

Article emphasizes the importance of students and faculty engaging in a critical analysis of family nursing theory and practice, including both ontological and epistemological inquiries. A critical pedagogy of family nursing that addresses both these factors is described (CR 2.6).

2.7.14   Hisama, K.K. (1999) Towards an international theory of nursing. *Nursing and Health Sciences* 1 (2) 77–81   10 References

Paper summarizes the development of nursing theories developed initially from North American nurses. It suggests how these might evolve into an international theory of nursing and future directions for such a theory (CR 3.1, 3.5, 3.22).

2.7.15   Holmes, C.A. & Warelow, P.J. (2000) Some implications of postmodernism for nursing theory, research and practice. *Canadian Journal of Nursing Research* 32 (2) 89–101   31 References

Paper explores ways in which some aspects of postmodernist thought impact upon nursing theory and research. The focus is on post-modernist accounts of epistemology and language, in particular notions such as multiple truths, uncertain and provisional knowledge, and claims as to the purposes of knowledge development. Common themes of post-modernism are articulated, including anti-foundationalism, the dissonance between competing discourses and the rejection of 'grand theories'. A short set of suggestions is given for a post-modern approach to nursing practice (CR 2.6).

2.7.16   Im, E. & Meleis, A.I. (1999) Situation-specific theories: philosophical roots, properties, and approach. *Advances in Nursing Science* 22 (2) 11–24   51 References

Authors believe it is imperative to develop further theoretical bases in nursing which incorporate diversities and complexities in nursing phenomena, and which consider socio-political, cultural and historic contexts of nursing encounters. Situation-specific theories are proposed, their philosophical roots and properties discussed, and an integrative approach to developing this type of theory is suggested.

2.7.17   Kenney, J.W. (2002) *Philosophical and theoretical perspectives for advanced nursing practice* (3rd edition). Sudbury, MA: Jones & Bartlett ISBN 0763718580   References

Book explores the healthy discourse surrounding nursing theory, research and practice. A collection of 26 classic and contemporary articles is divided into six parts that address the discipline and the development of nursing knowledge, the history and evolution of nursing science, the concepts of the meta-paradigm, contemporary perspectives of nursing, and the interrelationships between nursing theory, research and practice (CR 2.5, 2.6).

2.7.18   Kuokkanen, L. & Leino-Kilpi, H. (2000) Power and empowerment in nursing: three theoretical approaches. *Journal of Advanced Nursing* 31 (1) 235–41   52 References

Based on a literature review, this paper explores the uses of the empowerment concept as a framework for nurses' professional growth and development.

2.7.19   Layder, D. (1998) *Sociological practice: linking theory and social research*. London: Sage   ISBN 0761954309   References

Book offers a better understanding of the links between theory and research, and provides an analysis of the relationship between the two. Strategies are developed to encourage theory development, and a new approach called adaptive theory is discussed that can be used to generate new theory in conjunction with empirical research.

2.7.20   Lett, M. (2001) A case for chaos theory in nursing. *Australian Journal of Advanced Nursing* 18 (3) March–May 14–19   24 References

Paper addresses the question of why nurses should understand chaos theory. A critique of the literature shows how it has been used in a number of disciplines, including nursing. Possible applications of chaos theory in nursing are proposed in order to demonstrate where it might assist researchers, educators and policy-makers. The appropriateness of the application of chaos theory as a framework for knowledge generation is also discussed (CR 2.6, 2.12, 3.11).

2.7.21   Liehr, P. & Smith, M.J. (1999) Middle-range theory: spinning research and practice to create knowledge for the new millennium. *Advances in Nursing Science* 21 (4) 81–91   46 References

The foundation of middle-range theory reported during the 1990s is described and analysed. 22 such theories were identified which provide a firm base for theorizing, and recommendations are made as to how this may be carried forward.

2.7.22   Manias, E. & Street, A. (2000) Possibilities for critical social theory and Foucault's work: a toolbox approach. *Nursing Inquiry* 7 (1) 50–60   67 References

The benefits and constraints of philosophical frameworks, using the work of Michael Foucault and critical social theorists, such as Fay, Giroux and McLaren, are examined in the light of their traditions. The reasons nurse researchers adopt these frameworks are explored, as are the tensions between the respective theories. A complementary 'toolbox' approach to the research process addresses some of the theoretical and methodological challenges presented by each framework. By converging the two frameworks it is possible to examine or deconstruct existing practices, while also providing an avenue for nurses to reconstruct or change such practices (CR 2.6, 3.8).

2.7.23   Marriner-Tomey, A. & Alligood, M.R. (2001) *Nursing theorists and their work,* (5th edition). St Louis, MO: Mosby   ISBN 0323011934 References

This modern classic presents authoritative, up-to-date descriptions and analyses of 28 nursing theories. The book also covers the evolution of nursing theories, philosophies and the state of the art and science of nursing theory (CR 2.5, 3.6).

2.7.24   Meleis, A.I. (1997) *Theoretical nursing: development and progress* (3rd edition). Philadelphia, PA: Lippincott   ISBN 0397552599 References

A comprehensive text that explores, discusses, analyses, critiques, compares and contrasts different epistemologies, theories of truth and nursing theories. Although the focus is on nursing theories, the book emphasizes that nursing is based on philosophy, theory, practice and research. The theory–research/theory–strategy dichotomy is explained, abstracts of theoretical writing in nursing are given and there is an extensive bibliography on theory and meta-theory (CR 2.5, 2.6).

2.7.25 Mithaug, D.E. (2000) *Learning to theorize: a four-step strategy.* Thousand Oaks, CA: Sage ISBN 0761909X References

Through the use of questions and examples the author shows how to implement his four-step strategy to construct explanations for uncertainties about how things work, how they ought to work, and what should be done about them.

2.7.26 Moody, L.E. (1990) *Advancing nursing science through research.* Newbury Park, CA: Sage ISBN 080393811X (Volume 1) 0803938128 (Volume 2)

Intended for graduates and doctoral students, the two volumes cover major advances in theory and research. Many examples are given, together with questions for further study. Volume 2 discusses statistical approaches to theory-building and applications are described. Clinical trials, meta-analyses, causal modelling and time-series approaches are discussed. Non-statistical approaches include case studies, foundational, hermeneutical and sociolinguistic inquiry (CR 2.20, 2.29, 2.39, 2.92).

2.7.27 Morse, J.M. (1999) Exploring the theoretical basis of nursing using advanced techniques of concept analysis [French]. *Recherche en Soins Infirmiers* 58 September 35–45 References

The traditional methods of concept development are critiqued, and alternative methods that use qualitative methods of inquiry are presented. Variations of concept development techniques appropriate to the maturity of the concept being explored are then described, including methods for concept delineation, comparison, clarification, correction and concept identification. To illustrate the application of concept development methods to nursing theory, a research programme to delineate the construct of comfort is described.

2.7.28 Moynihan, C. (1998) Theories of masculinity. *British Medical Journal* 317 (7165) 17 October 1072–5 23 References

Paper shows how theories that underlie research influence the ways in which we perceive phenomena and how we deal with them. It questions assumptions about the concept of masculinity in medicine

and how these assumptions affect men. Alternative ways of seeing may widen our perceptions, but at the same time present us with more difficulties.

2.7.29 Nicoll, L.H. (ed.) (1992) *Perspectives on nursing theory* (2nd edition). Philadelphia, PA: Lippincott Williams & Wilkins ISBN 0397549105 References

An anthology of 80 articles on nursing theory, covering more than 40 years of writings. It includes classics and often-cited writings in the field. Bibliographical information provides insight into the authors' thoughts, experiences and purposes for writing the articles; commentaries introduce another perspective and represent current thinking.

2.7.30 Olszewski, L., Walker, R.N., Coalson, K. & Avant, R.N. (1999) *Strategies for theory construction in nursing.* (3rd edition). New York: Prentice-Hall ISBN 0838586880 References

This new edition features nursing theory development within the larger nursing context. Chapters discuss concept, statement and theory development with recently published examples of research strategies, emphasizing concept analytical work.

2.7.31 Parse, R.R. (1998) *The Human Becoming School of Thought: a perspective for nurses and other health professionals.* Thousand Oaks, CA: Sage ISBN 0761905839 References

Discusses Parse's Theory of Human Becoming, which has now evolved into a school of thought. This developed from philosophical foundations laid down by Martha Rogers and the existential phenomenologists. This concept enables nursing scholars to understand people and their universe in a unique way, thus providing a human science context for nursing and practice (CR 2.5, 2.6, 2.49).

2.7.32 Parse, R.R. (1999) *Illuminations: the Human Becoming Theory in practice and research.* Sudbury, MA: Jones & Bartlett ISBN 0763711101 References

Book explores a human science that reveals the eloquence of the nurse–person encounter. Parse and other nursing scholars provide a dynamic model for professional nurses, undergraduate and graduate students, and all others who believe that individuals know their own needs best (CR 2.5, 2.6).

2.7.33 Roberts, K.L. (1999) Through a looking glass: nursing theory and clinical nursing research. *Clinical Nursing Research* 8 (4) 299 1 Reference Editorial

Discusses the need for nursing theory to underpin clinical nursing research and urges prospective authors to develop the relationship between them.

2.7.34 Schwartz-Barcott, D., Patterson, B.J., Lusard, I.P. & Farmer, B.C. (2002) From practice to theory: tightening the link via three fieldwork strategies. *Journal of Advanced Nursing* 39 (3) 281–9   37 References

Paper presents a two-step fieldwork approach and three specific strategies that have been found useful for developing theory that is tightly aligned to nursing practice. These are theoretical selectivity, integration and creation. They are an extension of the Hybrid Model of Concept Development and each is described and an example given. They identify alternative paths for concept clarification and theoretical congruence through fieldwork in clinical settings.

2.7.35 Vehviläinen-Julkunen, K. (1998) The discipline of nursing: a journey from grand theories to situation specific theories. In: *Knowledge development: clinicians and researchers in partnership.* Helsinki: The Finnish Federation of Nurses   ISSN 0251–4753 Proceedings of the Workgroup of European Nurse Researchers (9th Biennial Conference 5–8 July 1998 Helsinki, Finland) Volume 1 88–93   27 References

Paper describes theory and knowledge development issues in nursing using Finland as an example. Similar issues around the world, such as methodological debate, concept analysis, philosophical aspects and middle-range theory-building, are noted.

2.7.36 Villarruel, A.M., Bishop, T.L., Simpson, E.M., Jemmott, L.S. & Fawcett, J. (2001) Borrowed theories, shared theories, and the advancement of nursing knowledge. *Nursing Science Quarterly* 14 (2) April 158–63 33 References

Despite the continued use of borrowed theories in nursing, little attention has been given to whether theories developed in other disciplines are empirically adequate descriptions, explanations or predictions of nursing phenomena. The authors demonstrate how a borrowed theory can be placed within a nursing context by linking it with two different conceptual models of nursing. Plans for research on condom use behaviour are outlined and results will be used to determine whether the borrowed theory can be a shared theory (CR 2.6).

2.7.37 Walker, L.O. & Avant, K.C. (1999) *Strategies for theory construction in nursing* (3rd edition). New York: Prentice-Hall ISBN 0838586880   References

This text places theory development within the nursing context. Chapters discuss concept, statement and theory development with recently published examples of theory strategies. Introductory chapters clarify the relevance of theory to nursing practice, while later material puts a greater emphasis on how these can be tested for validity.

2.7.38 Wang, Y. & Li, X. (2000) Cross-cultural nursing theory and Chinese nursing today [Chinese]. *Chinese Nursing Research* 14 (6) 231–2   10 References

Article discusses Leininger's concept and structure of cross-cultural nursing theory. Based on an analysis of Chinese culture, nurses' knowledge and the benefits of this theory, the authors believe that it has a positive influence on nursing today (CR 2.53).

2.7.39 Warms, C.A. & Schroeder, C.A. (1999) Bridging the gulf between science and action: the 'new fuzzies' of neopragmatism. *Advances in Nursing Science* 22 (2) 1–10   21 References

Rather than a philosophy, pragmatism is a way of doing philosophy that has major implications for solving disputes involving nursing science, theory and practice that may otherwise be interminable. Pragmatism weaves together theory and action so that one modifies the other continuously, but both maintain their mutual relevance. Authors believe that a better understanding of the history and utility of pragmatism will enhance both clinically relevant nursing theory and theoretically relevant nursing practice.

2.7.40 Watson, J. (1999) *Postmodern nursing and beyond.* Edinburgh: Churchill Livingstone ISBN 0443057443   References

Book re-establishes the critical balance between caring and curing. This theory blends the technical aspects of modern medicine with the holistic aspects traditionally associated with nursing, and serves as a model for nursing practice into the twenty-first century.

2.7.41 Wilde, M.H. (1999) Why embodiment now? *Advances in Nursing Science* 22 (2) 25–38 50 References

Embodiment is a promising new area for theory development, but several issues impair its evolution, including confusion over terminology and a lack of organization of existing literature. Embodiment is defined, based on the philosophy of Merleau-Ponty. Works of scholars and the current debate about embodiment are summarized. Embodied meanings of illness are explored in terms of their relevance for nursing.

2.7.42 Young, A., Taylor, S.G. & Renpenning, K.Mc. (2001) *Connections: nursing research, theory and practice.* St Louis, MO: Mosby ISBN 0323009484   References

Text discusses theory and research, the importance of the connections between the two, and the interlinking cyclical connection between clinical practice, research and theory. Core chapters review major nursing theories and research tools related to each, a review of research conducted to support or advance each theory, and ideas for continued research. It also includes select reliable and valid nursing theory research tools used for research (CR 2.24, 2.25).

2.8 SCIENCE AND THE SCIENTIFIC METHOD

The major components of the scientific method are asking questions, defining problems, obtaining and interpreting data and drawing conclusions. These allow researchers to complete work according to a set of rules so that a series of workable ideas and results are generated. Over time, more ideas and theories emerge which can be tested and retested using these same rules.

Definitions [See Appendix D for sources]

Applied science – that which is orientated towards the solution of practical problems

Basic science – study of phenomena from a purely epistemological viewpoint, regardless of any practical applications the findings might happen to have

Deductive reasoning – the process of developing specific predictions from general principles

Inductive reasoning – the process of reasoning from specific observations to more general rules

Objectivity – the claim to achieve a detached and independent point of view [Whether this ideal is attainable can be debated, and the term is often used tendentiously to recommend one's opinions as superior in debate with someone else]

Science – an activity that combines research (the advancement of knowledge) and theory (explanation for knowledge)

Scientific method – a way of pursuing knowledge that presumes a logical, observational and cautious approach

Scientism – uncritical or unsuitable application of scientific concepts or terms

Subjectivity – usually used in a dismissive way to indicate that something is based on a personal whim or fancy, without reference to public standards or without exposing your beliefs or actions to the criticism of others. However, all actions are obviously subjective insofar as they are the action of a subject

Annotations

2.8.1 Avis, M. (1998) Objectivity in nursing research. *International Journal of Nursing Studies* 35 (3) 141–5   30 References

Recent writing on nursing research methodology has introduced paradigms of research that challenge conventional notions about truth and objectivity, which hold that scientific research is the factual and value-free study of objective reality. Author questions this assumption by examining the objectivity in science and states that this does not permit fruitful research on human subjects. This relativistic view of the conventions of objectivity is rebutted and it is argued that a rejection of its conventions cannot license new paradigms of research.

2.8.2 Berman, H., Ford-Gilboe, M. & Campbell, J.C. (1998) Combining stories and numbers: a methodologic approach for a critical nursing science. *Advances in Nursing Science* 21 (1) 1–15   51 References

Article reviews the aims and assumptions of the critical paradigm and discusses the merits of combining stories and numbers for the agenda of change. Using their own examples, the authors describe three strategies for using this method.

2.8.3 Browne, A.J. (2000) The potential contribution of critical social theory to nursing science. *Canadian Journal of Nursing Research* 32 (2) 35–55 67 References

Article examines the potential contributions of critical social theory (CST) to nursing science and areas of philosophical compatibility and incongruity. The author argues that the most significant contribution of CST to nursing science may be achieved by critiquing the fundamental ideologies upon which nursing knowledge is developed. By interrogating these ideological assumptions, and by maintaining the integrity of our diverse epistemological requirements, CST can advance nursing science towards progressive, emancipatory objectives.

2.8.4 Chalmers, A. (1999) *What is this thing called science? An assessment of the nature and status of science and its methods.* (3rd edition). Buckingham: Open University Press ISBN 0335201091   References

This introduction to the philosophy of science surveys the answers of the past hundred years to this central question. The text has been brought up to date and is enriched by many new historical examples. Chapters are included on the new experimentalism, the Bayesian approach to science currently in vogue, the nature of scientific laws and recent developments in the realism/anti-realism debate.

2.8.5 Bush, C.T. (2001) Science and the scientific method. In K.K. Chitty (ed.) *Professional nursing: concepts and challenges* (3rd edition). Philadelphia, PA: W.B. Saunders ISBN 0721687113 Chapter 12 276–28 References

Chapter differentiates between pure and applied science, describes development of the scientific method, gives examples of inductive and deductive reasoning, explains its steps and highlights its limitations.

2.8.6 Clark, J.A. (2000) Hypothetico-deduction and educational research. *Educational Research* 42 (2) 183–91 11 References

Reconceptualizes hypothetico-deduction to provide a framework that accommodates both inductive and deductive inquiry. Uses an example from educational research (CR 2.6).

2.8.7 Couvalis, G. (1997) *The philosophy of science: science and objectivity*. London: Sage ISBN 0761951016 References

Provides a clear, non-technical guide to the philosophy of science. The works of key thinkers and debates that define the field are all discussed (CR 2.5).

2.8.8 Eriksson, E. & Lauri, S. (2000) From research to clinical practice – different perspectives on the philosophy of science in Finnish nursing research (Finnish). *Vard i Norden. Nursing Science and Research in the Nordic Countries* 20 (1) 50–5 51 References

Article describes research of nursing science in Finland, particularly in the 1990s. Research has been done based on different scientific philosophies: positivism, phenomenology and critical theory. This has resulted in different knowledge and theories. Positivistic and phenomenological-hermeneutical approaches have been widely used, whereas critical theory rarely so. The purpose of nursing science is to produce knowledge that develops the science itself, and which supports nursing practice in developing the quality of care. The integration of theory and practice demands active input from researchers and nurses (CR 2.5, 2.7, 3.3).

2.8.9 Fitzpatrick, J. & Martinson, I. (eds) (1996) *Selected writings of Rosemary Ellis: in search of meaning of nursing science*. New York: Springer ISBN 0826194001 References

This book is a collection of many previously unpublished writings, as well as several classic publications of Rosemary Ellis. She tried to get to the very essence of nursing science, and lay the philosophical groundwork for the development of theory and research to improve nursing practice.

2.8.10 Friesacher, H. & Rux-Haase, A. (1998) The concept of paradigm in nursing science (German). *Pflege* 11 (2) 61–70 88 References

Paper critically analyses the use of the term 'paradigm' in nursing science. The 'pre-Kuhnian' meaning of the paradigm is described and discussion of its application in nursing science, firstly in the USA and then in Germany. The insufficient extent of discussions on questions and problems regarding the philosophy of science is elucidated. Authors conclude that applying the term 'paradigm' to nursing science is neither possible nor is it sensible. A brief review on the prospects for nursing science is given.

2.8.11 Hawley, P., Young, S. & Pasco, A.C. (2000) Reductionism in the pursuit of nursing science: (in)congruent with nursing's core values? *Canadian Journal of Nursing Research* 32 (2) 75–88 58 References

Within nursing scholarship a critique has developed around the philosophy and approaches of traditional science. Its central theme is that the approaches of traditional science are antithetical to nursing's commitment to a humanistic philosophy, as reflected in the premise that reductionism is incongruent with nursing's core values. Several nurse scholars, believing that nursing's humanistic philosophy should guide the research efforts of the discipline, have advocated abandonment of the reductionist approaches of traditional science. The authors believe that adoption of such a position will have serious consequences for knowledge development and subsequently be detrimental to the advancement of nursing practice and the discipline of nursing (CR 2.5, 2.6).

2.8.12 Monti, E.J. & Tingen, M.S. (1999) Multiple paradigms of nursing science. *Advances in Nursing Science* 21 (4) 64–80 38 References

Discusses the concept of paradigm, explores those that influence nursing science, and compares the advantages and disadvantages of theoretical unification and multi-paradigmism. The implications and consequences for the present and future development of nursing as a science within a practice discipline are presented.

2.8.13 O'Meara, J.T. (2001) Causation and the postmodern critique of objectivity. *Anthropological Theory* 1 (1) 31–56 60 References

Debates the post-modern rejection of objective knowledge and critiques the notion that different types of fact require different approaches. This notion is applied to a survey of anthropological theory.

2.8.14   Omery, A., Kasper, C.E. & Page, G.G. (eds) (1995) *In search of nursing science*. Thousand Oaks, CA: Sage   ISBN 0803950942   References

Book analyses the major schools of thought in contemporary Western science in order to arrive at a philosophy (or philosophies) of science consistent with the discipline of nursing. The traditional views of science are examined and the contributors then focus on schools that challenge them, for example feminism, phenomenology, critical theory and post-structuralism. Each discussion is followed by an exploration of how particular tenets of the school have influenced the development of nursing knowledge and nursing science (CR 2.5, 2.6, 2.10, 2.49).

2.8.15   Rambihar, V., Wilson, J., Vali, Y., LeBlanc, L., Jagdeo, D., Caryer, C. & Howes, E. (1999) Chaos 2000: a new science of nursing for the new millennium … proceedings of non-linear dynamics in nursing conference. *Complexity and Chaos in Nursing* 4 Summer 35–8   17 References

Chaos has emerged in the second half of the twentieth century as a new science with widespread application. It has become a basic, physical, biological, behavioural, management, leadership and organizational science. An experience in Toronto utilized chaos in various interdisciplinary and nursing projects, taking it beyond new meanings, models and metaphors. It was used to bridge the gap between research and utilization, and as a creative tool for empowerment and change for nurses and nursing (CR 2.101, 3.8).

2.8.16   Rodgers, B.L. & Yen, W.-Y. (2002) Re-thinking nursing science through the understanding of Buddhism. *Nursing Philosophy* 3 (3) 213–21   35 References

Reflects on the Western narrow view on science and its failure to recognize the significance of Eastern philosophy. Examines how cross-cultural exchanges have encouraged the exploration of such philosophies, including Buddhism, and discusses the potential benefits to nursing science.

2.8.17   Schettini, B. (1997) Introductory remarks to an empirical science of care [Italian]. *Professioni Infermieristiche* 50 (1) 10–14   11 References

Nursing has traditionally been about caring. Nurses are now working with other disciplines to develop their own body of knowledge and creating a new professional identity relating in particular to man, life and health (CR 2.6).

2.8.18   Trigg, R. (2002) Does science deal with the real world? *Interdisciplinary Science Reviews* 27 (2) 94–9   6 References

Traces the origins of science and discusses its historical links with theology. Notes the growth of opposition to scientific inquiry by social scientists, who question its lack of 'real world' grounding and ponder whether science can ever regain its proper authority.

2.8.19   Whittemore, R. (1999) Natural science and nursing science: where do the horizons fuse? *Journal of Advanced Nursing* 30 (5) 1027–33   44 References

The natural sciences have an influential effect on society, contemporary worldviews and other scientific disciplines. A brief history of major advances in the natural sciences and the associated philosophies provides a platform for scholarly discourse regarding the subsequent influence on nursing epistemology. The concepts of knowledge and understanding are differentiated and a cautionary word is expressed not to cast aside the natural sciences and their corollary philosophies as nursing embarks upon its epistemological journey into the twenty-first century. Aesthetics is presented as a possible fusion of horizons of nursing and natural science (CR 2.6).

2.9   QUALITATIVE AND QUANTITATIVE RESEARCH METHODS

'The roots of the qualitative and quantitative quandary can be traced to two opposed Greek philosophical visions of human science that emphasize number (Pythagoras) and meaning (Socrates) as the essence of mind, and we may yet have something to learn about improving qualitative validity from the idiographic question-and-answer method of studying meaning systems by Socrates.' (Wakefield, 1995: 9)

Definitions [See Appendix D for sources]

Qualitative research – this is usually inductively derived and seeks to name and describe categories into which observations belong, e.g. grounded theory or ethnomethodology

Quantitative research – this mode of research is often deductively derived and seeks to confirm the construct validity and internal structure of a research instrument designed to measure a particular concept

Example

Chan, D.S.K. (2001) Combining qualitative and quantitative methods in assessing hospital-learning environments. *International Journal of Nursing Studies* 38 (4) August 447–59 46 References

Article describes nursing students' perceptions of the hospital-learning environment, which were assessed by combining qualitative and quantitative approaches. The Clinical Learning Environment Inventory, based on the theoretical framework of learning environment studies, was developed and validated. The qualitative and quantitative findings reinforced each other. It was found that there were significant differences in students' perceptions of the actual clinical learning and their preferred environment. Generally they preferred a more positive and favourable clinical learning environment than they perceived as being actually present (CR 2.55).

Annotations

2.9.1 Berger, A.A. (2001) *Media and communication research: an introduction to qualitative and quantitative approaches*. Thousand Oaks, CA: Sage ISBN 0761918531 References

Book combines a practical focus, the use of numerous examples, a step-by-step approach and humour to examine both qualitative and quantitative research methods.

2.9.2 Bernard, H.R. (2000) *Social research methods: qualitative and quantitative research approaches*. Thousand Oaks, CA: Sage ISBN 076191403X References

Outlines the origins of social science and research and explains all the important techniques, both qualitative and quantitative. Examples are included (CR 2.1, 2.29, 2.36).

2.9.3 Bryman, A. (2001) Breaking down the quantitative/qualitative divide. In Author *Social research methods*. Oxford: Oxford University Press ISBN 0198742045 Chapter 21 427–41 References

Chapter is concerned with the degree to which the quantitative/qualitative divide should be regarded as a hard-and-fast one. While there are many differences between the two research strategies, there are also many examples of research that transcend the distinction (CR 2.1.11).

2.9.4 Bryman, A. (2001) Combining quantitative and qualitative research. In Author *Social research methods*. Oxford: Oxford University Press ISBN 0198742045 Chapter 22 443–57 References

Chapter discusses multi-strategy research, i.e. research that combines both quantitative and qualitative

methods. The arguments for and against are discussed (CR 2.1.11).

2.9.5 Burman, E. (1997) Minding the gap: positivism, psychology and the politics of qualitative methodology. *Journal of Social Issues* 53 (4) Winter 785–802 62 References (Accessed 14/11/03)

Explores the politics and practices of qualitative research by examining the gap between qualitative and quantitative approaches. The problems, claims, ethics and arguments are all discussed (CR 2.17, 2.36).

2.9.6 Burnard, P. & Hannigan, B. (2000) Qualitative and quantitative approaches in mental health nursing: moving the debate forward. *Journal of Psychiatric and Mental Health Nursing* 7 (1) 1–6 25 References

Critiques the ongoing debate among mental health nursing researchers between quantitative and qualitative methods. Offers an opportunity for synthesis and reconciliation for both positions.

2.9.7 Burton, D. (ed.) (2000) *Research training for social scientists: a handbook for postgraduate researchers*. London: Sage ISBN 0761963510 References

Book follows the life-cycle of a research project and begins with a discussion of ethical issues. It presents guides to both quantitative and qualitative data techniques, gives help on using computers, together with advice on presentation (CR 2.17, 2.29, 2.36).

2.9.8 Campbell, D.T. & Russo, M.J. (1999) *Social experimentation*. Thousand Oaks, CA: Sage ISBN 0761904050 References

Book presents Donald T. Campbell's essential work in social experimentation. This includes exploration of the experimenting society; the compatibility of quantitative and qualitative methods of validity seeking; threats to validity of social experiments and how these may be controlled. Also discussed are the degree to which social sciences can achieve scientific status and whether the operations, products and consequences of science have a social impact (CR 2.8, 2.25, 2.29, 2.36).

2.9.9 Campbell, D.T. & Russo, M.J. (2001) *Social measurement*. Thousand Oaks, CA: Sage ISBN 0761904077 References

The essential work in measurement includes: arguments as to why qualitative approaches belong with quantitative ones; a debate with deconstructionists and social constructionists on measurement validity, and an expansion and further explanation of the multitrait–multimethod matrix (CR 2.17, 2.25).

2.9.10 Clark, A.M. (1998) The qualitative–quantitative debate: moving from positivism and confrontation to post-positivism and reconciliation. *Journal of Advanced Nursing* 27 (6) 1242–9   68 References

Paper highlights an alternative philosophy to positivism that can also underpin empirical inquiry, that of post-positivism. Though some acknowledgement of post-positivism has occurred in the nursing literature, this has yet to permeate into mainstream nursing research. Many still base their arguments on a positivistic view of science. Through a better understanding of post-positivism and a greater focus on explicating the philosophical assumptions underpinning all research methods, the distinctions that have long been perceived to exist between qualitative and quantitative methodologies can be confined to the past. Rather, methods will be selected solely on the nature of research questions (CR 2.5).

2.9.11 Corbetta, P. (2003) *Social research: theory, methods and techniques.* London: Sage ISBN 0761972536   References

Text offers students an understanding of social research practice through an appreciation of its foundations and methods. Stretching from the philosophy of science to detailed descriptions of both qualitative and quantitative techniques, it illustrates not only 'how to' do social research, but critically 'why' particular techniques are used today (CR 2.1, 2.5, 2.29, 2.36).

2.9.12 Cresswell, J.W. (2003) *Research design: qualitative, quantitative, and mixed methods approaches* (2nd edition). Thousand Oaks, CA: Sage ISBN 0761924426   References

In this new edition, each chapter shows how to implement a mixed method design as well as how to tackle qualitative and quantitative approaches. Ethical issues have been added, together with writing tips, and the latest developments in qualitative inquiry (advocacy, participatory and emancipatory approaches) (CR 2.9, 2.17, 2.29, 2.36, 2.97).

2.9.13 Darlington, Y. & Scott, D. (2002) Mixing methods. In Authors *Qualitative research in practice: stories from the field.* Buckingham: Open University Press ISBN 033521147X   Chapter 6 19–141   References

Chapter discusses studies that have used combined qualitative and quantitative methods of data analysis (CR 2.36, 2.86, 2.87).

2.9.14 DePoy, E. & Gitlin, L.N. (1998) *Introduction to research: understanding and applying multiple strategies* (2nd edition). St Louis, MO: Mosby ISBN 0815109792   References

Book addresses the challenge of explaining and integrating qualitative and quantitative approaches to clinical investigation (CR 2.29, 2.36).

2.9.15 Francisco, V.T., Butterfoss, F.D. & Capwell, E.M. (2001) Key issues in evaluation: quantitative and qualitative methods and research design. *Health Promotion Practice* 2 (1) 20–3   10 References

Article discusses the strengths and limitations of qualitative and qualitative designs, asks what questions it is possible to answer, and the influence of research designs on the inferences that can be drawn from data (CR 2.29, 2.36, 2.95).

2.9.16 Gill, J. & Johnson, P. (2002) *Research methods for managers* (3rd edition). London: Sage ISBN 0761940022   References

Book covers both qualitative and quantitative research methods and discusses how methodological choices are made, the philosophical basis for research and how to resolve the dilemmas in choosing a research strategy (CR 2.5, 2.29, 2.36).

2.9.17 Goding, L. & Edwards, K. (2002) Evidence-based practice. *Nurse Researcher* 9 (4) 45–7   30 References

Examines the philosophical assumptions behind evidence-based practice, comparing it to different research methodologies. Argues that nursing involves complex behaviour that requires holism rather than reductionism (CR 2.29, 2.36, 2.43).

2.9.18 Greenstein, T.N. (2001) *Methods of family research.* Thousand Oaks, CA: Sage ISBN 0761919481   References

Book covers specific methods that are appropriate when undertaking family research, including using the Internet (CR 2.85).

2.9.19 Greig, A.D. & Taylor, J. (1998) *Doing research with children.* London: Sage ISBN 0761955895   References

Book provides a comprehensive and practical introduction to undertaking a research project with children. Different frameworks and techniques for conducting both qualitative and quantitative methods are outlined. An important underlying theme of the book is the unique and vulnerable nature of children as research subjects and the ethical issues this raises (CR 2.17, 2.29, 2.36).

2.9.20 Harvey, L., MacDonald, M. & Hill, J. (2000) *Theories and methods.* London: Hodder & Stoughton ISBN 0340737387   References

Book outlines the main sociological perspectives and focuses on overcoming the problem of oppositional thinking (quantitative and qualitative). Three main approaches are discussed: positivism, phenomenology and critical social research (CR 2.5, 2.8, 2.10, 2.26, 2.29, 2.36, 2.49).

2.9.21 Jablin, F.M. & Putnam, L.L. (eds) (2000) *The handbook of organizational communication* (2nd edition). Thousand Oaks, CA: Sage ISBN 0803955030 References

Book comprises up-to-date information in this field, with leading scholars reviewing and synthesizing important developments in research and theory. Future directions are also suggested. Theoretical and methodological issues in both qualitative and quantitative research are covered (CR 2.29, 2.36).

2.9.22 Kelly, B. & Long, A. (2000) Quantity or quality? *Nurse Researcher* 7 (4) 53–67 27 References

Paper examines the methodological issues arising from the quantitative–qualitative debate and the nature and resolution of the perceived theory–practice gap (CR 2.14, 2.102, 3.8).

2.9.23 Larsson, N.O. (2001) A design view on research in the social sciences. *Systemic Practice and Action Research* 14 (4) 383–405 51 References

Reviews research methods used in the social sciences and compares their perceived worth with methods traditionally used in the natural sciences. Methods are assessed for their applicability to Human Activity Systems, and the possibility of incorporating action research methods are discussed (CR 2.37).

2.9.24 Marks, D.F. & Yardley, L. (2003) *Research methods for clinical and health psychology.* London: Sage ISBN 0761971904 References

Book provides a detailed, yet concise, explanation of both qualitative and quantitative approaches. It draws on case study examples to illustrate how they can be used in a variety of health care settings, with special relevance to clinical disorders, disease prevention and health promotion (CR 2.29, 2.36).

2.9.25 McPherson, K. & Leydon, G. (2002) Quantitative and qualitative methods in UK health research: now and …? *European Journal of Cancer Care* 11 (3) 225–31 17 References

Re-articulates the quantitative–qualitative debate with reference to cancer care, where it is argued that the psychological aspects of living with cancer, together with the complexities of care, require a repertoire of methods (CR 2.29, 2.36).

2.9.26 Mertens, D.M. (1997) *Research methods in education and psychology: integrating diversity with quantitative and qualitative approaches.* Thousand Oaks, CA: Sage ISBN 0803958285 References

Book explains both quantitative and qualitative methods and incorporates the view of various research paradigms into the descriptions of these methods. Included are the post-positivist and interpretative/constructivist paradigms and a relative newcomer, the emancipatory paradigm that includes the perspectives of feminists, ethnic/racial minorities and people with disabilities. In each chapter, a step of the research process is explained from the literature through to analysis and reporting (CR 2.9, 2.10, 2.29, 2.36).

2.9.27 Murdaugh, C.L. (1999) Relationships of research perspectives to methodology. In Hinshaw, A.S., Feetham, S.L. & Shaver, J.L.F. (eds) *Handbook of clinical nursing research.* Thousand Oaks, CA: Sage ISBN 080395784X Part 1 Chapter 4 61–70 82 References

Chapter provides an overview of the major paradigms that currently guide the two commonly preferred research methods chosen to investigate problems in nursing: empiricism, which emphasizes quantitative methods, and phenomenology, which stresses qualitative methods. Proposed solutions to accommodate the multiple paradigms suggested are described, including triangulation, critical multiplism and scientific pluralism (CR 2.26, 2.29, 2.36, 3.6.4).

2.9.28 Punch, K.F. (1998) *Introduction to social research: quantitative and qualitative approaches.* London: Sage ISBN 0761958134 References

Uses a common framework to give equal weighting to both quantitative and qualitative methods. Book describes the research process for each design, indicates further reading and incorporates a section on writing, including preparing research proposals (CR 2.29, 2.36, 2.96).

2.9.29 Rabinowitz, V.C. & Weseen, S. (1997) Elu(ci)d(at)ing epistemological impasses: re-viewing the qualitative/quantitative debates in psychology. *Journal of Social Issues* 53 (4) Winter 605–31 56 References

Article examines some of the reasons behind the difficulties with, and resistance to, integrating qualitative and quantitative approaches. It focuses on the psychological, social and political factors that are frequently glossed over in this debate. 20 doctoral students were interviewed and asked how they thought about and chose research methods for their own studies (CR 2.29, 2.36).

2.9.30 Rapley, M. (2003) *Quality of life research: a critical introduction.* London: Sage ISBN 0761954570 References

'Quality of life' is one of the fastest-growing areas of research and policy and this introductory text offers a critical overview of the concept and ways in which it is researched. Theoretical issues covered include: what does 'quality of life' (QOL) mean?, whose QOL is it anyway?, qualitative and quantitative approaches to QOL research. Practical aspects include: researching QOL as a cultural object, QOL in health and social care research, QOL research with special populations, researching QOL as a psychological object and should we 'hang up QOL as a hopeless term?' (CR 2.29, 2.36, 2.58, 2.61).

2.9.31 Roberts, A. (2002) A principled complementarity of method: in defence of methodological eclecticism and the qualitative–quantitative debate. *The Qualitative Report* 7 (3) 14pp. 5 References www.nova.edu/ssss/QR/QR7–3/roberts.html (Accessed 13/11/03)

Rehearses the arguments in the qualitative–quantitative debate and advocates using these methods in a complementary rather than integrated fashion (CR 2.29, 2.36).

2.9.32 Sandelowski, M. (2000) Focus on research methods: combining qualitative and quantitative sampling, data collection and analysis techniques in mixed-method studies. *Research in Nursing and Health* 23 (3) 246–55   36 References

Discusses mixed-method techniques, which advocates argue are required because the complexity of human phenomena needs more complex designs to capture them. This paper examines the where, what, why and how of combining qualitative and quantitative techniques (CR 2.22, 2.29, 2.36, 2.64, 2.79).

2.9.33 Shortell, S.M. (1999) The emergence of qualitative methods in health services research. *Health Services Research* 34 (5) 1083–8   11 References

Draws attention to the growing role of qualitative methods in health services research in response to developments in health policy. Discusses impediments to qualitative research and offers some solutions (CR 2.36, 3.12).

2.9.34 Tashakkori, A. & Teddlie, C. (eds) (2002) *Handbook of mixed methods in social and behavioral research.* Thousand Oaks: CA: Sage ISBN 0761920730   References

Handbook contains articles by leading scholars on what has become known as the third methodological movement in social research. It explores the differing viewpoints and disciplinary approaches of mixed methods and examines them from the research enterprise to paradigmatic issues to application. It discusses the strengths and weaknesses of mixed methods designs, and provides specific examples from a variety of disciplines, from psychology to nursing (CR 2.2, 2.15).

2.9.35 Thyer, B.A. (ed.) (2001) The *handbook of social research methods.* Thousand Oaks, CA: Sage   ISBN 0761919058   References

This edited book covers both qualitative and quantitative research methods, data collection, ethical issues, gender and ethnicity, and offers advice on how to write up and present research (CR 2.17, 2.29, 2.36, 2.64, 2.98, 3.13).

2.9.36 Yates, S.J. (2003) *Issues in social research.* London: Sage/Open University Press ISBN 0761967982   References

Book provides an introductory overview of the process of social research, and also includes some classic readings in research methods with which all students and researchers should be familiar. The text offers a comprehensive introduction to key areas of quantitative and qualitative research, such as survey research, experimental research, interviews, focus groups, fieldwork and discourse analysis (CR 2.29, 2.36, 2.52, 2.68, 2.69, 2.89).

2.10   FEMINIST RESEARCH

'Not only do men and women view a common world from different perspectives, they view different worlds as well' (Bernard, 1973: 782). Feminist research is multi-disciplinary in nature and is in the process of defining, gathering and making knowledge. It is rigorous because gender is taken into consideration and the experiences of women are deemed to be as important as those of men. As such it has much to offer the predominantly female nursing profession.

Definitions [See Appendix D for sources]

Feminism – may be understood as theory – systems of concepts, propositions and analysis that describe and explain women's situations and experiences and support recommendations about how to improve them

Feminist research – involves an epistemological stance ... that gives direction to the diversity of evolving research practices in the field. The goal is to entertain a critical dialogue that focuses on women's experiences in historical, cultural and socio-economic perspectives

---

Example

Kasper, A.S. (2002) A feminist qualitative methodology: a study of women with breast cancer. In Fielding, N.G. (ed.) *Interviewing.* London: Sage

ISBN 0761973397   Volume II Part 2 Section 12
Chapter 30 168–84   21 References

A feminist qualitative methodology was used to
study women who had lived through a breast cancer
crisis. The methodology that was developed drew
on elements of the unstructured sociological interview, oral history methods, the ethnographer's
account, the art of story-telling and its more contemporary form, consciousness-raising. Women
were placed at the centre of the inquiry, not as subjects of the research, but to capture the material
from their viewpoint. Author discusses the differences between traditional sociological perspectives
and those used in this study (CR 2.36, 2.42, 2.47,
2.68.12, 2.78).

Annotations

2.10.1   Allen, D.G. (2002) Feminism, relativism
and the philosophy of science: an overview. In
Rafferty, A.M. & Traynor, M. (eds) *Exemplary
research for nursing and midwifery.* London:
Routledge   ISBN 0415241634   Chapter 10 188–204
90 References

Chapter introduces some key issues in the feminist
philosophy of science and attempts to increase
understanding of what a body of research, based on
feminist philosophy, would look like (CR 3.21.5).

2.10.2   Anderson, J.M. (2000) Gender, 'race',
poverty, health and discourses of health reform in
the context of globalization: a post-colonial feminist perspective in policy research. *Nursing Inquiry*
7 (4) 220–9   52 References

Discusses the impact of globalization and health
care reform on the lives of women. Economic hard-
ships are identified, what global processes mean for
health, and how nurse scientists might develop
research agendas in the twenty-first century that
would foster social transformation and justice for
all people. Drawing on a post-colonial feminist
epistemology might help to define these agendas,
and express the multi-layered socio-political contexts of health and illness in advocacy with policy-
makers (CR 2.6, 3.11).

2.10.3   Anderson, J.M. (2002) Toward a post-
colonial feminist methodology in nursing research:
exploring the convergence of post-colonial and
black feminist scholarship. *Nurse Researcher: The
International Journal of Research Methodology
in Nursing and Health Care* 9 (3) 7–27   74
References

Explores post-colonial feminist scholarship, generated through the convergence of black feminist and
post-colonial scholarship, and examines its use as a
theory and methodology for nursing scholarship.

2.10.4   Andrist, L.C. & MacPherson, K.I.
(2001) Conceptual models for women's health
research: reclaiming menopause as an exemplar of
nursing's contributions to feminist scholarship.
Annual Review of Nursing Research 19 29–60
References

Paper reviews the birth of women's health scholarship, as it is the foundation for theory that underpins
feminist nursing research. The tenets of nursing
scholars are then discussed. Using the historical
context of the menopause to highlight the ways in
which it has been transformed from a normal physiological event to a disease, nursing studies were
reviewed in the areas of 'women reclaiming
menopause' and 'menopause across cultures'.
These studies demonstrated that similar to other
health issues, women's experiences cannot be uni-
versalized, and research must take into consideration the social, political, economic and cultural
factors that impact on their experience of the
menopause transition.

2.10.5   Banks-Wallace, J. (2000) Womanist ways
of knowing: theoretical considerations for research
with African American women. *Advances in
Nursing Science* 22 (3) 33–45   50 References

Many researchers are unfamiliar with womanist
thought, or are unsure how it can be used to inform
specific aspects of research design. This article
explicates a womanist epistemologic framework
that can undergird the development of intervention
designs aimed at assisting African-American
women to incorporate health-promoting behaviours
into their lives.

2.10.6   Brayton, J. *What makes feminist research
feminist? The structure of feminist research within
the social sciences* www.unb.ca/web/PAR-L/win/
feminmethod.htm (Accessed 08/02/03)

While there is no standard agreement over what
constitutes feminist research, many authors seem to
draw upon certain elements as defining features.
This essay acts as a starting point to discussing the
shape and forms of feminist research. The principal
concepts are defined, and the differences and similarities of qualitative and quantitative research,
feminist criticisms of the qualitative–quantitative
debate, and some of its limitations are all discussed.

2.10.7   Cooper, E.A. & Bosco, S.M. (1999)
Future research. In Powell, G.N. (ed.) *Handbook of
gender and work.* Thousand Oaks, CA: Sage   ISBN
0761913556   References

Authors discuss methodological issues in conducting research on gender in organizations.

2.10.8   Delamont, S. (2003) *Feminist sociology.*
London: Sage   ISBN 0761972552   References

Book explores the achievements of British sociology in theory, methods and empirical research. It outlines barriers to the development of feminism and explores contemporary challenges. It provides a guide to the origins of feminism in the discipline of sociology, analyses the uneasy relationships between feminists and the founding fathers, and elucidates the opportunities and challenges presented by post-modernism.

2.10.9 *Encyclopedia of feminist theories* (2000) Edited by Code, L. London: Routledge ISBN 0415132746 References

'The aims of this encyclopedia are to provide a resource for students and teachers across academic disciplines – both those already involved in feminist studies, and those interested in learning about this area of inquiry, and to produce a volume in accessible language and conceptual framing for scholars and activists everywhere. It is cross-disciplinary in scope, and [includes] mini-biographies of feminist theorists, designed to introduce readers to some of the makers of feminist theory, and to acknowledge the specifically located crafting process that makes feminist knowledge possible' (p. xxiv).

2.10.10 *Encyclopedia of women and gender* (2001) Editor-in Chief Worell, J. Oxford: Elsevier Science ISBN 0122272455 2 Volume Set

This resource brings together the latest information on theory, research and social policy concerning the psychology of women and gender. One area included is feminist perspectives on quantitative and qualitative research methods. Chapters are enhanced with outlines, glossaries of important terms and references (CR 2.2, 2.29, 2.36).

2.10.11 **Fisher, L. & Embree, L.** (eds) (2000) *Feminist phenomenology.* Dordrecht: Kluwer Academic Publishers ISBN 0792365801 References

A collection of original essays on the related issues of gender and feminism approached phenomenologically. Lived experience is gendered and especially women's experiences are not well reflected in ordinary language. To understand them, one must go beyond analysing language and study matters of gendered human life itself. The essays in this volume advance these investigations (CR 2.49).

2.10.12 **Francis, B.** (2000) Post-structuralism and nursing: uncomfortable bedfellows? *Nursing Inquiry* 7 (1) 20–8 60 References

The benefits and limitations of the application of post-structuralist theory in nursing research are discussed. Its use in feminist research is drawn on to argue a divergence between a deconstructionist post-structuralism and nursing aims. It is argued

that there are strong parallels between nursing and social movements such as feminism. Author believes that post-structuralism is useful for examining or deconstructing existing discourse and practice, but is incompatible and inadequate for research that aims to develop such discourses or practices (CR 2.7).

2.10.13 **Gillis, A. & Jackson, W.** (2002) New wave research: contemporary approaches. Feminist research. In Authors *Research for nurses: methods and interpretation.* Philadelphia, PA: F.A. Davis ISBN 0803608969 Part 2 Chapter 8 281–9

Discusses the philosophical tenets of feminist research, the application of method and methodology. An example is given (CR 2.1.34).

2.10.14 **Glass, N. & Davis, K.** (1998) An emancipatory impulse: a feminist postmodern integrated turning point in nursing research. *Advances in Nursing Science* 21 (1) 43–52 45 References

Article critiques the current debates regarding feminism, post-modernism and feminist/postmodernism within nursing research. These are classified as dissatisfaction, fragmentation and integration. Authors propose a solution from the integration debate that is within feminism and draws on the epistemological constructs of modernism and post-modernism. Nursing research is framed within the proposed ontological links that characterize the integrated solution.

2.10.15 **Gustafson, D.L.** (2000) Best laid plans: examining contradictions between intent and outcome in a feminist, collaborative research project. *Qualitative Health Research* 10 (6) 717–33 33 References

Article examines a feminist, collaborative research method that was intended to be political in standpoint, gendered in focus, reflexive in process and transformative in outcome. The author hoped to challenge what was known about nurses' job displacement and how that knowledge was produced. The contradictions between the author's best-laid plans and the actual process of discovery are described. Recommendations for future research include considerations about the social and political context in which research takes place, cautions about gender inclusivity in the research population and analytic frameworks (CR 2.6, 2.15, 2.16, 2.22, 3.11).

2.10.16 **Hall, A.** (1992) *Doing feminist research: an annotated bibliography* www.Inform.umd.edu/ EdRes/Topic/WomensStudies/Bibliographies/ research-methods (Accessed 23/01/03)

Books and articles from 1981 to 1991 are listed which may be useful in helping feminists sort out issues related specifically to methodology in their own subject area, or in topics common to all discussions of social science research methodology.

2.10.17 Holland, J., Blair, M. & Sheldon, S. (eds) (1995) *Debates and issues in feminist research and pedagogy (equality and difference: gender issues in education).* Plymouth, UK: Multilingual Matters ISBN 185359251X

Articles in this book engage with practical issues relating to teaching and feminist research.

2.10.18 Hughes, C. (2002) *Key concepts in feminist theory and research.* London: Sage ISBN 0761969888 References

Book addresses the implications of post-modernism and post-structuralism for feminist theorizing. It identifies the challenges of this through the development of 'conceptual literacy'. The text focuses on students' needs to understand that the meaning of concepts is linked to contexts and theoretical framing, and demonstrates how this is particularly important at the research design and analysis stage and when comparing research studies (CR 2.7).

2.10.19 Im, E. & Chee, W. (2001) A feminist critique of research on cancer pain. *Western Journal of Nursing Research* 23 (7) 726–52 105 References

In this article, nursing research on cancer pain is critiqued from a feminist perspective and directions for future research are proposed. 82 nursing articles are presented with four themes that may provide reasons why nursing research on cancer pain rarely incorporated gender and ethnic differences: absence of participants' own views and experiences, androcentrism and ethnocentrism, lack of consideration on contextual factors, and distant relationships between researchers and research participants. Six critical elements for inclusion in further studies are suggested.

2.10.20 Järviluoma, H., Moisala, P. & Vilkko, A. (2003) *Gender and qualitative methods.* London: Sage ISBN 076196584X References

Book outlines the practical and philosophical issues of gender in qualitative research. The authors emphasize that the task of the researcher is to investigate how gender(s) is/are defined, negotiated and performed by people themselves within specific situations and locations. Each chapter introduces a specific method and/or research subject and discusses gender as an analytical category in relation to it. Practical exercises are included that will teach methods of observation and analysis in various texts and contexts. Examples are taken from men's and women's studies as well as from feminist and other gender studies (CR 2.36).

2.10.21 Kitzinger, C. (2000) Doing feminist conversation analysis. *Feminism & Psychology* 10 (2) 163–93 95 References

Counters the debate regarding the alleged incompatibility of conversation analysis with feminism using two examples (CR 2.89).

2.10.22 Lather, P. (2002) Feminist perspectives on empowering research methodologies. In Fielding, N.G. (ed.) *Interviewing.* London: Sage ISBN 0761973397 Volume II Part 2 Section 12 Chapter 29 149–67 89 References

Paper addresses three questions: What does it mean to do feminist research? What can be learned about research as praxis and practices of self-reflexivity from looking at feminist efforts to create empowering research designs? And what are the challenges of post-modernism to feminist empirical work? (CR 2.68.12).

2.10.23 Letherby, G. (2003) *Feminist research in theory and practice.* Buckingham: Open University Press ISBN 0335200281 References

Book charts the debates concerned with the epistemological, political and practical issues involved in doing feminist research, and places it within a wider consideration of the status of knowledge. The main focus of the book is the practical issues for feminist researchers – how the process of research affects the results and the relationships between politics and practice in terms of research and knowledge production. Current theoretical debates are summarized and developed (CR 2.6).

2.10.24 Mauthner, M., Birch, M., Jessop, J. & Miller, T. (eds) (2002) *Ethics in qualitative research.* London: Sage ISBN 0761973095 References

Book addresses the gap between research practice and ethical principles that inform it, focusing on responsibility and accountability in applied feminist research practice (CR 2.17, 2.36, 3.8).

2.10.25 Miller, C. & Treitel, C. (eds) (1991) *Feminist research methods: an annotated bibliography.* Westport, CT: Greenwood Press ISBN 031326029X

A compilation of English language sources which help to answer the question 'what makes a research project feminist?' Each item addresses some aspect of feminist research and includes both general and specific literature.

2.10.26 Morawski, J. (1997) The science behind feminist research methods. (Transforming psychology: interpretive and participatory research methods). *Journal of Social Issues* 53 (4) Winter 667–81 91 References.

Author believes that acquaintance with the variety of feminist approaches towards science will enable feminist scholars to better configure their research and strategies. The science of feminism, remedial methods, transformative strategies, objectivity, subjectivity and challenges for researchers are all discussed.

2.10.27 Nelms, T.P & Lane, E.B. (1999) Women's ways of knowing in nursing and critical thinking. *Journal of Professional Nursing* 15 (3) 179–86   8 References

Reports a longitudinal qualitative study that aimed to extend previous work by interviewing female university students to determine their 'way of knowing', and determine what relationship this might have with critical thinking when accumulating a specific body of knowledge such as nursing. Results are discussed (CR 2.6, 2.36, 2.48).

2.10.28 Nielsen, J.McC. (1990) *Feminist research methods: exemplary readings in the social sciences.* Boulder, CO: Westview Press ISBN 0813305772 References

Goal of this book is to represent as many disciplines and methodological strategies in the social sciences as possible that will be meaningful to students who may not have a background in the discipline. An overview of what traditional social scientists mean by methods is given, and the author shows that there is an identifiable feminist approach that is grounded in an older positivist-empirical tradition, and in a newer post-empirical one. Examples of readings include feminist inquiry through oral history; a combination of anthropological fieldwork and feminist literary analysis; some unusual survey and interview work with women workers; re-analyses of existing data and two kinds of linguistic analysis (CR 2.42, 2.47, 2.52, 2.68, 2.89).

2.10.29 Oakley, A. (1999) People's ways of knowing: gender and methodology. In Hood, S., Mayall, B. & Oliver, S. (eds) *Critical issues in social research: power and prejudice.* Buckingham: Open University Press ISBN 0335201407 Chapter 11 154–70   73 Notes and References

Examines issues of power embedded in research methodologies themselves. Author argues that current choices between qualitative and quantitative methods reflect a gendered history in which different ways of knowing have been aligned with minority and majority groups. Cutting across the choice of research methods is the fundamental issue of tailoring the method to the research question, and of creating knowledge in a reliable and trustworthy way (CR 2.20).

2.10.30 Ozga, J. (2000) Feminist research on policy. In Author *Policy research in educational settings: contested terrain.* Buckingham: Open University Press ISBN 0335202950 Chapter 5 83–90   References

Author uses the example of feminist research to illustrate ways in which processes of knowledge production, including research, can themselves act as oppressive structures in the policy context on research in educational policy (CR 2.6, 3.11.14).

2.10.31 Rafael, A.R.F. (1997) Advocacy oral history: a research methodology for social activism in nursing. *Advances in Nursing Science* 20 (2) 32–44   44 References

Philosophies underpinning the research method of advocacy oral history and characteristics of feminist post-modern research are reviewed. Implications for the use of this methodology for social activism in nursing are discussed (CR 2.47).

2.10.32 Ramazanoglu, C. & Holland, J. (2002) *Feminist methodology: challenges and choices.* London: Sage ISBN 0761951237 References

Book demonstrates how feminist approaches to methodology engage with debates in Western philosophy to raise critical questions about knowledge production. Guiding the reader through the terrain of feminist methodology, the book shows that it has a distinct place in social research (CR 2.6).

2.10.33 Ribbens, J. & Edwards, R. (eds) (1997) *Feminist dilemmas in qualitative research.* London: Sage ISBN 0761956646 References

Book explores the key dilemma of producing work relevant to theoretical and formal traditions and the requirements of academic knowledge, while remaining faithful to the participants' experiences. The interplay between theory, epistemology and the detailed practice of research are all discussed (CR 2.6, 2.7, 2.36).

2.10.34 Ristock, J.L. & Pennell, J. (1997) *Research as empowerment: feminist links, postmodern interruptions.* Don Mills, Ontario: Oxford University Press ISBN 0195410807 References

Volume suggests ways of carrying out research for social action in order that power is both critically analysed and responsibly used at all stages of the research. Examples of research methods used by the author in various feminist situations are included (CR 2.2).

2.10.35 Roberts, H. (ed.) (1991) *Doing feminist research.* (2nd edition). London: Routledge & Kegan Paul ISBN 0415025478 References

Volume presents accounts of research where practical, methodological, theoretical and ethical issues are raised where the sociologist adopts, or is aware of, a feminist perspective.

2.10.36 Sangster, J. (1998) Telling our stories: feminist debates and the use of oral history. In

Perks, R. & Thomson, A. (eds) *The oral history reader*. London: Routledge ISBN 0415133521 Part I Chapter 8 87–100   52 Notes and References

Based on research undertaken in Canada, this chapter examines oral history and the construction of women's memories, together with ethical and theoretical dilemmas that historians may encounter (CR 2.17, 2.47.18).

2.10.37 Seibold, C. (2000) Qualitative research from a feminist perspective in the postmodern era: methodological, ethical and reflexive concerns. *Nursing Inquiry* 7 (3) 147–55   41 References

Paper describes the ongoing process of methodology development in a qualitative study of single midlife women. It describes reflexive concerns on the ethics of data collection and dissemination of research findings from a feminist post-modern perspective, as well as the way in which modification of analytic techniques occurred as the study progressed (CR 2.17, 2.36, 2.45, 2.64, 2.89, 2.98).

2.10.38 Sherwin, S. (2002) Towards a feminist ethics of health care. In Fulford, K.W.M., Dickenson, D.L. & Murray, T.H. (eds) *Healthcare ethics and human values: an introductory text with readings and case studies*. Malden, MA: Blackwell Publications ISBN 0631202242   Chapter 1 25–28 10 References

Discusses the areas of similarity between feminist and medical ethics in health care (CR 2.17).

2.10.39 Taylor, J.Y. (1998) Womanism: a methodologic framework for African American women. *Advances in Nursing Science* 21 (1) 53–64   60 References

Article presents an abbreviated review and synthesis of Afrocentric ways of knowing, which includes black feminist, womanist and Afrocentric perspectives. A developing methodology for use with African-American women is also described.

2.10.40   University of Oregon Library *Feminist research methods: a guide to library and internet sources*   libweb.uoregon.edu/subjquid/women/womenst.htm/. (Accessed 08/02/03)

This bibliography is for researchers interested in the literature of women's studies. It lists the key reference sources for identifying and locating information and special collections of material in the University of Oregon Library and throughout the World Wide Web.

2.10.41 Wilkinson, S. (ed.) (1996) *Feminist social psychologies: international perspectives*. Buckingham: Open University Press ISBN 0335193544   References

This collection reviews the growth and development of feminist social psychology over the last ten years, highlights theoretical and methodological advances and looks forward to the future. The papers demonstrate the use of a broad range of quantitative and qualitative methods in feminist research, including questionnaires and rating scales, voice-relational methods, discourse analysis, memory work, biography, focus groups, Q-methodology and meta-analysis (CR 2.69, 2.71, 2.74, 2.75, 2.92).

2.11   NEW PARADIGM RESEARCH

'New paradigm research is another way of doing research. It puts forward alternatives to "orthodox" research methods and capitalizes on the contributions of those who are normally just subjects. It is an approach to inquiry which is a systematic, rigorous search for truth but which does not kill off all it touches. It is a synthesis of naive inquiry and orthodox research.' (Reason & Rowan, 1981: xiii)

Definition [See Appendix D for source]

New paradigm research – research that is done with people rather than on people. It involves working with people so that they may discover some truth about themselves.

Example

Smith, P., Masterson, A. & Lask, S. (1995) Health and the curriculum: an illuminative evaluation – Part 1: Methodology. *Nurse Education Today* 15 (4) 245–9   22 References

AND

Part 2: Findings and recommendations. *Nurse Education Today* 15 (5) 317–22   10 References

Paper describes a 6-month exploratory study, which evaluated the integration of a philosophy of health within pre- and post-registration curricula in England. The principle of including such a philosophy is discussed together with the project's aims, methodology, relevant literature, findings and their implications.

Major Text

Reason, P. & Rowan, J. (eds) (1981) *Human inquiry: a sourcebook of new paradigm research*. Chichester: Wiley ISBN 0471279358   References

Annotations

2.11.1 Chappell, A.L. (2000) Emergence of participatory methodology in learning difficulty research: understanding the context. *British Journal of Learning Disabilities* 28 (1) 38–43 34 References

Examines participatory and emancipatory research and debates the growing acceptance that those with a learning difficulty need to be included in the research process. Discusses the role of non-disabled people in learning-difficulty research (CR 2.22).

2.11.2 Heron, J. (1981) Experiential research methodology. In Reason, P. & Rowan, J. (eds) *Human inquiry: a sourcebook of new paradigm research*. Chichester: Wiley ISBN 0471279358 Chapter 12 153–66   References

Traditional and experiential research methodologies are contrasted. Contributions of the latter to the body of knowledge are explored (CR 2.11.7).

2.11.3 Heron, J. (1996) *Co-operative inquiry: research into the human condition*. London: Sage ISBN 0803976844   References

Book explores the philosophical and methodological grounds of co-operative inquiry and gives practical advice on doing this type of work. Topics include: a critique of established research techniques; the underlying participative paradigm of co-operative inquiry; the epistemological and political aspects of participation; different types and range of inquiry studies; and ways of setting up groups and carrying out the necessary procedures to enhance validity (CR 2.25).

2.11.4 Heron, J. & Reason, P. (2001) The practice of co-operative inquiry: research 'with' rather than 'on' people. In Reason, P. & Bradbury, H. (eds) *Handbook of action research: participative inquiry and practice*. London: Sage ISBN 0761966455 Part 2 Chapter 16 179–88 50 References

Chapter gives examples, different forms of co-operative inquiry, investigating cultures, ways of knowing, skills and validation procedures, and initiating an inquiry group (CR 2.15, 2.37.19).

2.11.5 Kiernan, C. (1999) Participation in research by people with learning disability: origins and issues. *British Journal of Learning Disabilities* 27 (2) 43–5   24 References

Contrasts the traditional model of human inquiry with that of a new paradigm research and the issues arising out of the latter. Discusses participation by people with a learning disability and how this might be achieved (CR 2.15).

2.11.6 Reason, P. (ed.) (1994) *Participation in human inquiry*. London: Sage ISBN 080398832X References

Book provides a theoretical perspective and set of examples to give would-be researchers a range of possible research approaches. It is not a methods text, but is about research as a participative process with, rather than on, people (CR 2.15).

[This book is now out of print but is being made available by the editor on a website. The text may not be exactly as published so the printed copy should be consulted before quoting. See www.bath.ac.uk/~mnspwr/Participationinhumaninquiry/titlepage.htm]

2.11.7 Reason, P. & Rowan, J. (eds) (1981) *Human inquiry: sourcebook of new paradigm research*. Chichester: Wiley ISBN 0471279358 References

Sourcebook suggests a new paradigm for the philosophy and practice of research that is collaborative and experiential. New paradigm research means doing research with people rather than on people and seeks to develop new insights into the actions and behaviour of diverse groups. The book covers the philosophy, methodology, practice and prospects of new paradigm research. Many examples are included to illustrate these new approaches.

2.11.8 Reinhart, S. (1981) Implementing new paradigm research: a model for training and practice. In Reason, P. & Rowan, J. (eds) *Human inquiry: a sourcebook of new paradigm research*. Chichester: Wiley ISBN 0471279358 Chapter 36 415–35

Chapter presents a model of the process by which individuals may develop a commitment and the skills to carry out new paradigm research. An appendix suggests the elements needed in a training programme for researchers (CR 2.11.7).

2.11.9 Walters, M. (2000) The mature students' three Rs. *British Journal of Guidance and Counselling* 28 (2) 267–78   30 References

Using new paradigm methods, the study formulates a framework for determining mature students' expectations, motivations and outcomes in higher education. Author proposes that this framework is also useful outside educational settings.

2.12   SYSTEMATIC LITERATURE REVIEWING

Summarizing, analysing and evaluating current knowledge in the form of an integrative or systematic literature review, provides valuable information on a given topic. Reviews can either be developed as a discrete piece of work to inform practice or as a precursor to a research project in order to identify conceptual, methodological and practical issues that might affect the conduct and outcome of the research. It is acknowledged that a competent and critical review, which answers a specific research question, is less costly and more useful than undertaking primary research and can be invaluable to clinical decision-making. Reviews that highlight deficits in knowledge are also helpful because they identify methodological flaws that occur in studies and indicate the most appropriate strategies for future research.

Definitions [See Appendix D for sources]

Cochrane review – ... a systematic, up-to-date summary of reliable evidence of the benefits and risks of health care

ejournals – online journals

ezines – online magazines

Grey literature – literature that is not generally available, [not] published in large quantities, [not] readily distributed, [not] generally indexed in public-domain reference systems [and is] not necessarily peer reviewed

Integrative literature review – integration of a body of research findings (including theory, statistics) which concludes by addressing issues for future research

Literature review – scholarly analysis of a body of research about a specific issue or topic

Primary source – ... an account of a research study that has been written by the original researcher(s); in historical studies, primary sources consist of first-hand information or direct evidence of an event

Secondary source – ... an account of a research study that has been written by someone other than the study investigators; in historical studies, secondary sources are second-hand information provided by someone who did not observe the event

Systematic review – comprehensive, unbiased analysis of research findings on a specific topic that uses strict scientific design to select and assess various related scientific studies

Example

Evans D. & Land L. (2003) Topical negative pressure for treating chronic wounds: a Cochrane review. In: *The Cochrane Library* Issue 2. Oxford: Update Software.

Assesses the effectiveness of topical negative pressure (TNP) for the treatment of chronic wounds. Two small trials provide weak evidence that TNP may be superior to saline gauze dressings in healing human chronic wounds but concludes that further high-quality randomized, controlled trials are needed before further evaluation can take place.

Annotations

2.12.1 Altman, D.G. (2001) Systematic reviews of evaluations of prognostic variables. *British Medical Journal* 323 (7306) 28 July 224–8 39 References

The clinical importance of information on prognostic factors is discussed, detailing how these studies can aid decisions about treatment. The author considers the specific issues and processes to be addressed in producing a systematic review, while emphasizing the difficulties reviewers face in locating and synthesizing appropriately designed and conducted studies for inclusion (CR 2.43).

2.12.2 Carnwell, R. & Daly, W. (2001) Strategies for the construction of a critical review of the literature. *Nurse Education in Practice* 1 (2) 57–63 11 References

Paper describes the process of conducting a literature review. Its purpose is identified and the authors show how key words can be used to define the scope of the review. It also discusses how the literature can be organized into themes and conclusions drawn to inform further study.

2.12.3 Chalmers, I. & Altman, D.G. (eds) (1995) *Systematic reviews*. London: British Medical Journal Publishing Group ISBN 0727909045 References

Book, based on papers given at a BMJ/UK Cochrane Centre meeting in 1993, discusses the processes involved in undertaking systematic reviews. The identification of relevant studies, obtaining data from randomized controlled trials and meta-analysis data are all discussed. Guidelines are given for assessing reviews, how they may be prepared, updated and disseminated. A bibliography on the science of reviewing research is included. Updated versions of this will be disseminated on disk as the Cochrane Database of Systematic Reviews and also through the Internet using the FTP servers at the Canadian and UK Cochrane Centres. Addresses, telephone, fax and email addresses are included for the eight Cochrane Centres (CR 2.12.13, 2.29, 2.85, 2.92).

2.12.4 Ciliska, D., Cullum, N. & Marks, S. (2001) Evaluation of systematic reviews of treatment or prevention interventions. *Evidence Based Nursing* 4 (4) 100–4   11 References

Using the example of nocturnal eneuresis in children, the article examines the nature of systematic reviews, the validity of the results and whether they may help in caring for patients.

2.12.5   Clarke, M. & Oxman, A.D. (eds) (2003) *Cochrane reviewers' handbook Version* 4.1.6 [Updated January 2003]. In: The Cochrane Library. Oxford: Update Software. Updated quarterly www. update-software.com/ccweb/

Systematic reviews establish where the effects of health care are consistent and research results can be applied across populations, settings, and differences in treatment (e.g. dose); and where effects may vary significantly. The handbook aims to help reviewers make good decisions about the methods they use for examining the literature and the guidelines will enable them to be systematic and explicit. The focus is particularly on systematic reviews of randomized controlled trials, but issues are also addressed when reviewing other types of evidence, for example the inclusion of non-randomized studies in Cochrane reviews. Fuller guidance on such reviews may be found at: www.cochrane.dk/nrsmg/ The format of Cochrane reviews will help readers to find the results quickly and to assess the validity, applicability and implications of these results. It is also suited to electronic publication and updating, and it generates reports that are informative and readable when viewed on a computer monitor or printed. This book is now setting the standard for the systematic reviews of research literature (CR 2.2.4).

2.12.6   Cook, D.J. & Mulrow, C.D. (1998) *Systematic reviews: synthesis of best evidence for healthcare decisions.* Philadelphia, PA: American College of Physicians   ISBN 0943126665 References

Book aims to increase understanding of the important role that systematic reviews play in advancing knowledge and motivate more practitioners to conduct their own systematic reviews. A CD-ROM included with the book presents numerous interactive exercises (CR 2.2).

2.12.7   Cooper, H., Carlisle, C., Watkins, C. & Gibbs, T. (2000) Using qualitative methods for conducting a systematic review. *Nurse Researcher: The International Journal of Research Methodology in Nursing and Health Care* 8 (1) 28–38   21 References

Reports a study that developed strategies for systematically reviewing 'soft' data, i.e. data that is not rigorous or scientific. It describes methods used to review literature on inter-professional education,

designed to overcome the barriers currently associated with integrating narrative studies into a systematic review. This can be described as an alternative, but analogous, strategy to that developed for evidence-based practice.

2.12.8   Cooper, H., Carlisle, C., Gibbs, T. & Watkins, C. (2001) Developing an evidence base for interdisciplinary learning: a systematic review. *Journal of Advanced Nursing* 35 (2) 228–37   39 References

Review examined British and American literature from 1967 to 1999 in order to explore the feasibility of introducing interdisciplinary education within undergraduate health professional programmes. This paper reports on the first stage of the study and its outcomes, based on textual analysis, have provided guidelines for future interventions and recommendations for research (CR 2.89).

2.12.9   Cooper, H.M. (1998) *Synthesizing research: a guide for literature reviews* (3rd edition). Thousand Oaks, CA: Sage ISBN   0761913483   References

Book gives guidance on conducting an integrative research review in a systematic, objective way. The process of reviewing is carried out in six phases: problem formulation, data collection, data evaluation, analysis, interpretation and public presentation. This enables more rigorous reviews to be carried out with greater potential for creating consensus among scholars and focusing debate in a constructive fashion. This new edition includes the latest information on the use of electronic technology and the Internet to conduct literature searches. The American Psychological Association's most recent guidelines are also included (CR 1.2, 2.99).

2.12.10   Deeks, J.J. (2001) Systematic reviews of evaluations of diagnostic and screening tests. *British Medical Journal* 323 (7305) 21 July 157–62   24 References

Explains how systematic reviews of studies of diagnostic accuracy differ from other systematic reviews and, using examples, describes the processes involved in evaluating or constructing such a review.

2.12.11   Dickson, R. (1999) Systematic reviews. In Hamer, S. & Collinson, G. (eds) *Achieving evidence-based practice: a handbook for practitioners.* London: Ballière Tindall   ISBN 0702023493 Chapter 3 41–60   33 References

Chapter discusses systematic reviews, what they are (and are not), their key components and how to assess their quality (CR 2.102.20).

2.12.12   Doyle, J. (2001) Forensic nursing: a review of the literature. *Australian Journal of Advanced Nursing* 18 (3) 32–9   36 References

A review of the literature reveals that forensic nursing is an emergent specialist area of practice that has undergone substantive role development in recent years. Forensic nurses have begun to write about the challenging and distinctive nature of their practice and are seeking greater recognition of their particular skills. The problematic nature of caring for forensic clients in correctional and less restrictive contexts of care remains a prominent feature in their writing.

2.12.13   Egger, M., Smith, G.D. & Altman, D. (eds) (2001) *Systematic reviews in health care* (2nd edition of *Systematic reviews*). London: BMJ Books ISBN 072791488X   References

This new edition has been revised and expanded to reflect significant changes and advances made in systematic reviewing. New features include discussion of the rationale of systematic reviewing, meta-analyses of prognostic and diagnostic studies and software, and the use of systematic reviews in practice. For further information a website is available: www.systematicreviews.com (CR 2.12.3, 2.92).

2.12.14   Elphick, H.E., Tan, A., Ashby, D. & Smyth, R.L. (2002) Systematic review and lifelong disease. *British Medical Journal* 325 (7360) 17 August 381–5   23 References

Identifies the use of systematic reviews in the evaluation of effective interventions, but highlights the lack of structured information regarding the long-term outcomes or side-effects from treatments.

2.12.15   Evans, D. (2001) Systematic reviews of nursing research. *Intensive and Critical Care Nursing* 17 (1) 51–7   58 References

Systematic reviews are now accepted as the most reliable way by which large volumes of research evidence can be managed. The process included documentation of methods prior to commencement, a comprehensive search to identify all studies on the topic and the use of rigorous methods for the appraisal, collection and synthesis of data. On completion of the review, the methods used are reported to allow its validity to be evaluated by end users of the evidence.

2.12.16   Evans, D. & Kowanko, I. (2000/2001) Literature reviews: evolution of a research methodology. *Australian Journal of Advanced Nursing* 18 (2) 33–8   28 References

Because reviews, rather than primary research, are now being used as the basis for many health care decisions, it is important that they are conducted with the same rigour as the primary research. The past two decades have seen a progressive evolution in review methodology, to the point where reviews are now considered research in their own right.

Despite this development, the standard of many published reviews remains poor. This paper summarizes the development of literature review methodology and discusses some of the implications for nursing.

2.12.17   Evans, J. & Benefield, P. (2001) Systematic reviews of educational research: does the medical model fit? *British Educational Research Journal* 27 (5) 527–41   42 References

Article describes the process of review, the adaptations of the 'medical model' to educational settings and discusses some of the implications of these for researchers and policy-makers (CR 2.12.21).

2.12.18   Fairbrother, P. & Ford, S. (1998) Lecturer practitioners: a literature review. *Journal of Advanced Nursing* 27 (2) 274–9   70 References

Paper examines mainly British and American literature from 1984 to 1996 and reviews the literature of the multifaceted aspects of the lecturer/practitioner role. These include the need for such practitioners, their origin within nursing and midwifery education, development of the role, the debate surrounding academic and clinical credibility and the current situation for lecturer/practitioners.

2.12.19   Fink, A. (1998) *Conducting research literature reviews: from paper to the Internet.* Thousand Oaks, CA: Sage   ISBN 0761909052 References

Book shows readers how to identify, interpret and analyse published and unpublished research literature. It also gives information on using databases and Internet searches (CR 2.85, 2.95).

2.12.20   Forbes, D.A. (2003) An example of the use of systematic reviews to answer an effectiveness question. *Western Journal of Nursing Research* 25 (2) 179–92   23 References

Uses an example from a systematic review on behavioural symptoms in Alzheimer's disease to outline the steps involved in critically appraising or conducting a review (CR 2.18, 2.25).

2.12.21   Hammersley, M. (2001) 'Systematic' reviews of research literature: a narrative response to Evans and Benefield. *British Educational Research Journal* 27 (5) 543–54   57 References

The production of systematic reviews of research findings has recently come to be treated as a priority in education and other disciplines. Such reviews are believed to play an important role in making evidence for research available in a usable form to policy-makers and practitioners. This article examines the assumptions about research, and about the task of reviewing, which are built into the concept of the systematic review. In addition, attention is given to the likely consequences of the priority now being given to this type of review (CR 2.12.17).

2.12.22   Harcourt, D. & Rumsey, N. (2001) Psychological aspects of breast reconstruction: a review of the literature. *Journal of Advanced Nursing* 35 (4) 477–87   67 References

Study critically examined British, American and European literature from 1971 to 2000 relating to the psychological aspects of breast reconstruction and the role of specialist breast care nurses. Findings revealed a lack of theoretically-based studies and methodological flaws. There was reliance on retrospective designs and inappropriate use of randomized controlled trials (CR 2.29).

2.12.23   Hart, C. (1998) *Doing a literature review: releasing the social science imagination.* London: Sage   ISBN 0761959750   References

Book, intended for undergraduates and postgraduates, guides readers to researching, preparing and writing a literature review. Text offers advice on searching out existing knowledge, analysing arguments and ideas, mapping arguments and perspectives, producing a literature review and constructing a case for investigating a topic. Appendices include the content of a proposal, citing references, summary of standards required for the presentation of a master's dissertation, managing information, keeping records and a checklist of dos and don'ts for reviewing (CR 2.96).

2.12.24   Hek, G., Langton, H. & Blunden, G. (2000) Systematically searching and reviewing literature. *Nurse Researcher* 7 (3) 40–57   37 References

Paper is based on a one-year project commissioned by the English National Board for Nursing, Midwifery and Health Visiting in the area of cancer nursing education. The authors describe the principles of systematic reviewing and the processes involved in a literature review. It also outlines techniques of critically appraising all types of literature, including evidence that is 'opinion'-based rather than research-based.

2.12.25   Hopayian, K. (2001) The need for caution in interpreting high quality systematic reviews. *British Medical Journal* 323 (7314) 22 September 681–4   32 References

Assesses the validity of three systematic reviews and highlights their variable quality and differing conclusions. Advises that important clinical details should not be overlooked and suggests that trials should be assessed from both a clinician's and reviewer's viewpoint.

2.12.26   Jones, T. & Evans, D. (2000) Conducting a systematic review. *Australian Critical Care* 13 (2) 66–71   39 References

Describes the steps necessary when undertaking a systematic review. These include preparing a detailed research protocol, selecting criteria for inclusion of articles, systematically searching the published and unpublished literature, determining which articles meet the criteria, critically appraising the quality of the research, extracting outcome data and combining it statistically, where appropriate, in order to summarize the best available evidence. These processes are documented in the report and can be subject to peer review and critique.

2.12.27   Louw, G., Williams, J.E. & Towlerton, G. (2000) Quality of evidence: problems with analyzing 'low-grade' case series studies. *Nurse Researcher: The International Journal of Research Methodology in Nursing and Health Care* 8 (1) 39–46   25 References

Paper discusses the methodology used to score studies that formed the evidence in a systematic review of intra-thecal pump systems for chronic pain. The vast majority of literature in intra-thecal techniques is in the form of case reports and case series, the very type of 'low-grade' evidence that is placed at the bottom of the 'Hierarchy of Evidence'. The issue is the extent to which they can, or should, be validated.

2.12.28   Magarey, J.M. (2001) Elements of a systematic review. *International Journal of Nursing Practice* 7 (6) 376–82   40 References

Provides a history of the evidence-based movement and identifies differences between systematic and traditional literature reviews. Gives a step-by-step account of how reviews should be conducted.

2.12.29   Marshall, M.J. & Hutchinson, S.A. (2001) A critique of research on the use of activities with persons with Alzheimer's disease: a systematic literature review. *Journal of Advanced Nursing* 35 (4) 488–96   66 References

Study examined British and American Literature from 1983 to 1999 on the use of activities with people suffering from Alzheimer's disease. While researchers have shown interest in such therapy, theoretical and methodological difficulties exist, together with unclear findings, gaps and a lack of emphasis on gender, ethnic, racial or cultural differences. Other types of research designs are suggested.

2.12.30   McInnes, E., Duff, L. & McClarey, M. (1999) Challenges in updating a systematic review. *NT Research* 4 (1) 66–71   13 References

Paper provides a frank description of the difficulties encountered in updating a systematic review. These included different reviewers, literature searching and sifting, study appraisal and a lack of pre-determined 'acceptable' designs. Authors believe that all decisions associated with critical appraisal and synthesis should be clearly documented and all research journals should adopt a structured abstract format. Advice is given to those about to undertake this task and recommendations are made for further research.

2.12.31 Müller-Mundt, G., Brinkhoff, P. & Schaeffer, D. (2000) Pain management in nursing care – results of a literature review (German). *Pflege* 13 (5) 325–38   78 References

An analysis of German nursing textbooks and journals was carried out to determine the state of the art with regard to pain management. This showed that there is a wide gap between the state of the art and practice. Multidisciplinary role model programmes, where nurses play a major role as change agents, have proved to be an effective strategy to change the institutional practice of pain management. Enhancing knowledge and educative skills of nurses, now that pain research and therapy is included in academic courses, will promote the quality of care (CR 2.98, 3.8).

2.12.32 Murphy, E. (2000) Qualitative research methods in health technology assessment: a review of the literature. www.doh.gov.uk/research (Accessed 23/01/03) [Project-related website: www.hta. nhsweb.nhs.uk]

Review examines the nature and status of qualitative methods in relation to their potential uses in health technology assessment (CR 2.36).

2.12.33 Nixon, J., Khan, K. & Klejnen, J. (2001) Summarizing economic evaluations in systematic reviews: a new approach. *British Medical Journal* 322 (7302) 30 June 1596–8   10 References

Identifies the existing methods for summarizing the evidence on the effects and costs of competing interventions, and describes a new method for presenting the same information in a clear and concise manner to improve decision-making.

2.12.34 Petticrew, M. (2001) Systematic review from astronomy to zoology: myths and misconceptions. *British Medical Journal* 322 (7278) 13 January 98–101   24 References

Article answers common criticisms directed at systematic reviews. It explains that they do not have to adopt a biomedical model or entail some form of statistical analysis and can contain a wide range of methodologies.

2.12.35 Prescott, R. (2000) Factors that limit the quality, number and progress of randomized controlled trials www.doh.gov.uk/research (Accessed 23/01/03) [Project-related web site: www.hta. nhsweb.nhs.uk]

Literature from 1986 to 1996 was examined for factors limiting the quality, number and progress of randomized controlled trials. Issues included design, barriers to participation, conduct and structure, analysis, reporting and costs (CR 2.29).

2.12.36 Roe, B., Guiness, L. & Rafferty, A.M. (1999) A systematic search of the literature on effectiveness of alliances for health promotion: some methodological issues and their implications for research. *Health Education Journal* 58 78–90   57 References

Reports a systematic literature search and an annotated bibliography compiled on the effectiveness of alliances for health promotion. The methods used for searching are presented along with a preliminary description of the studies retrieved. The methodological issues are discussed together with their implications, and suggestions are made for research and health policy (CR 3.11).

2.12.37 Ross, S., Grant, A., Counsell, C., Gillespie, W., Russell, I. & Prescott, R. (1999) Barriers to participation in randomized controlled trials: a systematic review. *Journal of Clinical Epidemiology* 52 (12) 1143–56   86 References

A systematic review of three bibliographic databases from 1986 to 1996 identified 78 papers reporting barriers to recruitment of clinicians and patients to randomized controlled trials. These are all identified and suggestions are made as to how they may be overcome (CR 2.22, 2.29).

2.12.38 Schlomer, G. (1999) RCTs and systematic reviews in nursing literature: a comparison of German and international nursing research (German). *Pflege* 12 (4) 250–8   21 References

Author investigated whether there are randomized-controlled trials (RCTs) and systematic reviews on nursing care written in German that should be included in reviews of the effects of health care. 15 were identified but there were no nurse researchers as first authors. German nurse researchers are urged to adapt high-quality study designs to nursing intervention studies to achieve international research standards (CR 2.29, 3.3).

2.12.39 Shepperd, S. & Iliffe, S. (2001) Hospital at home versus in-patient hospital care. In: *The Cochrane Library* Issue 4 26 pages Oxford: Update Software   23 References

The objectives of this systematic review were to assess the effects of hospital at home compared with inpatient hospital care. The search strategy is described together with the reviewers' conclusions, and suggestions are made for future research.

2.12.40   Sleep, J. & Clark, E. (1999) Weighing up the evidence: the contribution of critical literature reviews to the development of practice. *NT Research* 4 (4) 306–13   42 References

Authors argue that health professionals should draw on evidence and insights from a broad range of research traditions, rather than just relying on synthesized evidence from randomized clinical trials. The potential of other types of literature are explored.

2.12.41   Sutton, A.J., Jones, D.R., Abrams, K.R., Sheldon, T.A. & Song, F. (1999) Systematic reviews and meta-analysis: a structured review of the methodological literature. *Journal of Health Services Research & Policy* 4 (1) 49–55   50 References

Assesses 1,000 papers to review the methodological and statistical methods used in systematic reviews and meta-analysis. Among other issues, the paper discusses methods for dealing with publication bias and economic evaluation. It provides a concise description of the methods available for the promotion of better quality reviews of health service research (CR 2.87, 2.92).

2.12.42   Swanson, K.M. (1999) What is known about caring in nursing science: a literary meta-analysis. In Hinshaw, A.S., Feetham, S.L. & Shaver, J.L.F. (eds) *Handbook of clinical nursing research.* Thousand Oaks, CA: Sage ISBN 080395784X   Part 1   Chapter 3   31–60   136 References

Chapter summarizes a literary meta-analysis of published nursing research on the concept of caring, and proposes a framework that adequately integrates the current state of substantive knowledge about this concept. Throughout the chapter issues pertaining to the syntax (methodology) are addressed (CR 2.92, 3.6.4).

2.12.43   Thompson, C. & Thompson, G. (2001) Support for carers of people with Alzheimer's type dementia. In: *The Cochrane Library* Issue 4   13 pages Oxford: Update Software   6 References

Paper provides an example of an updated systematic Cochrane Review, which aimed to provide an assessment of the effectiveness of health and/or social interventions designed to support the carers of people with Alzheimer's-type dementias. The original problem is identified, the search strategy and results are discussed, and suggestions are made for future areas of research (CR 2.29, 2.92).

2.12.44   Watts, T., Jones, M., Wainwright, P. & Williams, A. (2001) Methodologies analyzing individual practice in health care: a systematic review. *Journal of Advanced Nursing* 35 (2) 238–56   77 References

Article reviews US, UK, and European nursing and medical literature from 1967 to 2000. Its aim was to identify, explore and evaluate the current level of knowledge of methodologies used in the comparative analysis of the individual practice of doctors, nurses and midwives. Authors believe that the current level of knowledge is biased towards quantitative research and argue for a more balanced approach that recognizes the strengths of both quantitative and qualitative research methods (CR 2.29, 2.36).

2.12.45   Woodward, V. & Webb, C. (2001) Women's anxieties surrounding breast disorders: a systematic review of the literature. *Journal of Advanced Nursing* 33 (1) 29–41   49 References

Reports a review of literature published in English between 1990 and 1999 to discover whether women with benign breast disorders suffer similar amounts of anxiety to women with breast cancer in the time between discovery of the problem and receiving a diagnosis, to include the immediate post-diagnosis phase. The processes of reviewing are highlighted, the results are reported and the implications for practice are discussed.

2.13   REPLICATION RESEARCH

Replication of nursing research, particularly clinical studies, is an essential element of a sound, empirically-based body of knowledge that is fundamental to good nursing practice. Replication studies are infrequently found in the literature, but these are a vital step in the development of nursing science and should be supported and encouraged. 'As a result of nurses' reluctance to replicate studies, many isolated pieces of nursing research exist. Researchers must become convinced of the value of replication' (Nieswiadomy, 2002: 302).

Definition [See Appendix D for source]

Replication study – a research study that repeats or duplicates an earlier research study, with all of the essential elements of the original study held intact. A different sample or setting may be used

Example

Bajracharya, S.M. (1999) Employers' perceived importance and use of skills that are specific to health educators: a replication study in a rural setting. *International Electronic Journal of Health Education* 2 (2) 59–65   8 References

This study examined the perceptions of rural community health employees in regard to the importance of specific skills defined as the role of entry-level health educators. A survey undertaken in 1993 was modified and used and the results are reported (CR 2.52).

Annotations

2.13.1   Collins, H.M. (1992) *Changing order: replication and induction in scientific practice* (2nd edition). Chicago: University of Chicago Press ISBN 0226113760   References

Discusses the processes and outcomes of replication from a philosophical point of view and uses three field studies for illustration. These examined laser building, the detection of gravitational radiation and mind over matter. The complexities involved are explored.

2.13.2   Klein, J.G., Brown, G.T. & Lysyk, M. (2000) Replication research: a purposeful occupation worth repeating. *Canadian Journal of Occupational Therapy* 67 (3) 155–61   33 References

Although it is common for researchers at the end of their published studies, to suggest that further work is required, very few published studies have replicated original work. This article provides a framework for understanding issues related to replication research for all seeking to establish evidence-based practice.

2.13.3   Martin, P.A. (1995) More replication studies needed. *Applied Nursing Research* 8 102–3   References

'Replication studies should be a high priority for nursing research' – this is particularly true for clinical nursing research. Because of the small, non-random samples used in many studies, nurses need to conduct many similar studies on the same topic to allow generalization of findings. Nursing studies have generally been one-of-a-kind, with few replication or extension studies. It is rare that a single study is sufficient foundation for making decisions about nursing practice (CR 2.28).

2.13.4   Neuliep, J.W. (ed.) (1991) *Replication research in the social sciences*. Newbury Park, CA: Sage   ISBN 0803940920   References

Discusses all aspects of replication research, including the processes involved, its importance and editorial bias against it. Illustrative material is given from the literature of several disciplines (CR 2.27).

2.13.5   Nieswiadomy, R.M. (2002) Findings are not ready for use in practice. In Author *Foundations of nursing research* (4th edition). Upper Saddle River, NJ: Prentice-Hall   ISBN 0130339911   Chapter 16 323–4   60 References

Studies are cited that discuss research findings and the dangers of trying to apply them without replication. It would be appropriate for masters students to undertake such studies, and journal editors need to be willing to publish them (CR 2.1.55).

2.13.6   Nieswiadomy, R.M. (2002) Replication of the research study. In Author *Foundations of nursing research* (4th edition). Upper Saddle River, NJ: Prentice-Hall   ISBN   0130339911   Chapter 15 301–2   8 References

Author documents the paucity of replication studies and the problems this has for the body of nursing knowledge that must be based on research findings (CR 2.1.55).

2.13.7   Reese, H.W. (1999) Strategies for replication research exemplified by replications of the Istomina study. *Developmental Review* 19 (1) 1–30   75 References

Identifies strategies for undertaking replication research, including meta-analysis, using the often replicated work of Soviet psychologist Istomina as an example. A critique of several of the replication studies is included (CR 2.92).

2.14   RESEARCH PLANNING

Studies of previous research in nursing reveal that many have had both qualitative and quantitative components. In order to understand the complexity of nursing, with its wide range of problems and practices, a variety of research approaches may be required, including multi-methods.

Definitions [See Appendix D for sources]

Gatekeeper – a person whose permission must be sought by the researcher in order to gain access to the respondents

Research protocol – the overall plan or recipe for procedures to be carried out in a particular study

Annotations

2.14.1   Abbott, P. & Sapsford, R. (eds) (1997) *Research into practice: a reader for nurses and the caring professions* (2nd edition). Buckingham: Open University Press   ISBN 0335196950   References

This edition contains papers relating to nursing, health and community care, showing the types of research that may be undertaken by a small team or single researcher. Papers show a variety of approaches, the limitations typical of small-scale projects and how research works out in practice. Three major sections are: observing and participating; talking to people and asking questions; controlled trials and comparisons (CR 2.16, 2.29, 2.68, 2.72, 3.16).

2.14.2 American Sociological Association *Sociological methodology* weber.u.washington. edu/~socmeth2/ (Accessed 23/01/03)

This website provides information on research methods in the social sciences. It includes contents pages and abstracts of articles from 1994, together with subscription details and information for authors.

2.14.3 Barrett, E., Lally, V.E., Purcell, S. & Thresh, R. (1999) *Signposts for educational research CD-ROM: a multimedia resource for the beginning researcher.* London: Sage ISBN 076196245X

By using the metaphor of researcher as traveller, the beginning researcher can navigate his/her way through a research project.

2.14.4 Bickman, L. & Rog, D.J. (eds) (1998) *Handbook of applied social research methods.* Thousand Oaks, CA: Sage ISBN 076190672X References

Provides a practical guide to selecting the appropriate questions and procedures, from among the diverse perspectives available, for studying some of the highly complex areas within the real world (CR 2.9, 2.16, 2.18, 2.20, 2.29, 2.36).

2.14.5 Birley, G. & Moreland, N. (1998) *A practical guide to academic research.* London: Kogan Page ISBN 0749422777 References

Book is intended for all students and academic staff in the fields of education and the social sciences. It introduces the important methodologies and data collection techniques, provides a framework for the critical assessment of quality and role of existing research, and aims to support involvement in research (CR 2.64, 2.95).

2.14.6 Blaikie, N. (1993) *Approaches to social enquiry.* Cambridge: Polity Press ISBN 0745611737 References

Book is intended for experienced and novice researchers and covers science and social science, research strategies and some methodological issues.

2.14.7 Brink, P.J. & Wood, M.J. (2001) *Basic steps in planning research: from question to proposal* (5th edition). Sudbury, MA: Jones & Bartlett ISBN 0763715719 References

Book is an introduction to the research process and deals solely with the beginning phase of research – the research plan, from question to proposal (CR 2.96).

2.14.8 Chambliss, D.F. & Schutt, R.K. (2003) *Making sense of the social world: methods of investigation.* Thousand Oaks, CA: Pine Forge Press ISBN 0761987878 References

Authors present the logic and essential techniques of research methods with a light, readable style and without skimping on critical concepts or recent developments. The book focuses on validity as a unifying concept and supplies an integrated treatment of research ethics and practices with examples and exercises. A CD-ROM is included that comprises key concepts, qualitative data analysis software, data for SPSS analysis, and links to related websites. The latter includes activities to help students master the content while doing some web-based research (CR 2.17, 2.25, Appendix A).

2.14.9 Chapple, A. (2000) Managing a project under pressure: learning from experience. *Nurse Researcher* 7 (4) 4–13 17 References

Paper describes the difficulties faced when undertaking a large-scale survey on the potential use of 'walk-in' centres, which had to be planned and completed in four months. Suggested solutions are given for those who may find themselves in similar circumstances (CR 2.16, 2.68, 2.75).

2.14.10 Crotty, M. (1998) *The foundations of social research: meaning and perspective in the research process.* London: Sage ISBN 0761961062 References

Book links methodology with theory to guide students and researchers when navigating the maze of conflicting terminology during the planning stages of research (CR 2.2, 2.7).

2.14.11 Dennis, M.L., Perl, H.I., Huebner, R.B. & McLellan, A.T. (2000) Twenty-five strategies for improving the design, implementation and analysis of health services research related to alcohol and other drug abuse treatment. *Addiction* 95 (3) S281–S308 118 References

Discusses the challenge of undertaking research into alcohol and drug addiction and identifies 25 strategies encompassing the whole research process from identification of problems through to implementation of findings and organizational policy changes (CR 2.4, 2.21, 2.35, 2.54, 2.64, 2.95, 3.11, 3.20).

2.14.12 Denscombe, M. (2002) *Ground rules for good research: a 10 point guide for social researchers.* Buckingham: Open University Press ISBN 0335206514 References

Book is intended for those undertaking small research projects. It identifies key ideas and practices that underlie good research, and provides guidelines to help newcomers and experienced researchers alike.

2.14.13 Emden, C. & Borbasi, S. (2000) Programmatic research: a desirable (or despotic) nursing strategy for the future. *Collegian: Journal of the Royal College of Nursing, Australia* 7 (1) 32–7 20 References

Highlights the rationale and problems in conducting programmatic research within nursing and the resulting implications for nursing scholarship. Provides a definition and example and makes recommendations for research students, early-career and experienced researchers (CR 3.16, 3.19).

2.14.14 Fuller, R. & Petch, A. (1995) *Practitioner research: the reflexive social worker.* Buckingham: Open University Press ISBN 0335193226 References

Discusses the relationships between practice and research, how these can be married together and what types of research can realistically be undertaken by busy practitioners. It also provides a conceptual framework for practitioner research.

2.14.15 Granger, B. & Chulay, M. (1999) *Research strategies for clinicians.* London: Prentice Hall ISBN 0838515398 References

Text takes a pragmatic approach to research, providing theory and suggestions on how to carry out research when employed in a clinical setting. Its design as a text/workbook will encourage 'hands-on' use and provide a supplement to introductory texts.

2.14.16 Hannigan, B. (2000) Getting started in research. *Nurse Researcher* 7 (4) 31–9 14 References

This step-by-step guide is intended to help novice researchers explore and clarify some of the issues associated with getting started in research (CR 2.20).

2.14.17 Ibrahim, J.E. (2000) Translating quality into research: do we need more research into quality or should quality activities be conducted using the principles and methodological rigour of scientific research? Australasian Association for Quality in Health Care. *Journal of Quality in Clinical Practice* 20 (2–3) 63–4

Suggests that quality projects are implemented with the best intentions but often fall short of the rigour required to be 'scientific'. Conducting and presenting all quality activities in the standard scientific format will improve their design and provide clear and objective evidence about outcomes.

2.14.18 Knight, P.T. (2001) *Small-scale research: pragmatic inquiry in social science and the caring professions.* London: Sage ISBN 0761968628

Examines the whole research process, including anticipating common mistakes and 'times of trouble', and offers advice on making things easier.

2.14.19 Lewith, G., Jonas, W.B. & Walach, H. (eds) (2002) *Clinical research in complementary therapies: principles, problems and solutions.* Edinburgh: Churchill Livingstone ISBN 0443063672 References

Book describes and analyses general research issues, which may have a special significance in complementary therapy research. It suggests factors that need to be considered in planning projects, and pinpoints aspects that differ from orthodox medical research. It briefly reviews the types of research carried out in specific complementary therapies, and suggests ways in which future research should be approached.

2.14.20 Maxwell, J. (1996) *Qualitative research design: an interactive approach.* Thousand Oaks, CA: Sage ISBN 0803973292 References

Book emphasizes the components of a design together with how these interact with each other and the environment in which the study is situated. A clear strategy for creating coherent and workable relationships among these design components is provided and key design issues are highlighted. These include clarifying the purpose of the study, creating a theoretical context, formulating research questions, developing a relationship with the people being studied, making decisions about sampling, data collection and analysis, assessing validity threats and alternative explanations to the study's conclusions (CR 2.3, 2.7, 2.20, 2.22, 2.25, 2.64).

2.14.21 Moore, M., Beazley, S. & Maelzer, J. (1998) *Researching disability issues.* Buckingham: Open University Press ISBN 0335198031 References

Book provides illustrations of how to carry out research that seeks to explore disability issues. Both quantitative and qualitative frameworks are considered and a variety of studies, which examine different aspects of disabled people's lives, are reviewed. Substantive examples of dilemmas that face researchers in this field are highlighted (CR 2.9, 2.16, 2.29).

2.14.22   Potter, S. (ed.) (2002) *Doing postgraduate research*. London: Sage/Open University ISBN 0761947450   References

Book covers all aspects of planning and organizing a research project, the writing process, using computers in research, responsibilities, rights and ethics and the examination process and viva (CR 2.14, 2.17, 2.85, 2.97).

2.14.23   Pruitt, R.H. & Privette, A.B. (2001) Planning strategies for the avoidance of pitfalls in intervention research. *Journal of Advanced Nursing* 35 (4) 514–20   29 References

Study discusses some of the methodological challenges that may be encountered in intervention research. These include maintaining an adequate sample size, intervention demands, measuring variables, timing issues and experiencing unexpected results. Suggested strategies for maintaining the integrity of the study are addressed (CR 2.16, 2.19, 2.22, 2.43).

2.14.24   Roberts, J. & DiCenso, A. (1999) EBN notebook. Identifying the best research design to fit the question. Part 1: Quantitative designs. *Evidence Based Nursing* 2 (1) 4–6   3 References

The most rigorous quantitative designs to address questions of prevention or treatment, causation and prognosis are outlined (CR 2.20, 2.29).

2.14.25   Robertson, J. (ed.) (1994) *Handbook of clinical nursing research*. Melbourne: Churchill Livingstone   ISBN 044304866   References

Written primarily for facilitating the conduct of nursing research in the clinical setting, this book is intended to complement other methodology texts. The steps involved in undertaking research are described and some common problems encountered in clinical settings are discussed. Book includes standards for nursing research compiled in 1990 by members of the Western Australian Nurse Researchers' Network (CR 2.1, 2.101, 3.2).

2.14.26   Rothwell, H. (1998) A beginner's picture of research (II) Research methods: no short cuts. *The Practising Midwife* 1 (11) 16–18   8 References

Gives a broad outline of some of the issues to consider when choosing a research design (CR 2.4).

2.14.27   Saks, M., Williams, M. & Hancock, B. (eds) (2000) *Developing research in primary care*. Oxford: Radcliffe   Medical   Press   ISBN 1857753976   References

Primarily intended for the novice researcher, this book gives a clear understanding of what is involved

in research, together with some of the key knowledge necessary to undertake such studies.

2.14.28   Schostak, J.F. (2002) *Understanding, designing and conducting qualitative research in education: framing the project*. Buckingham: Open University Press   ISBN 0335205097   References

Book aims to help readers identify what is new and important about their project, how it relates to previous work and how it may be used to bring about change at individual, community, national or even international levels (CR 2.36).

2.14.29   Shipman, M. (1997) *The limitations of social research* (4th edition). London: Longman   ISBN 0582311039   References

Book examines the underlying assumptions of different traditions that justify different research methods, techniques for collecting evidence and preparing for publication. Each chapter is preceded by a controversy illustrating problems in the following text. This new edition is fully updated to take account of new developments in methodology and a chapter is included on designing research (CR 2.99).

2.14.30   Treacy, M.P. & Hyde, A. (1999) *Nursing research: design and practice*. Dublin: University College Dublin Press   ISBN 1900621290 References

Book introduces the strategies and processes of undertaking research including planning, quantitative and qualitative approaches, and utilizing research. Also included are papers on the application of research strategies (CR 2.9, 2.29, 2.36, 2.102).

2.14.31   Usherwood, T. (1996) *Introduction to project management in health research: a guide for new researchers*. Buckingham: Open University Press   ISBN 0335197078   References

Offers advice to first-time researchers on a systematic and structured approach to research project management.

2.14.32   Williams, M. (2002) *Making sense of social research*. London: Sage   ISBN 0761964223 References

Book identifies the essentials for undergraduates and graduates engaged in quantitative and qualitative research, and suggests how the gap between formulating a research question and carrying out research can be bridged. Key features include clarification of essential issues and problem-solving guidance, demonstration of the importance of interplay between theory and research, realism in defining research issues and the problems that researchers encounter (CR 2.1, 2.9, 2.16, 2.17, 2.20, 2.29, 2.36).

2.14.33 Wright State University Libraries
Guide to beginning the nursing research process
www.libraries.wright.edu/libnet/subj/nur/nursres.html (Accessed 20/01/03)

Provides an example of material available on the Internet that gives starting points for nursing students. Information makes reference to books on 'how to do' research, the writing process, statistics, locating theses and finding information on tests and measurements.

Designing Nursing Research

2.15   COLLABORATIVE/ INTERDISCIPLINARY RESEARCH

'In research partnerships ... individual personalities and interpersonal processes both play a crucial part. ... The complex interplay between institutions and individuals, personal and professional agendas are important variables to consider. ... [It is] through identifying ... the principles of formal and informal processes impacting upon research, complementarity and reciprocity [that the important aspects of a research partnership are identified].' (Mackenzie, Husband & Gerrish, 1995: 88–9) [adapted]

Definitions [See Appendix D for sources]

Collaborative research – to labour or co-operate with another, especially in ... scientific pursuits

Cross-disciplinary research – task requires a combination of disciplines for its achievement

Multi- and interdisciplinary research – organizational form used to carry out cross-disciplinary research

Networking – the establishing of professional contacts ... for such purposes as disseminating information ... or offering mutual guidance

Example

Underwood, F. & Parker, J. (1998/99) Developing and evaluating an acute stroke pathway through action research. *Nurse Researcher* 6 (2) 27–38   17 References

Reports an action research study focusing on acute stroke management by using the care pathway approach. After relocating an Acute Stroke Unit to a neurology ward, an opportunity was taken to question inherited practices. This led to the development of a multidisciplinary team with representatives from occupational therapy, physiotherapy, dietetics, speech and language therapy, nursing, pharmacy, consultant and stroke services co-ordinator. Results are reported which show many positive influences on the outcomes of care (CR 2.37).

Annotations

2.15.1   Barker, J. & Weller, S. (2003) 'Is it fun?' Developing children centred research methods. *International Journal of Sociology and Social Policy* 23 (1/2) 33–58   51 References

Identifies the shift in orientation towards conducting research with, rather than on, children. Reflects upon two studies that adopted child-centred methodologies, where techniques such as photographs and diaries were used to stimulate interest from the children (CR 2.67).

2.15.2   Bartunek, J.M. & Louis, M.R. (1996) *Insider/outsider team research*. Thousand Oaks, CA: Sage   ISBN 0803971591   References

Discusses the recent growth of research partnerships and identifies problems that occur at various stages of team research.

2.15.3   Bray, J.N., Lee, J., Smith, L.L. & Yorks, L. (2000) *Collaborative inquiry in practice: action, reflection, and making meaning*. Thousand Oaks, CA: Sage   ISBN 0761906479   References

The reader is guided step-by-step through the theory and practice of collaborative inquiry. Authors demonstrate how effective collaborative inquiry demystifies research and makes learning more accessible. The guidance provided is equally applicable to professional and academic settings.

2.15.4   Byrne-Armstrong, H. (2001) Whose show is it? The contradictions of collaboration. In Byrne-Armstrong, H., Higgs, J. & Horsfall, D. (eds) *Critical moments in qualitative research*. Oxford: Butterworth Heinemann   ISBN 0750651598   Chapter 8 106–14 14 References

Chapter explores collaboration in research from the viewpoint that 'everything is dangerous'. Inevitable power differences exist between those undertaking collaborative projects, but instead of being visible and overt, these may become invisible and covert. These ideas are discussed using three personal narratives (CR 2.36.17).

2.15.5   Campbell, M., Copeland, B. & Tate, B. (1998) Taking the standpoint of people with disabilities in research: experiences with participation.

Canadian Journal of Rehabilitation 12 (2) 95–104 13 References

Reports a participatory study of health experiences of people with disabilities. The research team included people with disabilities, health care providers, hired research staff and university faculty. There are differences between an intent to be inclusive and collaborative and what actually happens in practice. This is due to power differences among researchers in a participatory approach, the knowledge they bring and the authority afforded to different kinds of knowledge. Regardless of how challenging participation may be, success in the project depends on attending analytically and practically to the problems related to ruling relations that inevitably invade participatory research (CR 2.16).

2.15.6 Crabtree, B.F., Addison, R.B., Gilchrist, V., Kuzel, A. & Miller, W.L. (eds) (1994) *Developing collaborative research in primary care.* London: Sage ISBN 0803954891 References

Authors believe that multi-method research, moving beyond any particular discipline would enable more primary care research to be successful.

2.15.7 Downie, J., Orb, A., Wynaden, D., McGowan, S., Seeman, Z. & Ogilvie, S. (2001) A practice research model for collaborative partnership. *Collegian: Journal of the Royal College of Nursing, Australia* 8 (4) 27–32 14 References

Describes an initiative that developed a practice research model of collaboration between practitioners and academics in Western Australia. Changes, innovations and dissemination of best practice outcomes have arisen from the pursuit of research to support clinical practice (CR 2.98).

2.15.8 Dufault, M.A. (2001) A program of research evaluating the effects of collaborative research utilization model. *Online Journal of Knowledge Synthesis for Nursing* 8 (3) August 16 7 pages 29 References

Article describes a programme of research in which a collaborative research utilization (CRU) model was developed and tested in four clinical studies on pain management. The overall aim of the research programme was to decrease the long time lag from when innovations are developed to when they appear in clinicians' day-to-day care-giving activities. In the model, partnerships are formed between researchers, undergraduate and graduate students, and clinicians in academic and practice settings. The developmental process, structure, and steps of the model are described as well as the outcomes that have been achieved (CR 2.98).

2.15.9 Epton, S.R., Payne, R.L. & Pearson, A.W. (eds) (1983) *Managing inter-disciplinary research.*

Chichester: Wiley ISBN 0471903175 References [2nd International Conference on the Management of Inter-disciplinary Research held at Manchester Business School, England, July 1981]

Book contains chapters on nomenclature, where this type of research may provide the best approach to solving problems, consideration of institutional and personal barriers and extracting lessons for management. Editors suggest that it should not be read as a formal record of proceedings, but rather capture the main themes and illustrate the variety of activity taking place. Also reported are the deliberations of the first Interdisciplinary Research Management Conference held in Schloss Reisenburg in the Federal Republic of Germany, 22–28 April 1979.

2.15.10 Fishman, S.M. & McCarthy, L. (2000) *Unplayed tapes: a personal history of collaborative teacher research.* New York: National Council of Teachers of English and Teachers College Press ISBN 0807739677 References

Book explores three critical concerns for practitioner researchers: the nature of practitioner research itself in the field and in their own work; the use of theory to buoy, complement and complete research studies, and the overall picture of practitioner research as a helpful tool for improving teaching and learning and creating knowledge in the field of education (CR 2.78).

2.15.11 Fitzpatrick, J.F. (2002) Multidisciplinary and interdisciplinary research: what it is and what it is not. *Applied Nursing Research Online* 15 (2) May 59 Editorial www2.appliednursingresearch.org/scripts/om.dll/serve?action=searchDB&searchD… (Accessed 13/11/03)

Discusses two forms of collaboration and the circumstances in which they may be used most appropriately.

2.15.12 Gelling, L. & Chatfield, D. (2001) Research collaboration. *Nurse Researcher: The International Journal of Research Methodology in Nursing and Health Care* 9 (2) 4–16 25 References

Paper considers the nature of collaborative research, describes three models of collaboration and suggests some potential benefits of successful research collaboration to individuals, groups, organizations and consumers.

2.15.13 Grant, G., Guyton, O. & Forrester, R. (1999) Creating effective research compliance programs in academic institutions. *Academic Medicine* 74 (9) September 951–71 References

Authors believe that academic centres should expand their present compliance programmes (which are for their hospitals and faculty practice plans) into their other programmes, including research. Similarly, universities should expand or institute programmes of compliance for research. The reasons for this are given and key questions answered about the benefits and risks of such collaboration. Information on how to establish a programme, its elements, the experiences of institutions engaged in such work, and positive outcomes are all discussed.

2.15.14 Grundy, S. (1998) Research partnerships: principles and possibilities. In Atweh, B., Kemmis, S. & Weeks, P. (eds) *Action research in practice: partnerships for social justice in education.* London: Routledge   ISBN 0414171520   Chapter 3 37–46   13 References

Chapter explores some issues relating to the concept of professional partnerships, not so much in relation to teacher education, but to research partnerships (CR 2.37.2).

2.15.15 Hewison, A. & Sim, J. (1998) Managing interprofessional working: using codes of ethics as a foundation. *Journal of Interprofessional Care* 12 (3) 309–12   64 References

Paper considers the role of professional codes of ethics where working together requires co-operation and mutual understanding, and addresses their potential for both enhancing and compromising inter-professional working. Comparisons are made between codes and their moral status and the practical support they offer to health care practitioners is evaluated, with particular reference to the issue of 'whistleblowing'. Recommendations are made for refinement of the codes to make them more relevant to contemporary practice (CR 2.17).

2.15.16 Institute for Advanced Interdisciplinary Research *Mission statement* www.systems. org/html/framesetabout.html (Accessed 11/11/03)

The Institute for Advanced Interdisciplinary Research is a Texas-based non-profit organization that serves government, industry and the community by providing research, information and services designed to aid in anticipating and managing change. Its strategies include public education, client services and state-of-the-art communication of issues, ideas and knowledge.

2.15.17 Knight, T., Smith, J. & Cropper, S. (2001) Developing sustainable collaboration: learning from theory and practice. *Primary Health Care Research and Development* 2 (3) 139–48   24 References

Paper draws on the experience and observation of two forms of strategic collaborative ventures established with the ultimate purpose of improving the

nation's health. Using a specific framework, the development of these initiatives is evaluated and key lessons are identified for developing sustainable collaborative research.

2.15.18 Knox, M., Mok, M. & Parmenter, T.R. (2000) Working with the experts: collaborative research with people with an intellectual disability. *Disability and Society* 15 (1) 49–61 31 References

Analyses the collaborative approach adopted in a study about six people with an intellectual disability. The outcomes and implications are identified, including informed consent as a process and the informants as experts in their experience.

2.15.19 Krishnasamy, M. & Plant, H. (1998) Developing nursing research with people. *International Journal of Nursing Studies* 35 (1–2) 79–84   31 References

Paper explores issues surrounding the role and capacity of research to inform practice. Using three research projects undertaken by cancer nurses, some questions concerning nurse-led research and practice development issues are raised. The use of collaborative inquiry and action research forms the basis of the exploration (CR 2.3, 2.37).

2.15.20 Leighton-Beck, L. (2000) What is networking? *Nurse Researcher* 7 (3) 4–13   5 References

Article explores some of the potential benefits and pitfalls of the networking process and discusses its meaning in the context of nursing research (CR 2.98).

2.15.21 Mumford, R. & Sanders, J. (2000) Getting to the heart of the matter: making meaning – three challenges for family researchers. *Qualitative Health Research* 10 (6) 841–52   13 References

Discusses three challenges facing qualitative researchers when working in the family health and well-being field. These are the formulation of research questions, access and reciprocity, research partnerships and teams (CR 2.16, 2.20, 2.22, 2.36).

2.15.22 Northway, R. (2000) Finding out together: lessons in participatory research for the learning disability nurse. *Mental Health Care and Learning Disabilties* 3 (7) 229–32   35 References

Describes how participatory research provides a model for nurses to work with people with learning disabilities as equal partners. It discusses issues which they must be aware of if they are not to perpetuate disabling relationships with their co-researchers.

2.15.23 Northway, R. (2000) The relevance of participatory research in developing nursing research and practice. *Nurse Researcher* 7 (4) 40–52 35 References

Paper argues that participatory research has the potential to counter many of the problems identified within traditional research approaches that seek to determine the views of patients/clients. Its key features are discussed, together with organizational factors, the resources available, ethical aspects and the need for reflexivity (CR 2.11).

2.15.24 Northway, R., Parker, M. & Roberts, E. (2001) Collaboration in research. *Nurse Researcher: The International Journal of Research Methodology in Nursing and Health Care* 9 (2) 75–83 13 References

Paper provides an overview of how one university department worked in collaboration with a mental health user group to develop and undertake a research project. Five key stages in the process are discussed.

2.15.25 Robbins, D. (ed.) (2000) *Pierre Bourdieu.* London: Sage   ISBN 0761964657 References   4 Volumes

Pierre Bourdieu's work in post-war sociology covers many fields; the sociology of culture, research methods, higher education, social theory, power and stratification. The editor seeks to show the notable and, in some cases, seminal contributions Bourdieu has made. Volumes cover his life and career, philosophy of science/knowledge and his methodology, key concepts, intellectual fields, transnational transmission, applications and ways of reading Bourdieu. One of his major achievements has been to develop a blueprint for multidisciplinary research (CR 2.5, 2.6, 2.7, 2.8, 2.10, 2.53).

2.15.26 Ryan, S. & Hassell, A. (2001) Interprofessional research in clinical practice. *Nurse Researcher: The International Journal of Research Methodology in Nursing and Health Care* 9 (2) 17–28   21 References

Argues that the need for interdisciplinary participation has been recognized and endorsed in clinical practice, but has yet to impact fully on nursing research. An example of inter-professional research, led by a clinical nurse specialist and a consultant rheumatologist, illustrates how collaboration enhanced the research design and specific aspects of the research process are discussed.

2.15.27 Seng, J.S. (1998) Praxis as a conceptual framework for participatory research in nursing. *Advances in Nursing Science* 20 (4) 37–48   36 References

Article derives from praxis a conceptual framework for participatory nursing research. A praxis model cannot only guide research, but can also provide congruent ways to assess the quality of the project and ensure researchers are accountable to the needs of the groups they study. A definition is given and the components that are specific to the tasks of participatory research are described (CR 2.7, 2.10).

2.15.28 Sitthi-amorn, C. & Somrongthong, R. (2000) Strengthening capacity in developing countries: a critical element for achieving health equity. *British Medical Journal* 321 (7264) 30 September 18 References

Highlights the inequities in health within and between countries and discusses how international collaboration can assist developing countries in participating in health research.

2.15.29 Solomon, N., Boud, D., Leontios, M. & Staron, M. (2000) Tale of two institutions: exploring collaboration in research partnerships. *Studies in the Education of Adults* 33 (2) 135–42   8 References

Paper explores a particular research partnership and examines the realities of such collaboration, what is involved and how they are made to work.

2.15.30 Tetley, J. & Hanson, E. (2000) Participatory research. *Nurse Researcher: The International Journal of Research Methodology in Nursing and Health Care* 8 (1) 69–88   53 References

Discusses the growth, nature of and approaches to participatory research. The paper illustrates some of the issues that can arise in a participatory research project, providing concrete examples, from a multi-centre gerontechnology project (CR 2.15).

2.15.31 Thompson, C.J., McNeill, J.A. & Sherwood, G.D. (2001) Using collaborative research to facilitate student learning. *Western Journal of Nursing Research* 23 (5) 504–16   11 References

Article outlines the methodological steps in recruiting and training undergraduate students for clinical research teams. Student evaluation of the research experience is presented (CR 3.16, 3.17).

2.15.32 Ward, L. & Simons, K. (1998) Practising partnership: involving people with learning difficulties in research. *British Journal of Learning Disabilities* 26 (4) 128–31   35 References

Gives practical examples of how people with learning difficulties can help set a research agenda, advise and assist with projects and undertake research themselves.

2.15.33 Watkins, C., Gibbon, B., Leathley, M., Cooper, H. & Barer, D. (2001) Performing interprofessional research: the example of a team care project. *Nurse Researcher: The International Journal of Research Methodology in Nursing and Health Care* 9 (2) 29–48 22 References

Article examines the impact of a research project that focused on the effectiveness of interdisciplinary team working in a variety of settings.

2.16 THE REALITIES OF DOING RESEARCH

The conventions within research require authors to present their work in a particular order and format. This may give the impression that research is more 'tidy' than it actually is, and the difficulties may not be mentioned. Literature in this section highlights some of the problems that may be encountered.

Annotations

2.16.1 Adamson, J. & Donovan, J.L. (2002) Research in black and white. *Qualitative Health Research* 12 (6) 816–25 41 References

Authors consider the methodological, interpretative and practical issues that arise when there is a difference in ethnicity between researcher and informant in qualitative research.

2.16.2 Asmundson, G.J.G., Norton, G.R. & Stein, M.B. (2002) *Clinical research: a practical guide*. Thousand Oaks, CA: Sage ISBN 0761922105 References

Written with minimal use of scientific jargon, this book provides thorough coverage of clinical research issues with real-life examples.

2.16.3 Barakat, S., Chard, M., Jacoby, T. & Lume, W. (2002) The composite approach: research design in the context of war and armed conflict. *Third World Quarterly* 23 (5) 991–1003 25 References

Presents the particular challenges that arise when researching situations of armed conflict and examines the methods that might be applicable. Introduces the idea of a composite approach that might be effective in overcoming difficulties.

2.16.4 Bass, M.J., Dunn, E.V. & Norton, P.G. (eds) (1993) *Conducting research in the practice setting*. London: Sage ISBN 0803951264 References

Discusses some of the practical considerations necessary when conducting primary care research.

2.16.5 Beale, B., Martin, K. & Jarvis, L.A. (1999) Locked up: researching in an unfamiliar environment. *International Journal of Nursing Practice* 5 (3) 137–42 9 References

Describes the personal experiences of researchers involved in a project with juvenile detainees in Australia. Debates the implications for working in secure and threatening environments.

2.16.6 Bell, C. & Encel, S. (eds) (1978) *Inside the whale: ten personal accounts of social research*. Rushcutters Bay, New South Wales: Pergamon ISBN 0080222447 References

This collection of papers allows a view into a normally closed world. They discuss many of the activities and factors that take place behind and around the methodology of research. The political and social issues which lie behind much research are highlighted and a wide range of styles are included to illustrate the problems, issues and constraints.

2.16.7 Buckeldee, J. & McMahon, R. (eds) (1994) *The research experience in nursing*. London: Chapman & Hall ISBN 0412441101 References

Book explores many of the realities of doing research through the experience of ten researchers. Examples of dilemmas, compromises, failure and solutions are all discussed which bring the joys and sorrows of doing research alive (CR 2.20, 2.22, 2.23, 2.26, 2.29, 2.37, 2.54, 2.68, 2.86, 2.98, 2.102, 3.8).

2.16.8 Craig, G., Corden, A. & Thornton, P. (2000) Safety in social research. *Social Research Update* Issue 29. Guildford: University of Surrey, Department of Sociology 8 References www.soc.surrey.ac.uk/sru/SRU29.html (Accessed 15/11/03)

Discusses the elements of risk associated with undertaking research, who should be concerned with safety, race, culture and gender, and who pays for safety. Suggestions for a code of practice and its development are made.

2.16.9 Dadds, M. & Hart, S. (2001) *Doing practitioner research differently*. London: Routledge/Falmer ISBN 0415237580 References

Authors aim to show that research should not just be a technical activity, but a living process that contributes to the quality of life experience for researchers and those who read their accounts. This book is an account of a project that presents the professional learning stories of seven educators, together with the authors' learning as supporters of higher degrees (CR 2.78).

2.16.10 Dolan, B. (2000) *The nurse practitioner: real world research in the A & E*. London: Whurr Publishers ISBN 1861561415 References

Examines the practicalities of undertaking research in the Accident and Emergency Department. The three initial stages are described: the literature review, methodology and pilot studies. The conclusions concentrate on methodological issues rather than the findings (CR 2.12, 2.14, 2.23).

2.16.11 Elsbach, K.D. (2000) Six stories of researcher experience in organizational studies. In Moch, S.D. & Gates, M.F. (eds) *The researcher experience in qualitative research*. Thousand Oaks, CA: Sage ISBN 0761913424 Chapter 6 54–74 23 References

Chapter discusses qualitative research in organizations and the literature on qualitative researchers' experiences. It is illustrated by using stories, together with the changes reported in attitude and ability by the researchers themselves (CR 2.16.29, 2.36, 3.16).

2.16.12 Evans, M.E., Mejía-Maya, L.J., Zayas, L.H., Boothroyd, R.A. & Rodriguez, O. (2001) Conducting research in culturally diverse inner-city neighbourhoods: some lessons learned. *Journal of Transcultural Nursing* 12 (9) 6–14 32 References

Article discusses several problems that confronted a research team trying to secure the participation of inner-city children discharged from home-based, family-oriented mental health crisis intervention programmes. It is hoped that other investigators may be able to anticipate problems, avoid mistakes and reduce logistical difficulties when undertaking similar fieldwork (CR 2.22, 2.53).

2.16.13 Frost, P. & Stablein, R. (eds) (1992) *Doing exemplary research*. Newbury Park, CA: Sage ISBN 0803939094 References

Book takes readers on seven 'journeys' using excerpts from selected articles. It focuses on research processes rather than content in order to understand phenomena relevant to organizational life. Contributions feature recollections by researchers on the origins, experiences and outcomes of research. The accounts and commentaries aim to demystify the research process and provide inspiration for future research (CR 2.43).

2.16.14 Fuller, M.L. (1999) Becoming a researcher: it's the trip not the destination and studying the mono-cultural pre-service teacher. In Grant, C.A. (ed.) *Multi-cultural research: a reflective engagement with race, class, gender and sexual orientation*. London: Falmer ISBN 0750708808 Chapter 18 240–63 33 References

The two perspectives covered in this chapter are the nature and effect of her research, and the influences of research on the researcher (CR 2.53.5).

2.16.15 Griffiths, M. (1998) *Educational research for social justice: getting off the fence*. Buckingham: Open University Press ISBN 0335198597 References

Book addresses some of the questions researchers have to face. Will a prior political or ethical commitment bias the research? How far can the ideas of empowerment or 'giving voice' be realized? How can researchers who research communities to which they belong deal with the ethical issues of being an insider and an outsider? It provides a set of principles that are rooted in considerations of methodology, epistemology and power relations, and give a framework for dealing with the practical issues (CR 2.6, 2.14, 2.15, 2.17, 2.27, 2.36, 2.98).

2.16.16 Hanrahan, M. (1998) Academic growth through action research: a doctoral student's narrative. In Atweh, B., Kemmis, S. & Weeks, P. (eds) *Action research in practice: partnerships for social justice in education*. London: Routledge ISBN 0415171520 Chapter 15 302–25 28 References

Describes the personal journey of learning and exploration of one PhD student. Chapter takes the form of a narrative and highlights the highs and lows of her academic growth (CR 2.37.2, 3.17).

2.16.17 Hardey, M. & Mulhall, A. (eds) (1994) *Nursing research: theory and practice*. London: Chapman & Hall ISBN 0412498502 References

Book gathers together material reflecting the diversity and richness of research in nursing. Opportunities and constraints of different approaches are discussed and illustrated by authors' own experiences (CR 2.1, 2.12, 2.29, 2.36, 2.52, 2.91, 2.98, 2.102).

2.16.18 Hayes, P. (2001) The research time line. *Clinical Nursing Research* 10 (4) 343–6 Editorial

Discusses reasons for the length of time taken to undertake research and the problems this may bring to policy-makers and bureaucrats. Also the time-consuming nature of research dissemination that is part of the scholarly development of knowledge is often not understood (CR 2.98, 3.11).

2.16.19 Hockey, L. (1985) *Nursing research: mistakes and misconceptions*. Edinburgh: Churchill Livingstone ISBN 0443028621 References

Discusses in a light-hearted way some of the pitfalls encountered by nurse researchers and how they might be avoided.

2.16.20 Hunt, J.C. (1989) *Psychoanalytic aspects of fieldwork*. Newbury Park, CA: Sage ISBN 0803934734 References

Author discusses her own experiences when interviewing colleagues and reports on the unconscious strivings, aversions and emotional conflicts that arise. The roles that these factors play when selecting, studying and constructing hypotheses about target populations are examined (CR 2.20, 2.22, 2.68).

2.16.21   James, T. & Whittaker, D. (1998) Researching hidden worlds: dilemmas for nurse researchers. In Smith, P. (ed.) *Nursing research: setting new agendas*. London: Arnold   ISBN 0340661941   Chapter 7 139–59   14 References

Chapter focuses on the content and method for researching sensitive topics. Using examples from their own research, issues raised are ethics, its emotional impact on participants, the interface with practice, research as a collective process, confidentiality and ownership of findings (CR 2.14, 2.17, 3.7.7).

2.16.22   Johnson, B. & Clark, J.M. (2003) Collecting sensitive data: the impact on researchers. *Qualitative Health Research* 13 (3) March 421–34 46 References

Authors identified issues that arose when conducting fieldwork. Ten researchers were interviewed and the difficulties reported were: lack of training, confidentiality, role conflict, costs to participants, the desire for reciprocity and feelings of isolation (CR 2.68, 3.16).

2.16.23   Kanuha, V.K. (2000) 'Being native' versus 'going native': conducting social work research as an insider. *Social Work* 45 (5) October 439–47   59   References

Article reports the work of a native social work researcher who conducted an ethnographic study with her social identity group. The complex and inherent challenges of being an insider with intimate knowledge of one's study population and an outsider as researcher are explored. Implications for social work research and practice with regard to native social work perspectives and methods are also discussed (CR 2.42).

2.16.24   Kayser-Jones, J. (2003) Continuing to conduct research in nursing homes despite controversial findings: reflections by a nurse scientist. *Qualitative Health Research* 13 (1) 114–28   7 References

Illustrates the potential controversial nature of research findings by providing data from an ongoing study on care of the terminally ill in nursing homes. This keynote address responded to the question 'how can you go into nursing homes, find out all you do, publish the findings and

continue to gain access afterwards?' The author believes that controversial findings should be presented to advocates and policy-makers who are in a position to bring about changes in the quality of care.

2.16.25   Langford, D.R. (2000) Pearls, pith and provocation. Developing a safety protocol in qualitative research involving battered women. *Qualitative Health Research* 10 (1) 133–42   20 References

Presents a safety protocol developed for a study of battered women's perceptions of danger in their relationships. Issues relating to safety, contacting participants, conducting the interviews, and protecting data are discussed.

2.16.26   Lee, R.M. (1995) *Dangerous fieldwork*. London: Sage   ISBN 0803956614   References

Book explores the contexts, settings and situations that pose high physical risks to the fieldworker and presents strategies for maintaining personal safety (CR 2.36).

2.16.27   Lee-Treweek, G. & Linkogle, S. (eds) (2000) *Danger in the field: risk and ethics in social research*. London: Routledge   ISBN 0415193222 References

Book analyses the experience of different forms of danger in various qualitative research settings. Researchers' own reflexive accounts of 'danger' are discussed, which include physical, emotional, ethical and professional difficulties. These give thought-provoking insights into the importance of well-chosen research designs (CR 2.36).

2.16.28   Mellor, N. (2001) Messy method: the unfolding story. *Educational Action Research* 9 (3) 465–84   65 References

Article outlines an attempt to develop a method of inquiry that takes a fresh look at the untidy realities of research. During a practitioner-based PhD, the author was mainly working without rules. New understandings of concepts such as analysis, data theory and writing began to evolve as a positive view of the 'mess' was gradually embraced. Over the six years of study the author made many errors, but wanted to be honest about them and eventually began to see an 'honesty trail', together with clear communication, as essential parts of the project's 'strength' (a term offered in place of validity).

2.16.29   Moch, S.D. & Gates, M.F. (eds) (2000) *The researcher experience in qualitative research*. Thousand Oaks, CA: Sage   ISBN 0761913424 References

Aims of this book are to describe various researcher experiences, give novices some insight in choosing research settings, dealing with personal issues and reporting research accurately (CR 2.36).

2.16.30 Morse, J.M. (2000) Researching illness and injury: methodological considerations … keynote address presented at the 5th Qualitative Health Research Conference, the University of Newcastle, Australia, 8 April 1999. *Qualitative Health Research* 10 (4) 538–46   14 References

Discusses the methodological problems that may arise when obtaining data from sick people. These include the lack of everyday language to describe their experiences, the instability of the participants' reality, and the instability of self. Decisions about the timing of data collection, challenges to validity and reliability and debates about who should be conducting the research are all discussed (CR 2.24, 2.25, 2.64).

2.16.31 Orna, E. & Stevens, G. (1995) *Managing information for research.* Buckingham: Open University Press   ISBN 0335193978   References

Text provides practical information for first-time researchers, that is often omitted from conventional books on research methods. Examples from real projects are used and students are encouraged to question their work, make their own decisions and move forward at each stage in the project.

2.16.32 Patton, C. (2000) Helping ourselves: research after (the) enlightenment. *Health* 4 (3) 267–87   13 References

Discusses some of the difficulties encountered while working as a field ethnographer in a large prospective study on the implementation of HIV counselling and testing at methadone clinics in the northeastern USA (CR 2.42).

2.16.33 Punch, M. (1986) *The politics and ethics of fieldwork.* Newbury Park, CA: Sage   ISBN 0803925174   References

Discusses many points relating to the practical, political and ethical aspects of fieldwork, which are not often found or explored in conventional research texts (CR 2.11, 2.17, 3.11).

2.16.34 Reed, J. & Procter, S. (eds) (1995) *Practitioner research in health care: the inside story.* London: Chapman & Hall Publishing   ISBN 0412498103   References

Explores important elements of research processes which face health care practitioners when conducting research into their own practice as a serious gap in methodological literature has been identified. Basic issues are explored, including the nature of practitioner knowledge, how this may be used and the contribution of quantitative and qualitative approaches. Several studies are reported which illustrate some difficulties encountered. Evaluating and developing practitioner research forms the final chapter (CR 2.6, 2.9, 2.25, 2.27, 2.29, 2.36, 2.42, 2.72, 2.86, 2.87, 2.98).

2.16.35 Romm, N.R.A. (2001) *Accountability in social research: issues and debates.* Dordrecht: KluwerAcademic/Plenum   Publishers   ISBN 0306465647   References   [Also available as eBook (2002) ISBN 030647199X]

Book considers issues relating to accountability in social research by juxtaposing seven ways of approaching the issues and moving towards the development of trust. The focus of the book is on reviewing discourses around the practice of 'professional' inquiry, with a view to highlighting differing arguments around the question of what it might mean to assess researchers' accountabilities.

2.16.36 Rosnow, R.L. & Rosenthal, R. (1997) *People studying people: artefacts and ethics in behavioral research.* New York: W.H. Freeman & Co.   ISBN 0761730715   References

Book discusses how unintended or uncontrolled factors, known as artefacts, can confound the outcome of behavioural research. Examples are given from actual experiments that show how things can go wrong when real people are involved. Ways of overcoming these difficulties are discussed (CR 2.17).

2.16.37 Roth, J. (1970) Hired hand research. In Denzin, N.K. (ed.) *Sociological methods: a sourcebook.* London: Butterworths   ISBN 0408701250   Part XIII Chapter 35 540–57   References

Section discusses some of the disadvantages and problems relating to the use of additional researchers in a project. Using three case studies of his own, the author shows how observers may cheat in their record keeping, coders can be inconsistent in analysing questionnaire responses, and interviewers may fill in or fabricate answers for respondents (CR 2.17, 2.68, 2.75, 3.16).

2.16.38 Shakespeare, P., Atkinson, D. & French, S. (eds) (1993) *Reflecting on research practice: issues in health and social welfare.* Buckingham: Open University Press   ISBN 0335190383   References

Book covers some of the 'hidden from view' aspects of social research and explores many of the complex processes involved. Specially written accounts by ten researchers tell real stories about undertaking research.

2.16.39 Silverman, D. (1987) *Communication and medical practice: social relations in the clinic.* London: Sage   ISBN 0803981090   References

An account of several research studies which examined doctor–patient interactions in hospital clinics. Author believes that many research reports are too 'polished' and do not necessarily reflect reality, so the book includes detailed accounts of his feelings as a researcher, and how apparently disparate work can be woven into a whole. Key themes are how doctor–patient talk varies according to the trajectory of the patient's medical career, the method of payment for treatment, the problems implicit in paediatric medicine with children and parents as actors, and the intrinsic difficulties in reforming medical practice and making it more patient-centred. Attention is given to three types of assumptions: paradigmatic, prescriptive and causal. The specific strategies discussed are examining the gap between conclusions and reasons, analysing the ideas that support reasons, identifying with the researcher's point of view, identifying with opposing viewpoints, learning more about relevant issues, and considering barriers in current thinking.

2.16.40   Strean, W.B. (1998) Identifying what we take for granted in our research: suggestions for assumption hunters. *Adapted Physical Activity Quarterly* 15 (3) 278–84   10 References

In order to assess the validity of assumptions, they must first be identified, and this paper describes how researchers can set about locating what they take for granted in their work (CR 2.25).

2.16.41   Tarling, M. & Crofts, L. (2002) *The essential researcher's handbook for nurses and health care professionals* (2nd edition). London: Ballière Tindall   ISBN 0702026360   References

Book addresses the practical problems encountered in doing research. Authored by experienced nurse researchers, the text draws and reflects upon the day-to-day experiences of doing research, allowing the reader to learn from mistakes and avoid the common pitfalls. Practical issues addressed are: access to data, IT problems, ethics committees, literature searching and publication. A checklist of dos and don'ts are also included. New to this edition is the latest information on searching the World Wide Web and on the R&D strategy in the NHS. A chapter on a career in research is also included (CR 2.12, 2.14, 2.17, 2.99, 3.16).

2.16.42   Walford, G. (2001) *Doing qualitative educational research: a personal guide to the research process*. London: Continuum   ISBN 0826447023   References

Describes the processes of doing research from 'behind the scenes'. Some of the problems and dilemmas encountered are discussed (CR 2.36).

2.16.43   Whyte, W.F. (1997) *Creative problem solving in the field: reflections on a career*. Thousand

Oaks, CA: AltaMira Press   ISBN 0761989218   References

Book guides researchers through the practical problems and conceptual complexities associated with fieldwork, and suggests how they were overcome (CR 2.36).

2.17   ETHICS, THE LAW AND RESEARCH

'Health care research is central to the quest for an increased understanding, improved knowledge and generalized explanation of the complexities of all health related issues ... research and ethical considerations are inextricably linked. The researcher must consider the implications of the proposed research, primarily for the participating subjects, but also the resulting status of knowledge and its relevance to society as a whole.' (Apps & Yeomans, 1995: 55)

Definitions [See Appendix D for sources]

Anonymity – assurance that subjects' identities will not be disclosed in any way

Autonomy – a condition of moral or personal independence

Beneficence – the principle that we should do good to others rather than harm, means responsible care or having a duty of care

Confidentiality – a subject's right to privacy ... anonymity and non-disclosure of information

Covert research – carrying out research without the knowledge or consent of those being studied or by misrepresenting the role of the researcher

Deception – involves the intentional misleading of prospective subjects or withholding information from them, so that subjects believe that the procedures or objectives of the research are different from what they actually are. Deception may include deliberate presentation of false information, suppression of material information, or selection of revealed truths in a way designed to mislead

Equipoise – a lack of consensus among the expert community on the relative efficacy of ... treatment

Ethics – moral principles which, in the context of research, pertain to treating subjects fairly and responsibly throughout the research process

Informed consent – ... the extent to which prospective participants are aware of the exact nature of the research and their right to agree or decline to participate without fear of loss or reprisal

Institutional Review Boards – a group of individuals who convene to review proposed and ongoing studies with respect to ethical considerations

Interference – an investigator or reviewer shall not intentionally and without authorization take or sequester or materially damage any research-related property of another, including without limitation the apparatus, reagents, biological materials, writings, data, hardware, software, or any other substance or device used or produced in the conduct of research

Justice – the moral principle by which actions are determined as just or unjust

Maleficence – evil doing

Misappropriation – an investigator or reviewer shall not intentionally or recklessly: (a) plagiarize, which shall mean the presentation of the documented words or ideas of another as his or her own, without attribution appropriate for the medium or presentation: or (b) make use of any information in breach of any duty of confidentiality associated with the review of any manuscript or grant application

Misrepresentation – an investigator or reviewer shall not with intent to deceive, or in reckless regard for the truth, (a) state or present a material or significant falsehood; or (b) omit a fact so that what is stated or presented as a whole states or presents a material or significant falsehood

Research misconduct – ... significant misbehaviour that improperly appropriates the intellectual property or contributions of others, that intentionally impedes the progress of research, or that risks corrupting the scientific record, or compromising the integrity of scientific practices. Such behaviours are unethical and unacceptable in proposing, conducting or reporting research, or in reviewing the proposals or research reports of others.

Annotations

2.17.1 Alderson, P. & Goodey, C. (1998) Theories of consent. *British Medical Journal* 317 (7168) 7 November 1313–15 18 References

Article reviews the advantages and limitations of theories about real consent, constructed consent, functionalist and critical consent, and post-modern choice. The authors demonstrate how an analysis of theories can clarify practical knowledge about the advantages and problems in obtaining consent, which will help everyday practice and research.

2.17.2 Amdur, R.J. & Bankert, E.A. (2002) *Institutional Review Board: management and function*. Sudbury, MA: Jones & Bartlett ISBN 0763716863 References

Book is designed as an instructional manual that gives Institutional Review Board (IRB) members and administrators the information they need to run an efficient and effective system of protecting human subjects in compliance with federal research regulations.

2.17.3 Amdur, R.J. (2003) *Institutional Review Board member handbook*. Sudbury, MA: Jones & Bartlett ISBN 076372257X References

Handbook is designed to give IRB members the information they need to protect the rights and welfare of research subjects in a way that is both effective and efficient. Much of the book is devoted to topic-specific chapters that list the criteria they should use to determine how to vote on specific kinds of study.

2.17.4 American Medical Association (2000) *Code of medical ethics: current opinions and annotations 2000–2001*. Chicago, IL: AMA Press ISBN 1579470777

Provides physicians and patients with critical guidance on current issues in medical ethics.

2.17.5 Anonymous (2001) Death of a volunteer at Johns Hopkins. *Bulletin of Medical Ethics* 171 September 3–7 News

Reports the death of a 24-year-old technician who had volunteered for a non-therapeutic study of underlying mechanisms in asthma. The subsequent investigation is outlined and its findings discussed. This article gives a rare insight into the work of an ethics committee, and lessons for such groups in the UK and elsewhere are highlighted.

2.17.6 Arndt, H.M. (1998) Ethical issues in knowledge development – objects and objectives. In: *Knowledge development: clinicians and researchers in partnership*. Helsinki: The Finnish Federation of Nurses ISSN 0251–4753 Proceedings of the Workgroup of European Nurse Researchers (9th Biennial Conference 5–8 July 1998 Helsinki Finland) Volume 1 1–12 16 References

Paper focuses on the general problem of research-based practice and the specific problem of a principle-guided ethics in its application to qualitative research (CR 2.6, 2.9, 2.36, 3.8).

2.17.7 Ashcroft, R. & Pfeffer, N. (2001) Ethics behind closed doors: do research ethics committees need secrecy? *British Medical Journal* 322 (7297) 26 May 1294–6 34 References

Contends that there is poor justification for the secrecy that surrounds ethics committees apart from significant areas such as medical, commercial and academic confidentiality, the privacy of researchers and the maintenance of independence within committees. Discusses the need for more transparency in ethical decision-making.

2.17.8   Ashcroft, T. (2002) An ethical perspective – nursing research. In Tingle, J. & Cribb, A. (eds) *Nursing law and ethics* (2nd edition). Oxford: Blackwell Science   ISBN 0632055073   Sections 12.8–12.15 278–86

Covers sources of nursing ethics, ethics and research design, the competence of research staff and research governance, recruitment and consent, research and care.

2.17.9   Benatar, D. & Benatar, S.R. (1998) Informed consent and research. *British Medical Journal* 316 (7136) 28 March 1008–10   2 References

Authors discuss a particular South African HIV study and the questions surrounding consent from the subjects involved.

2.17.10   Benatar, S.R. & Singer, S. (2000) A look at the new international research ethics. *British Medical Journal* 321 (7264) 30 September 824–6 29 References

Examines the failure to address standards of care in clinical trials which may differ from country to country and requests that researchers examine the context in which their research takes place. Contends that the greatest ethical challenge is the inequity in global health (CR 2.9, 3.22).

2.17.11   Berwick, D., Davidoff, F., Hiatt, H. & Smith, R. (2001) Refining and implementing the Tavistock Principles for everybody in health care. *British Medical Journal* 323 (7313) 15 September 616–20   5 References

Describes the origins of the Tavistock Principles as an ethical compass for those involved in health care, including patients and owners of health systems. Discusses each principle and illustrates these with case studies.

2.17.12   Bindless, L. (2000) Identifying ethical issues in nursing research. *Journal of Community Nursing* 14 (4) 26, 28, 30   17 References

Article shows that ethical issues can be identified by considering the extent to which respect is shown for the four prima facie principles – autonomy, beneficence, non-maleficence and justice. A good understanding of these and their implications for practice will help to expose the issues.

2.17.13   Boman, J. & Jevne, R. (2000) Ethical evaluation in qualitative research. *Qualitative Health Research* 10 (4) 547–54   13 References

Article explores the experience of being charged with an ethical violation for disclosing the identity of a study participant in a qualitative research project. A narrative account gives the researcher's point of view and looks at different ways in which the situation might be judged. It raises questions about what constitutes ethical conduct in qualitative research and how these decisions are made. Authors believe that such difficulties and problems should be shared so that all can learn (CR 2.16, 2.36).

2.17.14   Broome, M.E. (1999) Consent (assent) for research with pediatric patients. *Seminars in Oncology Nursing* 15 (2) 96–103   23 References

The participation of children in research is complex. Developmental limitations, the imbalance of power between children and adults, and, in some cases, their compromised health status can influence their willingness to participate in clinical research. Those wishing to encourage children to participate in research must be aware of their need to have full disclosure and clear descriptions about research in an age-related language (CR 2.22).

2.17.15   Brownlow, C. & O'Dell, L. (2002) Ethical issues for qualitative research in on-line communities. *Disability and Society* 17 (6)   24 References

Reflecting upon online discussion forums with people with autism, protection of participants is discussed, including informed consent, privacy and power differentials (CR 2.85).

2.17.16   Brykczynska, G. (1998) Can nursing research be a caring process? In Smith, P. (ed.) *Nursing research: setting new agendas*. London: Arnold   ISBN 0340661941   Chapter 6 108–38 76 References

Chapter examines some of the more neglected aspects of nursing research: the inherent moral values manifest in the intention to undertake research, the clarity of motivation behind the research process and the resultant moral obligations on the profession if it wishes to engage in research. The moral significance of disseminating research findings and publication processes are also discussed (CR 2.98, 2.99, 3.7.7).

2.17.17   Canadian Institutes of Health Research *Ethics – useful links* www.cihr-rsc.gc.ca/about_ cihr/organization/ethics/useful_links_e.shtml (Accessed 24/01/03)

Website provides lists of useful links for ethical issues under the headings of: guidelines for health research; relevant agencies and organizations; academic bioethics and health law centres/institutes; and bioethics information resources on the World Wide Web.

2.17.18   Center for the Study of Ethics in the Professions – Illinois Institute of Technology *Codes of ethics online* www.iit.edu/departments/csep/PublicWWW/codes/health.html (Accessed 02/03/03)

Website includes over 850 codes of ethics of professional societies, corporations, government and academic institutions. Earlier versions of some organizations' codes are included so researchers may study their development. It also provides links to a growing list of health care sites that have developed codes of ethics.

2.17.19   Center for the Study of Ethics in the Professions – Illinois Institute of Technology *Introduction to CSEP* www.iit.edu/departments/csep (Accessed 02/03/03)

Introduces the Center for Study of Ethics, and makes reference to the codes of ethics online, publications, other links and resources for ethics on the World Wide Web, its library, a workshop, projects and events, a bibliography and information on those who helped develop this resource.

2.17.20   Central Office for Research Ethics Committees (COREC) *UPDATE – Changes affecting procedures for applications to NHS research ethics committees* (04/03/03) www.corec.org.uk/ (Accessed 02/06/03)

Provides information on interim arrangements being made to standardize applications to research ethics committees. Initially, applications made to multi-centre research committees only will need to use the new procedure. Further guidance will be issued later on this website.

2.17.21   Cerinus, M. (2001) The ethics of research. *Nurse Researcher: The International Journal of Research Methodology in Nursing and Health Care* 8 (3) 72–89   18 References

Paper makes a contribution to the attention, debate and discourse of the ethics of research by presenting some of the issues of ethical significance that emerged in the process of conducting a doctoral research study.

2.17.22   Coyne, I.T. (1998) Researching children: some methodological and ethical considerations. *Journal of Clinical Nursing* 7 (5) 409–16   31 References

Examines the ethical issues surrounding children as research participants, including informed consent.

Discusses the need to be flexible, build a rapport and strategies to enhance the quality of responses from children.

2.17.23   David, M., Edwards, R. & Alldred, P. (2001) Children and school-based research: 'informed consent' or 'educational consent'? *British Educational Research Journal* 27 (3) 347–65   26 References

Authors discuss informed consent in relation to children and young people in educational settings. They reflect on issues that arose while obtaining consent from the children rather than from their parents.

2.17.24   Davis, A.J. (1999) Global influence of American nursing: some ethical issues. *Nursing Ethics* 6 (2) 118–25   17 References

Raises the issues that American values embedded in nursing and ethics can be exported to other countries with differing cultures and values. An example is Japan, where these imported ideas can create ethical problems.

2.17.25   de Laine, M. (2000) *Fieldwork, participation and practice: ethics and dilemmas in qualitative research*. London: Sage   ISBN 0761954872 References

Book aims to promote an understanding of the harmful possibilities of fieldwork and suggests ways of dealing with real ethical problems and dilemmas (CR 2.36).

2.17.26   de Raeve, L. (ed.) (1996) *Nursing research: an ethical and legal appraisal*. London: Ballière Tindall   ISBN 0702018880   References

Using case studies, this book explores ethical issues by analysing and synthesizing material from various perspectives (CR 2.39).

2.17.27   Department of Health and Human Services, Office of Inspector General (1998) *Institutional review boards: a time for reform*. OEI–01–97–00193   53 Notes and References

Summarizes the challenges facing institutional review boards and makes recommendations for federal oversight.

2.17.28   Dolan, B. (1999) The impact of local research ethics committees on the development of nursing knowledge. *Journal of Advanced Nursing* 30 (5) 1009–10   7 References   Guest Editorial

Discusses problems in the UK arising from the historical, medical dominance of research ethics committees. The inculcation of positivist ideology has led some doctors to a narrowness of vision concerning other research approaches. Because of the nature of nursing, qualitative techniques have been used in many instances, although not exclusively. These projects, seen as 'soft', have often been rejected, and this has a direct impact on the development of nursing knowledge. Suggestions are made as to how the processes and attitudes of some committee members can change and develop for the benefit of patients (CR 2.6, 2.36).

2.17.29 Doyal, L. & Tobias, J. (eds) (2000) *Informed consent in medical research.* London: BMJ Books   ISBN 0727914863   References

Book contains a comprehensive discussion of the ethical issues involved in informing patients of their rights, and of participation in medical research by internationally recognized specialists.

2.17.30 Earl-Slater, A. (2002) Institutional review board. In Author *The handbook of clinical trials and other research.* Oxford: Radcliffe Medical Press   ISBN 1857754859   163–5 www.fda.gov/ (Accessed 13/11/03)

Outlines the structure and functions of Institutional Review Boards in the United States (CR 2.2.13)

2.17.31 Earl-Slater, A. (2002) Local/multi-centre research ethics committees. In Author *The handbook of clinical trials and other research.* Oxford: Radcliffe Medical Press   ISBN 1857754859   186–8/198–207 www.corec.org.uk (Accessed 13/11/03)

Outlines the purposes of both local and multi-centre ethics committees, together with their membership, activities and procedures (CR 2.2.13).

2.17.32 Earl-Slater, A. (2002) Medical Research Council guidelines for good practice in clinical trials. In Author *The handbook of clinical trials and other research.* Oxford: Radcliffe Medical Press ISBN 1857754859   191–4

Presents a set of guidelines from the UK's Medical Research Council (MRC) purporting good practice in clinical trials (CR 2.2.13).

2.17.33 Earl-Slater, A. (2002) Patient information sheet and consent forms. In Author *The handbook of clinical trials and other research.* Oxford: Radcliffe Medical Press   ISBN 1857754859 236–42

Gives guidance on consent, and includes a list of specific questions that participants in any research programme will need answers to (CR 2.2.13).

2.17.34 Edwards, S.J.L., Braunholtz, A.D., Lilford, R.J. & Stevens, A.J. (1999) Ethical issues in the design and conduct of cluster randomised controlled trials. *British Medical Journal* 318 (7195) 22 May 1407–9   35 References

Explains the need for cluster randomization when individual randomization is not possible and highlights the ethical difficulties that may arise (CR 2.29).

2.17.35 *Encyclopedia of applied ethics* (1997) Edited by Chadwick, R. New York: Academic Press   ISBN 0122270657   4 Volumes

International experts have contributed to this major resource which includes theories and concepts of ethics, and articles, glossaries and brief bibliographies relating to the following disciplines: medical, scientific, environmental, legal, education, politics, business and economics, media, social services and social ethics (CR 2.2).

2.17.36 Erlen, J.A., Sauder, R.J. & Mellors, M.P. (1999) Ethics. Incentives in research: ethical issues. *Orthopaedic Nursing* 18 (2) 84–7   6 References

Authors ask whether the use of monetary or other non-monetary incentives are ethical when recruiting subjects for research. Some relevant ethical questions are suggested. There is also discussion of implications for nurses, such as acquiring knowledge of research and ethics, creating an environment in which patient's questions and any issues can be discussed, being an advocate for the patient who is being asked to participate, and the nurse's responsibilities when asked to help with recruitment efforts (CR 2.22).

2.17.37 Erlen, J.A. (2000) Ethics. Clinical research: what do patients' understand? *Orthopaedic Nursing* 19 (2) 95–9   8 References

Author discusses clinical research, patients as vulnerable subjects, the therapeutic misconception and informed consent. A series of potential questions to consider and ask are listed, and recommendations are provided to help assure the rights of patients are protected (CR 2.22).

2.17.38 Erlen, J.A. (2000) Ethics. 'Conflicts of interest': an ethical dilemma for the nurse researcher. *Orthopaedic Nursing* 19 (4) 74–7 References

Article discusses instances where there may be conflicts of interest, for example, if a corporation is interested in particular projects because the investigator's interest fits with the company's product. Recommendations are made to help nurses avoid and address this potential ethical problem (CR 2.16, 3.13).

2.17.39 Foster, C. (2001) *The ethics of medical research on humans.* Cambridge: Cambridge University Press   ISBN 0521645735   References

Book examines three main approaches to moral decision-making: goal-based, duty-based and rights-based. The underlying philosophical arguments of each, and their relative strengths and weaknesses are identified, and suggestions are made as to how they may be applied. Case studies are also included (CR 2.5).

2.17.40   Fox, M. (2002) Clinical research and patients: the legal perspective. In Tingle, J. & Cribb, A. (eds) *Nursing law and ethics* (2nd edition). Oxford: Blackwell Science ISBN 0632055073 Sections 12.1–12.7 252–77   113 References

Chapter defines clinical research and covers its regulation. An ethical review is given and how to care for vulnerable groups. A case study is included.

2.17.41   Fry, S. & Johnstone, M.J. (2002) *Ethics in nursing practice: a guide to ethical decision making* (2nd edition). Oxford: Blackwell Publishing/ International Council of Nurses   ISBN 0632059354 References

Comprehensive in scope and addressing a broad range of ethical issues, this book guides readers towards ethical decision-making. Offering an expanded view of ethics, it now includes Islamic and Hindu perspectives. Real-life dilemmas in health care today are presented, including HIV/AIDS, abortion, caring for the terminally ill and victims of violence.

2.17.42   Gallagher, S.M. (1999) Barriers to informed consent in clinical trials. *Ostomy Wound Management* 45 (11) November 14–16   References

Informed consent is a key element in clinical research but one concern is the confusion between therapeutic intervention and experimental treatment. This paper includes a case study to illustrate the misunderstandings that might arise from the patient who is compelled to consent to clinical trials because of his/her sense of hopelessness from a chronic health condition and the traditional medical intervention he/she is receiving (CR 2.29).

2.17.43   Greenwood, J., Holmes, C. & Bidewell, J. (2001) Developing best practice guidelines for institutional ethics committees (IECs) in Greater Sydney: mission impossible? *Collegian: Journal of the Royal College of Nursing, Australia* 8 (1) 8–13   28 References

Authors submitted to the local Health Research Ethics Committee (HREC) a research proposal to investigate Institutional Ethics Committee policies and practices in Greater Sydney, Australia. It had previously received approval from the Scientific Advisory Committee, which is a sub-committee of the HREC and the IEC of the University of Western Sydney. The local HREC refused to approve the proposal. The study's background is described, together with its aims, expected outcomes and design. The scientific and ethical review process to which the proposal had been subjected is also described. Authors speculate on the reasons why the proposal had been impeded. These illustrate with pressing irony precisely those issues the research sought to explore and address (CR 2.96).

2.17.44   Grinyer, A. (2002) The anonymity of research participants: assumptions, ethics and practicalities. *Social Research Update* 36 Guildford: Department of Sociology, University of Surrey   11 References   www.soc.surrey.ac.uk/sru/SRU36.html

Author suggests that anonymity is assumed to be an integral feature of ethical research, and this is a requirement of the Data Protection Act. Most researchers go to considerable lengths to protect respondents' identities, but sometimes participants may feel they have lost ownership of the data when it is anonymized. The allocation of pseudonyms to protect identity can cause unanticipated distress and the practicalities of mixing real names and pseudonyms in publication can be complex. These problems arose in a study with parents of young adults with cancer and are not usually mentioned in orthodox guidelines or texts on the practice of research.

2.17.45   Haggman-Laitila, A. (1999) The authenticity and ethics of phenomenological research: how to overcome the researcher's own views. *Nursing Ethics: An International Journal for Health Care Professionals* 6 (1) 12–22   37 References

Author assumes that it is difficult to detach oneself from personal views in phenomenological research. The purpose of the article is to describe practical aspects and their theoretical grounds which are of crucial importance in overcoming these views in data gathering and analysis (CR 2.49).

2.17.46   Hendrick, J. (2000) *Research, law and ethics in nursing and health care.* Cheltenham: Nelson Thornes   ISBN 0748733213   Chapter 8 196–217   37 References

Chapter covers types of research, ethical principles, ethical codes and professional guidelines. Ethical committees are also discussed, together with the legal aspects and regulation of research. Case studies are included.

2.17.47   Hermann, D.H.J. (2000) Lessons taught by Miss Evers' boys: the inadequacy of benevolence and the need for legal protection of human subjects in medical research. *Journal of Law and Health* 15 (2) 147–64   8 References

Provides a detailed account of the Tuskegee syphilis study and discusses the subsequent legal repercussions and ethical implications.

2.17.48   Hudson, S. (1999) Ethics for alternative paradigms: an exploration of options. *Graduate Nursing Research* 1 (2) October–November (11pp)   34 References

Paper examines concepts of ethics in qualitative research. It begins with an exploration of traditional Western moral thought on which conventional bioethics is based. Author then argues that this model is unsuited to qualitative research, and proposes an alternative ethics for these paradigms (CR 2.36).

2.17.49   Im, E.-O. & Chee, W. (2002) Issues in protection of human subjects in Internet research. *Nursing Research* 51 (4) July/August 266–9   22 References

Issues in the protection of human subjects in Internet research are explored by analysing an international study. Based on a discussion of five issues (anonymity and confidentiality; security; self-determination and authenticity; full disclosure; and fair treatment) the development of standard guidelines, investigator triangulation and information sharing are proposed as safeguards for protecting human subjects. (CR 2.26, 2.85).

2.17.50   International Centre for Nursing Ethics *Index* www.freedomtocare.org/iane.htm (Accessed 21/05/03)

Gives links to ICNE basic information, news, *Nursing Ethics* journal, the students' gopher, spiritual care, and other health care and nursing websites.

2.17.51   Jacobson, A.F. & Winslow, E.H. (1998) Clinical nurse researchers' perceptions of hospital nursing research committees: results of a national survey. *Applied Nursing Research* 11 (3) 122–9 16 References

A growing body of literature portrays sharpening controversy over the appropriate roles and functions of hospital nursing research committees (HNCRs). This study examined the experiences of 139 nurse researchers. Responses differed, largely according to the nurses' level of academic attainment, with non-doctorally prepared researchers perceiving the assistance of some HNCRs as helpful, whereas doctorally prepared nurses tended to perceive them as obstacles (CR 3.11).

2.17.52   Jeffers, B.R. (2001) Human biological materials in research: ethical issues and the role of stewardship in minimizing research risks. *Advances in Nursing Science* 24 (2) 32–46   39 References

A new model of stewardship is described that can be used as a guide for protecting research participants who are involved in studies which include collecting and handling human biological samples.

Nursing implications to ensure protection of human research participants are discussed.

2.17.53   Jokinen, P., Lappalainen, M., Meriläinen, P. & Pelkonen, M. (2002) Ethical issues in ethnographic nursing research with children and elderly people. *Scandinavian Journal of Caring Sciences* 16 (2) 165–70   34 References

Based on the authors' experiences, the article debates the need for extra protection for children and elderly people as informants to qualitative research (CR 2.36, 2.42).

2.17.54   Kellett, M. & Nind, M. (2001) Ethics in quasi-experimental research on people with severe learning disabilities: dilemmas and compromises. *British Journal of Learning Disabilities* 29 (2) 51–5   24 References

Using their own study as an example, the authors debate the ethics of doing research on, rather than with, people with learning disabilities (CR 2.35).

2.17.55   King, N.M. & Henderson, G. (eds) (1999) *Beyond regulations: ethics in human subjects research.* Chapel Hill, NC: University of North Carolina Press   ISBN 0807847704   References

Book is a re-examination of research ethics across a broad range of disciplines. It combines case studies and commentaries to explore such issues as informed consent, conflict of interest, confidentiality and research on illegal behaviour.

2.17.56   Kite, K. (1999) Anonymizing the subject: what are the implications? *Nurse Researcher* 6 (3) 77–84

Cites a seminar paper that is a reflexive account of research undertaken to investigate the intensive care unit as a learning environment for registered nurses. Discusses some difficulties associated with anonymity and believes that it is not without implications for the researcher, the researched and the impact of the report (CR 2.16, 2.22).

2.17.57   Koivisto, K., Janhonen, S., Latvala, E. & Väisänen, L. (2001) Applying ethical guidelines in nursing research on people with mental illness. *Nursing Ethics: An International Journal for Health Care Professionals* 8 (4) 328–39   35 References

Identifies various guidelines published to protect vulnerable people, but notes the absence of guidelines regarding those people who have a mental impairment. Describes how the authors helped participants to understand their role in a research study and the ethical dilemmas that this raised.

2.17.58   Latvala, E., Janhonen, S. & Moring, J. (1998) Ethical dilemmas in a psychiatric nursing study. *Nursing Ethics: An International Journal for Health Care Professionals* 5 (1) 27–35 33 References

Article describes the ethical dilemmas encountered while conducting qualitative research with psychiatric patients as participants. These conflicts are explored in terms of the principles of personal autonomy, voluntariness and awareness of the purpose of the study, with illustrations from the authors' experience. The data were collected in a university hospital in northern Finland, using videotaped observations and recorded interviews. Although no definitive resolutions are proposed to the conflicts, the authors endeavour to enhance awareness of potential ethically-perplexing situations. Some solutions to problems encountered during this particular study are suggested (CR 2.36, 2.68, 2.72).

2.17.59 Lemmens, T. & Freedman, B. (2000) Ethics review for sale? Conflict of interest and commercial research review boards. *The Millbank Quarterly* 78 (4) 547–84 68 References

Traces the development and regulation of commercial research review boards and focuses on the potential financial conflicts of interest that might arise from such boards.

2.17.60 Lewis, A. & Lindsay, G. (eds) (1999) *Researching children's perspectives.* Buckingham: Open University Press ISBN 0335202799 References

Book addresses issues and practicalities surrounding the obtaining of children's views, particularly in the research context. Section 1 of the book examines ethical issues and codes of conduct, children's rights, the legal perspective, developmental dimensions and sociological issues. Section 2 illustrates these aspects by focusing on methods and applications in obtaining children's views in specific projects (CR 2.22).

2.17.61 Little, M. (2000) Conflict of interests, vested interests and health research. *Journal of Evaluation in Clinical Practice* 6 (4) 413–20 23 References

Explains the difference between vested interest and conflict of interest arising from the activities of research advisory and ethical review committees.

2.17.62 Lock, S., Wells, F. & Farthing, M.J.G. (eds) (2001) *Fraud and misconduct in biomedical research* (3rd edition). London: BMJ Books ISBN 00727915088 References

Fraud and misconduct in biomedical research have become increasingly recognized and reported, placing these problems high on the agenda in research

ethics. This new edition gives a historical overview from 1974 to 1990, the role of research ethics committees, a pharmaceutical company's approach to the threat of research fraud, and the activities for prevention in the US, Norway, Finland, Denmark, France and Germany. The founding of the Committee on Publication Ethics (COPE) has also increased exposure of fraud (CR 2.99.11).

2.17.63 Marjut, N. & Sirpa, J. (1998) The choice of informants from an ethical viewpoint. In: *Knowledge development: clinicians and researchers in partnership.* Helsinki: The Finnish Federation of Nurses ISSN 0251–4753 Proceedings of the Workgroup of European Nurse Researchers (9th Biennial Conference 5–8 July 1998 Helsinki, Finland) Volume 3 1221–30 14 References

Outlines ethical viewpoints in research and discusses the responsibilities of the researcher, institution and the profession. The publication of sensitive subject matter is briefly mentioned (CR 2.22).

2.17.64 Mastroianni, A. & Kahn, J. (2001) Swinging on the pendulum: shifting views of justice in human subjects research. *Hastings Center Report* 31 (3) 21–8 23 References

Federal policies on human subjects research have performed a near about-face. In the 1970s, policies were motivated chiefly by a belief that subjects needed protection from the harms and risks of research. Now the driving concern is that patients, and the populations they represent, need access to the benefits of research.

2.17.65 Matthews, J. (2000) *Introduction to randomised controlled trials.* London: Arnold ISBN 0340761431

Text introduces students to the basics of trial design and relevant methods of analysis. Medical examples are used to ensure a real-world approach to the subject (CR 2.29).

2.17.66 McCabe, M.S. (1999) The ethical foundation of informed consent in clinical research. *Seminars in Oncology Nursing* 15 (2) 76–80 18 References

Provides a foundation for understanding the ethical concept of informed consent with particular emphasis on the characteristics that make it a moral imperative. Understanding the theory and practice of informed consent is every nurse's responsibility. This is to ensure that decision-making is properly informed because of the severity of malignant disease and complexity of research in which the patient may become involved.

2.17.67 Meade, C.D. (1999) Improving understanding of the informed consent process and document. *Seminars in Oncology Nursing* 15 (2) 124–37   135 References

Article reviews theoretical perspectives, relating to the communication of informed consent, and describes research efforts and strategies to enhance the informed consent process. Documenting information given during the informed consent process may be difficult to understand, raising ethical concerns about whether informed decision-making has taken place. Several communication strategies are suggested.

2.17.68   Mill, J.E. & Ogilvie, L.D. (2002) Ethical decision-making in international nursing research. *Qualitative Health Research* 12 (6) 807–15   37 References

Balances perspectives of ethical universalism against ethical relativism in respect of research undertaken in Ghana with HIV positive women (CR 3.22).

2.17.69   Moreno, J.D. (2001) Goodbye to all that: the end of moderate protectionism in human subjects research. *Hastings Center Report* 31 (3) 9–17 29 References

Federal policies on human subjects research have undergone a progressive transformation. Initially these policies relied on the discretion of investigators to decide when and how to conduct research, and then policies were introduced that augmented investigator discretion with externally imposed protections. Researchers may now be entering an era of even more stringent controls.

2.17.70   Nelson-Marten, P. & Rich, B.A. (1999) A historical perspective of informed consent in clinical practice and research. *Seminars in Oncology Nursing* 15 (2) 81–8   22 References

Consent as a fundamental principle of clinical ethics has developed within the last 50 years and authors review its history in relation to human subjects. As full disclosure and shared decision-making have not come naturally to clinicians, so respecting the autonomy of patients and research subjects requires a conscious, sustained effort. It is therefore important for cancer nurses to understand the significance of this and act as advocate for the patient and research subject at all times.

2.17.71   *New dictionary of medical ethics* (1997) Edited by Boyd, K.M., Higgs, R. & Pinching, A. London: BMJ Books   ISBN 0727910019

Book informs the increasingly complex area of ethical issues in health care.

2.17.72   NHMRC National Health and Medical Research Council *Advice from CEO on New Committee Structures for NHMRC* www.health. gov.au/nhmrc/aboutus/adviceceo.htm (Accessed 18/04/03)

Outlines the rationale for having one ethics research committee in the next triennium, its composition and functions. Members will need to address national research priorities and other matters associated with the whole government approach to research funding and outcomes (CR 2.43, 3.13).

2.17.73   Noble-Adams, R. (1999) Ethics and nursing research 2: examination of the research process. *British Journal of Nursing* 8 (14) 22 July 956–60   12 References

States that nurses need to understand their own ethical beliefs and standpoint before embarking on a research project. The key principles of ethics and its relationship to the research process must also be considered (CR 2.14).

2.17.74   O'Donohue, W. & Ferguson, K.E. (eds) (2003) *Handbook of professional ethics for psychologists: issues, questions, and controversies.* Thousand Oaks, CA: Sage   ISBN 0761911898   References

Book reviews the philosophical issues and unanswered questions raised by the Code of Ethics of the American Psychological Association. The key areas covered are moral reasoning and the ethics of professional licensing, confidentiality in psychotherapy, fees and financial arrangements, the termination and referral of clients, the use of deception in research, ethnic minority issues, consent to treatment and research involving children.

2.17.75   Oliver, P. (2003) *The student's guide to research ethics.* Buckingham: Open University Press   ISBN 0335210872   References

Book identifies ethical issues that arise throughout research, from the design stage through to data collection and analysis. It discusses consent, confidentiality, research dissemination and ethical theories. Examples of ethical dilemmas and case studies are given throughout the text (CR 2.14, 2.98).

2.17.76   Olsen, D.P. (2000) Equipoise: an appropriate standard for ethical review of nursing research? *Journal of Advanced Nursing* 31 (2) 267–73   22 References

When using control group methodologies, the provision of different forms of treatment, which may vary in efficacy, to similar groups of research subjects must be ethically justified. The conventional justification is the existence of a state of clinical equipoise. Control groups are justified when the profession does not know which treatment confers more benefit; otherwise, the provision of treatment known to be less effective than other available treatment is unethical. The concept of equipoise was developed to justify clinical trials of medical interventions, and has proved a durable standard in studies that confer benefit, regardless of the subject's perception. However, equipoise does not apply when a substantive benefit is conferred by the subject's perception. In psychosocial interventions, a subject's experience of the intervention confers benefit and is used to evaluate benefit. Therefore the subject is in a valid position to prefer one treatment to the other and equipoise does not apply (CR 2.29).

2.17.77 Olsen, D.P. & Mahrenholz, D. (2000) IRB-identified ethical issues in nursing research ... institutional review board. *Journal of Professional Nursing* 16 (3) May/June 140–8   18 References

Ethical issues in nursing research protocols, submitted to a School of Nursing Institutional Review Board, were identified by examining the letters sent to researchers whose protocols required revision or were not approved. Themes were extracted and categorized as follows: the informed consent document, barriers to informed consent, subject benefit, subject risk, confidentiality, and problems with specific populations. A total of 157 protocols were examined and the results are reported. They were found to be more vulnerable to ethical problems arising from the relationship between the researcher and subject than from physical harm. Nurses are advised to give extra care to issues of coercion, deception and attention to problems uncovered in the research process.

2.17.78 O'Neill, P. (1998) Communities, collectivities and the ethics of research. *Canadian Journal of Community Mental Health* 17 (2) 67–78   36 References

Discusses a new code of ethics that will give unprecedented power to 'collectivities'. Some see this as a long-overdue corrective to hit-and-run research, while others see it as a threat to unfettered inquiry. The paper argues a different point: involvement of collectivities is essential for ethical research relationships, but it ought not to limit the sort of questions studied or publication of answers found. The difference is illustrated by two examples in which aboriginal communities asserted their collective rights against researchers.

2.17.79 Orb, A., Eisenhauer, L. & Wynaden, D. (2000) Ethics in qualitative research. *Journal of Nursing Scholarship* 33 (1) 93–6   17 References

Paper examines the common ethical concerns that qualitative researchers confront and highlights the principles that can guide research and researchers (CR 2.36).

2.17.80 Padberg, R.M. & Flach, J. (1999) National efforts to improve the informed consent process. *Seminars in Oncology Nursing* 15 (2) 138–44   16 References

A federally-funded research programme, conducted by the National Cancer Institute, aimed to improve informed consent documents in cancer clinical trials, and a model consent document developed by the National Action Plan on breast cancer are presented. These will assist investigators and Institutional Review Boards when presenting relevant and understandable information to potential clinical trial participants (CR 2.29).

2.17.81 Peter, E. (2000) The politicization of ethical knowledge: feminist ethics as a basis for home care nursing research. *Canadian Journal of Nursing Research* 32 (2) 103–18   77 References

Author believes that because much health care is now being provided in patients' homes there are largely unexplored ethical concerns for nurses. The current state of ethical knowledge in nursing is not adequate to address these issues, and a new method to develop this knowledge is proposed. Phenomenological approaches and feminist ethics are examined and an alternative method is described which could be applied to home care ethics research (CR 2.10, 2.49).

2.17.82 Ramcharan, P. & Cutcliffe, J.R. (2001) Judging the ethics of qualitative research: considering the 'ethics as process' model. *Health and Social Care in the Community* 9 (6) 358–66   76 References

Discusses health/medical and social research ethical models and proposes a system for monitoring qualitative research (CR 2.36).

2.17.83 Randall, F. & Downie, R.S. (1999) *Palliative care ethics: a companion for all specialities* (2nd edition). Oxford: Oxford University Press ISBN 0192630687 Chapter 11 236–47 References

Chapter considers why research in palliative medicine gives rise to particular ethical problems. It discusses codes of ethics, randomized double-blind clinical trials, local research ethics committees and their role in giving consent (CR 2.29).

2.17.84 Redsell, S.A. & Cheater, F.M. (2001) The Data Protection Act (1998): implications for health researchers. *Journal of Advanced Nursing* 35 (4) 508–13   12 References

Amendments to the United Kingdom Data Protection Act (1998) are causing confusion within the health service and academic institutions. This paper reports on methods used to obtain access to subjects which comply with the common law duty of confidence laid down in the Act. There is a need to balance patient confidentiality with the requirement to conduct vital, unbiased research in which professionals are not subject to ethical dilemmas. Methodological problems are discussed and the authors urge that clarity should be sought to solve the issues raised (CR 2.16, 2.22, 2.27, 2.29).

2.17.85   Roberts, L.W., Warner, T.D. & Brody, J.L. (2000) Perspectives of patients with schizophrenia and psychiatrists regarding ethically important aspects of research participants. *American Journal of Psychiatry* 157 (1) January 67–74   31 References

Few data have been gathered to improve our understanding of how individuals with serious mental illness and psychiatrists view ethically important aspects of biomedical research participation. Structured interviews and written surveys were used to collect data. Both groups supported schizophrenia research and saw helping others and science as important reasons for protocol participation. Previously neglected attitudes of psychiatric patients and clinicians towards ethically important aspects of biomedical research participation were identified.

2.17.86   Rolph, S. (1998) Ethical dilemmas in historical research with people with learning difficulties. *British Journal of Learning Disabilities* 26 (4) 135–9   32 References

Discusses the ethical issues that may arise, in both oral and archival historical research, when involving people with learning difficulties. As there is now a growing interest in their own views, new issues have arisen which are highlighted and solutions suggested (CR 2.46, 2.47, 2.71).

2.17.87   Rosse, P.A. & Krebs, L.U. (1999) The nurse's role in the informed consent process. *Seminars in Oncology Nursing* 15 (2) 116–23   28 References

Authors review the informed consent process in relation to oncology nursing roles and responsibilities, patient comprehension, cultural sensitivity and qualitative methodologies. Nursing is involved in almost every aspect of the informed consent process so they must be knowledgeable about fundamental concepts and their responsibilities, and be willing to address the complexities of the process.

2.17.88   Ruiz-Canela, M., de Irala-Estevez, J., Martinez-González, M.A., Gómez-Gracia, E. & Fernández-Crehuet, J. (2001) Methodological quality and reporting of ethical requirements in clinical trials. *Journal of Medical Ethics* 27 172–6   27 References

Reports a study that assessed the relationship between the approval of trials by a research ethics committee and the fact that informed consent was obtained from participants, with the quality of study design and methods. Authors concluded that trials of higher methodological and scientific quality were more likely to provide information about their ethical aspects (CR 2.29).

2.17.89   Schüklenk, U. & Ashcroft, R. (2000) International research ethics. *Bioethics* 14 (2) 158–72   27 References

Provides a critical overview of international research ethics, focusing on the conduct of therapeutic trials in developing countries. It is argued that research participants in these countries are not subject to the same ethical regulations demanded in developed countries and discusses the difficulty in developing international ethical principles to protect human rights.

2.17.90   Schwartz, L., Preece, P. & Hendry, R. (2002) *Medical ethics*. Philadelphia, PA: W.B. Saunders   ISBN 0702025437   References

Book was developed specifically for medical students. Realistic case studies introduce the discussion in each chapter, together with coverage of informed consent and refusal of treatment, confidentiality, euthanasia, advanced directives, negligence and malpractice, the new genetics, abortion and the rationing of care.

2.17.91   Seedhouse, D. (1998) *Ethics: the heart of health care* (2nd edition). Chichester: Wiley   ISBN 0471975923   References

A classic ethics text that demonstrates how ethics and health care are inextricably bound together, and creates a firm theoretical basis for practical decision-making. The Ethical Grid, which teaches a practical skill, and two further decision-making tools – the Rings of Uncertainty and Autonomy Test – are all discussed.

2.17.92   Seymour, J.E. & Ingleton, C. (1999) Research issues. Ethical issues in qualitative research at the end of life. *International Journal of Palliative Nursing* 5 (2) 65–73   38 References

Discusses the specific ethical challenges, present at all stages of the research process, which arose during the conduct of two doctoral studies in a palliative care department. The authors propose a guide for the conduct of ethically-responsible research (CR 2.36).

2.17.93   Seymour, J.E. & Skilbeck, J. (2002) Ethical considerations in researching user views. *European Journal of Cancer Care* 11 (3) 215–19   24 References

Examines the process of accessing users' views when researching those receiving cancer and palliative care. Highlights the need to balance achieving the outcomes of the research and the duty to provide support and care.

2.17.94 Sharp, S.M. (2000) Issues in human subject research: reliability of informed consent documents in medical device trials. *Research Practitioner* 1 (6) 211–14 17 References

Reports a study that evaluated the readability of informed consent documents used in recent clinical trials of a variety of investigational medical devices. The results showed that a majority of adults in the United States would not be able to comprehend the information included in these forms (CR 2.29).

2.17.95 Silva, M.C. (1995) *Ethical guidelines in the conduct, dissemination and implementation of nursing research*. Washington, DC: American Nurses' Association ISBN 1558101098

Provides a useful framework for conducting ethical nursing research. Each of the current principles presented includes historical commentary and research guidelines.

2.17.96 Simons, H. & Usher, R. (eds) (2000) *Ethics in educational research*. London: Falmer ISBN 0415206677 References

Book aims to show how ethical decisions are made within particular fields and practices of educational research. Some examples include the concept of ethical integrity in health care practitioner research, an overview of feminist approaches to research ethics, ethical and political dilemmas, ethical space, educational issues in quantitative research and research on educational 'markets' (CR 2.10).

2.17.97 Skene, L. & Smallwood, R. (2002) Informed consent: lessons from Australia. *British Medical Journal* 324 (7328) 5 January 39–41 11 References

In the past decade both English and Australian courts have adopted a more patient-centred standard in deciding what risks doctors must disclose to patients. Professional bodies have issued guidelines, yet in Australia many doctors still do not understand their legal duties and are being held liable for their failure to inform. The authors suggest that an empirical study of doctors' understanding and practices might be useful in the UK.

2.17.98 Slowther, A., Bunch, C., Woolnough, B. & Hope, T. (2001) Clinical ethics support services in the UK: an investigation of current provision of ethics support to health professionals in the UK. *Journal of Medical Ethics* 27 (Supplement 1) i2–i8

Paper identifies and describes the current state of clinical ethics support services in the UK. Many clinical ethics committees have been in existence for a relatively short time and are still defining their role. Issues that need to be discussed from this questionnaire survey are highlighted so that support services can develop appropriately.

2.17.99 Stalker, K. (1998) Some ethical and methodological issues in research with people with learning difficulties. *Disability and Society* 13 (1) 5–19 49 References

Discusses ethical and methodological issues that arose in a study examining the choice exercised by people with learning difficulties, including gaining access and informed consent, avoiding the risk of intrusion and expectations of a continuing friendship. Also considers the process of research, including dissemination (CR 2.22, 2.36, 2.42, 2.78, 2.98).

2.17.100 Sugarman, J., McCrory, D.C., Powell, D., Krashny, A., Adams, B., Ball, E. & Cassell, J. (1999) Empirical research on informed consent: an annotated bibliography. *Hastings Center Report Special Supplement* 29 (1) S1–S42

377 abstracts are included, covering the topics of authorization, consent forms, decision-making capacity, disclosure, policies, recruitment, understanding and voluntariness.

2.17.101 Tadd, W. (ed.) (2002) *Ethics in nursing education, research and management: perspectives from Europe* (Volume 2). Basingstoke: Palgrave ISBN 0333749944 References 3 Volumes

This second volume in a series of three on European Nursing focuses on ethical considerations. Authors give a multinational overview of European traditions in moral philosophy to provide increased awareness of the differing perspectives to be found across Europe.

2.17.102 Taylor, H.A. (1999) Barriers to informed consent. *Seminars in Oncology Nursing* 15 (2) 89–95 35 References

Identifies barriers as patient-centred (such as age, education, illness) and process-centred (content and readability of the consent form, timing of the discussion, and amount of time allotted to the process) that can both affect an individual's ability to provide informed consent. Nurses must be aware of these in order to improve and facilitate the consent process.

2.17.103 Thiroux, J.P. (2001) Bioethics – ethical Issues in medicine. In Author *Ethics: theory and practice* (7th edition). Upper Saddle River, NJ: Prentice-Hall ISBN 0130314080 Chapter 13 362–93 References

Chapter discusses the rights and obligations of health care professionals, patients and their families when participating in research. The importance of truth-telling, confidentiality and informed consent, and some of the ethical issues involved in human experimentation, are considered.

2.17.104 Thomas, N. & O'Kane, C. (1998) The ethics of participatory research with children. *Children and Society* 12 (5) 336–48 38 References

Explores the ethical problems that arise from research involving children and describes a study where children were given the opportunity to choose topics, methods of data collection and interpretation of the data. Suggests that this participatory approach can also assist with validity and reliability (CR 2.11, 2.15, 2.24, 2.25).

2.17.105 Thombs, D.L., Mahoney, C.A. & Olds, R.S. (2001) Balancing risks and benefits of deception in assessing genetic screening utilization. *American Journal of Health Behavior* 25 (2) 100–5 17 References

Authors argue that research using intentional deception is sometimes appropriate. A deception paradigm, created to assess utilization of genetic screening for alcohol susceptibility, generated useful knowledge, and authors state that participants were exposed to no more than minimal risk.

2.17.106 Thompson, I.E., Melia, K.M. & Boyd, K.M. (2000) Conflicting demands in nursing groups of patients. In Authors *Nursing ethics* (4th edition). Edinburgh: Churchill Livingstone ISBN 0443061475 Chapter 7 172–6

Chapter includes a section on persuading patients to 'volunteer' as research subjects. The ethics of this and other issues, including consent, use of minors or other vulnerable individuals, are explored. The functions of research ethics committees and Institutional Review Boards in the United States are outlined. The book also includes appendices containing traditional codes of medical and nursing ethics, Patients' Rights and the Ottawa Charter for Health Promotion (CR 2.2, 2.22).

2.17.107 Tollman, S.M. (2001) Fair partnerships support ethical research. *British Medical Journal* 323 (7326) 15 December 1417–20 15 References

Discusses clause 29 of the Declaration of Helsinki, arguing that although it is intended to protect participants in developing countries with regard to the best alternative treatment, it may actually cause harm. Author calls for research strategies that are based upon mutually beneficial partnerships between and within countries.

2.17.108 Ulusoy, M.F. & Ucar, H. (2000) An ethical insight into nursing research in Turkey. *Nursing Ethics: An International Journal for Health Care Professionals* 7 (4) July 285–95 14 References

An increasing number of research studies are now being undertaken, causing a rise in ethical problems. This study examined problems which had occurred in 169 Master of Science and 66 doctoral theses written between 1972 and 1998 in the Department of Nursing, Institute of Health Sciences, Hacettepe University, Ankara, Turkey. The ethical rules used as criteria were: that no harm should be caused; the subject was informed about the research topic; their permission was obtained and the subject's privacy was maintained. Results are reported and the problems found are discussed (CR 2.97, 3.3).

2.17.109 US Department of Health and Human Services (1995) *Integrity and misconduct in research*. Report of the Commission on Research Integrity. Washington, DC: US Department of Health and Human Services

Report of a commission created by Congress in response to continuing controversy concerning the apparent inability of the scientific community and the federal government to deal adequately with misconduct in scientific research. The major problems are identified, discussed and recommendations are made to guide states, institutions and individuals.

2.17.110 University of Newcastle – Australia, Faculty of Health *Human Research Ethics* www.newcastle.edu.au/faculty/health/research/ethics.html (Accessed 01/05/03)

Provides information on the necessary processes prior to submitting a research proposal to the ethics committee, together with a list of suitable links.

2.17.111 Upvall, M. & Hashwani, S. (2001) Negotiating the informed-consent process in developing countries: a comparison of Swaziland and Pakistan. *International Nursing Review* 48 (3) 188–92 9 References

Article reports a study that compared and contrasted the process of obtaining informed consent in Swaziland and Pakistan. The data are based on qualitative collaborative research between nurses and healers. Results demonstrated the inadequacy and complexity of applying Western-based concepts to developing countries (CR 2.15, 2.36).

2.17.112 Verdú-Pascual, F. & Castelló-Ponce, A. (2001) Randomized clinical trials: a source of ethical dilemmas. *Journal of Medical Ethics* 27 177–8 8 References

Advances in medicine are closely linked to clinical research, but certain study procedures may be in conflict with the fundamental principles of ethics and codes of conduct in medicine. Following an analysis of two studies involving treatments for acute myocardial infarction, the admissibility of continuing a study was questioned after the initial results for two types of treatment showed that one was significantly better than the other. Also considered doubtful was the information provided to patients with the object of obtaining their informed consent (CR 2.29).

2.17.113 Wang, C.H. & Huch, M.H. (2000) Protecting human research subjects: an international perspective. *Nursing Science Quarterly* 13 (4) 293–8   20 References

Article explores ethical standards, their applications and the challenges in protecting human subjects in an international arena (CR 3.22).

2.17.114 Weijer, C. (1999) Selecting subjects for participation in clinical research: one sphere of justice. *Journal of Medical Ethics* 25 31–6   34 References

Recent guidelines from the US National Institutes of Health mandate the inclusion of adequate numbers of women in clinical trials. Author asks whether these standards should apply internationally. Walzer's theory of justice is introduced (its first use in research ethics), and it argues for broad application of the theory of adequate representation. A number of practical questions for research ethics committees are outlined (CR 2.22, 2.29).

2.17.115 Weijer, C. & Anderson, J.A. (2001) The ethics wars: disputes over international research. *Hastings Center Report* 31 (3) 18–20   12 References

The effort to revise the Declaration of Helsinki and the Council of International Organizations for Medical Sciences (CIOMS) Guidelines has sparked a sometimes vitriolic debate centring on the use of placebo controls (CR 2.29).

2.17.116 West, E. & Butler, J. (2003) An applied and qualitative LREC reflects on its practice. *Bulletin of Medical Ethics* 185 February 13–20   17 References

Describes how one NHS local research ethics committee critically reviewed its practice with a view to increasing awareness of its decision-making processes and the ethical frameworks on which they were based.

2.17.117 Whitaker, B., van der Arend, A. & Harman, G. (1998) Factors affecting the timing of ethical approval of research in humans: a survey of hospital and university ethics committees in Australia and the Netherlands. In: *Knowledge development: clinicians and researchers in partnership*. Helsinki: The Finnish Federation of Nursing ISSN 0251–4753 Proceedings of the Workgroup of European Nurse Researchers (9th Biennial Conference 5–8 July 1998 Helsinki, Finland) Volume 1 134–45   9 References

Reports a study that identified factors that cause delay in granting ethical approval of research in Australia and the Netherlands and the extent to which human research ethics committees are concerned with matters regarding methodology in quantitative and qualitative research. It also raised awareness in both novice and experienced researchers about the ethical implications of research in humans, and identified factors regarding ethical approval of nursing research as perceived by hospital and university ethics committee members in Australia and the Netherlands (CR 2.9).

2.18   DEFINING THE PROBLEM

'The term problem may be a misnomer…rather than calling it the "problem statement" it might be clearer if we call it "the need for study"… these needs may be based on personal experience with an issue, job-related problems, an adviser's research agenda, and/or the scholarly literature… the strongest and most scholarly rationale for a study… follows from a documented need in the literature for increased understanding and dialogue about an issue.' (Cresswell, 1998: 94)

Definition [See Appendix D for source]

Problem statement – the statement of the research problem that identifies the key research variables, specifies the nature of the population and suggests the possibility of empirical testing

Example

Moody, L., Vera, H., Blanks, C. & Visscher, M. (1989) Developing questions of substance for nursing science. *Western Journal of Nursing Research* 11 (4) 393–404   15 References

Describes a study undertaken to establish from leading nurse researchers the sources and origins of their ideas, devices for finding and developing researchable questions or hypotheses and how they decided which were significant for the discipline. Focused interviews were conducted by telephone and data was analysed by computer. Data showed that the significant questions are those aimed at nursing intervention and clinical research and that students need to be guided early to find those important to nursing (CR 2.20, 2.70, 2.84).

Annotations

2.18.1 Baldamus, W. (1979) Alienation, anomie and industrial accidents. In Wilson, M. (ed.) *Social and educational research in action: a book of readings*. London: Longman/Open University Press ISBN 058229004X Section 2 Reading 6 104–40 References

This paper, by a social scientist, is rare in that it reports the very early stages of a major research project. It takes the reader to the position where an idea begins, before it is known whether there is a problem worth researching or what it might be. The focus is on the startling rise in industrial accidents reported to the Factory Inspectorate in the 1960s and the similarity between the variation by days of the week in the patterns of absenteeism and industrial accidents. More widely, methodological issues in studies on social change are explored, and a preliminary assessment of the use and limitations of sociological time-series studies is made.

2.18.2 Butterworth, T. (1994) Developing research ideas: from theory to practice. *Nurse Researcher* 1 (4) 78–86 24 References

Discusses the development of a research idea that took place over many years. The subject of psychosocial intervention in schizophrenia is used to illustrate some of the processes involved in translating theory to practice.

2.18.3 Campbell, J.P., Daft, R.L. & Hulin, C.L. (1982) *What to study: generating and developing research questions*. Beverly Hills, CA: Sage ISBN 0803918720 References

This book is a teaching device, intended to examine what is being investigated versus what should be. It discusses how research questions are developed, gives a list of ideas for consideration, suggests ways of reformulating research questions and how difficulties may be avoided. Some resource materials are also included.

2.18.4 Cresswell, J.W. (1998) Introducing and focusing the study. In Author *Qualitative inquiry and research design: choosing among five traditions*. Thousand Oaks, CA: Sage ISBN 0761901442 Chapter 6 93–107 References

Chapter discusses the problem and purpose of statements and research questions (CR 2.36.25).

2.18.5 Fleming, J.W. (1984) Selecting a clinical nursing problem for research. *Image: Journal of Nursing Scholarship* 16 (2) 62–4 5 References

A series of questions are identified which will assist in the appropriate selection of problems.

2.18.6 Hinds, P.S., Gattuso, J.S., Norville, R., Oakes, L. & Prichard, L. (1992) Bedside clinical research: a new category of research. *Clinical Nursing Research* 1 (2) 169–79 12 References

Describes a type of clinical research which authors label bedside nursing research. Features that characterize and separate it from the traditional view between research and practice are outlined. Examples and limitations are discussed, together with issues that affect its conduct (CR 2.102).

2.18.7 Jorgensen, D.L. (1989) Defining a problem. In Author *Participant observation: a methodology for human studies*. Newbury Park, CA: Sage ISBN 0803928777 Chapter 2 26–39

Chapter illustrates the logic and process of defining a problem. Procedures for formulating concepts and specifying indicators are outlined and exemplified. The process of problem definition is located within the human context of values, politics and ethics of research (CR 2.17, 2.72.10).

2.18.8 Liehr, P. (1992) Prelude to research. *Nursing Science Quarterly* 5 (3) 102–3 6 References

Discusses where ideas may come from for subsequent research. Two examples show how some initial observations developed into researchable questions.

2.18.9 Martin, P.A. (1994) The utility of the research problem statement. *Applied Nursing Research* 7 (1) 47–9 6 References

Discusses the value of a carefully formatted research problem statement and identifies the root of confusion which exists. Some helpful approaches are suggested.

2.18.10 Miles, J. (1994) Defining the research question. In Buckeldee, J. & McMahon, R. (eds) *The research experience in nursing*. London: Chapman & Hall ISBN 0412441101 Chapter 3 31–46 12 References

Identifies some of the processes required when defining and developing appropriate, researchable questions in a project investigating creativity in nursing (CR 2.16.7).

2.18.11 Vaughan, B. (1991) Identifying clinical problems for research. *Surgical Nurse* 4 (4) 10–12 10 References

Examines sources of research questions, discusses where to start, how to refine the question and clarify the purpose of a study.

2.19 IDENTIFICATION OF VARIABLES

Variables are those factors, events or behaviour about which information is desired, and which may be studied in isolation or in combination. They can be examined in their natural setting, or be manipulated to see if a particular response is evoked. During a study unknown variables may arise which may affect the data collected.

Definitions [See Appendix D for sources]

Construct – a hypothetical term designed to clarify and give meaning to behaviour. A construct cannot be observed but must be operationally defined by either an independent or dependent variable

Dependent variable – dependent upon or caused by another variable. It is *not* controlled by the researcher

Extraneous variable – when some factor produces error that becomes systematic and directional in nature

Independent variable – believed to cause or influence the dependent variable. In experimental studies it is manipulated by the researcher

Intervening variable – a third variable in a trivariate study that logically falls in a time sequence between the independent and dependent variables

Mediating variable – other variables which could affect the dependent variable or outcome which the research tries to control for in design or in statistical analysis

Variable – factor within a situation which can change or be changed

---

Annotations

2.19.1 Bennett, J.A. (2000) Focus on research methods. Mediator and moderator variables in nursing research: conceptual and statistical differences. *Research in Nursing & Health* 23 (5) October 415–20 9 References

Mediators and moderators are variables that affect the association between an independent variable and an outcome variable. Mediators provide additional information about how or why two variables are strongly associated. In contrast, moderators explain the circumstances that cause a weak or ambiguous association between two variables that were expected to have a strong relationship. This article summarizes the differences between them. Their statistical analysis in multiple regression is briefly described and two examples are given (CR 2.87).

2.19.2 Burgess, R.G. (ed.) (1986) *Key variables in social investigation*. London: Routledge & Kegan Paul ISBN 0710099010 References

Book comprises a series of papers that examine the relationship between theory and research, the identification of concepts and their translation into variables. Health and illness are two of the key variables explored (CR 2.7).

2.19.3 Drevdahl, D., Taylor, J.Y. & Phillips, D.A. (2001) Race and ethnicity as variables in nursing research, 1952–2000. *Nursing Research* 50 (5) September–October 305–13 References

Although the use of race and ethnicity as variables in nursing research has increased over the past five decades, there is confusion regarding the meaning of the terms, as well as how they are defined and determined in scientific inquiry. Results in this study showed that these variables present nurses with many challenges. Although they were widely used in the 337 articles examined from the journal *Nursing Research*, the categories were not defined in the majority of papers, and methods used to determine a participant's race or ethnicity were unclear. Nurses are urged to be explicit when using these variables.

2.19.4 Hayes, P. (2002) The complexity of multiple variables. *Clinical Nursing Research* 11 (3) 239–41 Editorial

Discusses the multiplicity of variables that practising nurses encounter as they provide care and the difficulty of understanding patterns in the interactions among multiple variables are explored.

2.20 FORMULATING HYPOTHESES OR RESEARCH QUESTIONS

A frequent goal in scientific research is to test a hypothesis that may be concerned with explaining relationships between observations or differences between groups. Some projects do not have hypotheses as they have different objectives. These may be guided by research questions and/or objectives.

Definitions [See Appendix D for sources]

Alternative hypothesis – a hypothesis that is pitted against the null hypothesis. It usually emerges from theory and is the hypothesis that the investigator usually believes to be true prior to carrying out the research [also called research hypothesis]

Conceptual definition – an abstract, dictionary-type definition (as contrasted with an operational definition)

Critical multiplism – the philosophy that researchers should use many ways of obtaining evidence regarding a particular hypothesis rather than relying on a single approach

Hypothesis – a conjecture about the relationships between two or more concepts

Hypothetico-deductive method – ... an approach to research that begins with a theory about how things work and derives testable hypotheses from it

Null hypothesis – ... states that the results observed in a study are no different from what might have occurred as a result of the play of chance

Operational definition – defining a construct by specifying precisely how it is measured or manipulated in a particular study

Research hypothesis – an alternative hypothesis to the statistical null hypothesis; predicts the researcher's actual expectations about the outcome of a study [also called alternative, scientific, substantive or theoretical]

Research objective – states the goal(s) of a study which is intended to describe rather than predict

Annotations

2.20.1   Booth, A. (2001) Turning research priorities into answerable research questions. *Health Information and Libraries Journal* 18 (2) 130–2 10 References

Discusses the responsibilities researchers have in formulating clinically applicable questions (CR 3.20).

2.20.2   Clark, A. (2000) Hypothetico-deduction and educational research. *Educational Research* 42 (2) 183–91   References

Paper suggests that the classic account of hypothetico-deduction in educational research needs to be replaced by a more adequate model that distinguishes between the logic of hypothetico-deduction and its methodological application. A reconceptualization entails exploration of the logical relationship between three levels of explanation: observation sentences, observation categoricals and theory formulations. Taken together these provide a framework to accommodate all inquiry. An educational example is included to show how this may be applied to educational research.

2.20.3   Earl-Slater, A. (2002) Types of research questions. In Author *The handbook of clinical trials and other research*. Oxford: Radcliffe Medical Press   ISBN 1857754859   334–5

A table gives the types of research question that may be asked, together with examples and suggestions for improvement (CR 2.2.13).

2.20.4   Griffin-Sobel, J.P. (2002) Formulating a research question. *Gastroenterology Nursing* 25 (2) 72–3   1 Reference

Using the author's Delphi Study as an example, the process of generating a research question is discussed (CR 2.66).

2.20.5   Hockey, L. (1999) Research questions and themes in district nursing. In McIntosh, J. (ed.) *Research issues in community nursing*. Basingstoke: Macmillan   ISBN 0333735048 Chapter 3 53–69 40 References

Chapter describes the early history of research in District Nursing and the author's programme of research is outlined, together with her reflections. Some recent developments are also described, together with potential new avenues for future research (CR 2.20.8).

2.20.6   Leary, M.R. (2001) Getting ideas for research. In Author *Introduction to behavioural research methods*. Boston, MA: Allyn & Bacon   ISBN 0205322042   Chapter 1 18–19 References

Author lists some ways of stimulating ideas for research which will help students at the beginning of their quest for suitable subject areas (CR 2.1.45, 2.2).

2.20.7   Luft, H.S. (2000) Identifying and assessing the null hypothesis. *Health Services Research* 34 (6) 1265–72   5 References

Discusses the issues arising from hypothesis testing, including statistical significance and clinical significance (CR 2.82, 2.83).

2.20.8   McIntosh, J. (ed.) (1999) *Research issues in community nursing*. Basingstoke: Macmillan Press   ISBN 0333735048   References

Book is an addition to the relatively sparse research literature on community nursing which discusses the conceptualization and elucidation of ideas that drive research questions. Themes in the book include the analysis of the evolution of research questions concerning role definition, detailed discussion of method and the meaning of evidence, together with its value and application to practice.

2.20.9 McKibbon, K.A. & Marks, S. (2001) Posing clinical questions: framing the question for scientific inquiry. *AACN Clinical Issues* 1 12 (4) 477–81   19 References

Advises on the formulation of clinical questions in order to be able to identify appropriate research questions for best practice.

2.20.10 Playle, J. (2000) Developing research questions and searching the literature. *Journal of Community Nursing* 14 (2) 20, 22, 24   14 References

Examines the first two stages of the research process – developing research questions and establishing current knowledge through searching the literature (CR 1.2, 2.12).

2.20.11 Stone, P. (2002) Deciding upon and refining a research question. *Palliative Medicine* 16 (3) 265–68   11 References

Highlights the importance of defining and refining a research question, gives points to consider in doing so and advises on how to pose a well-structured question.

2.20.12 Wyatt, J. & Guly, H. (2002) Identifying the research question and planning the project. *Emergency Medicine Journal* 19 (4) 318–21   21 References

With reference to accident and emergency, the article summarizes what constitutes a good research question and describes approaches that could be used to plan a project (CR 2.14, 2.18).

2.21   SELECTING A RESEARCH DESIGN

'The design is a blueprint for conducting research. It contains plans for collecting, organizing and analysing the data. The choice of design depends on the purposes of the study but it is generally approached from a descriptive or experimental perspective. Research is never as perfect as we would like, every type of design involves compromise and error.' (Phillips, L.R.F., 1986: xiii)

Definition [See Appendix D for source]

Research design – the overall plan of research intended to yield specific, unambiguous answers to research questions or to allow useful hypotheses to emerge

Annotations

2.21.1 Bechhofer, F. & Paterson, L. (2000) *Principles of research design in the social sciences.* London: Routledge   ISBN 0415214424   References

Book is intended as preliminary reading for students who have decided on their area of investigation but have little experience of designing social research. It discusses ideas rather than technicalities to encourage students to consider appropriate designs for their questions (CR 2.14, 2.29, 2.39, 2.42, 2.52).

2.21.2 Bickman, L. (ed.) (2000) *Research design: Donald Campbell's legacy.* Thousand Oaks, CA: Sage   ISBN 0761910867   References 2 Volumes

Applied researchers who want to improve their research designs will find this book a thought-provoking and compelling read (CR 2.25.4, 2.29, 2.35, 2.43, 2.51).

2.21.3 Douglas, J. (1998) Developing appropriate research methodologies with black and minority ethnic communities. Part 1: Reflections on the process. *Health Education Journal* 57 (4) 329–38 29 References

Outlines and reviews research methodologies developed in a Heart Action Research Project to ascertain and document the needs and experiences of black and ethnic minority communities. A number of areas were explored in developing anti-oppressive and participatory methodologies, in particular strategies for sampling black and ethnic minority populations, matching interviewers to respondents for language and ethnicity, and the effect of the 'race' of the interviewer (CR 2.22, 2.37, 2.68, 2.75).

2.21.4 Hakim, C. (2000) *Research design: successful designs for social and economic research* (2nd edition). London: Routledge   ISBN 041522313X   References

Provides a practical overview of the central issues involved in the design of social and economic research. The key features, strengths and limitations of eight main types of study are included, with examples and strategies for choosing designs. A chapter on cross-national studies is also included (CR 3.22).

2.21.5 McPherson, K. & Lord, S. (2000) Clinician's guide to research. Part 2: Matching the method to the question. *New Zealand Journal of Physiotherapy* 28 (2) 20–8   33   References

Considers a number of approaches to answering research questions and discusses common flaws that can weaken a study design (CR 2.20).

2.21.6 Nahin, R.L. & Straus, S.E. (2001) Research into complementary and alternative medicine: problems and potential. *British Medical Journal* 322 (7279) 20 January 161–4 22 References

'The National Center for Complementary and Alternative Medicine at the National Institutes of Health aims to explore complementary and alternative healing practices in the context of vigorous science, to educate and train researchers, and disseminate authoritative information to the public and professionals.' This article discusses allocation of resources, problems with research design and suggests approaches to good design in this field of study (CR 2.14).

2.21.7 Ploeg, J. (1999) Identifying the best research design to fit the question. Part 2: Qualitative designs. *Evidence-Based Nursing* 2 (2) 36–7   16 References

Provides an overview of three types of qualitative research and the types of question that are most usefully addressed by a qualitative approach (CR 2.42, 2.45, 2.49).

2.21.8 Roberts, J. & DiCenso, A. (1999) Identifying the best research design to fit the question. Part 1: Quantitative designs. *Evidence-Based Nursing* 2 (1) 4–6   3 References

Identifies the range of quantitative designs that can be used to answer research questions involving diagnosis, prognosis, prevention, treatment and economic evaluation (CR 2.29).

2.21.9 Whitney, J.D. (1999) Moving from concept to research design. *Journal of Wound Care Nursing* 26 (6) 290–1   7 References

Identifies seven research designs and discusses their application to research into wound care.

2.22   POPULATIONS AND SAMPLES

Nursing research is usually concerned with people and the intention of researchers is to say something about them and their responses to a health care system. Careful identification and description of the population, together with appropriate sample selection techniques, are important steps in any research design. Researchers are not entirely in agreement about the language used to define 'populations' but the following set of definitions is listed in descending order of size.

Definitions [See Appendix D for sources]

Populations:

Population – the portion of the universe to which the researcher has access

Population element – a single member of a population

Population stratum – a population contained within another population

Subject – ... the person who is being studied

Target population – all the cases that meet a designated set of criteria

Universe – all possible respondents or measures of a certain kind

Sampling:

Sampling – the process of selecting a few elements from a population. These elements are expected to stand for all those within the population. The way in which this is done allows one to generalize the sample findings to a population, or does not allow one to do so

Sampling error – ... the probability that any particular sample is not fully representative of the population from which it is drawn

Non-probability sampling techniques:

Convenience (accidental) sample – sample obtained by accessing individuals who are easy to identify and contact

Purposive sample – cases to be included are hand-picked for their experience or knowledge or some other characteristic of interest to the researcher

Quota sample – sample aimed at ensuring adequate representation of underlying groups e.g. age or ethnic groups

Snowball sample – selection is carried out by word of mouth. The first people contacted are asked to name others with similar characteristics

Probability sampling techniques:

Cluster sample – groups of population elements with the same characteristics are chosen rather than individuals

Simple random sample – sample obtained using a table of random numbers, or some other means, and each population element has an equal probability of being selected

> Stratified random sample – population divided into sub-groups called strata [from which] a simple random sample is obtained
>
> Systematic random sample – obtained by taking every nth (selection interval) name on a population list

Annotations

2.22.1 Anderson, D.G. & Hatton, D.C. (2000) Accessing vulnerable populations for research. *Western Journal of Nursing Research* 22 (2) 244–51 10 References

Article discusses methods of accessing vulnerable populations for research. Particular points considered are how to invite participants into a research project and respect their input, how to care for oneself as a researcher, how to reciprocate with staff and organizations where studies take place and how to obtain approval from an institutional review board (CR 2.16, 2.17, 3.16).

2.22.2 Barnitt, R. & Partridge, C. (1999) The legacy of being a research subject: follow-up studies of participants in therapy research. *Physiotherapy Research International* 4 (4) 250–61 19 References

Few researchers have reported carrying out follow-up studies of their subjects, so the ethical effects of research are not known. Follow-up studies were conducted on 87 (56%) subjects who had participated in research interviews, or were sent a letter and questionnaire – some with physical disabilities who lived in residential care, physical therapists and occupational therapists. Some subjects later had concerns about their involvement in the research that included confidentiality, expectations that had not been met, anger, disappointment, and loss of face. Others reported positive outcomes (CR 2.16, 2.17).

2.22.3 Bebout, R.R., Becker, D.R. & Drake, R.E. (1998) Brief report. A research induction group for clients entering a mental health research project: a replication study. *Community Mental Health Journal* 34 (3) 289–95 14 References

Through education and discussion, a research induction group was established to encourage prospective mental health clients to participate in a research study. Its purpose was to help clients understand the clinical and research procedures so that they could make a fully informed decision about whether or not to participate. This replication study showed similar results to a previous one that demonstrated that informed decision-making led to high rates of participation and satisfaction with both vocational and research procedures (CR 2.13).

2.22.4 Bragadottir, H. (2000) Children's rights in clinical research. *Journal of Nursing Scholarship* 32 (2) 2nd Quarter 179–84 72 References

Paper addresses the use of children and children's genetic information in research, analyses Icelandic laws, reviews existing literature on children in clinical research and describes nurses' actions as children's advocates (CR 2.17).

2.22.5 Britton, A., McKee, M., Black, N., McPherson, K., Sanderson, C. & Bain, C. (1999) Threats to applicability of randomized trials: exclusions and selective participation. *Journal of Health Service Research Policy* 4 (2) 112–21 63 References

A systematic review of cited references to assess the extent, nature and importance of excluding potential participants. The review concludes that while narrow inclusion criteria may have benefits, it may also result in the denial of effective treatment to groups who might benefit.

2.22.6 Brown, B.A., Long, H.L., Weitz, T.A. & Milliken, N. (2000) Challenges of recruitment: focus groups with research study recruiters. *Women & Health* 31 (2/3) 153–66 30 References

Regulations have been promulgated by the National Institutes of Health requiring the inclusion of women and minorities in research studies. While these have resulted in more inclusive research, their unintended consequences are discussed in this article (CR 2.69).

2.22.7 Carlin, J.B. & Doyle, L.W. (2002) Statistics for clinicians. 7: sample size. *Journal of Paediatric Child Health* 36 (5) 502–5 6 References

Provides a detailed explanation of the effect on outcomes of different sample sizes and suggests that an a priori sample size calculation can reduce uncertainty.

2.22.8 Champ, S. (2002) Questionnaires from the heart: national agendas and private hopes. *Nurse Researcher: The International Journal of Research Methodology in Nursing and Health Care* 9 (4) 20–9 7 References

Article reflects on issues in mental health from the user's perspective. The author discusses the frustrations felt by consumers of mental health services in Australia at their lack of involvement in research, and puts forward an argument for developing a greater partnership between consumers and researchers.

2.22.9 Davis, L.L., Broome, M.E. & Cox, R.P. (2002) Maximizing retention in community-based clinical trials. *Journal of Nursing Scholarship* 34 (1) 1st Quarter 47–53 54 References

Study identifies and discusses retention strategies and their effectiveness in clinical trials in the last decade. Nine strategies were identified and each is discussed (CR 2.29).

2.22.10 Draucker, C.B. (1999) The emotional impact of sexual violence research on participants. *Archives of Psychiatric Nursing* 13 (4) 161–9 36 References

Based on a literature review, this article explores the emotional impact on participants of undertaking research on sexual violence. A framework for understanding the responses of research subjects who write or talk about traumatic experiences is discussed (CR 2.16, 2.17).

2.22.11 Flaskerud, J.H. & Nyamathi, A.M. (2000) Attaining gender and ethnic diversity in health intervention research: cultural responsiveness versus resource provision. *Advances in Nursing Science* 22 (4) 1–15 50 References

Although mandated by the National Institutes of Health to include women and diverse ethnic groups in all their funded projects, these groups are still excluded as participants in health intervention research. They have thus been denied access to state-of-the-art treatments and prevention strategies, making them more vulnerable to increased morbidity and mortality and decreased longevity. This article compares two conceptual approaches to inclusion, cultural responsiveness and resource provision. Suggestions are made as to how this situation may be changed.

2.22.12 Grieg, A.D. & Taylor, J. (1998) *Doing research with children*. London: Sage ISBN 0761955909 References

Introduces themes and approaches when doing research with children and details frameworks for both qualitative and quantitative research methods. The unique nature of children as research subjects is discussed, together with the ethical issues involved (CR 2.9, 2.17).

2.22.13 Hagino, C. & Lo, R.J. (1998) Random versus systematic sampling from administrative databases involving human subjects. *Journal of Manipulative and Physiological Therapeutics* 21 (7) 454–9 4 References

Random and systematic sampling is compared to determine whether they yield similar and accurate distributions for the following factors: age, gender, geographic location and years in practice. The sampling frame was from the entire database of the Canadian Chiropractic Association. Authors conclude that both methods for different sample sizes yield similar results.

2.22.14 Hall, J.M., Stevens, P.E. & Pletsch, P.K. (2001) Team research using qualitative methods: investigating children's involvement in clinical research. *Journal of Family Nursing* 7 (1) 7–31 25 References

With changes in US federal guidelines mandating inclusion of children in clinical research, more and more children are being sought as subjects in clinical trials. As participants, children are more vulnerable than adults because of cognitive and emotional development, legal capacity, level of autonomy, and dependence on family influence. This article describes the methods and process of a family-focused qualitative study of the clinical research experiences of ill children and their families. Its aim was to understand the family's perspectives on research and recommend ways to obtain informed consent and conduct clinical research on children (CR 2.17, 2.36).

2.22.15 Harden, J.T. & McFarland, G. (2000) Avoiding gender and minority barriers to NIH funding. *Journal of Nursing Scholarship* 32 (1) 1st Quarter 83–6 11 References

Article informs investigators of the National Institutes of Health (NIH) guidelines for the inclusion of women and minorities as subjects in clinical research, and provides tips on avoiding barriers to federal funding. Applications for funding are being barred because the plan for inclusion of these groups is judged to be unacceptable, which is unnecessary and avoidable (CR 3.13).

2.22.16 Heptinstall, E. (2000) Gaining access to looked after children for research purposes: lessons learned. *British Journal of Social Work* 30 (6) 867–72 9 References

Gives an account of the process and difficulties of gaining access to children for research purposes.

2.22.17 Johnson, M., Marsden, J. & Day, E. (1998) Practical issues in survey sampling. *Australian Journal of Advanced Nursing* 15 (3) 38–45 28 References

Paper reviews the principles of survey sampling and applies these principles in a study examining the skills of 15,540 nurses. Three major facets of sampling are outlined – the sample frame, size and specific designs of the selection procedures, and how these may be used. The authors also recommend how to obtain assistance with these complex procedures and some steps in problem-solving (CR 2.52).

2.22.18 Klesges, R.C., Williamson, J.E., Somes, G.W., Talcott, W.G., Lando, H.A. & Haddock, C.K. (1999) A population comparison of participants and non-participants in a health survey. *American Journal of Public Health* 89 (8) 1228–31 9 References

Study examined the characteristics of Air Force recruits willing to take part in a health survey versus those who were unwilling to participate. Results suggest that, despite some low estimates of health behaviours due to response bias, relationships between most risk factors are generally unaffected by those who did not respond (CR 2.27, 2.52).

2.22.19 MacDougall, C. & Fudge, E. (2001) Planning and recruiting the sample for focus groups and in-depth Interviews. *Qualitative Health Care* 11 (1) January 117–26 17 References

Authors propose a checklist summarizing a strategy involving three stages of preparation, contact and follow-up. Each step is described and suggestions are made when research deals with sensitive issues (CR 2.68, 2.69).

2.22.20 Moorman, P.G., Newman, B., Millikan, R.C., Tse, C.-K. & Sandler, D.P. (1999) Participation rates in a case-control study: the impact of age, race and race of interviewer. *Annals of Epidemiology* 9 (3) April 188–95 References

This report describes factors associated with non-participation in a population-based, case-control study of breast cancer and discusses ways to overcome these barriers (CR 2.41).

2.22.21 Morse, J.M. (2000) Determining sample size. *Qualitative Health Research* 10 (1) January 3–5 Editorial 2 References

Discusses the factors to be considered when determining sample size, scope of the study, nature of the topic, quality of data, study design and the use of shadowed data (CR 2.36).

2.22.22 Murray, J.S. (2000) Clinical methods. Conducting psychosocial research with children and adolescents: a developmental perspective. *Applied Nursing Research* 13 (3) 151–6 19 References

In the past, adults who were thought to know their children best, provided representative accounts of a child's world. Literature suggests that in the past children have been perceived mainly as objects rather than subjects of research interest. This perhaps reflects the viewpoint held by many that children are unable to comprehend and describe their world because of developmental immaturity and/or that there are intrinsic difficulties in researching children. This article describes how a child's developmental level affects the research process, specifically those in response to psychosocial research methods, assent and consent with children (CR 2.17).

2.22.23 Neufeld, A., Harrison, M.J., Hughes, K.D., Spitzer, D. & Stewart, M.J. (2001) Participation of immigrant women family caregivers in qualitative research. *Western Journal of Nursing Research* 23 (6) 575–91 49 References

Article presents the authors' experience in recruiting immigrant women of Chinese and South Asian origin in an ethnographic study. They discuss issues related to the recruitment and participation of immigrant women in research, including establishing access to diverse groups of women, benefits for immigrant women, and placing the researcher and research process on the same level (CR 2.36, 2.42).

2.22.24 Oliver, M. (1998) Theories of disability in health practice and research. *British Medical Journal* 317 (7170) 21 November 1446–9 29 References

Paper considers the influence of implicit and explicit theories on interventions and research on disabled people. Another important influence is the experience of disabled people, and their increasing insistence that their voices be heard at all stages of research about their lives. The rise of various theories is posing important questions for health care and research and these are discussed.

2.22.25 Ory, M.G., Lipman, P.D., Barr, R., Harden, J.T. & Stahl, S.M. (2000) A national program to enhance research on minority aging and health promotion. *Journal of Mental Health & Aging* 6 (1) 9–18 6 References

Article addresses the importance of minority aging research for understanding and reducing health differentials found in older minority/ethnic populations. It highlights a national effort, the Exploratory Centers for Minority Aging and Health Promotion (MAHP), and reviews their projects and lessons learned about outreach, recruitment and retention that are critical for conducting research in older minority populations.

2.22.26 Outlaw, F.H., Bourjolly, J.N. & Barg, F.K. (2000) A study on recruitment of black Americans into clinical trials through a cultural competence lens. *Cancer Nursing* 23 (6) 444–51 27 References

Black Americans are stricken disproportionately with cancer and continue to be underrepresented in clinical trials that could offer them state-of-the-art therapy in a research context. This article describes findings from the first phase of a two-phase project on recruitment of black Americans into clinical trials. Findings are reported and the second phase proposed to examine the knowledge, beliefs, attitudes and behaviours of the potential subjects (CR 2.29).

2.22.27   Peruga, A., Maria Leon, E., Child, R., Cruz, A., Hernandez, M., Arredondo, A., Hernandez, C., Cuchi, P. & Zacarias, F. (2000) Analysis of participation in surveys in five countries: the importance of public health research. *Pan American Journal of Public Health* 7 (4) 249–54 12 References

Study compares participation rates and reasons for non-response in surveys conducted in five countries of Latin America and the Caribbean. The study objective was to measure the prevalence of risk behaviours affecting the transmission of human immunodeficiency virus. Results are discussed and will provide useful information for future research (CR 2.52).

2.22.28   Playle, J. (2000) Sampling issues in research. *Journal of Community Nursing* 14 (5) 22, 24, 27   13 References

Explores the principles and rationale behind sampling, describes the different stages and techniques, including probability and non-probability sampling, and discusses some issues involved in arriving at a sample size.

2.22.29   Pletsch, P.K. & Stevens, P.E. (2001) Inclusion of children in clinical research: lessons learned from mothers of diabetic children. *Clinical Nursing Research* 10 (2) May 140–62 20 References

Nine mothers of diabetic children were asked in a qualitative study about the factors that influenced them to consent to have their children involved in clinical research. They were asked to describe how they made such decisions, what motivated them to keep the children in the programme once enrolled, and how they evaluated the studies afterwards. Results suggest that mothers engage in a personal calculus before making a choice to consent (CR 2.17, 2.36).

2.22.30   Porter, E.J. (1999) Defining the eligible, accessible population for a phenomenological study. *Western Journal of Nursing Research* 21 (6) 796–804   26 References

The author reports the development of a method for estimating the eligible, accessible population in a phenomenological study that aimed to examine older widows' experience of home care. The philosophical rationale is explained and the procedures detailed. Suggestions are given for adapting the method in keeping with the aims of a particular phenomenological study (CR 2.17, 2.49).

2.22.31   Rhodes, P., Nocon, A., Wright, J. & Harrison, S. (2001) Involving patients in research: setting up a service users' advisory group. *Journal of Management in Medicine* 15 (2) 167–71   References

Paper examines some of the issues raised by patients' involvement in the research process. It uses as an example a users' group involved in a diabetes service evaluation in the north of England. The key conclusions are that a precise role should be specified at the outset, genuine user involvement is needed, wide and accurate representation of all relevant groups is essential, and researchers must approach users with an open mind with a view to shared decision-making rather than control (CR 2.16).

2.22.32   Ross, F., Triggs, E., Cadbury, H., Axford, J. & Victor, C. (1998) Evaluation of education for people with osteoarthritis of the knee: recruitment and retention in study design. *Nurse Researcher* 6 (1) 49–59   7 References

The aim of this study was to compare patient outcomes in practices using structured education group sessions, with those given usual care in a randomized control trial. The paper addresses some of the methodological issues arising from undertaking this trial in primary care and discusses in particular recruitment and retention of the sample (CR 2.14, 2.29).

2.22.33   Ross, S., Grant, A., Counsell, C., Gillespie, W., Russell, I. & Prescott, R. (2001) Barriers to participation in randomized controlled trials: a systematic review. *Journal of Clinical Epidemiology* 54 (3) March 323–4   References

Paper discusses reported barriers to recruitment of clinicians and patients to randomized controlled trials. Suggestions are made as to how these may be overcome (CR 2.12, 2.29).

2.22.34   Sturm, R., Unützer, J. & Katon, W. (1999) Effectiveness research and implications for study design: sample size and statistical power. *General Hospital Psychiatry* 21 (4) 274–83   31 References

Highlights that while clinical differences in treatments can be observed by relatively small sample sizes, studies requiring quality of life and cost measures usually require much larger samples. Publications that are based on small but significant clinical findings may mislead readers as to the true value of treatments.

2.22.35   Taber, K.S. (2002) 'Intense, but it's all worth it in the end': the co-learner's experience of the research process. *British Educational Research Journal* 28 (3) 435–57   65 References

Article describes one aspect of a research project that investigated learning in science, but its concerns are those of any researcher (especially teacher researcher) using learners as sources of data. Such research involves a considerable time commitment, as well as risking exposure of their personal limitations as learners. The author describes some ethical concerns in using learners as research subjects (CR 2.16, 2.17).

2.22.36 Thompson, C. (1999) If you could provide me with a sample: examining sampling in qualitative and quantitative research papers. *Evidence-Based Nursing* 2 (3) 68–70   10 References

Uses an example from a randomized controlled trial and a study using grounded theory to highlight the general principles of sampling and issues surrounding sampling characteristics (CR 2.29, 2.36, 2.45, 2.95).

2.22.37 Torgerson, D.J. & Campbell, M.K. (2000) Cost-effectiveness calculations and sample size. *British Medical Journal* 321 (7276) 16 September 697   7 References

Urges researchers to consider the cost-effectiveness of treatments as well as clinical differences when calculating sample size.

2.22.38 White, A. & Johnson, M. (1998) The complexities of nursing research with men. *International Journal of Nursing Studies* 35 (1/2) 41–8   32 References

Because research into men's health has been comparatively neglected, the authors explore the issues that need to be taken into consideration when conducting research with (or on) men. It outlines the current thinking on men and masculinity and the social development of male stereotypes. The position of men with regard to feminist thinking is also explored. Examining the stages of the research process develops the argument, and consideration also needs to be given to the gender of both researched and researcher (CR 2.10).

2.22.39 Wilson, K. & Rose, K. (1998) Patient recruitment and retention strategies in randomized controlled trials. *Nurse Researcher* 6 (1) 35–46   25 References

Paper aims to share the authors' experience of research to increase awareness of issues surrounding recruitment and retention strategies in randomized controlled trials. The ethical issues involved are also discussed (CR 2.14, 2.17, 2.29).

2.22.40 Wilson-Barnett, J. & Griffiths, P. (2002) The disappearing sample: researcher and research ability. *International Journal of Nursing Studies* 39 (4) May 365–7   12 References   Editorial

One of the commonest barriers to completing clinical research is the inadequacy of patient numbers recruited to the sample within the allotted timescale. Factors include those related to the context of

the research and those related to the researcher's decisions and approaches. The authors map out some of the potential problems using examples from their own teams' work.

2.22.41 Wood, J. & Lambert, M. (1999) Sample size calculations for trials in health service research. *Journal of Health Service Research Policy* 4 (4) 226–9   8 References

Argues that confidence intervals are replacing significance tests in summarizing the results of clinical trials and therefore estimation of sample size using a power calculation needs to be reconsidered. Provides an example of how to calculate sample size on the basis of measurement error.

2.23   PILOT STUDIES

'Pilot studies fulfil a range of important functions and can provide valuable insights for other researchers. There is a need for more discussion amongst researchers of both the process and outcome of pilot studies.' (van Teijlingen & Hundley: 1)

Definitions [See Appendix D for sources]

Feasibility study/tests – any equipment or procedures that are unique to [a] major study and new to [a] research team

Pilot study – a small-scale preliminary study undertaken to test the feasibility of the proposed research and to improve the procedures and methods of measurement

Example

Whyte, R. & Watson, H. (1998) Developing research methods in qualitative research: using a radio microphone in a pilot study. *Nurse Researcher* 6 (1) 60–71   18 References

Paper describes the use of a radio microphone in a pilot study in which verbal interactions between diplomate nurses and patients in hospital were recorded. The development of the research approach is explored, and practical information is given on using this method of data collection. Ethical implications are considered, together with the lessons learned during the pilot study (CR 2.14, 2.17, 2.36, 2.72).

Annotations

2.23.1 Hall, J. (2001) A qualitative survey of staff responses to an integrated care pathway pilot study in a mental healthcare setting ... including commentary by von Degenberg, K. *NT Research* 6 (3) 696–706   53 References

Reports a study that explored participants' beliefs about the effectiveness and limitations of a pilot and its impact on practice, and to use these findings to develop recommendations for the future of integrated care pathways within the clinical area (CR 2.36, 2.88, Appendix A).

2.23.2 Lackey, N.R. & Wingate, A.L. (1998) The pilot study: one key to research success. In Brink, P.J. & Wood, M.J. (eds) *Advanced design in nursing research* (2nd edition). Thousand Oaks, CA: Sage   ISBN 0803958005   Chapter 15 375–86 25 References

Chapter defines a pilot study, its philosophies and purposes. It discusses conducting the study and evaluating the results (CR 2.36.15).

2.23.3 Ort, S.V. (1981) Research design: pilot study. In Krampitz, S.D. & Pavlovich, N. (eds) *Readings for nursing research*. St Louis, MO: Mosby   ISBN 0801627478   Chapter 6 49–53 References

Discusses the purposes and characteristics of a pilot study, its design and implementation. Ethical aspects, reliability and validity of instruments, potential difficulties and guidelines are all discussed (CR 2.17, 2.24, 2.25).

2.23.4 Prescott, P.A. & Soeken, K.L. (1989) The potential uses of pilot work. *Nursing Research* 38 (1) 60–2   3 References

Following a review of published studies and research texts, the authors reported that pilot studies are under-discussed, under-used and under-reported. The article focuses on the separate components within a main study, and highlights the contribution of pilot work to each. Although increasing the time spent in preparation for a study, it enables defects to be corrected that cannot be removed or remedied after the study has commenced.

2.23.5 van Teijlingen, E.R. & Hundley, V. *The importance of pilot studies*. Social Research Update Issue 35 1–7   26 References Guildford: Department of Sociology, University of Surrey www.soc. surrey.ac.uk/sru/SRU35.html (Accessed 13/11/03)

Paper gives many reasons for conducting pilot studies, their problems and limitations and the reasons why they may not be reported in the literature. The authors urge researchers to report their pilot studies, and in particular to give more details of the actual improvements made to the study design and the research process as a result of their preliminary work.

2.23.6 van Teijlingen, E.R., Rennie, A., Hundley, V. & Graham, W. (2001) The importance of conducting and reporting pilot studies: the example of the Scottish Births Survey. *Journal of Advanced Nursing* 34 (3) 289–95   35 References

In many research papers, pilot studies are only reported as a means of justifying the methods, and it is unusual for these to include practical problems faced by the researcher(s). This study aimed to identify the most appropriate method for conducting a national survey of maternity care. Pilot studies were carried out in five hospitals to establish the best of four possible methods. These studies raised a number of fundamental issues relating to the process of conducting a large-scale survey. Lessons learned are reported and may assist others in avoiding similar pitfalls and mistakes (CR 2.52).

2.24 RELIABILITY

'Reliability and validity are two major characteristics that need to be considered when undertaking both quantitative and qualitative research. The criteria for these need to be differentiated as the purpose, goals and intent of each type of research are different. Many students are taught to use quantitative reliability and validity criteria for qualitative studies. This is inappropriate and results in confusion.' (Leininger, 1985: 35)

[The item below outlines the essential difference between the focus of reliability in qualitative and quantitative research.]

Qualitative research – Focus is on identifying and documenting features and phenomena in similar and different contexts.

Quantitative research – Focus is on the measuring tool or its ability to assess the degree of consistency or accuracy with which it measures an attribute.

Definitions [See Appendix D for sources]

Inter-rater (inter-observer)reliability – the degree to which two raters or observers, operating independently, assign the same ratings or values for an attribute being measured

Intra-observer (rater) reliability – ... reproducibility of a set of observations on one variable made by the same observer at different times

Reliability – the extent to which a test would give consistent results if applied more than once to the same people under standard conditions

Split-half reliability – a set of items is divided in half and the two halves are correlated

Test–retest reliability – an approach to reliability that compares two administrations of the same measuring instrument

Annotations

2.24.1   Carmines, E.G. & Zeller, R.A. (1979) *Reliability and validity assessment.* Beverly Hills, CA: Sage   ISBN 0803913710   References

This basic text introduces the issues in measurement theory. The concepts of reliability and validity are thoroughly discussed in light of current debate (CR 2.25).

2.24.2   Kirk, J. & Miller, M.L. (1986) *Reliability and validity in qualitative research.* Beverly Hills, CA: Sage   ISBN 0803924704   References

Book concerns itself with the issues surrounding the scientific status

2.24.3   Peräkylä, A. (1997) Reliability and validity in research based on tapes and transcripts. In Silverman, D. (ed.) *Qualitative research: theory, method and practice.* London: Sage   ISBN 0803976666   Part VI Chapter 13 201–20   68 References

Chapter deals with issues of reliability and validity in research based upon tapes and transcripts, and in conservation analysis (CR 2.25, 2.28, 2.36.127, 2.89).

2.24.4   Thompson, B. (ed.) (2002) *Score reliability: contemporary thinking on reliability issues.* Thousand Oaks, CA: Sage   ISBN 0761926267

Book is aimed at helping researchers create and evaluate scores in a more appropriate way, and this reader presents the basic concepts of classical ('true score') and modern ('generalizability') test theory (CR 2.28).

2.24.5   Traub, R.E. (1994) *Reliability for the social sciences: theory and applications.* Thousand Oaks, CA: Sage   ISBN 0803943253   References

Integrates theory and application of classic approaches to measurement reliability. Practical advice is given on the estimation of reliability and its statistics.

2.24.6   Yen, M. & Lo, L.-H. (2002) Examining test–retest reliability: an intra-class correlation approach. *Nursing Research* 51 (1) January–February 59–62   8 References

Authors suggest that intra-class correlation is an alternative to test the reliability of an instrument and is more sensitive to the detection of systematic error.

2.25   VALIDITY

The second major property required in any measuring instrument, in addition to reliability, is that of validity. The researcher should try to ensure that any existing tools used fulfil the required criteria, and information on this should be sought prior to their use.

[The item below outlines the essential difference between the focus of validity in qualitative and quantitative research.]

Qualitative research – Focus is on gaining knowledge and understanding of the phenomena under study

Quantitative research – Focus is on measurement

Definitions [See Appendix D for sources]

Concurrent validity – a test or question is said to have concurrent validity if it correlates well with other measures of the same concept

Construct validity – the degree to which a test measures the desired characteristic or construct of interest. It is estimated by validating the theory underlying the instrument

Content validity – the degree to which the desired domain (content) is adequately sampled and represented in the instrument. Also considered is the adequacy of the operational definition of the domain being sampled

Convergent validity – a test or question has convergent validity when several dissimilar measures of the same concept correlate well with it

Criterion-related validity – the degree to which the instrument correlates with external variables or criteria believed to measure the concept under investigation. Concurrent and predictive validity are two types

External validity – the ability to generalize or frame a single study to other populations and conditions

Face validity – ... [will] subjects perceive [an] instrument as being valid

Internal validity – the ability to believe in the conclusion drawn based on the design of the study.

To assess this, one asks if the treatment did indeed make a difference

Member validation – an array of techniques that purport to validate findings by demonstrating a correspondence between the researcher's analysis and collectively members' descriptions of their social worlds

Predictive validity – the degree to which an instrument can predict some criterion observed at a future time

Qualitative validity – is concerned with confirming the truth or understandings associated with phenomena

Validity – the degree to which an instrument measures what it is intended to measure (in qualitative research, validity refers to the extent to which the research findings represent reality)

Annotations

2.25.1 Andrews, M., Lyne, P. & Riley, E. (1996) Validity in qualitative health research: an exploration of the impact of individual researchers' perspectives within collaborative enquiry. *Journal of Advanced Nursing* 23 (3) 441–7   19 References

Paper explores the problem of validity in qualitative inquiry and reports a review of published strategies for analysing interview data (CR 2.15, 2.36, 2.68).

2.25.2 Angen, M.J. (2000) Pearls, pith and provocation. Evaluating interpretive inquiry: reviewing the validity debate and opening the dialogue. *Qualitative Health Research* 10 (3) May 378–95   73 References

Article reviews the various approaches to the problem of validity in the hope of turning the debate into a dialogue. Validity is traced from its origins in realist ontology and foundational epistemology of quantitative inquiry to its reformulations within the lifeworld ontology and non-foundationalism of interpretative human inquiry. Various recent qualitative approaches to validity are considered, and interpretative reconfigurations of validity are reviewed. Interpretative approaches to validity are synthesized as ethical and substantive procedures of validation.

2.25.3 Benfer, R.A., Brent, E.E. Jr. & Furbee, L. (1991) *Expert systems*. Newbury Park, CA: Sage   ISBN 080394036X   References

Discusses the process of expert systems development as a model for acquiring, representing and validating knowledge about relatively limited domains.

2.25.4 Bickman, L. (ed.) (2000) *Validity and social experimentation: Donald Campbell's legacy*. Thousand Oaks, CA: Sage   ISBN 0761911618   References   2 Volumes

Leading social research methodologists and evaluators address the issues of validity, research design and social experimentation in the first of two volumes inspired by the work of Donald Campbell (CR 2.21.2, 2.29, 2.43).

2.25.5 Bloor, M. (1997) Techniques of validation in qualitative research: a critical commentary. In Miller, G. & Dingwall, R. (eds) *Context and method in qualitative research*. London: Sage   ISBN 0803976321   Part 1 Chapter 3 37–50   References

Discusses the problems inherent in validating qualitative research, including triangulation and member validation. Examples are given examining these attempts to validate data and the difficulties that ensued. Author believes that neither technique can validate findings but are relevant to the issue of validity (CR 2.26, 2.36.88).

2.25.6 Fogg, L. & Gross, D. (2000) Focus on research methods: threats to validity in randomized clinical trials. *Research in Nursing and Health* 23 (1) 79–87   45 References

Article presents an overview of randomized clinical trials, describes five threats to validity that increase the likelihood of making invalid conclusions about intervention efficacy, and offers three strategies to overcome these problems (CR 2.29).

2.25.7 George, K., Batterham, A. & Sullivan, I. (2000) Research without tears. Validity in clinical research: a review of basic concepts and definitions. *Physical Therapy in Sport* 1 (1) 19–27   18 References

Paper addresses the concept of validity in clinical research. Key components of validity are defined with regard to the general aims of research and research design.

2.25.8 Kapborg, I. & Berterö, C. (2002) Using an interpreter in qualitative interviews: does it threaten validity? *Nursing Inquiry* 9 (1) 52–6   19 References

Discusses the threats to validity using an interpreter when accommodating three language changes. Suggests that the interpreter needs to possess research skills in addition to linguistic abilities (CR 2.68).

2.25.9 Lummis, T. (1998) Structure and validity in oral evidence. In Perks, R. & Thomson, A. (eds) *The oral history reader*. London: Routledge   ISBN 0415133521   Part IV Chapter 23 273–83   22 Notes and References

The validation of oral evidence can be divided into two main areas: the degree to which any individual interview yields reliable information on the historical experience, and whether that experience is typical of its place and time. Two examples are given and ways suggested in which simple aggregation can be used to assess validity. The process of structuring data should be part of the interpretative process and may be used to elucidate some of the wider problems of omission and distortion in oral evidence (CR 2.47.18).

2.25.10   Maxwell, J.A. (2002) Understanding and validity in qualitative research. In Huberman, A.M. & Miles, M.B. (eds) *The qualitative researcher's companion*. Thousand Oaks, CA: Sage   ISBN 076191191X   Chapter 2 37–64   79 References

Article is a reformulation of the categorization of validity in qualitative research, and gives an account of the way in which researchers think about and deal with validity in actual practice (CR 2.36.62).

2.25.11   Nanda, S.K., Rivas, A.L., Trochim, W.M. & Deshler, J.D. (2000) Emphasis on validation in research: a meta-analysis. *Scientometrics* 48 (1) 45–64   References

The emphasis of validation as a publication content was investigated in dissertations and articles. The longitudinal data suggested three fields (agricultural science, applied science and social science) showed consistent differences among groups and similarities within groups in their emphasis on validity-related content. Adoption of such content in dissertations always preceded adoption in journal articles. Findings support the hypothesis that validity has been introduced and disseminated within fields predicted by the diffusion of innovations theory. It is argued that this pattern is inconsistent with an efficient and interdisciplinary utilization of available knowledge. Policy recommendations are made for developing strategic communication and educational programmes for academicians and journal reviewers (CR 2.92).

2.25.12   Papadopoulos, I., Scanlon, K. & Lees, S. (2002) Reporting and validating research findings through reconstructed stories. *Disability and Society* 17 (3) 269–81   17 References

Describes the use and rationale for reconstructed stories as a method for validating findings from interview data with visually impaired people. The use of this method is advocated as a user-friendly and effective means of presenting and validating qualitative research data.

2.25.13   Reason, P. & Rowan, J. (eds) (1981) Issues of validity in new paradigm research. In Authors *Human inquiry: a sourcebook of new paradigm research*. Chichester: Wiley   ISBN 0417279358   Chapter 21 239–50   References

Chapter gathers together material from a number of sources in order to create a coherent statement about the principles and practices that lead to a more valid inquiry within new paradigm research (CR 2.11.7).

2.25.14   Seale, C. (2001) Forum for applied cancer education and training. Qualitative methods: validity and reliability. *European Journal of Cancer Care* 10 (2) 131–6   11 References

Provides an overview of the need to improve the rigour of qualitative research and outlines the qualitative researcher's position on the substitution of qualitative criteria to replace validity and reliability (CR 2.24, 2.36).

2.25.15   Whitley, G.G. (1999) Processes and methodologies for research validation of nursing diagnoses. *Nursing Diagnosis* 10 (1) January–March 5–14   52 References

Provides a historical review of processes and methodologies for research validation of nursing diagnoses and makes suggestions for future research (CR 3.20).

2.25.16   Winter, G. (2000) A comparative discussion of the notion of 'validity' in qualitative and quantitative research. *The Qualitative Report* [Online serial] 4 (3/4) March [58 paragraphs]   18 References   www.nova.edu/ssss/QR/QR4-3/winter.html (Accessed 13/11/03)

Author aims to establish the use and nature of the term 'validity' in qualitative research and believes that it is not a single fixed or universal concept, but rather a contingent construct, inescapably grounded in the processes and intentions of particular research methodologies and projects. Problems of definition are discussed, the claims made by qualitative and quantitative researchers are compared and an attempt is made to establish an understanding of the nature of 'truth' that is central to any theorization of 'validity' (CR 2.36).

2.26   TRIANGULATION

'The purpose of using triangulation is to provide a basis for convergence on truth. By using multiple methods and perspectives it is hoped that "true" information can be sorted from "error" information. In the final analysis this is not conceptually different from the process of estimating reliability and validity by quantitative researchers.' (Polit & Hungler, 1995: 362)

Definitions [See Appendix D for sources]

Analysis triangulation – ... the use of two or more approaches to the analysis of the same set of data for the purpose of validation

Between-methods triangulation – the combination of research strategies using different methods

Data triangulation – use of a variety of multiple data sources in a study (e.g. interviewing multiple key informants about the same topic)

Interdisciplinary triangulation – ... using other disciplines ... to inform research processes ... which may broaden ... understanding of method and substance

Investigator triangulation – use of many individuals to collect and analyse a single set of data

Methodological triangulation – use of multiple methods to study a single problem (e.g. observation, interviews, inspection of documents)

Multiple triangulation – ... a complex form of triangulation that combines more than one type of triangulation into a study design

Theory triangulation – use of multiple perspectives to interpret a single set of data

Triangulation – the use of different research methods or sources of data to examine the same problem

Example

Campbell, S. & Whyte, F. (1999) The quality of life of cancer patients participating in phase 1 clinical trials using SEIQOL–DW. *Journal of Advanced Nursing* 30 (2) 335–43   29 References

Aim of this study was to examine the quality of life of cancer patients participating in phase 1 clinical trials. A descriptive triangulation approach was used. A secondary aim was to determine the acceptability of the Schedule for the Evaluation of Individual Quality of Life – Direct Weighting which is a new tool investigating the areas identified by individual patients as important to their quality of life (CR 2.17, 2.29, 2.55, 2.61, 2.68).

Annotations

2.26.1 Bechtel, G.A., Davidhizar, R. & Bunting, S. (2000) Triangulation research among culturally diverse populations. *Journal of Allied Health* 29 (2) 61–3   18 References

Triangulation offers an alternative for investigators studying transcultural health by integrating the inherent strengths of both quantitative and qualitative data while minimizing their limitations. This article discusses six approaches for employing triangulation research in transcultural health (CR 2.9, 2.53).

2.26.2 Campbell, D.T. & Fiske, D.W. (1959) Convergent and discriminant validation by the multitrait-multimethod matrix. *Psychological Bulletin* 56 (2) 81–105   References

This seminal paper advocates use of cumulative evaluations rather than single methods of measurement.

2.26.3 Docherty, B. (2000) Using triangulation in health-care research. *Professional Nurse* 16 (2) 926–7   11 References

Author suggests that combining research methods can be a useful approach to complex subjects. For example, using questionnaires, interviews and focus groups will provide robust study data (CR 2.68, 2.69, 2.75).

2.26.4 Foss, C. & Ellefsen, B. (2002) The value of combining qualitative and quantitative approaches in nursing research by means of method triangulation. *Journal of Advanced Nursing* 40 (2) 242–8   38 References

Article contributes to the debate on epistemological grounds of triangulation in nursing research (CR 2.6, 2.9, 2.29, 2.36).

2.26.5 Rees, C.E. & Bath, P.A. (2001) The use of between-methods triangulation in cancer nursing research: a case study examining information sources for partners of women with breast cancer. *Cancer Nursing* 24 (2) 104–11   68 References

The use of between-methods triangulation is illustrated by a case study that identified information sources for partners of women with breast cancer. By combining both qualitative and quantitative data, the study was found to have good convergent validity. It also provided a more complete picture of the topic than that supplied by either method alone (CR 2.9, 2.29, 2.36, 2.39).

2.26.6 Risjord, M., Moloney, M. & Dunbar, S. (2000) Methodological triangulation in nursing research. *Philosophy of the Social Sciences* 31 (1) 40–59   29 References

Nurse researchers investigate health phenomena using methods drawn from the natural and social sciences. The methodological debate concerns the possibility of confirming a single theory with different kinds of method. The nursing debate parallels the philosophical debate about how the natural and social sciences are related. The article critiques the suppositions of the nursing debate and suggests alternatives. The consequence is a view of triangulation that permits different methods to confirm a single theory. Also explored are the consequences for the philosophy of social science (CR 2.5, 2.9).

2.26.7 Risjord, M.W., Dunbar, S.B. & Moloney, M.F. (2002) A new foundation for methodological triangulation. *Journal of Nursing Scholarship* 34 (3) 269–75   22 References

Authors discuss how triangulation with qualitative and quantitative methods can confirm a theory to a greater degree than using either method alone (CR 2.29, 2.36).

2.26.8   Speziale, H.J.S. & Carpenter, D.R. (2003) Triangulation as a qualitative research strategy. In Authors *Qualitative research in nursing: advancing the humanistic imperative* (3rd edition). Philadelphia, PA: Lippincott Williams & Wilkins ISBN 0781734835 Chapter 15 299–308   20 References

Discusses the use of triangulation as a strategy and describes four types: data, investigator, theory and methodological triangulation (CR 2.36.132).

2.26.9   Thurmond, V.A. (2001) The point of triangulation. *Journal of Nursing Scholarship* 33 (3) 3rd Quarter 253–8   41 References

Author explores various types of triangulation strategy and indicates when different types should be used in research.

2.26.10   Wendler, M.C. (2001) Triangulation using a meta-matrix. *Journal of Advanced Nursing* 35 (4) 521–5   9 References

Purpose of this paper is to introduce and describe a meta-matrix method as a tool for triangulation in nursing research. Its value is demonstrated for complex data management, and secondary analysis of qualitative and quantitative data, in a study testing the impact of an emerging nursing therapeutic intervention (CR 2.29, 2.36, 2.91).

2.27   BIAS

A major consideration at many stages in any research project is the possibility of bias. If this factor is not taken into account, then the results may be distorted.

Definitions [See Appendix D for sources]

Attrition bias – ... systematic differences between comparison groups in the loss of participants from [a] study

Bias – ... a preference or predisposition to favour a particular conclusion

Detection bias – ... systematic differences between ... comparison groups in outcome assessment

Methodological quality – the extent to which the design and conduct of a study are likely to have prevented systematic errors (bias)

Observational bias – ... suggest[s] that observations are informed, even contaminated, by the beliefs, prejudices, and background assumptions of the observer(s)

Performance bias – ... systematic differences in the care provided to ... participants in ... comparison groups other than the intervention under investigation

Research bias – ... the systematic distortion of research conclusions

Selection bias – systematic differences in comparison groups

Example

Peeters, F. & Meijboom, A. (2000) Electrolyte and other blood serum abnormalities in normal weight bulimia nervosa: evidence for sampling bias. *International Journal of Eating Disorders* 27 (3) 358–62   12 References

Study examined the role of sampling bias in research settings, and results were compared with previous reports that showed that they had probably been affected. Authors conclude that it is therefore not necessary to perform routine laboratory studies in ambulatory patients with normal weight.

Annotations

2.27.1   Clarke, M. & Oxman, A.D. (eds) (2002) Bias in non-experimental studies. In Authors *Cochrane reviewers handbook*. Version 4.1.5 [Updated April 2002]. In: The Cochrane Library Issue 2 6.8 44–5 Oxford: Update Software

Section describes some issues that should be considered in assessing the validity of non-randomized studies. Four sources of bias are identified and discussed (CR 2.12).

2.27.2   Clarke, M. & Oxman, A.D. (eds) (2002) Sources of bias in trials of healthcare interventions. In Authors *Cochrane reviewers handbook*. Version 4.1.5 [Updated April 2002]. In: The Cochrane Library Issue 2 6.2 40–3 Oxford: Update Software

Discusses selection, performance, attrition and detection bias (CR 2.12, 2.29).

2.27.3 Day, S.J. & Altman, D.G. (2000) Blinding in clinical trials and other studies. *British Medical Journal* 321 (7259) 19–26 August 504   4 References

Explains why treatment allocation should not be revealed in randomized controlled trials in order to prevent selection bias (CR 2.29).

2.27.4 Drapeau, M. (2002) Subjectivity in research: why not? but ... *The Qualitative Report* 7 (3) 14 pp 58 References www.nova.edu/ssss/QR/QR7–3/drapeau.html (Accessed 13/11/03)

Discusses the use of peer debriefing as a strategy for dealing with subjectivity in qualitative research and gives an example to illustrate the approach (CR 2.36).

2.27.5 Earl-Slater, A. (2002) Types of bias and meaning. In Author *The handbook of clinical trials and other research*. Oxford: Radcliffe Medical Press ISBN 1857754859 39–43

Section contains an extensive list of types of bias, together with their meaning (CR 2.2.13).

2.27.6 Egger, M. & Smith, G.D. (1998) Bias in location and selection of studies. *British Medical Journal* 316 3 January 61–66 53 References

Examines various aspects of bias in relation to meta-analysis, but it also applies to all research studies. Elements discussed are bias in publication, location of studies, articles in the English language, databases, citations, multiple publication and provision of data. Ways of testing for bias are outlined (CR 2.92).

2.27.7 Gillis, A. & Jackson, W. (2002) Understanding bias. In Authors *Research for nurses: methods and interpretation*. Philadelphia, PA: F.A. Davis Co ISBN 0803608969 Part 3 Chapter 9 297–321 References

Chapter discusses the nature of bias, how it affects the research process, advocacy versus pure research, guidelines for minimizing bias and the gap between myth and reality (CR 2.1.34).

2.27.8 Hammersley, M. & Gomm, R. (1997) Bias in social research. *Sociological Research Online* 2 (1) 73 References www.socresonline.org.uk/socresonline/2/1/2.html (Accessed 13/11/03)

Discusses the ambiguous nature of the term 'bias' and the problems that result from this. Authors see the growing threat of bias in the present state of social research (CR 2.27.11).

2.27.9 Hewstone, M., Rubin, M. & Willis, H. (2002) Intergroup bias. *Annual Review of Psychology* 53 575–604 References

Chapter reviews the extensive literature on bias in favour of in-groups at the expense of out-groups. It focuses on five issues and identifies areas for future research (CR 2.12).

2.27.10 Roberts, C. & Torgerson D.J. (1999) Baseline imbalance in randomised controlled trials. *British Medical Journal* 319 (7203) 17 July 185   6 References

Explains how differences in in-group characteristics at the start of a study can produce bias in the results (CR 2.29).

2.27.11 Romm, N. (1997) Becoming more accountable: a comment on Hammersley & Gomm. *Sociological Research Online* 2 (3) 33 References www.socresonline.org.uk/socresonline/2/3/2.html (Accessed 13/11/03)

Author responds to Hammersley and Gomm's article entitled 'Bias in social research'. Their proposed conception of bias is rooted in a particular view of the pursuit of scientific knowledge, a view they call foundationalist. The way in which they arrive at this view is challenged as Romm believes their account excludes a serious consideration of alternative epistemological orientations (CR 2.6, 2.27.8).

2.27.12 Sadler, D.R. (2002) Intuitive data processing as a potential source of bias in naturalistic evaluations. In Huberman, A.M. & Miles. M.B. (eds) *The qualitative researcher's companion*. Thousand Oaks, CA: Sage ISBN 076191191X Chapter 6 123–35 47 References

Article classifies potential sources of bias. It draws the attention of naturalistic evaluators to some common failings that can serve as a checklist in reducing, integrating and drawing inferences from field data (CR 2.36.62).

2.27.13 Song, F., Eastwood, A., Gilbody, S., Duley, L. & Sutton, A. (2001) Publication and related biases. In Stevens, A., Abrams, K., Brazier, J., Fitzpatrick, R. & Lilford, R.J. (eds) *The advanced handbook of methods in evidence-based health care*. London: Sage ISBN 0761961445 Chapter 21 371–90 157 References

Chapter presents the results of studies that have examined methodological issues or provided empirical evidence concerning publication and related biases. Potential sources of bias are discussed and methods of dealing with them are described. Recommendations are made for future research (CR 2.43.69, 2.99).

2.27.14 Spiegelman, D. & Valanis, B. (1998) Correcting for bias in relative risk estimates due to exposure measurement error: a case study of occupational exposure to antineoplastics in pharmacists. *American Journal of Public Health* **88** (3) 406–12   36 References

Paper describes two statistical methods designed to correct for bias from exposure measurement error in point and interval estimates of relative risk.

2.28   GENERALIZABILITY

Generalizability refers to our efforts to compare the results of studies. An important research goal is to try to understand what is taking place in a general way during a series of events. One isolated event may have considerable importance, particularly in qualitative research, but the ability to extrapolate beyond the specifics is a characteristic of the scientific method.

Definitions [See Appendix D for sources]

Empirical generalization – ... the application of findings from qualitative studies to populations or settings beyond the particular sample of the study

Fuzzy generalization – ... a kind of statement which makes no absolute claim to knowledge, but hedges its claims and uncertainties [...it arises from studies of singularities and typically claims that 'it is possible, or likely, or unlikely that' what was found in the singularity will be found in similar studies elsewhere – it is a qualitative measure]

Generalizability (applicability) – ... the degree to which the results of a study or systematic review can be extrapolated to other circumstances, in particular to routine health care situations

Inferential generalization – ... generalizing from the context of the research study itself to other settings or contexts

Representational generalization – ... the extent to which findings can be inferred to the parent population that was sampled

Scientific generalization – ... a statement that had to be absolutely true [the basis of the concept of scientific method ... in which a hypothesis stands as a generalization (or law) only if it withstands all attempts at refutation]

Statistical generalization – ... expresses the chance that something will be the case [...it arises from samples of populations and typically

claims that 'there is an x per cent or y per cent chance that' what was found in the sample will also be found throughout the population – it is a quantitative measure]

Theoretical generalization – ... draws theoretical propositions, principles or statements from the findings of a study for more general application

Theory building – ... the generation of theoretical concepts or propositions which are deemed to be of wider or even universal application

Example

Geertzen, J.H.B., Dijkstra, P.U., Stewart, R.E., Groothoff, J.W., ten Duis, H.J. & Eisma, W.H. (1998) Variation in measurements of range and motion: a study in reflex sympathetic dystrophy patients. *Clinical Rehabilitation* 12 (3) 254–64   25 References

Study aimed to quantify the amount of variation attributed to different sources in measurement results of upper extremity range of motion, and to estimate the smallest detectable differences in reflex sympathetic dystrophy patients. The measurement results were analysed using an analysis of variance according to the generalizability theory. Results are reported (CR 2.36).

Annotations

2.28.1 Brennan, R.L., Fienberg, S., Lievesley, D. & Rolph, J. (2001) *Generalizability theory.* New York: Springer Verlag   ISBN 0387952829 References

This book provides an up-to date treatment of generalizabilty theory. In addition, it provides a synthesis of those parts of the statistical literature that are directly applicable to this theory.

2.28.2 Fuller, B.F. & Neu, M. (2001) Generalizability and clinical utility of a practice-based infant pain assessment. *Clinical Nursing Research* 10 (2) May 122–39   30 References

Study aimed to determine the clinical usefulness and generalizability of an infant pain assessment tool. The ways in which this was determined is discussed and results showed it was excellent (CR 2.61).

2.28.3 Hayes, P. (1998) The issue of generalizability. *Clinical Nursing Research* 7 (3) 227–9 Editorial

Discusses the issues of generalizability and replication studies in nursing research. Nurses are urged to consider undertaking more replication research projects (CR 2.13).

2.28.4   Myers, M. (2000) Qualitative research and the generalizability question: standing firm with Proteus. *The Qualitative Report* [Online serial] 4 (3/4) 30 Paragraphs www.nova.edu/ssss/QR/QR4-3/ myers.html (Accessed 13/11/03)

Discusses criticisms of qualitative research studies, generalizations and demands for justification. Paper acknowledges that small-scale qualitative studies are not generalizable in the traditional sense, yet have redeeming qualities that set them above that requirement (CR 2.36).

2.28.5   Ozga, J. (2000) Resources for policy research. In Author *Policy research in educational settings: contested terrain*. Buckingham: Open University Press   ISBN 0335202950   Chapter 5 90–4   References

Discusses the process of generalization, and literature is examined that highlights its appropriate use, or otherwise, in both qualitative and quantitative research (CR 3.11.14).

2.28.6   Ritchie, J. & Lewis, J. (2003) Generalising from qualitative research. In Authors (eds) *Qualitative research practice: a guide for social science students and researchers*. London: Sage   ISBN 0761971106   Chapter 10 263–86 References

Provides definitions of generalization, approaches to it, reliability and validity, generalizing from qualitative data and discusses its associated complexities (CR 2.24, 2.25, 2.36.113).

2.28.7   Robinson, J.E. & Norris, N.P.J. (2001) Generalisation: the lynchpin of evidence-based practice? *Educational Action Research* 9 (2) 303–9 27 References

Authors discuss several ways of understanding the concept of generalization. Until recently, only conventional understandings were used in determining the best evidence to underpin policy and practice. However, this notion of the 'best evidence', or discrimination on the basis of perceived quality, has been central to the ideological notion of evidence-based practice. If generalizability is to remain a central criterion for establishing the quality of evidence, as is the case for medicine and much health care research, then alternative ways of understanding

generalization must be considered at the same time (CR 2.102).

2.28.8   Schofield, J.W. (2002) Increasing the generalizability of qualitative research. In Huberman, A.M. & Miles, M.B. (eds) *The qualitative researcher's companion*. Thousand Oaks, CA: Sage   ISBN 076191191X   Chapter 8 171–203   77 References

Paper suggests that there are three useful targets for generalizability: what is, what may be and what could be. It gives examples of how qualitative research can be designed in a way that increases its ability to fit with each of these situations (CR 2.36.62).

2.28.9   Sharp, K. (1998) The case for case studies in nursing research: the problem of generalization. *Journal of Advanced Nursing* 27 (4) 785–9   14 References

Paper examines the logic of generalizing from case studies and other non-representative samples. It is argued that the generalizability is often underestimated because of a fundamental confusion about two distinct logical bases upon which generalizations can be made – empirical and theoretical. Once it is accepted that theoretical generalizations do not depend on representativeness for their validity, the full value of case study and other small-scale qualitative research can be appreciated.

2.28.10   Shavelson, R.J. & Webb, N.M. (1991) *Generalizability theory: a primer*. Newbury Park, CA: Sage   ISBN 0803937458   References

Discusses the underlying concepts and development of genaralizability theory, and assists readers in applying measurement methods that will encourage consistency.

2.28.11   Trochim, W. *The generalizability of research data: a guide for the novice researcher* trochim.human.cornell.edu/tutorial/ward/tutorial. htm (Accessed 12/03/03)

Tutorial explores the meaning of generalizability and how it can best be understood in the social sciences.

2.28.12   Writing @ CSU *Writing guide* writing. colostate.edu/references/research/gentrans/ (Accessed 07/05/03)

Provides an overview of generalizability, transferability, synthesis and applications to research.

Experimental/Quantitative Designs

2.29 EXPERIMENTAL DESIGNS – GENERAL

Experimental research involves the active manipulation of variables under the control of the researcher. This approach attempts to study how subjects will react to the manipulated conditions through monitoring one or more outcome measure(s). If an experiment is well designed, the experimenter may, in principle, detect causal relationships between variables. However, there are many threats to the satisfactory detection of such relationships.

Definitions [See Appendix D for sources]

CONSORT – ... an acronym for Consolidated Standard of Reporting Trials

Control group – the subjects who are not exposed to the experimental treatment

Controlled clinical trial – ... a study that compares one or more intervention groups to one or more comparison (control) groups. [While not all controlled studies are randomised, all randomised trials are controlled]

Cross-over trial – a type of clinical trial comparing two or more interventions in which the participants, upon completion of the course of one treatment, are switched to another

Double-blind trial – an experimental procedure, used particularly in drug trials, to guard against bias ... neither the subjects nor the person gathering the data are aware which treatments are being given to which subjects

Dual-blind – a methodological alternative [to double-blind trial] in which the caregiver is not blind but the patient and an external evaluator/ investigator are [The term 'double-blind' should be used strictly to describe a methodology in which both the patient and the caregiver are blind]

Experiment – ... is characterized by randomisation, manipulation and control

---

Multi-centre trials – the replication of a randomised clinical trial in several different settings to increase the level of confidence in research findings

Placebo – an inactive substance or procedure administered to a patient, usually to compare its effect with those of a real drug or other intervention, but sometimes for the psychological benefit to the patient through a belief that he/she is receiving treatment

Placebo effect – a favourable response to an intervention, regardless of whether it is the real thing or a placebo, attributable to the expectation of the effect, i.e. the power of suggestion [The effects of many health care interventions are attributable to a combination of both placebo and 'active' (non-placebo) effects]

Randomised clinical trial – ... a form of experimental research in which the effects of one or more treatments (interventions) are compared with a control 'treatment' by randomly assigning study subjects to the groups and measuring the differences in effects (outcomes) of the alternative treatments over time

Run-in period – a period before a trial is commenced when no treatment is given [The data from this stage of the trial are only occasionally of value but can serve to screen out ineligible or non-compliant participants, ensure that participants are in a stable condition, and provide baseline observations. A run-in period is sometimes called a washout period if treatments that participants were using before entering the trial are discontinued]

Sequential trial – a trial in which data are analysed after each participant's results become available, and the trial continues until a clear benefit is seen in one of the comparison groups, or it is unlikely that any difference will emerge [The main advantage of sequential trials is that they will be shorter than fixed-length trials when there is a large difference in the effectiveness of the interventions being compared. Their use is restricted to conditions where the outcome of interest is known relatively quickly]

Single-blind trial – the investigator is aware of the treatment/intervention the participant is getting, but the participant is unaware

Tracker trials – ... trials which start early on in periods of rapid technological change and which follow and inform developments

Trials register – in the Cochrane Collaboration, this is a database of bibliographic references to randomized controlled trials and controlled clinical trials relevant to a Collaborative Review Group of Field, which is maintained at the editorial base

Zelen consent design – participants are randomly allocated prior to seeking consent [Also known as pre-randomization/post-randomization design]

Annotations

2.29.1 Adèr, H.J. & Mellenbergh, G.J. (eds) (1999) *Research methodology in the social, behavioural and life sciences: designs, models and methods.* London: Sage ISBN 0761958843 References

Text for advanced courses in research methods and experimental design. Leading experts explain the fundamentals of the research process to enable students to understand the broader implications and unifying themes.

2.29.2 Altman, D.G. & Bland, M.J. (1999) How to randomise. *British Medical Journal* 319 (7211) 11 September 703–4 3 References

Describes the process of generating random allocation sequences and explains how stratified randomization can assist the researcher in achieving a balance of important characteristics between groups.

2.29.3 Altman, D.G. & Bland, M.J. (1999) Treatment allocation on controlled trials: why randomise? *British Medical Journal* 318 (7192) 1 May 1209 7 References

Identifies the problems that occur when researchers fail to randomize or do not randomize properly.

2.29.4 Altman, D.G. & Schulz, K.F. (2001) Concealing treatment allocation in randomised trials. *British Medical Journal* 323 (7310) 25 August 446–7 8 References

Considers the importance of concealing treatment allocation until the subject is entered into the trial and explains the difference between this and double-blinding.

2.29.5 Andrews, G. (1999) Randomized controlled trials in psychiatry: important but poorly accepted. *British Medical Journal* 319 (7209) 28 August 562–4 19 References

Paper states that there are good randomized controlled trials in psychiatry, but as psychological treatments are difficult to standardize, and disability is a difficult endpoint to measure, small trials are susceptible to bias. In Australia, evidence-based guidelines in mental health have been developed but psychiatry seems nervous about proceeding with the implementation of clinical practice guidelines on the evidence from randomized controlled trials. This dilemma is discussed (CR 2.27).

2.29.6 Benson, K. & Hartz, A.J. (2000) A comparison of observational studies and randomized controlled trials. *New England Journal of Medicine* 342 (25) 1878–86 79 References

Paper investigated the claim that observational studies produce stronger treatment effects than randomized controlled trials. The study combined the magnitude of effects for each on a total of 136 studies comparing 19 treatments and found that there was little evidence to support any difference in reporting (CR 2.72).

2.29.7 Black, T.R. (1999) *Doing quantitative research in the social sciences: an integrated approach to research design, measurement and statistics.* London: Sage ISBN 0761953531 References

Book focuses on the design and execution of research, including the key topics of planning, sampling, design of measuring instruments, choice of statistical test and interpretation of results (CR 2.14, 2.22, 2.83, 2.93).

2.29.8 Blackwood, B. & Lavery, G. (1998) The crossover study design and its clinical application. *Nurse Researcher* 5 (4) 5–14 13 References

Paper describes the cross-over design as used in a study on an intensive care unit. The design is described and problems with its use discussed. The authors believe that it is a serious option for nurse researchers working with small sample sizes.

2.29.9 Braunstein, M.S. (1998) Evaluation of nursing practice: process and critique. *Nursing Science Quarterly* 11 (2) Summer 64–8 16 References

Article describes the difficulties in conducting clinical trials to evaluate nursing practice models. A trial of a nursing practice model, based on a synthesis of Aristotelian theory with Rogers' science, is described. The rationale for decisions regarding research procedures and methodological limitations of the study design are examined. Clear specification of theoretical relationships within a practice model and clear identification of key intervening variables will enable researchers to better connect the treatment with the outcome (CR 2.7, 2.19).

2.29.10   Canadian Institutes of Health Research
National placebo initiative/www.cihr-irsc.gc.ca/services/initiatives/placebo/about_e.shtml (Accessed 24/01/03)

Reports on the establishment of a joint initiative to determine appropriate placebo use in clinical trials in Canada. Its objectives are: to advance the debate on placebos both nationally and internationally; to conduct stakeholder and public consultations on what constitutes appropriate placebo use; to reach a Canadian consensus on what constitutes ethical and scientifically appropriate use of placebos; to make a report that reflects that debate and consensus; and to make recommendations to Health Canada and CIHR regarding a common placebo policy. The final report will be posted on the website (CR 2.17).

2.29.11   Caspi, O., Millen, C. & Sechrest, L. (2000) Integrity and research: introducing the concept of dual blindness. How blind are double-blind clinical trials in alternative medicine?*Journal of Alternative and Complementary Medicine* 6 (6) 493–8   43 References

Double-blind methodology is used to maintain as much objectivity as possible on the part of researchers. Despite not being feasible in all medical disciplines, numerous studies spuriously claim its use. A new term ('dual-blind') is suggested to describe a methodological alternative in which the caregiver is not blind but the patient and an external evaluator/investigator are. Making this distinction should result in more reliable reports of clinical trials and will support integrity in research.

2.29.12   *Clinical trials dictionary: terminology and usage recommendations* (1996) Edited by Meinert, C.L. Baltimore, MD: Meinert Curtis ISBN 0964642409

This dictionary defines a large and complex vocabulary used to describe the methods and results of clinical trials. An index to the main entries facilitates the finding of terms associated with particular concepts and steps occurring during clinical trials. A section on usage provides illuminating discourse on nuances in the rhetoric of scientific speech and writing (CR 2.2).

2.29.13   ClinicalTrials.gov *An Introduction to clinical trials: linking patients to medical research* clinicaltrials.gov/ct/gui.info/whatis;jsessionid=E0F4AEFAE876DCE56D938008C

Paper presents questions that are frequently asked by patients who are invited to participate in a clinical trial. A glossary of clinical trials terms, general information, and links to specific websites are also included (CR 2.2, 2.17).

2.29.14   Concato, J., Shah, N. & Horwitz, R.I. (2000) Randomized, controlled trials, observational studies and the hierarchy of research designs. *New England Journal of Medicine* 342 (25) 1887–92   32 References

Authors used published meta-analyses to identify randomized controlled trials and observational studies that examined the same clinical topics. A comparison of the results led to the conclusion that well-designed observational studies do not systematically overestimate the magnitude of treatment effects compared with randomized controlled trials (CR 2.72, 2.92).

2.29.15   Conn, V.S., Rantz, M.J., Wipke-Tevis, D.D. & Maas, M.L. (2001) Designing effective nursing interventions. *Research in Nursing and Health* 24 (5) 433–22   58 References

Explains the conceptual basis of nursing interventions, highlighting their potential inadequacy and lack of validity. Eight developmental issues are discussed, and strategies are recommended for designing effective experimental interventions.

2.29.16   Cox, K. (1999) Researching research: patients' experiences of participation in phase 1 and 2 anti-cancer drug trials. *European Journal of Oncology Nursing* 3 (3) 143–52   37 References

Despite the ethical and practical dilemmas associated with early anti-cancer drug trials, little is known about their impact from the participant's perspective. The key findings from a one-year study that examined the views of 55 patients are reported. The consequences of trial involvement, previously hidden, are examined and findings can be used to guide and inform clinical practice (CR 2.16, 2.22).

2.29.17   Day, S.J. & Altman D.G. (2000) Blinding in clinical trials and other studies. *British Medical Journal* 321 (7259) 19–26 August 504   4 References

Explains the purpose and use of blinding in research studies.

2.29.18   *Dictionary for Clinical Trials* (1999) Edited by Day, S. Chichester: Wiley ISBN 0471986119

This dictionary provides a comprehensive guide to clinical trial terminology. Explanations and definitions normally found in clinical trial protocols, reports, regulatory guidelines and published manuscripts are given in jargon-free language (CR 2.2).

2.29.19   Duley, L. & Farrell, B. (eds) (2001) *Clinical trials.* London: BMJ Books ISBN 0727915991   References

Book covers the major issues involved in conducting of clinical trials.

2.29.20   Earl-Slater, A. (2001) The new CONSORT system. *British Journal of Clinical Governance* 6 (3) 211–17   23 References

The framework for the consolidated standard of reporting trials is outlined, together with its key strengths and limitations. The author suggests that around 80 journals will adopt this style of reporting (CR 2.2.13).

2.29.21   Earl-Slater, A. (2002) History of clinical trials.In Author *The handbook of clinical trials and other research.* Oxford: Radclife Medical Press ISBN 1857754859   158

Lists materials on a website (www.rcpe.org) for those interested in the history of clinical trials (CR 2.2.13). www.rcpe.org

2.29.22   Faithfull, S. (1999) Randomized trial, a method of comparisons: a study of supportive care in radiotherapy nursing. *European Journal of Oncology Nursing* 3 (3)176–84   30 References

Article explores some of the advantages and difficulties that can be encountered when undertaking a randomized trial, and reflects on its practical implications. This trial was used to evaluate the effectiveness of a nursing intervention relating to the side-effects of radiotherapy and results were compared with conventional medical care.

2.29.23   Field, A. & Hole, G.J. (2002) *How to design and report experiments.* London: Sage.   ISBN 0761973834   References

Textbook guides readers through the often bewildering process of experimental design and statistics. It provides a map of the entire process, beginning with how to get ideas about research, how to refine the research question, and the actual design of the experiment, leading on to statistical procedure and assistance with writing up results (CR 2.4, 2.14, 2.20, 2.97).

2.29.24   Field, D. & Elbourne, D. (2003) The randomized controlled trial. *Current Paediatrics* 13 (1) 53–7   17 References

Outlines the process of conducting a randomized controlled trial, including issues of blinding, sampling and ethics. Discusses the organization and reporting of trials (CR 2.17, 2.22).

2.29.25   Gatchel, R. J. & Maddrey, A.M. (1998) Clinical outcome research in complementary and alternative medicine: an overview of experimental design and analysis. *Alternative Therapies in Health and Medicine* 4 (5) 4 September 36–42   40 References

Provides an overview of the important experimental design and statistical issues of which those in the field of complementary and alternative medicine must be aware when attempting to demonstrate the effectiveness of particular treatment modalities. Key concepts, such as internal validity, statistical conclusion validity and the appropriate measurement and operational definitions of outcomes, are discussed. New scientific approaches that are evolving because of paradigm shifts in science (e.g. chaos theory) are also reviewed (CR 2.7, 2.20, 2.25, 2.43).

2.29.26   Getliffe, K. (1998) Developing a protocol for a randomized controlled trial: factors to consider. *Nurse Researcher* 6 (1) 5–17   15 References

Article discusses the issues involved in developing a robust randomized controlled trial (CR 2.14).

2.29.27   Giffels, J.J. (1996) *Clinical trials: what you should know before volunteering to be a research subject.* New York: Demos ISBN 1888799021

This booklet is designed for use in clinical trials of all new therapies. It will help patients to understand some of the basics of clinical research, providing answers to all key questions (CR 2.17, 2.22).

2.29.28   Gross, D. & Fogg, L. (2001) Clinical trials in the 21st century: the case for participant-centered research. *Research in Nursing & Health* 24 (6) 530–9   49 References

Advises that informed consumers will not be as willing to enter randomized controlled trials (RCTs) and, in order to remedy this, suggestions are made concerning how to make them more participant-centred. The suggestions include revising notions of validity, involving consumers in construction of studies and offering alternatives to randomization (CR 2.25).

2.29.29   Guess, H., Kleinman, A., Kusek, J. & Engal, L. (eds) (2002) *The science of the placebo*: *towards an inter-disciplinary research agenda.* London: BMJ Books   ISBN 0727915940   References

World-renowned researchers examine the biological, behavioural, cultural, social and ethical aspects of the placebo effect, and its place in clinical trials (CR 2.15, 2.17).

2.29.30   Hart, A. (2001) Randomized clinical trials: the control group dilemma revisited. *Complementary Therapies in Medicine* 9 (1) 40–4 31 References

In some clinical trials the nature of therapy means that subjects cannot and should not be blinded and such studies need very careful design. Particular attention should be given to the choice of control group and the nature of informed consent because these affect the precise research questions being addressed. A survey was carried out to investigate how these issues had been tackled and key findings are summarized. If the research question is about a specific effect of the therapy, a good case can be made for a second control group that is 'attention-controlled' (CR 2.17, 2.52).

2.29.31 Haslam, A. & McGarty, C. (2003) *Research methods and statistics in psychology.* London: Sage ISBN 0761942939 References

Book provides an introduction to the principal research methods and statistical procedures that underpin psychological research. Key features of this edition are: chapters on ANOVA, Chi-square and distribution-free tests, qualitative methods and analysis; an accompanying website; checklists, discussion questions and exercises; further reading; writing lab reports and multiple-choice questions (CR 2.36, 2.87).

2.29.32 Hicks, C. (1998) The randomized controlled trial: a critique. *Nurse Researcher* 6 (1) 19–32   24 References

Article questions the frequent uncritical attitude towards randomized controlled trials, seen as the unquestioned 'gold standard' for evidence-based health care. Author suggests a more balanced appraisal of their strengths and weaknesses, relative to non-experimental and quasi-experimental designs, as these methods also have a considerable contribution to make to investigations of nursing care (CR 2.35, 2.36).

2.29.33 Hicks, C. (1999) *Research methods for therapists: applied project design and analysis* (3rd edition). Edinburgh: Churchill Livingstone ISBN 0443062668 References

Book provides a jargon-free introduction to a number of research methods, mainly quantitative, directly related to the clinical situation (CR 2.2).

2.29.34 Holden, J.D. (2001) Hawthorne effects and research into professional practice. *Journal of Evaluation in Clinical Practice* 7 (1) 65–70   21 References

Suggests that there is no single phenomenon called the Hawthorne effect and poses that triangulation processes could be used more effectively. It includes a history of the seven studies conducted at the Hawthorne telephone equipment plant (CR 2.26).

2.29.35 Homer, C.S.E. (2002) Using the Zelen design in randomized controlled trials: debates and controversies. *Journal of Advanced Nursing* 38 (2) 200–7   43 References

The use of randomized consent (Zelen) design is explained, together with its advantages and disadvantages, ethical considerations and the controversy surrounding it.

2.29.36 Hubbard, S.M. & Setser, A. (2001) The cancer informatics infrastructure: a new initiative of the National Cancer Institute. *Seminars in Oncology Nursing* 17 (1) 55–61   16 References

Clinical trials represent the primary mechanism for evaluating promising new strategies to prevent, diagnose and treat cancer. Advances in information technology and the exponential increase in the use of the Internet are providing opportunities to streamline the operation and administration of the clinical trials supported by the National Cancer Institute. The revitalized system will facilitate input from oncology nurses and others committed to improving cancer care (CR 2.85).

2.29.37 Jadad, A.R. (1998) *Randomised controlled trials.* London: BMJ Books ISBN 0727912089 References

Text is written for those interested in the use of clinical trials in clinical, research or policy decisions. It includes answers to the 100 most frequently asked questions and has a non-statistical approach (CR 3.11).

2.29.38 Jüni, P., Altman, D.G. & Egger, M. (2001) Assessing the quality of controlled clinical trials. *British Medical Journal* 323 (7303) 7 July 42–6   37 References

The quality of controlled trials is of obvious relevance to systematic reviews. If the 'raw material' is flawed, then the conclusions of systematic reviews cannot be trusted. This article discusses the concept of study quality and the methods used to assess quality (CR 2.12, 2.24, 2.25, 2.27, 2.92).

2.29.39 Kerlinger, F.N. & Lee, H.B. (1999) *Foundations of behavioural research* (4th edition). Belmont, CA: Wadsworth ISBN 0155078976 References

Text examines the fundamentals of solving a scientific research problem, focusing on the relationship between the problem and research design. New information is included about computer statistical software, multivariate statistics, research ethics and writing reports (CR 2.17, 2.97, Appendix A).

2.29.40 Kienle, G.S. & Kiene, H. (1998) The placebo effect: a scientific critique … adapted from a paper published in the *Journal of Clinical Epidemiology* 1997 50 (12) 1311–18. *Complementary Therapies in Medicine* 6 (1) 14–24 90 References

The existence of so-called placebo effects, where the administration of an inert substance or imitation therapy brings about therapeutic change, seems to have been accepted without question in the biomedical community. Seminal review articles, such as Henry Beecher's *The Powerful Placebo*, are often said to constitute the scientific basis of a belief in placebo effects. The authors believe that these studies do not provide evidence of a placebo effect (CR 2.27).

2.29.41   Kirk-Smith, M.D. & Stretch, D.D. (2001) Evidence-based medicine and randomised double-blind clinical trials: a study of flawed implementation. *Journal of Evaluation in Clinical Practice* 7 (2) May 119–23   References

The randomized double-blind clinical trial (RDBCT) can have anomalous and inexplicable results, which have prompted suggestions that 'unknown and unidentifiable biases' may exist. The paper identifies a possible flaw that may account for this and suggests how it may be overcome (CR 2.27).

2.29.42   Knapp, T.R. (1998) *Quantitative nursing research*. Thousand Oaks, CA: Sage   ISBN 0761913637   References

This textbook on quantitative research methods is intended for masters and doctoral students. Numerous examples, guides for further reading and exercises are included.

2.29.43   Lilford, R.J., Braunholtz, D.A., Greenhalgh, R. & Edwards, S.J.L. (2000) Trials and fast-changing technologies: the case for tracker studies. *British Medical Journal* 320 (7226) January 1 43–6   32 References

Evaluating treatments is difficult when developments or variants arise frequently. In these circumstances randomized controlled trials should not await stability, but should track progress over time, providing unbiased comparisons at each stage. These 'tracker trials' should be guided by flexible protocols, without prefixed sample size (or duration), and will require sophisticated interim analyses. They will ensure the maximum use of information after it has stabilized, and monitor treatments and centres to detect poor performance quickly and to provide an effective early warning system.

2.29.44   Martin, C.R. & Thompson, D.R. (2000) *Design and analysis of clinical nursing research studies*. London: Routledge   ISBN 041522599X References

Text explains the basics of experimental design and statistics in a way that is sensitive to the clinical context within which nurses work. Data from actual studies are used and the authors show how qualitative data can be approached quantitatively, and how the advantages of using quantitative methodology can help nurses develop a common language with other disciplines (CR 2.9, 2.36).

2.29.45   Maxim, P.S. (1999) *Quantitative research methods in the social sciences*. New York: Oxford University Press   ISBN 0195114655 References

Designed for first-year undergraduates, this text reviews general statistical theory and methods, and explores potential problems.

2.29.46   National Institutes of Health (2002) *Clinical trials: linking patients to medical research.* Bethesda, MD: National Library of Medicine   www. ClinicalTrials.gov (Accessed 21/08/02)

Website provides answers to frequently asked questions for patients who may be asked or wish to participate in clinical trials (CR 2.2, 2.17).

2.29.47   Oakley, A. (2000) A historical perspective on the use of randomised trials in social science settings. *Crime and Deliquency* 46 (3) 315–29   93 References

Discusses the quantitative–qualitative debate in relation to medicine and sociology and traces the development of quantitative sociology in North America. It illustrates how experimental studies retain importance within the social sciences (CR 2.9).

2.29.48   O'Connell, D., Glasziou, P., Hill, S., Sarunac, J., Lowe, J. & Henry, D. (2001) Results of clinical trials and systematic reviews: to whom do they apply? In Stevens, A., Abrams, K., Brazier, J., Fitzpatrick, R. & Lilford, R. (eds) *The advanced handbook of methods in evidence-based health care.* London: Sage   ISBN 0761961445   Chapters 4 56–72   92 References

Chapter defines the methods currently suggested for applying clinical trial results in clinical practice. It assesses the strengths and weaknesses of these approaches and develops an appropriate method for applying results to individual patients, based on consideration of benefit and risk. The implications for design and reporting of clinical trials are discussed, together with the development of clinical guidelines (CR 2.12, 2.43.69).

2.29.49   Peat, J. (2002) *Health science research: a handbook of quantitative methods*. London: Sage/ Allen & Unwin   ISBN 0761974032   References

Book covers the planning, execution and appraisal of quantitative research studies. It also includes advice on preparing a grant application (CR 2.41, 2.96).

2.29.50 Pennings, P., Keman, H. & Kleinnijenhuis, J. (1999) *Doing research in political science: an introduction to comparative methods and statistics*. London: Sage   ISBN 0761951032   References

This introduction to methods and statistics gives a step-by-step guide to undertaking political research and incorporates summary questions, practice exercises, a glossary and further reading (CR 2.2).

2.29.51 Playle, J. (2000) Experimental designs in research. *Journal of Community Nursing* 14 (7) 6, 8, 10, 13   17 References

Explains the nature of experiments, manipulation, randomization, control and measurement, and provides an overview of some common experimental designs used in social research (CR 2.3, 2.31, 2.32, 2.33).

2.29.52 Prescott, R. (2001) Factors that limit the quality, number and progress of randomized controlled trials www.doh.gov.uk/research (Accessed 30/07/01) [Project-related website: www.hta.nhsweb.nhs.uk]

Literature from 1986 to 1996 was examined for factors limiting the quality, number and progress of randomized controlled trials. Issues covered included design, barriers to participation, conduct and structure, analysis, reporting and costs (CR 2.12).

2.29.53 Raven, A. (1997) *Consider it pure joy: an introduction to clinical trials*. Cambridge: Cambridge Healthcare Research Ltd.   ISBN 0951739611

Defines terms, processes, regulatory bodies and general concepts (CR 2.2).

2.29.54 Reiffel, J.A. (2000) The importance of considering trial design when interpreting clinical trial results. *Journal of Cardiovascular Pharmacological Therapy* 5 (1) January 17–25 References

The results of clinical trials are often affected by biases or design issues that may overtly or covertly alter the results or the way they should be evaluated. In addition, these biases and design analysis issues are rarely evident in abstracts or key figures and tables in the publications reporting the trials that may be all that busy people read. The author discusses the issues involved in optimally understanding clinical trial design and interpretation so that practitioners can better understand how to apply results to clinical practice (CR 2.27, 2.95).

2.29.55 Rothwell, H. (1999) A beginner's picture of research (iv): experimental research methods. *Practising Midwife* 2 (3) 32–5   4 References

Uses a practical example from midwifery to explain the experimental approach (CR 2.14, 2.24).

2.29.56 Shuldham, C. (1999) Pre-operative education: a review of research design. *International Journal of Nursing Studies* 36 (2) 179–87   61 References

Paper examines the research literature on pre-operative education in the light of modern standards in design and reporting of randomized controlled trials. Features considered were patient assignment, blinding of participants and researchers, follow-up procedures, statistical analysis, theoretical frameworks and ethical issues. The author believes that there is room for improvement in trial design as a basis for promoting evidence-based nursing. (CR 2.12, 2.14, 2.17).

2.29.57 Sims, J. & Miracle, V.A. (2002) Phases of a clinical trial. *Dimensions of Critical Care Nursing* 21 (4) 152–3   4 References

Explains the nature of clinical trials and the four phases used to introduce new treatments into practice (CR 2.102).

2.29.58 Thompson, D. & Martin, C.R. (2000) *Design and analysis of clinical nursing research studies*. London: Routledge   ISBN 041522599X   References

Text explains the basics of experimental design and statistics in a way that is sensitive to the clinical context within which nurses work. Data from actual studies are used, and the authors show how qualitative data can be approached quantitatively, and how the advantages of using quantitative methodology can help nurses develop a common language with other disciplines (CR 2.9).

2.29.59 Tonks, A. (1999) Registering clinical trials. *British Medical Journal* 319 (7224) 11 December 1565–8   9 References

Existing trial registers are not standardized, it is argued, and there are few incentives for researchers to register. The author demands the registration of clinical trials to promote openness and collaboration and prevent duplication and bias (CR 2.27).

2.29.60 Venkatraman, P., Anand, S., Dean, C. & Nettleton, R. (2002a) Clinical trials in wound care I: the advantages and limitations of different trial designs. *Journal of Wound Care* 11 (3) 91–4   16 References

Explains the major designs in clinical trials and how choice of design depends on the research question. Examines common mistakes in studies, such as population and sampling bias, loss of blinding and choice of statistical testing (CR 2.27).

2.29.61   Venkatraman, P., Anand, S., Dean, C. & Nettleton, R. (2002b) Clinical trials in wound care ll: achieving statistical significance. *Journal of Wound Care* 11 (4) 156–60   23 References

Outlines the steps required to design an appropriate trial in order to produce statistically and clinically significant results, including randomization, blinding, effect size, sample size, and type l and type ll error (CR 2.87).

2.29.62   Watson, R. (1998) Longitudinal quantitative research designs. *Nurse Researcher* 5 (4) 41–54   12 References

Presents the advantages and problems associated with longitudinal quantitative research designs. Paper argues that the effects of time on the subjects can be studied better than in cross-sectional designs, but there is also the problem of keeping subjects in the study (CR 2.48).

2.29.63   Whitney, J.D. (2000a) Spotlight on research basics of designing a clinical trial: Part 1 *Journal of WOCN* 27 (5) 257–9   5 References

Provides a background to clinical trials and discusses issues of sample size, eligibility, randomization and masking (CR 2.22).

2.29.64   Whitney, J.D. (2000b) Spotlight on research basics of designing a clinical trial: Part 2. *Journal of WOCN* 27 (6) 293–5   5 References

Explores the issues of outcome measures, adherence to treatment and data analysis.

2.29.65   Wolff, N. (2001) Randomised trials of socially complex interventions: promise or peril? *Journal of Health Service Research and Policy* 6 (2) 123–6   9 References

Examines the use of a randomized controlled trial where the interventions are complex and socially derived. It advocates that more attention is needed to avoid selection bias and awareness of unmeasured contextual variables and uncontrolled interaction effects. It recommends that where complex social interventions are evaluated, complex contextual evaluation using multiple sites should be utilized.

Experimental Designs

Sections 2.30–2.34 illustrate four types of experimental design. The use of standard notation is helpful in understanding alternative experimental designs.

R = Random assignment of subjects to experimental and control groups
O = Observation or measurement (O1 pre-test/O2 post-test)
X = Treatment or intervention

2.30 PRE-TEST/POST-TEST DESIGN

Measurements of the outcomes or dependent variables are taken both before and after the intervention. This allows the measurement of change in individual cases.

R O1 X O2 Experimental group
R O3 O4 Control group

The measurement process may influence change, thereby introducing difficulties in attributing this to the intervention on its own.

Example

de Rond, M., de Wit, R. & van Dam, F. (2001) The implementation of a pain monitoring programme for nurses in daily clinical practice: results of a follow-up study in five hospitals. *Journal of Advanced Nursing* 35 (4) 590–8   34 References

Using a pre-test–post-test design, this study investigated whether implementing a Pain Monitoring Programme is feasible in clinical practice. In addition, nurses' and physicians' pain knowledge and attitudes were studied as well as change in nurses' pain knowledge after implementation of the programme. Results are reported.

Annotations

2.30.1 Dixon, J. (1984) Effects of nursing intervention on nutritional and performance status in cancer patients. *Nursing Research* 33 (6) 330–5   30 References

Cancer patients were assigned to a control group or one of four intervention groups receiving (a) nutritional supplementation, (b) relaxation training, (c) both (a) and (b), and (d) neither (a) nor (b). Findings suggested that the cachexia of cancer may be slowed or reversed through non-invasive interventions.

2.30.2 Wong, K.N., Hills, E.C. & Strax, T.E. (1994) Rotating stations: an innovative approach to third year medical student education in physical medicine and rehabilitation. *American Journal of Physical Medicine and Rehabilitation* 73 (1) 23–6   3 References

Reports a study where students were pre- and post-tested about their knowledge of physical medicine and rehabilitation. A one-day combined lecture/rotating stations conference was held as a way of introducing students to this field and testing showed it to be a cost-effective way.

2.31 POST-TEST CONTROL DESIGN

This design may be useful in situations where it is not possible to pre-test the participants or where they have been randomly assigned.

R X O Experimental Group
R O Control Group

Example

Semple, M., Cook, R., Moseley, L. & Torrance, C. (2001) Social influences and the recording of blood pressure by student nurses. *Nurse Researcher: The International Journal of Research Methodology in Nursing and Health Care* 8 (3) 60–71   18 References

Authors discuss an experiment to investigate the influence of previously charted blood pressure recordings on the recording of blood pressure by student nurses. The results suggest that previously charted recordings exert a social influence that alters the judgement of student nurses when recording blood pressure.

Annotation

2.31.1 Kerr, S.M., Jowett, S.A. & Smith, L.N. (1996) Preventing sleep problems in infants: a randomized controlled trial. *Journal of Advanced Nursing* 24 (5) 938–42   25 References

Research aimed to examine the efficacy of health education in reducing the incidence of sleep problems. Results showed that a preventive approach produced a significant improvement in infant sleep behaviour.

2.32   SOLOMON FOUR GROUP DESIGN

A complex design useful in studies of developmental phenomena that permits the investigator to differentiate between many effects. Two experimental and two control groups are used.

R	01 X	02	Experimental Group 1
R	03	04	Control Group 1
R	X	05	Experimental Group 2
R		06	Control group 2

This design has potential for generating information about differential sources of effect of the dependent variable.

Example

Aschen, S.R. (1997) Assertion training therapy in psychiatric milieus. *Archives of Psychiatric Nursing* 11 (1) 46–51   13 References

Using a Solomon Four Group Design, author reports an attempt to develop a clinical procedure to decrease anxiety and increase responsiveness (assertion) of psychiatric inpatients of both sexes, in mixed diagnostic categories. The effectiveness of the procedure is reported.

Annotations

2.32.1 Malotte, C.K. & Morisky, D.E. (1994) Using an unobtrusively monitored comparison study group in a longitudinal design. *Health Education Research* 9 (1) 153–9   22 References

Study describes how a non-contact comparison group receiving treatment for tuberculosis, followed through medical records, can be used in combination with a randomized control design to assess pre-test and monitoring effects. Results and their implications are reported (CR 2.48).

2.32.2 Michel, Y. & Haight, B.K. (1996) Using the Solomon Four design. *Nursing Research* 45 (6) 367–9   5 References

Uses an example of caring for preventing depression in the elderly in a nursing home to explain the Solomon Four Group Design.

2.33   FACTORIAL DESIGNS

Factorial designs allow the researcher to analyse the effects of two or more factors simultaneously. They also provide information on whether factors interact to produce differences in the outcome that would not have occurred if each factor were considered separately.

Definition [See Appendix D for source]

Factorial design – research design with two or more categorical independent variables (factors), each studied at two or more levels

Example

Lauder, W., Scott, P.A. & Whyte, A. (2001) Nurses' judgements of self-neglect: a factorial survey. *International Journal of Nursing Studies* 38 (5) October 601–8   20 References

The notion of self-neglect as a social construction is the theoretical perspective that provides the framework for this study. Judgements made about self-neglect may be social judgements influenced by professional socialization and cultural values. The beliefs of different groups of nurses were investigated, together with the factors that influenced them. Including nursing students allowed a picture to emerge as to whether judgements develop over time or are relatively constant across a career path, albeit within the limitations of a non-longitudinal design.

Annotations

2.33.1 Gilmour, S.G. & Mead, R. (1995) Stopping rules for sequences of factorial designs. *Applied Statistics* 44 (3) 343–55   References

Reports on stopping rules for sequentially designed factorial experiments used in Monte Carlo simulation.

2.33.2 Ludwick, R. (1999) Taking the mystery out of research: factorial surveys. *Orthopaedic Nursing Journal* 18 (1) 66–7   4 References

Outlines the use and characteristics of factorial designs.

2.34   SINGLE-CASE DESIGN

'Single-case experiments are scientific investigations in which the effects of a series of experimental manipulations on a single subject are examined. ... [This type of research] should not be confused with case studies – [they] are retrospectively written reports of observations on individuals, which may raise questions that initiate research; single-case experiments are, of course, prospectively planned' (Wilson in Breakwell, Hammond & Fife-Schaw, 2000: 60). Examples of this design include the evaluation of behaviour modification and skill training programmes, assessment of the effects of drugs and the examination of treatments in physical rehabilitation.

[A number of terms are used to describe or name small sample research. These are single-case design, intensive research, N=1 design, ideographic research, experimental analysis of behaviour, applied analysis of behaviour and case study designs (Woods & Catanzaro, 1988: 558).]

Definition [See Appendix D for source]

Single-case design – an examination of a single subject in order to understand the specific cause of problems and the effectiveness of treatment applied to that individual

Example

Martini, R. & Polatajko, J. (1998) Verbal self-guidance as a treatment approach for children with developmental coordination disorder: a systematic replication study. *Occupational Therapy Journal of Research* 18 (4) 157–81   66 References

A new approach, verbal self-guidance, appears to have potential in helping children with developmental co-ordination disorder to become competent in occupations of their choice. This replication study with a different therapist, using a single-case study design, showed the technique's ability to enable children to surmount their motor challenges (CR 2.13).

Annotations

2.34.1   Bailey, J.S. & Burch, M.R. (2002) *Research methods in applied behavior analysis.* Thousand Oaks, CA: Sage   ISBN 0761925562   References

Text covers all the elements of single-subject research design and provides practical information for designing, implementing and evaluating studies.

2.34.2   Barlow, D.H. & Hersen, M. (1992) *Single case experimental designs.* New York: Pergamon ISBN 0080301355   References

Book provides a historical overview of the single case in basic and applied research and discusses general issues, procedures and assessment strategies. Different designs are covered and examples are given. Methods of statistical analysis are included, together with examples of direct, systematic and clinical replication (CR 2.13).

2.34.3   Gray, M. (1998) Introducing single case research design: an overview. *Nurse Researcher* 5 (4) 15–24   31 References

Author gives an overview of case study research, its types and uses. Single case studies are discussed together with their strengths and weaknesses (CR 2.39).

2.34.4   Kazdin, A.E. (1982) *Single case research designs: methods for clinical and applied settings.* New York: Oxford University Press   ISBN 0195030214   References

Provides a concise description of single-case experimental designs and places this methodology in the context of applied research in general. Examples are given from clinical psychology, psychiatry, education, counselling and other disciplines. The methodology covers assessment, design and data analysis.

2.34.5   La Grow, S. & Hamilton, C. (2000) The use of single-case experimental designs to evaluate nursing interventions for individual clients. *Australian Journal of Advanced Nursing* 18 (2) 39–43   18 References

Argues that single-case research offers nurses a practical strategy for assessing the efficacy of individualized interventions, using the control of an experimental design with the flexibility to apply interventions to particular settings. It outlines the basic principle of the design and illustrates its application.

2.34.6   Newell, R. (1998) Single case experimental design: controlling the study. *Nurse Researcher* 5 (4) 25–39   12 References

Explores some of the issues surrounding the introduction of experimental control in single-case research. A series of methods is examined which should increase its rigour when studying everyday practice. It may then be possible to apply research findings based on large group studies to the needs of the individual.

2.34.7   Ottenbacher, K.J. & Hinderer, S.R. (2001) Evidence-based practice: methods to evaluate individual patient improvement. *American*

Journal of Physical Medicine and Rehabilitation 80 (10) 786–96   66 References

Traditional research methods, including randomized clinical trials, are powerful techniques for determining rehabilitation interventions. However, they do have some practical and ethical limitations when examining the effectiveness of treatment techniques for individual patients and documenting clinical accountability. This paper examines the use of single-system designs and N of 1 research strategies. Their advantages and limitations are described, and examples relevant to the documentation of clinical outcomes in medical rehabilitation are given (CR 2.29, 2.43).

2.34.8   Wilson, S.L. (2000) Single case experimental designs. In Breakwell, G.M., Hammond, S. & Fife-Schaw, C. (eds) *Research methods in psychology* (2nd edition). London: Sage   ISBN 0761965912 Part II Chapter 5 59–74   References

Chapter discusses problems with the group comparison approach, general issues in single-case research, preparing and performing a single-case experiment and data analysis (CR 2.1.7).

2.35   QUASI-EXPERIMENTAL DESIGNS

Quasi-experimental designs are a compromise between a true experiment with random assignment and a pre-experiment. They also represent a compromise between maximizing internal and external validity.

Definitions [See Appendix D for sources]

Interrupted time-series designs – effects of a treatment are inferred from comparing measures of performance taken at many time intervals

Non-equivalent control group – those in which the responses of a treatment group and a comparison group are measured before and after the treatment

Quasi-experiment – a research design that has the features of manipulation and control, but in which the participants are not randomly assigned to the treatment and control groups

Example

Achterberg, W.P., Holtkamp, C.C.M., Kerkstra, A., Pot, A.M., Ooms, M.E. & Ribbe, M.W. (2001) Improvements in the quality of co-ordination of nursing care following implementation of the resident assessment instrument in Dutch nursing homes. *Journal of Advanced Nursing* 35 (2) 268–75   14 References

Using a quasi-experimental approach, an assessment instrument was designed to examine and improve the quality of care and quality of life in nursing homes. Results which showed that use of this tool might be capable of improving care for residents are reported.

Annotations

2.35.1   Cook, T.D. & Campbell, D.T. (1990) *Quasi-experimentation: design and analysis issues for field settings.* West Markham, Ontario, Canada: Houghton Mifflin Co.   ISBN 0395307902 References

Volume covers some quasi-experimental designs that can be used in many social research settings. The literature on causation is reviewed, aspects of validity are explored and the two major categories of quasi-experimental designs, non-equivalent group and interrupted time series are covered in detail. Further chapters on inferring cause from passive observation and the conduct of randomized experiments are included (CR 2.21, 2.25).

2.35.2   Cook, T.D., Campbell, D.T. & Shadish, W. (2001) *Experimental and quasi-experimental designs for generalized causal inference.* West Markham, Ontario, Canada: Houghton Mifflin Co. ISBN 0395615569   References

This book represents updates in the field over the last two decades. It covers four main topics in field experimentation: theoretical matters, quasi-experimental design, randomized experiments and generalized causal inference.

2.35.3   Fife-Schaw, C. (2000) Quasi-experimental designs. In Breakwell, G.M., Hammond, S. & Fife-Schaw, C. (eds) *Research methods in psychology* (2nd edition). London: Sage   ISBN 0761965912 Part II 7 Chapter 6 75–87   References

Discusses pre- and quasi-experiments, non-equivalent control group, time series and modifications to basic designs (CR 2.1.7).

2.35.4   Trochim, W. (ed.) (1986) Advances in quasi-experimentation. In Author *Advances in quasi-experimental design and analysis.* New directions for program evaluation Series No. 31. San Francisco, CA: Jossey-Bass   Editor's Notes [reprint]   trochim.human.cornell.edu/kb/advquasi. htm (Accessed 11/02/03)

This paper makes the case that researchers have moved beyond the traditional thinking on quasi-experiments as a collection of specific designs and threats to validity towards a more integrated, synthetic view of quasi-experimentation as part of a general, logical and epistemological framework for research. A number of themes are discussed that cut across validity typologies and design taxonomies. These themes may also be seen as a tentative description of the advances in thinking about quasi-experimentation in social research.

Non-Experimental/Qualitative Designs

2.36 NON-EXPERIMENTAL DESIGNS – GENERAL

'...[Q]ualitative researchers seek to preserve the form and content of human behaviour and to analyse its qualities, rather than subject it to mathematical or other formal transformations.' (Lindlof, 1995: 40)

[This section includes texts on qualitative research. Those including both quantitative and qualitative research methods may be found in sections 2.1 and 2.9.]

Definitions [See Appendix D for sources]

Bricolage – multiple methodologies used in qualitative inquiry

Bricoleur – the qualitative inquirer ... one who is adept at performing a large number of diverse tasks

Field- experiment – an experiment taking place in a real-world environment, where it is more difficult to impose controls

Field notes – notes taken by researchers regarding the unstructured observations they have made in the field, and their understanding of these observations

Field study – a study in which the data are collected 'in the field' from people in their normal roles with the aims of understanding the practices, behaviours and beliefs of individuals or groups as they normally function in real life

Fieldwork – an anthropological research approach that traditionally involves prolonged residence with members of the culture that is being studied

Imagework method – ... an active process in which the person 'actively imagining' lets go of the mind's normal train of thoughts and images and goes with a sequence of imagery that arises spontaneously from the unconscious

---

Interactionism – the theory that physical occurrences are the causes of mental modifications and that mental modifications give rise to physical changes

Naturalistic inquiry – ... the investigation of the phenomena within and in relation to their naturally occurring contexts

Qualitative research – is multi-method in focus, involving an interpretive, naturalistic approach to its subject matter

Queer theory – an approach to issues of sex and gender which has primarily arisen out of postmodernist thought

Theme – a theme is an abstract entity that brings meaning and identity to a recurrent experience and its variant manifestations. As such, a theme captures and unifies the nature or basis of the experience into a meaningful whole

Trajectory model – posits that human beings and things have biographies and histories that serve as context for each other

---

Annotations

2.36.1 Adamson, J. & Donovan, J.L. (2002) Research in black and white. *Qualitative Health Research* 12 (6) 816–25 41 References

Explores the methodological standpoints of 'researching others,' including interpretative and practical issues. Authors argue that such research should be judged by its plausibility, critical evaluation and the reflexivity of the researcher.

2.36.2 Agency for Healthcare Research and Quality *Research methodology* www.ahcpr.gov/research/dec99/1299ra18.htm (Accessed 05/05/03)

A supplement of the journal *Health Services Research* (December 1999) which includes papers and discussion papers given at a conference that explored the use of qualitative methods in health services research. Website lists the included articles. (CR 3.12).

2.36.3 Alasuutari, P. (1998) *An invitation to social research.* London: Sage ISBN 0761957375 References

Book aims to fill the gap between introductory sociology texts and practical 'how to' methods texts. Parallels are drawn between detective stories and research, how facts are gathered, using them as clues, and solving the case to present them as evidence. The novice student is drawn into a forceful argument based on compelling examples.

2.36.4 Albrecht, G.I., Fitzpatrick, R. & Scrimshaw, S. (eds) (1999) *The handbook of social studies in health and medicine.* London: Sage ISBN 0761956174 References

This resource book on social science, health and medicine identifies the focal issues of research and debate in one volume. Material is organized into three sections: social and cultural frameworks and analysis; the experience of health and illness; and health care systems and practices. Readers are provided with an authoritative guide to methodologies, key concepts, central theoretical traditions and an agenda for future research and practice.

2.36.5 Alvesson, M. & Deetz, S. (2000) *Doing critical management research.* London: Sage ISBN 0761953337 References

Provides a detailed discussion of the practice of doing critical research in organizations, utilizing both qualitative research processes and critical theories.

2.36.6 Alvesson, M. & Sköldberg, K. (2000) *Reflexive methodology: new vistas for qualitative research.* London: Sage ISBN 0803977077 References

Makes explicit links between techniques used in empirical research and different research traditions, giving a theoretically informed approach to qualitative research. The major schools of grounded theory, ethnomethodology, hermeneutics, critical theory, post-modernism, post-structuralism, discourse analysis, genealogy and feminism are covered. An extensive chapter is included on post-structuralism and post-moderism (CR 2.5, 2.10, 2.42, 2.45, 2.89).

2.36.7 Atkinson, P. & Housley, W. (2003) *Interactionism.* London: Sage ISBN 0761962700 References

Book provides readers with a guide to the essential thinking, research and concepts in interactionism, demonstrates use of the interactionist approach, and explains why the interactionist influence has not been fully acknowledged in Britain.

2.36.8 Banks, M. (2001) *Visual methods in social research.* London: Sage ISBN 0761963642 References

Written primarily for students in the social sciences, this book combines the theoretical and practical elements for those who wish to use visual materials in the course of empirical, qualitative field research.

2.36.9 Barbour, R.S. (2000) The role of qualitative research in broadening the 'evidence base' for clinical practice. *Journal of Evaluation in Clinical Practice* 6 (2) 155– 63 46 References

Defines qualitative research and its contribution to the evidence base for clinical practice. Discusses appropriate ways of incorporating qualitative findings into practice (CR 2.43, 2.95, 2.102).

2.36.10 Barbour, R.S. (2001) Checklists for improving rigour in qualitative research: a case of the tail wagging the dog. *British Medical Journal* 322 (7294) 5 May 1115–17 23 References

Argues against the use of checklists for the critical appraisal of qualitative research, stressing that adherence to the systematic application of qualitative principles is sufficient to maintain rigour (CR 2.22, 2.26, 2.45, 2.86).

2.36.11 Bauer, M.W. & Gaskell, G. (eds) (2000) *Qualitative researching with text, image and sound: a practical handbook for social research.* London: Sage ISBN 0761964819 References

This practical handbook provides a comprehensive and accessible introduction to a broad range of research methods with the objective of clarifying procedures, good practice and public accountability (CR 2.2, 2.64, 2.68, 2.71, 2.88, 2.99).

2.36.12 Bentz, V.M. & Shapiro, J.J. (1998) *Mindful inquiry in social research.* Thousand Oaks, CA: Sage ISBN 0761904093 References

Book aims to guide students through the maze of research traditions, cultures of inquiry and epistemological frameworks. Conceptual and intellectual traditions in research are classified and ten cultures of inquiry are introduced through their underlying logic rather than through detailed methods and techniques. These are: ethnomethods, phenomenology, action research, hermeneutics, evaluation research, feminist research, critical social science, historical, comparative and theoretical research (CR 2.5, 2.10, 2.37, 2.42, 2.46, 2.49).

2.36.13 Boudon, R., Cherkaoui, M. & Demeulenaere, P. (eds) (2003) *The European tradition in qualitative research.* London: Sage ISBN 0761974385 References 4 Volumes

These four volumes include contributions from the classic tradition to contemporary work. They are organized as: Volume 1: Collecting data; Volume 2: Selecting a type of approach; Volume 3: Building concepts; and Volume 4: Building theories.

2.36.14   Braud, W. & Anderson, R. (1998) *Transpersonal research methods for the social sciences.* Thousand Oaks, CA: Sage ISBN 0761910131   References

Book aims to assist researchers to develop new ways of knowing and methods of inquiry (CR 2.6, 2.25).

2.36.15   Brink, P.J. & Wood, M.J. (eds) (1998) *Advanced design in nursing research* (2nd edition). Thousand Oaks, CA: Sage   ISBN 0803958005 References

An advanced text focusing on research designs for students and teachers who have a basic knowledge of the research process. Three major designs – exploratory/descriptive, survey and experiential – are subdivided into further levels and fully discussed. Each one is contrasted with experimental design, and its strengths and weaknesses are reviewed (CR 2.29, 2.52, 2.96, 2.97).

2.36.16   Bryman, A. & Burgess, R.G. (eds) (1999) *Qualitative research.* London: Sage   ISBN 0761962433   References   4 Volumes

Volumes provide an overview of general issues in qualitative research, including epistemology, discussions on the different methods employed, information on the analysis and interpretation of data, discussions of ethical and cultural issues in research and new techniques. Each volume has an extensive introduction that places the examination of qualitative research issues in the appropriate historical and intellectual context (CR 2.6, 2.17, 2.79, 2.93).

2.36.17   Byrne-Armstrong, H., Higgs, J. & Horsfall, D. (eds) (2001) *Critical moments in qualitative research.* Oxford: Butterworth-Heinemann ISBN 0750651598   References

Book deals with some of the issues not talked about or mentioned in published research. These include finding a voice among the multitude of methodologies and methods, working through relationship conflicts, fighting battles with structural constraints, crises of confidence, writing blocks and the difficulties of being a student or supervisor (CR 2.16, 2.97, 3.17, 3.18).

2.36.18   Carson, D., Gilmore, A., Perry, C. & Gronhaug, K. (2001) *Qualitative marketing research.* London: Sage   ISBN 0761963669   References

Book explains the use and importance of qualitative methods, clarifying the theories behind the

methodology and giving examples and exercises that illustrate management studies and marketing.

2.36.19   Chao, Y.Y., Chiang, H., Chen, Y., Su, T. & Liou, Y. (1999) Quantification and interpretation of qualitative data: an exploration of research method and epistemology based on empirical nursing research. Part 1: methodological and epistemological issues in conducting qualitative clinical nursing research (Chinese). *Nursing Research (China)* 7 (3) 276–88   41 References

AND

2.36.20   Chao, Y.Y., Chiang, H., Chen, Y., Su, T. & Liou, Y. (1999) Quantification and interpretation of qualitative data: an exploration of research method and epistemology based on empirical research. Part 2: analysis and interpretation of empirical nursing research (Chinese). *Nursing Research (China)* 7 (4) 376–92   25 References

The purpose of this study was to explore an approach to research methodology that can better reconcile nursing research to the empirical world. The first part reviewed the development of qualitative research and the use of inductive and deductive data analysis approaches in a clinical nursing situation. Paper also reports the method and findings of the qualitative data obtained by participatory observation on 20 new mothers while feeding their newborn babies. A discussion of empirical validation, proper paradigm in nursing science and practice from the perspective of symbolic interactionism is also presented (CR 2.6, 2.8, 2.9, 2.86, 2.95).

2.36.21   Chow, J.D. (1999) Interruption to research design: substance-driven research. *Advances in Nursing Science* 22 (2) 39–48   49 References

When adolescent women met individually and in focus groups to talk about health messages, in particular teen magazines, their responses did not fit the feminist, critical theory and media reception analysis methods used to guide the study. The undisputed acceptance of research methods as the sole means to knowledge and truth was interrupted by the voices of adolescents that resisted methodological codification. Hermeneutics or interpretative inquiry transformed the study to one that became substantively driven and contributes to the qualitative approaches in the human sciences (CR 2.6, 2.10, 2.69).

2.36.22   Clegg, C. & Walsh, S. (1998) Soft systems analysis. In Symon, G. & Cassell, C. (eds) *Qualitative methods and analysis in organizational research: a practical guide.* London: Sage   ISBN 0761953515   Chapters 11 211–33   12 References

Soft systems analysis is primarily a method for investigating problems located within a system. The method is used to plan and implement change, although it can also be used to design new systems. This chapter describes soft systems analysis, gives some examples of its application and comments on its strengths and weaknesses (CR 2.36.135, 2.86).

2.36.23   Cowling, W.R. (2001) Unitary appreciative inquiry. *Advances in Nursing Science* 23 (4) 32–48   31 References

Describes unitary appreciative inquiry as a mode of inquiry that seeks to capture the essence of human life. Provides a full account of the approach and its potential for advancing nursing science and practice.

2.36.24   Crabtree, B.F. & Miller, W.L. (eds) (1999) *Doing qualitative research* (2nd edition). Thousand Oaks, CA: Sage   ISBN 0761914986 References

Spanning the spectrum of primary care research, this book illustrates when methods are appropriate and how to use them. New material includes additional collection methods, analysis and interpretation, participatory strategies and suggestions for evaluating quality and enhancing reflexivity (CR 2.64, 2.93).

2.36.25   Creswell, J.W. (1998) *Qualitative inquiry and research design: choosing among five traditions*. Thousand Oaks, CA: Sage   ISBN 0761901442   References

Book explores the philosophical underpinnings, history and key elements of each of five qualitative traditions: biography, phenomenology, grounded theory, ethnography and case study. Research designs are related to each tradition and each research strategy is compared for theoretical frameworks, writing introductions to studies, collecting and analysing data, writing the narrative, employing standards of quality and verifying results. Five articles in an appendix give examples of the five qualitative designs and a chapter shows how a case study can be re-interpreted using each of the other four traditions. Individual glossaries are given for each tradition (CR 2.2, 2.39, 2.42, 2.45, 2.49, 2.71).

2.36.26   Cutcliffe, J.R. & McKenna, H.P. (1999) Establishing the credibility of qualitative research findings: the plot thickens. *Journal of Advanced Nursing* 30 (2) 374–80   43 References

Paper explores issues relating to the representativeness or credibility of qualitative research findings. It critiques the existing distinct philosophical and methodological positions concerning the trustworthiness of qualitative research findings (CR 2.5).

2.36.27   Cutcliffe, J.R. & Goward, P. (2000) Mental health nurses and qualitative research methods:

a mutual attraction? *Journal of Advanced Nursing* 31 (3) 590–8   63 References

Paper examines why psychiatric/mental health nurses seem to gravitate towards the qualitative paradigm. The authors believe that this apparent synchronicity and linkage appears to centre around three themes: the purposeful use of self, the creation of an interpersonal relationship, and the ability to accept ambiguity and uncertainty. Reasons are suggested and discussed (CR 2.9).

2.36.28   Darlington, Y. & Scott, D. (2002) *Qualitative research in practice: stories from the field*. Buckingham: Open University Press   ISBN 033521147X   References

Book bridges the gap between theory and practice. Qualitative research is explored through actual projects that illustrate key stages in the research process (CR 3.8).

2.36.29   Denzin, N.K. (2001) *Interpretive interactionism*, (2nd edition). Thousand Oaks, CA: Sage ISBN 0761915141   References

Book includes information on how interpretative work can be used to further the workings of a free, democratic society; a new chapter on interpretative criteria in the Seventh moment; a re-examination of the key notion of thick description, in light of the narrative and performance turns in the social sciences; multi-sited ethnographies, the politics of place, the ethnoscapes of group life; links made with recent qualitative turns, from literary ethnography to feminist, cultural, critical race, interpretative and Foucauldian studies; and new coverage of narratives, sacred places and new writing forms (CR 2.10, 2.42, 2.78).

2.36.30   Denzin, N.K. & Lincoln, Y.S. (eds) (1998) *Collecting and interpreting qualitative materials*. Thousand Oaks, CA: Sage   ISBN 076191434X

Introduces researchers to basic methods of gathering, analysing and interpreting qualitative empirical materials (CR 2.86).

2.36.31   Denzin, N.K. & Lincoln, Y.S. (eds) (2000) *Handbook of qualitative research* (2nd edition). Thousand Oaks, CA: Sage   ISBN 0761915125   References (extensive)

This major handbook attempts to synthesize the world of qualitative research. It progresses from the theoretical to the specific, examining the various paradigms for doing qualitative research. Strategies are developed for studying people in their own settings and a variety of techniques for collecting, analysing, interpreting and reporting data are included. Contributors come from many disciplines and three continents. This new edition has been substantially revised, featuring 33 new chapter authors or co-authors. New topics included are queer theory, performance ethnography, testimony, focus groups in feminist research, applied ethnography and anthropological poetics. All returning authors have revised their original contributions (CR 2.10, 2.64, 2.86, 2.97).

2.36.32 Denzin, N.K. & Lincoln, Y.S. (eds) (2001) *The American tradition in qualitative research.* Thousand Oaks, CA: Sage ISBN 0761969802 References 4 Volumes

This book of intellectual craftsmanship provides an authoritative delineation of the field of qualitative research and refreshes discussion and understanding of the American tradition. Volumes cover a wide span from the classic to the neglected, and editors revive the field by including contributions by women, persons of colour, post-colonial writers, gays and lesbians. The history, techniques and future of qualitative research are all discussed.

2.36.33 Denzin, N.K. & Lincoln, Y.S. (eds) (2002) *The qualitative inquiry reader.* Thousand Oaks, CA: Sage   ISBN 0761924922   References

Reader offers a selection of landmark articles from the journal *Qualitative Inquiry*. These collected works introduce the necessary critical framework that will allow scholars and students to interpret cutting-edge work in the field of qualitative inquiry.

2.36.34 Denzin, N.K. & Lincoln, Y.S. (eds) (2003) *The landscape of qualitative research: theories and issues* (2nd edition). Thousand Oaks, CA: Sage   ISBN 0761926941

Book attempts to put the field of qualitative research in context and looks at it from a broadly theoretical perspective. Part 1 locates the field, starting with history, then action research and the academy, research for whom? and the politics and ethics of qualitative research. Part 2 isolates the major historical and contemporary paradigms (positivist, post-positivist, constructivist, critical theory) to specific interpretative perspectives, feminisms, racialized discourses, cultural studies, and queer theory. Part 3 considers the future of qualitative research (CR 2.10, 2.17, 2.37).

2.36.35 Denzin, N.K. & Lincoln, Y.S. (eds) (2003) *Strategies of qualitative inquiry* (2nd edition). Thousand Oaks, CA: Sage ISBN 0761926917

This new edition isolates the major strategies – historically, the research methods – that researchers can use in conducting concrete qualitative studies. Issues discussed include research design, and matters of money and funding. Chapters cover performance ethnography, case studies and issues of ethnographic representation, grounded theory strategies, testimonies, life histories, participatory action research and clinical research (CR 2.37, 2.42, 2.45, 2.71, 3.13).

2.36.36 Department of Sociology, University of Surrey *Social Research Update* www.soc.surrey, ac.uk/sru/ (Accessed 11/02/03)

Social Research Update is published quarterly and this website lists all the previous 37 issues that cover various aspects of qualitative research.

2.36.37 DeSantis, L. & Ugarriza, D.N. (2000) The concept of theme as used in qualitative nursing research. *Western Journal of Nursing Research* 22 (3) 351–72   70 References

A literature review revealed considerable diversity in the identification of themes, the interpretation of the concept and its function in data analysis. This article explores the concept of 'theme' as used in qualitative nursing research and develops a definition of the term. Assumptions are made that a basic definition is applicable to all qualitative research methods and will bring increased rigour to data collection and analysis (CR 2.12).

2.36.38 Devers, K.J. (1999) How will we know 'good' qualitative research when we see it? Beginning the dialogue in health services research. *Health Services Research* 34 (5) 1153–88   90 References

Debates the purpose and place of qualitative approaches and discusses the philosophical and theoretical assumptions underpinning this perspective. Provides a set of criteria for evaluating qualitative research in health services research.

2.36.39 Duffy, M. (2001) Getting qualitative research ideas and help on-line. In Munhall, P.L. (ed.) *Nursing research: a qualitative perspective* (3rd edition). Sudbury, MA: Jones & Bartlett and National League for Nursing   ISBN 0763711357 Chapter 25 639–45

Chapter lists several websites containing information on qualitative research (CR 2.36.98, 2.85).

2.36.40 Easton, K.L., McComish, J.F. & Greenberg, R. (2000) Avoiding common pitfalls in qualitative data collection and transcription. *Qualitative Health Research* 10 (5) 703–7   7 References

Article presents three of the pitfalls that can occur in qualitative research during data collection and transcription: equipment failure, environmental hazards and transcription errors (CR 2.64).

2.36.41   Edgar, I.R. (1999) The imagework method in health and social science research. *Qualitative Health Research* 9 (2) 198–211 39 References

Author states that alongside the traditional forms of qualitative social science research, there is a set of potential research methods that derive from experiential group work and the 'humanistic human potential' movement. Article locates these methods within the qualitative research domain and proposes a novel view of their value. The actual and potential use of one method, imagework, is discussed in detail. References to the use of artwork, sculpting, psychodrama, gestalt and dreamwork are also made.

2.36.42   Emden, C. & Sandelowski, M. (1999) The good, the bad and the relative. Part two: goodness and the criterion problem in qualitative research. *International Journal of Nursing Practice* 5 (1) 2–7   24 References

Analyses the way in which criteria may be applied to qualitative research in order to represent the reality of qualitative research demands, while acknowledging the value placed on validity and reliability in positivist research (CR 2.24, 2.25, 2.29).

2.36.43   Ereaut, G., Imms, M. & Callingham, M. (eds) (2002*) Qualitative market research: principle and practice*. London: Sage   ISBN 0761972722 References   7 Volumes

These seven volumes provide complete coverage of qualitative market research practice, written by experienced practitioners, for both a commercial and academic audience. Each book cross-references with others in the series, but can also be used as a stand-alone resource on a key topic.

2.36.44   Chandler, J. & Owen, M. (2002) *Developing brands with qualitative market research*. Book 5

2.36.45   Chrzanowska, J. (2002) *Interviewing groups and individuals in qualitative market research*. Book 2

2.36.46   Desai, P. (2002) *Methods beyond interviewing in marketing research*. Book 3

2.36.47   Ereaut, G. (2002) *Analysis and interpretation in qualitative market research*. Book 4

2.36.48   Imms, M. & Ereaut, G. (2002) *An introduction to qualitative market research*. Book 1

2.36.49   Lillis, G. (2002) *Delivering results in qualitative market research*. Book 7

2.36.50   Wardle, J. (2002) *Developing advertising with qualitative market research*. Book 6

2.36.51   Flick, U. (2002) *An introduction to qualitative research* (2nd edition). London: Sage ISBN 0761974369   References

Book provides students with a systematic structure for comparing qualitative methods, designing research, collecting and dealing with data. It also includes a chapter on visual research methods (CR 2.7, 2.14, 2.45).

2.36.52   Freebody, P.R. (2003) *Qualitative research in education: interaction and practice*. London: Sage   ISBN 0761961410   References

Book provides a thorough explanation of the complexities of educational research, and demonstrates the importance of placing this knowledge within cultural, linguistic and sociological contexts.

2.36.53   Gbrich, C. (1999) *Qualitative research in health: an introduction*. London: Sage   ISBN 0761961046   References

Provides an introduction to the main theories and methods of qualitative research for the health sciences (CR 2.10, 2.37, 2.42, 2.45, 2.46, 2.49, 2.71, 2.89).

2.36.54   Gilgun, J.F. & Sussman, M.B. (eds) (1997) *The methods and methodologies of qualitative family research*. Binghampton, NY: Haworth Press Inc   ISBN 0789003058   References

This volume pulls together a rich and diverse group of essays that teach readers about the complexities and challenges of qualitative inquiry. Sections cover a look at the mosaic of qualitative family research, learning to be qualitative and essays on methodologies (CR 2.49, 2.68, 2.72, 2.76, 2.89).

2.36.55   Glassner, B. & Hertz, R. (eds) (1999) *Qualitative sociology as everyday life*. Thousand Oaks, CA: Sage   ISBN 0761913696   References

This volume examines how sociological understanding helps with the experience of everyday life, how the observation of everyday life affects research agendas and vice versa, and how the qualitative approach helps the understanding of experiences in a broader sense rather than as random or isolated events.

2.36.56   Graue, M.E. & Walsh, D.J. (1998) *Researching children in context: theories, methods and ethics*. Thousand Oaks, CA: Sage   ISBN 0803972571   References

The art and science of doing qualitative research involving children is the subject of this book. The authors discuss the research process, dealing succinctly with generic issues, but emphasizing where work with children presents its own particular challenges.

2.36.57 Hammell, K.W. (2001) Using qualitative research to inform the client-centred evidence-based practice of occupational therapy. *British Journal of Occupational Therapy* 64 (5) 228–34 51 References

Paper explores the philosophical underpinning of methods used to develop theory, proposing that occupational therapy's evidence-based practice must be ethically consistent with its espoused client-centred philosophy to avoid a tendency towards hypocrisy. While traditional quantitative research approaches render client voices silent, qualitative methods may enable therapists to explore the complexities of clinical practice and of living with a disability (CR 2.5, 2.7).

2.36.58 Heinz, W.R & Krüger, H. (2001) Life course: innovations and challenges for social research. *Current Sociology* 49 (2) 29–53 109 References

Traces the history of life-course research and its contribution to the understanding of social change. Identifies the conceptual and methodological issues underpinning this type of research and the extent to which it crosses sociological boundaries.

2.36.59 Hollway, W. & Jefferson, T. (2000) *Doing qualitative research differently: free association, narrative and the interview method.* London: Sage ISBN 0761964266 References

Book critically reviews many of the assumptions, claims and methods of qualitative research. Authors believe that both researcher and researched are co-producers of meanings in the research relationship. To interpret interviewees' responses they describe a method in which narratives are central and their free associations should be given precedence over narrative coherence. This approach is demonstrated through the phases of empirical research practice. Examples are included, together with an extended case study (CR 2.17, 2.28, 2.71).

2.36.60 Holmes, R.M. (1998) *Fieldwork with children.* Thousand Oaks, CA: Sage ISBN 0761907556 References

Author overviews the study of children, discussing basic methodology and considering the school as the primary site for studying children. She examines how a researcher's personal attributes, such as gender and ethnicity, can and do affect the fieldwork process with children.

2.36.61 Horsburgh, D. (2003) Evaluation of qualitative research. *Journal of Clinical Nursing* 12 (2) 307–12 24 References

Examines the distinctive features of qualitative research using key writers in the field, and posits a formal evaluation framework for qualitative research as distinct from that used for quantitative research (CR 2.9).

2.36.62 Huberman, A.M. & Miles, M.B. (eds) (2002) *The qualitative researcher's companion.* Thousand Oaks, CA: Sage ISBN 076191191X References

Book introduces or reintroduces readers to papers that provide a solid intellectual grounding in qualitative research. They examine the theoretical underpinnings, methodological perspectives and empirical approaches that are crucial to the understanding and practice of qualitative inquiry. It includes seminal papers, persistent problems and documents the use of long-standing methods in social anthropology, linguistics, narratology and as yet 'undiscovered' classics.

2.36.63 International Institute for Qualitative Methodology www.ualberta.ca/~iiqm/ (Accessed 12/02/03)

The primary goal of this multidisciplinary institute at the University of Alberta, Edmonton, Alberta, Canada is to facilitate the development of qualitative research methods across a wide variety of disciplines. The website includes information about the staff and their research, publications, conferences and workshops.

2.36.64 Janesick, V.J. (1998) *'Stretching' exercises for qualitative researchers.* Thousand Oaks, CA: Sage ISBN 0761902562 References

Developing the skills necessary to become an effective qualitative researcher involves more than simply learning rules, tools and formats. The author argues that tapping into one's artistic side is a fundamental prerequisite for realizing one's potential as a researcher. A series of exercises are given, which can be used inside and outside the classroom, that are both artistically inspired and immensely practical (CR 3.16).

2.36.65 Jaye, C. (2002) Doing qualitative research in general practice: methodological utility and engagement. *Family Practitioner* 19 (5) October 557–62 References

This paper suggests that the value of in-depth engagement with theory and methodology when conducting qualitative research results in creative and innovative ways that are consonant with the nature of general practice and strengthens research findings. The importance of encouraging GPs in their postgraduate research dissertations and theses to engage with both theory and method are discussed (CR 2.7).

2.36.66 Johnson, M. (1999) Observations on positivism and pseudoscience in qualitative nursing research. *Journal of Advanced Nursing* 30 (1) 67–73   25 References

Paper examines the boundaries between positivism, interpretativism and pseudoscience, arguing that some qualitative researchers may risk the credibility of nursing research by utilizing concepts from the margins of science. Two major threats to the perceived rigour of qualitative research are discussed. The first is the trend in some work towards a mystical view of both the methods and content of the qualitative enterprise, and the second is almost its epistemological opposite, towards excessive reliance on precise procedures, strict definitions and verification. The author urges caution in uncritical acceptance of theories and 'research' which approach the boundaries of pseudoscience on the one hand, and 'hard' science on the other.

2.36.67 Johnson, M., Long, T. & White, A. (2001) Arguments for 'British pluralism' in qualitative health research. *Journal of Advanced Nursing* 33 (2) 243–9   33 References

Paper examines the argument that certain qualitative methods can be used in 'pure' forms. While rigid adherence to particular published procedures might be possible, it is argued that in many cases this is neither necessary nor more likely to increase the validity of the research outcome. Analysis of varied examples of qualitative research shows methods to be more flexible than is often admitted. 'British Pluralism' is an attempt to accept this reality while maintaining rigour through integrity, clear accounts, reflexivity and constructive criticism of one's own work and that of others.

2.36.68 Kendall, G. & Wickham, G. (1998) *Using Foucault's methods.* Thousand Oaks, CA: Sage   ISBN 0761957170   References

Authors address the thorny question of how-to-Foucault in a clear and distinctive manner.

2.36.69 Kincheloe, J.L. (2001) Conceptualizing a new rigor in qualitative research. *Qualitative Inquiry* 7 (6) 679–92   References

Picking up on Denzin and Lincoln's articulation of the concept of bricolage, this essay describes a critical notion of this research orientation. As an interdisciplinary approach, bricolage avoids both the superficiality of methodological breadth and the parochialism of unidisciplinary approaches. It employs historiographical, philosophical and social theoretical lenses to gain a more complex understanding of the intricacies of research design.

2.36.70 Kirkham, S.R., Smye, V., Tang, S., Anderson, J., Blue, C., Browne, A., Coles, R., Dyck, I., Henderson, A., Lynam, M.J., Perry, J., Semeniuk, P. & Shapera, L. (2002) Rethinking cultural safety while waiting to do fieldwork: methodological implications for nursing research. *Research in Nursing and Health* 25 (3) 222–32   41 References

Reflects upon the complexity of cultural safety, which, it is argued, comprises far more than an acknowledgement of cultural diversity. It draws upon New Zealand and Canadian perspectives to highlight the methodological implications of doing fieldwork in this area of research.

2.36.71 Koch, T. & Harrington, A. (1998) Reconceptualizing rigour: the case for reflexivity. *Journal of Advanced Nursing* 28 (4) 882–90   46 References

Paper is a critical review of recent discussions of rigour in nursing research. Authors argue that 'borrowing' evaluation criteria from one paradigm of inquiry and applying them to another is problematic. An attempt is made to map the 'rigour' field and add a dimension to the existing debate about rigour and qualitative research through inclusion of reflexivity guided by philosophical hermeneutics. Reflexivity is described as well as the valuable part it can play in making research more explicit (CR 2.6).

2.36.72 Kopala, M. & Suzuki, L.A. (eds) (1999) *Using qualitative methods in psychology.* Thousand Oaks, CA: Sage   ISBN 0761910379

The contributors to this volume address topics such as: reliability and validity, training issues, ethics and use of qualitative computer programmes. Issues related to the application of qualitative methods are discussed, for example HIV/AIDS, feminist perspectives, vocational and adolescent development (CR 2.6, 2.9, 2.10, 2.17, 2.24, 2.25, 2.37, 2.69, 2.85, 3.16).

2.36.73 Lambert, H. & McKevitt, C. (2002) Anthropology in health research: from qualitative methods to multidisciplinarity. *British Medical Journal* 325 (7357) 27 July 210–14   24 References

Discusses how the field of anthropology can contribute to understanding others' cultural beliefs and how medicine might use this to overcome miscommunication.

2.36.74 Latimer, J. (ed.) (2003) *Advanced qualitative research for nursing.* Oxford: Blackwell Science   ISBN 063205946X   References

Book brings together contributions from Australia, Canada, the UK and the USA. It is a collection of empirically-based articles presenting and explaining approaches to qualitative research. Its aim is to show how qualitative methodologies can produce rigour and relevant understandings about nursing practice and patienthood.

2.36.75 Learmonth, A. & Cheung, P. (1999) Evidence-based health promotion: the contribution of qualitative research. *International Journal of Health Promotion and Education* 37 (1) 11–15 23 References

Authors present a series of qualitative sociological research methods and highlight some potential applications to health promotion. The methods discussed are observation, conversational analysis and action research (CR 2.37, 2.68, 2.72, 2.89).

2.36.76 Lee, T.W. (1998) *Using qualitative methods in organizational research.* Thousand Oaks, CA: Sage ISBN 0761908064 References

Book examines the methods and tactics for both generating and testing management theories, including guidelines for deciding whether to use qualitative methods, and overviews four specific research designs. Data collection and analysis, reliability and viability are all discussed (CR 2.24, 2.25).

2.36.77 Lindlof, T.R. & Taylor, B.C. (2002) *Qualitative communication research methods* (2nd edition). Thousand Oaks, CA: Sage ISBN 0761924949 References

This new edition offers updated coverage of such topics as naturalistic inquiry, interpretative paradigm, ethnomethodology, symbolic interactionism, sampling and linearity, with new studies in the areas of culture analysis and cyberspace ethnography. Numerous examples are given that show how studies are designed, carried out, written, evaluated and applied to theory (CR 2.22, 2.45).

2.36.78 Lofland, J. & Lofland, L.H. (1995) *Analyzing social settings: a guide to qualitative observation and analysis* (3rd edition). Belmont, CA: Wadsworth ISBN 0534247806 References

Book teaches the techniques of gathering, focusing and analysing qualitative data in step-by-step discussions. Examples and applications are given throughout (CR 2.39, 2.42, 2.68, 2.72, 2.86).

2.36.79 Maggs-Rapport, F. (2001) 'Best research practice': in pursuit of methodological rigour. *Journal of Advanced Nursing* 35 (3) 373–83 63 References

Paper examines the different qualities of four major qualitative methodologies: ethnography, descriptive phenomenology, interpretative phenomenology/hermeneutics and critical social theory. A critical overview of methodological decision-making is given and the need for rigour is stressed (CR 2.5, 2.43, 2.49).

2.36.80 Mariampolski, H. (2001) *Qualitative market research: a comprehensive guide.* Thousand Oaks, CA: Sage ISBN 0761969454 References

Book follows through a complete research project from the perspective of both user and practitioner. It can be used as a continuous teaching text and training manual, or individual sections can be consulted to enhance knowledge of best practice.

2.36.81 Marshall, C. & Rossman, G.B. (1999) *Designing qualitative research* (3rd edition). Thousand Oaks, CA: Sage ISBN 0761913408 References

Book discusses the 'how' and 'what' of the research study, data collection methods, recording, managing and analysing data, planning one's time and defending the value and logic of qualitative research (CR 2.37, 2.64, 2.68, 2.69, 2.79).

2.36.82 Mason, J. (2002) *Qualitative researching* (2nd edition). London: Sage ISBN 0761974288 References

Book provides an introduction to the practice of qualitative social research for students and first-time researchers. This new edition has expanded coverage of observation, documents, visual data, CAQDAS and writing qualitative research (CR 2.72, 2.76, 2.97).

2.36.83 May, T. (ed.) (2002) *Qualitative research in action.* London: Sage ISBN 0761960686 References

Rather than being a 'how to' book, this volume should prove useful for advanced students and researchers who wish to study ideas and practices relevant to the place of qualitative research in the social sciences. Leading scholars make original contributions to the subject (CR 2.42, 2.72, 2.78).

2.36.84 Mays, N. & Pope, C. (2000) Assessing quality in qualitative research. *British Medical Journal* 320 (7226) 1 January 50–2 12 References

Challenges the view held by anti-realists that qualitative research cannot be judged by conventional criteria such as validity and reliability, by discussing the need to operationalize them differently in assessing qualitative work.

2.36.85 McLeod, J. (2000) *Qualitative research in counselling and psychotherapy.* London: Sage ISBN 0761955062 References

Readers are taken through each stage of the research process and qualitative method is clearly described and critically assessed in terms of its strengths and weaknesses. Examples are given to show how the methods work in practice.

2.36.86   McReynolds, C.J., Koch, L.C. & Rumrill, P.D. Jr (2001) Speaking of research. Qualitative research strategies in rehabilitation. *Work: A Journal of Prevention, Assessment & Rehabilitation* 16 (1) 57–65   36 References

Article presents an overview of the qualitative research methods used by social scientists to explore human phenomena. The authors describe the philosophical and historical foundations of qualitative research, coupled with illustrations of specific qualitative designs (CR 2.5).

2.36.87   Mill, J.E. & Ogilvie, L.D. (2002) Establishing methodological rigour in international qualitative nursing research: a case study from Ghana. *Journal of Advanced Nursing* 41 (1) 80–7   38 References

Reviews the literature in relation to rigour in qualitative research, highlights the methodological decisions enhancing research in this project, and describes the criteria used to assess research during the process of the study (CR 3.22).

2.36.88   Miller, G. & Dingwall, R. (eds) (1997) *Context and method in qualitative research.* London: Sage   ISBN 0803976321   References

Book addresses a range of methodological and practical issues central to the concerns of qualitative researchers. Major themes are validity and credibility, problems encountered using particular techniques in different social settings and moral issues raised in qualitative research (CR 2.17, 2.25).

2.36.89   Morse, J.M. & Field, P.A. (1996) *Nursing research: the application of qualitative approaches* (2nd edition). London: Chapman & Hall   ISBN 0412605104   References

Book is intended as an introductory text on research methods for undergraduates and graduates. It presents a broad view of qualitative methodologies and discusses their history and subsequent development.

2.36.90   Morse, J.M. (ed.) (1997) *Completing a qualitative project: details and dialogue.* Thousand Oaks, CA: Sage   ISBN 0761906010   References

With a contributor panel of 22 renowned qualitative research authors, this book addresses a wide range of topics from basics to the publishing process, and methodology to application. Each article is followed by dialogue resulting from brainstorming sessions between the contributors.

2.36.91   Morse, J.M. (1999) Qualitative generalizability. *Qualitative Health Research* 9 (1) 5–6   2 References   Editorial

Editor believes that qualitative research is generalizable, citing a particular example. Once qualitative researchers recognize that findings can be generalized, then this type of research will be considered appropriately and be more useful, powerful and significant (CR 2.25, 2.28).

2.36.92   Morse, J.M. (2000) Making qualitative research visible. *Qualitative Health Research* 10 (4) 437–9   Editorial

Reports the success of the International Institute for Qualitative Methodology (IIQM), now two years old, located in Alberta, Canada. Addresses of its seven affiliated international sites, located worldwide, are given and institutions are invited to join their nearest site so that a set of interlinking websites can be created (CR 2.36.63, 2.85, 3.5, 3.15).

2.36.93   Morse, J.M. (2000) Researching illness and injury: methodological considerations. *Qualitative Health Research* 10 (4) 538–46   14 References

When researching critically ill people, the injured and dying, methodological problems extend from the participants' condition, including the lack of everyday language to describe their experiences, the instability of the participants' reality and of the researcher. These problems result in decisions about the timing of data collection, challenges to reliability and validity and debates about who should be conducting the research. The article discusses these and makes suggestions about how to move forward (CR 2.24, 2.25, 2.64).

2.36.94   Morse, J.M. (2001) Are there risks in qualitative research? *Qualitative Health Research* 11 (1) 3–4   3 References   Editorial

Discusses risks to patients of qualitative inquiry itself.

2.36.95   Morse, J.M., Swanson, J. & Kuzel, A.J. (eds) (2001) *The nature of qualitative evidence.* Thousand Oaks, CA: Sage   ISBN 0761922857   References

Book provides urgently needed standards for qualitative inquiry while tackling the significant issues of what constitutes qualitative evidence. The book addresses the place of qualitative evidence in the planning, delivery and evaluation of health care.

2.36.96   Morse, J.M. & Richards, L. (2002) *ReadMe first for a user's guide to qualitative methods.* Thousand Oaks, CA: Sage   ISBN 0761918914   References

Offering a map to show readers how some methodological choices lead more directly than others to particular goals, this book provides novice researchers with an overview of techniques for creating data, and an explanation of the ways different tools fit different purposes and provide different research experiences and outcomes.

2.36.97 Mukherji, P.N. (ed.) (2000) *Methodology in social research: dilemmas and perspectives: essays in honour of Ramkrishna Mukherjee.* New Delhi, India: Sage   ISBN 0761994408

Volume contains an introduction to methodology in social research and will enable researchers trained in a particular field to look beyond and relate to other methodological domains.

2.36.98 Munhall, P.L. (ed.) (2001) *Nursing research: a qualitative perspective* (3rd edition). Sudbury, MA: Jones & Bartlett and National League for Nursing   ISBN 0763711357   64 References

Book continues to define the qualitative perspective as it relates to continuing progress in nursing research today. It includes research language, epistemology, qualitative paradigms, methods and exemplars, together with other considerations in qualitative research (CR 2.2, 2.5, 2.6, 2.17, 2.37, 2.39, 2.42, 2.45, 2.46, 2.49).

2.36.99 Murphy, E. (2000) *Qualitative research methods in health technology assessment: a review of the literature* www.ncchta.org/project.asp?pjtld=929 (Accessed 13/11/03)

Review examines the nature and status of qualitative methods in relation to their potential uses in health technology assessment (CR 2.12).

2.36.100 Murray, M. & Chamberlain, K. (eds) (1999) *Qualitative health psychology: theories and methods.* Thousand Oaks, CA: Sage   ISBN 0761956611   References

Constructing health and illness through language, conversing about health and illness and transforming talk into text are all addressed in this volume (CR 2.10, 2.45, 2.49, 2.53).

2.36.101 Myers, M.D. & Avison, D. (eds) (2002) *Qualitative research in information systems: a reader.* London: Sage   ISBN 0761966323   References

Information systems and qualitative research articles are now widely used for teaching in upper-level courses and this book fulfils the demand for a definitive collection of readings and teaching text. Seminal works in the field are brought together and editorial introductions assist the reader in understanding the essential principles of qualitative research.

2.36.102 O'Connor, D. (2001) Journeying the quagmire: exploring the discourses that shape the qualitative research process. *Affilia – Journal of Women & Social Work* 16 (2) 138–58   33 References

Author chronicles the pragmatic and ethical struggles encountered as her own ideas, reflecting the developing status of qualitative research perspectives, gradually shifted during the process of conducting a doctoral study. The purpose is to open for discussion the implications associated with contradictory discourses around qualitative research (CR 2.9, 2.16, 2.17).

2.36.103 Padgett, D.K. (1998) *Qualitative methods in social work research: challenges and rewards.* Thousand Oaks, CA: Sage   ISBN 0761902015   References

The author introduces and then dispels commonly-held misconceptions about qualitative methods, discusses the origins and basic components of methods, and presents a four-phase approach to conducting a study. The book concludes with a discussion of the challenges and rewards of using qualitative methods.

2.36.104 Parse, R.R. (2001) *Qualitative inquiry: the path of sciencing.* Sudbury, MA: Jones & Bartlett   ISBN 0763715654   References

Because human experience cannot be quantified or held captive in reports with digital measures, finding answers to research questions about lived experiences requires the use of rigorous qualitative methods. The author describes these rigorous methods, examines existing qualitative approaches from both the human science and nursing disciplines, as well as established and emerging nursing methods from the science of unitary human beings (CR 2.6).

2.36.105 Patton, M.Q. (2002) *Qualitative research and evaluation methods* (3rd edition). Thousand Oaks, CA: Sage   ISBN 0761919716   References

This resource and training manual for researchers, evaluators and graduate students has been completely revised. It is a 'tour de force' of the field of qualitative research in terms of its theoretical, conceptual, methodological, normative dimensions and foundations (CR 2.43).

2.36.106 Payne, J. (1999) *Researching health needs: a community-based approach.* London: Sage   ISBN 0761960848   References

This introduction to social science research techniques used in gathering evidence about the health of local communities takes the reader through each stage of the research process, getting the message across and trying to influence policy and practice. Key features include social survey and qualitative approaches, review of methods for investigating health status and community profiling. A section on using the Internet, visual techniques for collecting data, case studies and practical exercises are also included (CR 2.39, 2.72, 2.85, 2.86, 2.87, 2.94).

2.36.107 Pentland, W.E., Lawton, M.P., Harvey, A.S. & McColl, M.A. (eds) (1999) *Time-use research in the social sciences*. Dordrecht: Kluwer Academic/Plenum Publishers ISBN 030645951 References [Also available: eBook (2002) ISBN 0306471558]

This collection demonstrates the use and variety of applications of time-use methodology from multidisciplinary, multinational and multicultural perspectives. The fields of psychology, occupational therapy, sociology and economics are used to examine the complex relationship between human time utilization and health, and the future of time-use analysis as a research tool is discussed.

2.36.108 Piirto, J. (2002) The question of quality and qualifications: writing inferior poems as qualitative research. *Qualitative Studies in Education* 15 (4) 431–45 32 References

Addresses the question of skill and quality needed to produce data in the form of a novel or poems, and analyses the notion of art forms as qualitative research.

2.36.109 Playle, J. (2000) Qualitative approaches to research. *Journal of Community Nursing* 14 (9) 4–8 39 References

Article outlines some characteristics of qualitative research and discusses assumptions surrounding this approach. Data collection methods, observation, data analysis, credibility and authenticity are all considered (CR 2.64, 2.72, 2.86).

2.36.110 Pope, C. & Mays, N. (eds) (2000) *Qualitative research in health care* (2nd edition). London: BMJ Books ISBN 0727913964 References

This new edition includes developments in the field of qualitative research. New chapters on action research and analysing qualitative data are included (CR 2.37, 2.86).

2.36.111 Qualpage *Resources for qualitative research* www.ualberta.ca/~jrnorris/qual.html (Accessed 11/02/03)

This website lists information and resources of interest to qualitative researchers.

2.36.112 Rice, P.L. & Ezzy, D. (1999) *Qualitative research methods: a health focus*. Melbourne: Oxford University Press ISBN 0195506103 References

Book is a practical guide to conducting qualitative research, with an emphasis on health-related examples. It covers interviewing, focus groups, ethnography, narrative method, memory-work and participatory-action research. Detailed examples of each method are provided (CR 2.37, 2.42, 2.68, 2.69, 2.78).

2.36.113 Ritchie, J. & Lewis, J. (eds) (2003) *Qualitative research practice: a guide for social science students and researchers*. London: Sage ISBN 0761971106 References

Illuminating the possibilities of qualitative research, this textbook presents a sequential overview of the process by practising researchers active in the field of social and public policy. Numerous case studies are included, together with chapter summaries, explanations of key concepts, reflective points for seminar discussion and further reading.

2.36.114 Rose, G. (2001) *Visual methodologies: an introduction to interpreting visual objects*. London: Sage ISBN 076196665X

Book explains the methods that may be used when reading visual culture. The strengths and weaknesses of each method are illustrated with a detailed case study (CR 2.88, 2.89).

2.36.115 Rossman, G.B. & Rallis, S.F. (2003) *Learning in the field* (2nd edition). Thousand Oaks, CA: Sage ISBN 0761926518 References

Book aims to help readers visualize and grasp the concepts, issues and complexities of qualitative inquiry. The authors introduce each chapter with discussions among three 'characters' – students whose research projects demonstrate the challenges and excitement of qualitative research.

2.36.116 Sandelowski, M. (1999) Time and qualitative research. *Research in Nursing and Health* 22 (1) 79–87 31 References

Author believes that temporal concerns are integral to qualitative research, whether the focus is on disciplines in which qualitative methods are largely used, paradigms of inquiry that are primarily associated with qualitative methods, or on qualitative methods themselves. Temporal factors play a critical role in purposive sampling, the content and structure of data collection and analysis techniques, and in the re-presentation of the data in a qualitative research report. The Trajectory Model and Storyline Graph are discussed (CR 2.22, 2.45, 2.49, 2.64, 2.78, 2.79).

2.36.117   Sandelowski, M. (2000) Focus on research methods. Whatever happened to qualitative description? *Research in Nursing and Health* 23 (4) 334–40   37 References

Author describes qualitative description as a method that researchers can claim unashamedly without resorting to methodological acrobatics. This is the method of choice when straight descriptions of phenomena are desired and so is especially useful for researchers wanting to know the who, what and where of events. Although foundational to all qualitative research methods, these descriptive studies comprise a valuable methodologic approach in their own right.

2.36.118   Sandelowski, M. (2001) Focus on research methods. Real qualitative researchers do not count: the use of numbers in qualitative research. *Research in Nursing and Health* 24 (3) 230–40   29 References

The author focuses on the uses of numbers in analysing, interpreting and re-presenting qualitative data in primarily qualitative studies. Specifically, the uses of numbers to generate meaning from qualitative data, to document, verify and test researcher interpretation or conclusions, and to re-present target events and experiences are all discussed (CR 2.86).

2.36.119   Sandelowski, M. (2002) Re-embodying qualitative inquiry. *Qualitative Health Research* 12 (1) 104–15   71 References

Author discusses the problems of emphasizing interviews as the chief method of obtaining data in qualitative research. The primary reasons and potentially negative consequences of this choice are discussed, and recommendations are made for achieving more robust and full-bodied qualitative research by also using other data collection methods.

2.36.120   Sandelowski, M. & Barroso, J. (2002) Finding the findings in qualitative research. *Journal of Nursing Scholarship* 34 (3) 213–19   32 References

Authors describe the challenge of finding the findings in qualitative studies. Factors complicating the issues include varied reporting styles, misrepresentation of data and analytic procedures as findings, misuse of quotes and theory, and lack of clarity concerning patterns and themes. Theses and dissertations present special challenges because they often contain several of these problems.

2.36.121   Sayre, S. (2001) *Qualitative methods for marketplace research.* Thousand Oaks, CA: Sage   ISBN 0761922709   References

Book covers all key topics and borrows techniques from a wide variety of fields to present specific examples that illustrate how they may be adapted for marketplace research. Chapters draw from expert studies to provide a guide of the methods needed to develop, execute and analyse state-of-the-art marketplace studies.

2.36.122   Scott, D. (2002) Adding meaning to measurement: the value of qualitative methods in practice research. *British Journal of Social Work* 32 (7) 923–30   20 References

Discusses ways in which social work practitioners might develop research from questions that arise in practice and suggests the use of qualitative methods for such a purpose.

2.36.123   Seale, C. (ed.) (1998) *Researching society and culture.* London: Sage   ISBN 0761952772 References

Provides a comprehensive, definitive, introductory textbook on methods and methodology for students in the social sciences and cultural studies. It includes a full overview of, and introduction to, research methods used in these disciplines, examples from actual research, and methodological and theoretical issues in doing research (CR 2.5, 2.10, 2.42, 2.46, 2.52, 2.68, 2.86, 2.95, 2.96, 2.97).

2.36.124   Seale, C. (1999) *The quality of qualitative research.* London: Sage   ISBN 0761955984 References

Textbook is designed to help students and practising researchers improve the quality of their research. Practical examples and exercises demonstrate how to evaluate qualitative research, plan and collect good-quality data, do thoughtful analyses, write up and report on qualitative research (CR 2.13, 2.24, 2.28, 2.45, 2.95, 2.97, 2.100).

2.36.125   Shaw, I.F. & Gould, N.G. (eds) (2001) *Qualitative research in social work.* London: Sage ISBN 0761961828   References

Book examines epistemological and methodological issues in a context whereby the agenda is set by, and is relevant to, social work (CR 2.6, 2.78).

2.36.126   Sikes, P. (2000) 'Truth' and 'lies' revisited. *British Educational Research Journal* 26 (2) 257–70   33 References

Anecdotal evidence suggests that many qualitative researchers have had the experience of discovering that their informants have told them lies. The article draws on two examples in order to explore some of the questions and issues that may arise (CR 2.17).

2.36.127   Silverman, D. (ed.) (1997) *Qualitative research: theory, method and practice.* London: Sage   ISBN 0803976666   References

Contains chapters written by an international team of researchers under the major headings of observation, texts, interviews, audio and video, validity and social problems (CR 2.25, 2.68, 2.72).

2.36.128 Silverman, D. (1999) *Doing qualitative research: a practical handbook.* London: Sage ISBN 0761958231 References

Intended for all levels of users, this book presents the world of qualitative research and how it is done. Sections cover starting out, analysing the data, keeping in touch, writing up, the aftermath and an epilogue which discusses the contested character of qualitative research.

2.36.129 Slevin, L. & Sines, D. (1999/2000) Enhancing the truthfulness, consistency and transferability of a qualitative study: utilizing a manifold of approaches. *Nurse Researcher* 7 (2) 79–97 39 References

Paper describes criteria one of the authors used within a doctoral study to increase the truthfulness, consistency and transferability of a qualitative study that involved an investigation to explicate the role of community nurses for people with learning difficulties. Transferability rather than generalizability was felt to be a more appropriate term for qualitative findings that may have applications to other sites or situations (CR 2.24, 2.25, 2.28, 2.45, 2.68, 2.78).

2.36.130 Smith, J.A. (2003) *Qualitative psychology: a practical guide to research methods.* London: Sage ISBN 0761972307 References

Book covers all the main qualitative approaches now used in psychology and each chapter offers readers a step-by-step guide to these methods.

2.36.131 Smith, M.J. (1998) *Social science in question: towards a postdisciplinary framework.* London: Sage/Open University ISBN 0761960414 References

Book discusses the story of science and the emergence of the social sciences with all its complexities. Its paradigms, conventions, relativism, language, discourse and culture are all considered. It outlines current rethinking on representation, knowledge and reality in the social sciences (CR 2.8).

2.36.132 Speziale, H.J.S. & Carpenter, D.R. (2003) *Qualitative research in nursing: advancing the humanistic imperative* (3rd edition). Philadelphia, PA: Lippincott Williams & Wilkins ISBN 0781734835 References

Covers principle qualitative methods in current use. Chapters give an overview of each method, step-by-step guidance on implementation and application to nursing education, administration and practice. New

material is included on ethical issues, action research and triangulation as a qualitative research strategy. It includes an example of a funded grant proposal (CR 2.2, 2.17, 2.26, 2.29, 2.37, 2.42, 2.46, 2.96).

2.36.133 Stebbins, R.A. (2001) *Exploratory research in the social sciences.* Thousand Oaks, CA: Sage ISBN 0761923993 References

Author takes the reader through the process of exploratory research, providing the student or researcher with a complete reference for carrying out this type of research.

2.36.134 Sword, W. (1999) Accounting for presence of self: reflections on doing qualitative research. *Qualitative Health Research* 9 (2) 270–8 23 References

Provides an account of the author's experiences of doing qualitative research, including feelings, motives, challenges and strategies to make meaning from the research.

2.36.135 Symon, G. & Cassell, C. (eds) (1998) *Qualitative methods and analysis in organizational research: a practical guide.* London: Sage ISBN 0761953515 References

Bringing together a wide range of qualitative methods in organizational research, this book shows how they may be used in practice. The diversity of organizational contexts examined highlights the breadth of work issues and environments to which qualitative methods have been applied (CR 2.65, 2.71, 2.89).

2.36.136 Temple, B. (2002) Crossed wires: interpreters, translators and bilingual workers in cross language research. *Qualitative Health Research* 12 (6) 844–54 22 References

Describes how English-speaking researchers carry out research with people who do not, or prefer not, to speak English. Discusses the issues that arise from conducting cross-language research using two methodological models.

2.36.137 Travers, M. (2001) *Qualitative research through case studies.* London: Sage ISBN 0761968067 References

Introduces a wide range of traditions, including grounded theory, dramaturgical analysis, ethnomethodology, conversation analysis, critical discourse analysis, feminism and post-modern ethnography. Each chapter introduces the theoretical assumptions of the tradition and uses case studies for illustration (CR 2.10, 2.39, 2.42, 2.45, 2.89).

2.36.138 University of Missouri – Ward E. Barnes Library *Qualitative research subject*

guide-books www.umsl.edu/services/scampus/
ERSubGqualresbk.html (Accessed 22/01/03)

Provides an example of a qualitative research bibliography developed by a university library.

2.36.139   Weinberg, D. (ed.) (2002) *Qualitative
research methods.* Oxford: Blackwell   ISBN
0631217622   References

This edited book provides a definitive collection of
readings for students undertaking any kind of social
inquiry, and represents the finest classic and contemporary scholarship in the field. An overview is
given of qualitative research methods and the five
parts cover: the legacy of qualitative research methods; qualitative interviewing; life history and narrative analysis; observational fieldwork, conversation
and discourse analysis; and research using artefacts
as primary sources (CR 2.68, 2.71, 2.72, 2.89, 2.90).

2.36.140   Willig, C. (2001) *Introducing qualitative research in psychology: adventures in theory
and method.* Buckingham: Open University Press
ISBN 0335205356 References

Introduces students to the rationale behind qualitative research methods and gives guidance on six
different approaches: grounded theory, interpretative
phenomenology, case studies, discursive psychology, Foucauldian discourse analysis and memory
work (CR 2.39, 2.45, 2.49, 2.89).

2.36.141   Wright, K. & Flemons, D. (2002)
Dying to know: qualitative research with terminally
ill persons and their family. *Death Studies* 26 (3)
255–71   45 References

Illustrates the use of qualitative research in thana-
tology (death studies) and provides an explanation
of the decision-making process underpinning all
sections of the research, from question formulation
to data analysis. Includes reflections on the challenges faced by the researcher conducting this type
of research (CR 2.4, 2.16).

2.36.142   Zoucha, R. (1999) Using qualitative
methods in research [Spanish]. *Cultura De Los
Cuidados* 3 (6) 80–90   27 References

Purpose of this paper is to discuss the benefits
and usefulness of conducting qualitative research
studies, and to present an overview of four
methods frequently used in nursing (CR 2.29, 2.42,
2.45).

Non-Experimental Designs

2.37 ACTION RESEARCH/ PARTICIPATIVE INQUIRY

'The participatory action research strategy has a double objective. One aim is to produce knowledge and action directly useful to a group of people. ... [A further] aim is to empower people at a second and deeper level through the process of constructing and using their own knowledge.' (Denzin & Lincoln, 1994: 328)

Definitions [See Appendix D for sources]

Action research – research, where instead of minimizing the impact of the investigations on the subjects or individuals under study, changes are purposefully introduced in order to study what, if any, effects occur

Participatory action research – ... engages people in examining their knowledge (understandings, skills and values) and interpretive categories (the ways they interpret themselves and their action in the social and material world)

Example

Meyer, J., Bridges, J. & Spilsbury, K. (1999) Caring for older people in acute settings: lessons learned from an action research study in accident and emergency. *NT Research* 4 (5) 327–9 51 References

Paper reports the findings of a study that explored the organization of care for older people in an accident and emergency department. Authors believe that nurses may need to work together more closely to foster the much-needed improvements in the care of older people.

Annotations

2.37.1 Alvarez, A.R. & Gutierrez, L.M. (2001) Choosing to do participatory research: an example and issues of fit to consider. *Journal of Community Practice* 9 (1) 1–20 34 References

Article describes a participatory research process through which community members collaborated in the design and implementation of a project to identify, learn about the work of, and develop training on the perspectives of people doing multicultural community organizing in Detroit. Suggestions are made for those considering similar research (CR 2.15).

2.37.2 Atweh, B., Kemmis, S. & Weeks, P. (eds) (1998) *Action research in practice: partnerships for social justice in education.* London: Routledge ISBN 0414171520 References

Book presents a compilation of action research projects in schools and a university. The collection shows how projects that differ on a wide variety of dimensions can raise similar themes, problems and issues. Theme chapters discuss action research, social justice and partnerships, followed by case studies (CR 2.39).

2.37.3 Badger, T.G. (2000) Action research, change and methodological rigour. *Journal of Nursing Management* 8 (4) July 201–7 49 References

Examines action research in relationship to its potential for instigating change and provides an explanation of the various philosophical/methodological approaches that fall within it. Ethical issues and validity and reliability are discussed, and comments on the utility of the approach are made (CR 2.17, 2.24, 2.25, 2.101).

2.37.4 Balcazar, F.E., Keys, C.B., Kaplan, D.L. & Suarez-Balcazar, Y. (1998) Participatory action research and people with disabilities: principles and challenges. *Canadian Journal of Rehabilitation* 12 (2) 105–12 31 References

Participatory action research (PAR) provides a framework in which people with disabilities can take an active role in designing and conducting research. Four principles are discussed, together with some of the challenges of conducting participatory research.

2.37.5 Blenkin, G.M., Kelly, A.V. & Rose, J. (2001) *Action research for professional development: an early years perspective.* London: Paul Chapman ISBN 1853964204 References

Book describes and evaluates the work of Phase 2 of the Principles and Practice Project. This aimed to promote the professional development of all kinds of practitioners working with children under the age of eight, and to explore the effectiveness of an action research approach.

2.37.6　Coghlan, D. & Brannick, T. (2000) *Doing action research in your own organization.* London: Sage　ISBN 0761968873　References

Book addresses the advantages and potential pitfalls, the politics and ethics of researching your own organization. Each chapter includes examples and exercises (CR 2.17).

2.37.7　Dickson, G. & Green, K.L. (2001) The external researcher in participatory action research. *Educational Action Research: An International Journal* 9 (2) 243–60　31 References

Article addresses questions to be considered by a researcher who is external to the participants but wants to use participatory action research. Roles played, challenges faced and lessons learned illuminate the reality of an alluring yet complex approach to research (CR 2.16).

2.37.8　Earl-Slater, A. (2002) The superiority of action research? *British Journal of Clinical Governance* 7 (2) 132–5　5 References

Describes the features of action research and what use has been made of it in fields other than health (CR 2.2.13).

2.37.9　Greenwood, D.J. & Levin, M. (1998) *Introduction to action research: social research for social change.* Thousand Oaks, CA: Sage　ISBN 0761916768　References

Provides an overview of different approaches to action research. Authors introduce the history, philosophy, social change agenda, methodologies, ethical arguments for and fieldwork tools for action research. An extensive range of cases is included, some of which failed while others succeeded (CR 2.17).

2.37.10　Hampshire, A.J. (2000) What is action research and can it promote change in primary care? *Journal of Evaluation In Clinical Practice* 6 (4) 337–43　42 References

Outlines action research and its use in promoting individual and organizational change.

2.37.11　Hart, E. & Bond, M. (1995) *Action research for health and social care: a guide to practice.* Buckingham: Open University Press　ISBN 0335192629　References

Book is designed for students at undergraduate and postgraduate level and others undertaking professional courses. It describes the processes of action research and how it may be used to solve problems and improve care. Five case studies of action research are described from the researcher's perspective. A tool kit is included which will assist in preparing research proposals, thinking about problems and formulating strategies (CR 2.14, 2.16, 2.20, 2.96).

2.37.12　Hope, K. (1998/99) Starting out with action research. *Nurse Researcher* 6 (2) 16–26　23 References

The author draws parallels between the process of action research and its instigation. Both are characterized by decision trails and logistics that are context-bound, complex and open to confusion. Using the analogy of a journey, the processes that need to be undertaken when considering this type of research are discussed.

2.37.13　Kelly, D. & Simpson, S. (2001) Methodological issues in nursing research. Action research in action: reflections on a project to introduce clinical practice facilitators to an acute hospital setting. *Journal of Advanced Nursing* 33 (5) 652–9　35 References

The process and philosophical basis of action research are discussed by reviewing the insights gained from a study designed to enhance the support available to junior nursing staff in an acute hospital setting (CR 2.5).

2.37.14　Lilford, R., Warren, R. & Braunholtz, D. (2003) Action research: a way of researching or a way of managing? *Journal of Health Services Research and Policy* 8 (2) 100–4　14 References

Argues that action research is a misnomer and that it does not differ significantly from change methodologies. Compares the approach with total quality management, noting that in terms of its ultimate aim of effecting change, it is irrelevant which methodology is used.

2.37.15　Lyon, J. (1998/99) Applying Hart and Bond's typology: implementing clinical supervision in an acute setting. *Nurse Researcher* 6 (2) 39–56　18 References

Article describes how Hart and Bond's action research typology was used to clarify the process of implementing clinical supervision. The seven criteria listed by Hart and Bond are discussed in relation to the four action research approaches they describe (CR 2.37.11).

2.37.16　Meyer, J. (2000) Using qualitative methods in health-related action research. *British*

Medical Journal 320 (7228) 15 January 178–81 23
References

Describes the fundamentals of action research, its typologies and potential application to health care.

2.37.17 Meyer, J., Spilsbury, K. & Prieto, J. (1999/2000) Comparison of findings from a single case in relation to those from a systematic review of action research. *Nurse Researcher* 7 (2) 37–59 37 References

Paper presents the results of a systematic review of action research that aimed to identify those factors that facilitate and inhibit change in health care practice. These findings are compared with the findings of a single case study. The comparative results of these two studies suggest it may be possible to generalize more widely from action research (CR 2.12, 2.28, 2.34).

2.37.18 Morrison, B. & Lilford, R.J. (2001) How can action research apply to health services? *Qualitative Health Research* 11 (4) 436–49 20 References

Article identifies the principles of action research and its stated philosophical position. Action research is hailed as pioneering, imaginative and flexible but the authors argue that it is not so very different from other, mainstream approaches. They suggest that both action and mainstream researchers reconsider their stances towards each other.

2.37.19 Reason, P. & Bradbury, H. (eds) (2001) *Handbook of action research: participative inquiry and practice*. London: Sage ISBN 0761966455 References

Handbook explores the latest approaches in social inquiry and moves the field forward. The contributors grapple with questions of how to integrate knowledge with action, how to collaborate with other researchers and how to present the necessarily disparate components in a coherent fashion (CR 2.15).

2.37.20 Stringer, E.T. (1999) *Action research* (2nd edition). Thousand Oaks, CA: Sage ISBN 0761917136 References

Book provides a simple but highly effective model for approaching action research. This new edition has been broadened in scope to include university and other bureaucratic settings. End of chapter summaries provide checklists for researchers and an appendix of electronic resources is included.

2.37.21 Wallis, S. (1998/99) Changing practice through action research. *Nurse Researcher* 6 (2) 5–15 31 References

Author explains why nurses should use action research approaches and how such approaches may contribute to changes in practice (CR 2.102, 3.7).

2.37.22 Wang, C.C. (1999) Photovoice: a participatory action research strategy applied to women's health. *Journal of Women's Health* 8 (2) March 185–92 References

Photovoice is a process by which people can identify, represent and enhance their community through a specific photographic technique. This paper gives an overview of the origins, key concepts, methods and uses of photovoice as a strategy to improve women's health.

2.37.23 Waterman, H., Tillen, D., Dickson, R. & de Koning, K. (2001) Action research: a systematic review and guidance for assessment. *Health Technology Assessment* 5 (23) References 166 pages

A systematic review that defines action research and identifies action research projects conducted in UK health care settings. It provides guidance on the assessment of action research proposals and reports (CR 2.12).

2.37.24 Winter, R. & Munn-Giddings, C. (2001) *A handbook for action research in health and social care*. London: Routledge ISBN 0415224845 References

Book describes the nature of action research and gives a series of examples. It provides practical guidance on undertaking an action research project and justifies this type of research as a form of social inquiry. Authors believe that action research is not a way of 'ignoring the challenges' of conventional inquiry, but is a way of addressing real philosophical difficulties. Action research and relativism and critical realism are both explored.

2.38 ATHEORETICAL RESEARCH

'Some purists may regard research which is not based on theoretical frameworks or conceptual orientations as problem-solving rather than scientific research. However, early studies in clinical nursing research tended to be problem solving endeavours, rather than scientific research. More recently, emphasis has been put on the use of theory as the appropriate grounding, but there is still room for work to be done in nursing while a theoretical base is being discovered.' (Phillips, L.R.F., 1986: 87)

Example

Mills, C.M., McSweeney, M. & Lavin, M.A.
(1998) Characteristics of patient visits to nurse
practitioners and physician assistants in hospital
outpatient departments. *Journal of Professional
Nursing* 14 (6) 335–43   35 References

This exploratory, atheoretical research, using the
1992 National Hospital Ambulatory Medical Care
Survey data set, examined which of the following
characteristics predicted patients being seen by
nurse practitioners and physician assistants: patient
and hospital demographics, diagnosis, diagnostic/
screening services, therapeutic services and disposi-
tion of the visit. Results are reported and the authors
believe these may assist with understanding the
utilization of nurse practitioners and physician
assistants in primary care (CR 2.91).

Annotations

**2.38.1 Brack, C.J., Brack, G., Brogan, R. &
Edwards, D.** (1996) Mental health consultation: in
defence of merging theory and practice. *Journal of
Mental Health Counseling* 18 (4) 347–57

Consultation based on a systematic approach
grounded in theory categorizes information, antici-
pates difficulties and frames interventions, whereas
atheoretical or unsystematic approaches tend to lack
direction and deal with problem-solving in a haphazard manner. This article explores the obstacles
in merging theory and practice in consultation and
illustrates the effect of theory on practice with a
consultation case.

2.38.2 Carson, D.K. (1999) The importance of
creativity in family therapy: a preliminary consideration. *Family Journal: Counseling and Therapy for
Couples and Families* 7 (4) 326–34

Experimental therapy, though often labelled as
atheoretical, facilitates creative, spontaneous, non-
rational experiencing in families, in part due to the
therapist's own creativity. The stages of the creative
process are described and some of the blocks that
may be encountered are discussed.

2.38.3 Chwalisz, K. (1996) The perceived stress
model of caregiver burden: evidence from spouses

of persons with brain injuries. *Rehabilitation
Psychology* 41 (2) 91–114

Study investigated the efficacy of the Perceived
Stress Model of Caregiver Burden (PSB) with 135
caregivers of brain-injured people. A theoretical
model was tested against an atheoretical model containing relationships among variables previously
reported in burden literature. By combining both
models, results showed a more parsimonious representation of the relationships among variables.

2.38.4 Corcoran, J. (2000) Family interventions
with child physical abuse and neglect: a critical
review. *Children and Youth Services Review* 22 (7)
563–91

Article reviews the research on family treatments for
child physical abuse and neglect. Studies are
organized according to theoretical, cognitive-
behavioural, family therapy, social network and atheoretical treatments. A critique is offered, together
with suggestions for strengthening future research.

2.39   CASE STUDY RESEARCH

The term 'case study' does not denote a single specific technique, but rather a general strategy for
research. Typically, a case study involves one or
several cases that are studied over time by multiple
data-gathering methods. They have a contemporary,
rather than historical focus, are naturalistic and conducted in a setting that is not controlled by the
researcher.

Example

Holroyd, E., Twinn, S. & Shiu, A. (2001)
Evaluating psychosocial nursing interventions for
cardiac clients and their caregivers: a case study of
the community rehabilitation network in Hong
Kong. *Journal of Advanced Nursing* 35 (3)
393–401   29 References

Using a two-phase case study design and telephone
interviews, this study describes the type and nature
of psychosocial nursing interventions for cardiac
clients. Findings showed that the nurses' interpersonal skills were highly valued but there was a
concern about the lack of individual care (CR 2.70).

Annotations

2.39.1 Bassey, M. (1999) *Case study research in educational settings*. Buckingham: Open University Press ISBN 0335199844 References

Book offers new insights into the case study as a tool of educational research and suggests how it can be a prime research strategy for developing educational theory that illuminates policy and enhances practice. Different kinds of case study are identified, examples are given and readers are taken through each stage of conducting the research.

2.39.2 Bryar, R.M. (1999/2000) An examination of case study research. *Nurse Researcher* 7 (2) 61–78 35 References

Article explores the significant features, history and application of case study research in nursing research and in relation to aspects of research and development.

2.39.3 Gomm, R., Hammersley, M. & Foster, P. (eds) (2000) *Case study method: key issues, key texts*. London: Sage ISBN 0761964142 References

Editors bring together key contributions from the field that reflect the different interpretations of the purpose and capacity of case study research. They offer in-depth assessment of the main arguments. An annotated bibliography of the literature relating to case study research is also included (CR 2.28, 2.34).

2.39.4 Gummesson, E. (1999) *Qualitative methods in management research* (2nd edition). Thousand Oaks, CA: Sage ISBN 0761920145 References

Book presents a fresh approach to case study research, stressing the need for involved rather than detached researchers. Author links quality assessment of case study research to current total quality management thinking, and proposes the concept of management action science in which the researcher is both actor and student (CR 2.36).

2.39.5 Pegram, A. (1999/2000) What is case study research? *Nurse Researcher* 7 (2) 5–16 27 References

Discusses the nature of case study research, its validity, multiple meaning and its use in nursing (CR 2.9, 2.25, 2.86, 2.87).

2.39.6 Ritchie, J.E. (2001) Case series research. a case for qualitative method in assembling evidence. *Physiotherapy Theory and Practice* 17 (3) 127–35 32 References

Although the hierarchy of evidence favours quantitative methods in evidence-based practice, there is a place for rigorous, systematically undertaken qualitative research methods in physiotherapy and other health care disciplines. The author argues that in some instances the use of case series research can stand alone. Inductively derived findings from a series of carefully and systematically undertaken case studies have an important role in the assembling of evidence for more effective practice, especially in a discipline such as physiotherapy where interventions are more often context-dependent and complex (CR 2.36, 2.43).

2.39.7 Scholz, R.W. & Tietje, O. (2001) *Embedded case study methods: integrating quantitative and qualitative knowledge*. Thousand Oaks, CA: Sage ISBN 0761919465 References

In an embedded case study, the starting and end point is the comprehension of the case as a whole in its real-world context. The authors emphasize that a qualitative analysis starting from the real-world level is an indispensable part of case analysis. The book bridges the gap between quantitative and qualitative approaches to complex problems when using case study methodology (CR 2.9).

2.39.8 Vallis, J. & Tierney, A. (1999/2000) Issues in case study analysis. *Nurse Researcher* 7 (2) 19–35 31 References

Paper provides a realistic, first-hand account of undertaking case study research in the context of a four-centre investigation of hip fracture care. Practical and methodological issues, techniques of analysis and the difficulties of using both qualitative and quantitative methods in this type of research are all discussed (CR 2.29, 2.36, 2.86, 2.87).

2.39.9 Yin, R.K. (1999) Enhancing the quality of case studies in health services research. *Health Services Research* 34 (5) 1209–24 19 References

Gives advice on how to improve the quality of case study research (CR 3.12).

2.39.10 Yin, R.K. (2003) *Applications of case study research* (2nd edition). Thousand Oaks, CA: Sage ISBN 0761925511 References

Written to augment *Case Study Research: Design and Methods* (2003), this new edition presents and discusses new case studies offering a wide variety of examples. These applications demonstrate specific techniques or principles that are integral to the method. Through these, the reader will be able to identify solutions to problems encountered during this type of research (CR 2.39.11).

2.39.11 Yin, R.K. (2003) *Case study research: design and methods* (3rd edition). Thousand Oaks, CA: Sage ISBN 0761925538 References

Focuses on case study design and analysis as a distinct research tool with wide applicability. It has been revised, updated and expanded to include recent developments in the field. The book refers to case studies in many different fields, illustrating points made in the text, and includes 44 boxes describing real case studies, paying particular attention to design and analysis.

2.39.12 Zucker, D.M. (2001) Using case study methodology in nursing research. *The Qualitative Report* 6 (2) 12 pp   23 References www.nova.edu/ssss/QR/QR6–2/zucker.html (Accessed 11/11/03)

Defines case study research and outlines the origins of its approach, method and analysis using a case study of men with coronary heart disease. Discusses its usefulness for theory generation and practice (CR 2.7).

2.40   CORRELATIONAL RESEARCH

Correlational research aims to describe the relationship between two naturally occurring events.

Definitions [See Appendix D for sources]

Causal comparative – a type of correlational research in which two or more groups are compared with one another, either prospectively or retrospectively, to generate hypotheses regarding relationships between non-experimental variables

Correlational research – investigations that explore the interrelationships among variables of interest without any active intervention on the part of the researcher

---

Example

Chapman, K.J. & Pepler, C. (1998) Coping, hope, and anticipatory grief in family members in palliative home care. *Cancer Nursing* 21 (4) 226–34   59 References

Article describes an exploratory, cross-sectional, correlational study designed to examine the relationships among general coping style, hope and anticipatory grief in a convenience sample of 61 family members of people with terminal cancer. Findings showed that family members experienced individual anticipatory grief patterns and these are described.

Annotations

2.40.1   Davis, J. (1997) *Correlational research methods.* Department of Psychology, Metropolitan State College of Denver clem.mscd.edu/~davisj/prm2/correl_1.html (Accessed 11/02/03)

These notes are intended as a brief introduction and overview for undergraduate students in psychological research methods courses.

2.40.2   LaMar, Y.L. *Correlational research designs* trochim.human.cornell.edu/tutorial/lamar/ylamar.htm (Accessed 01/05/03)

Tutorial covers the uses, planning and interpretation of correlational research designs.

2.41   EPIDEMIOLOGICAL RESEARCH

Epidemiological researchers have a special interest in data that may be retrospective in terms of diseases, epidemics or disasters; or prospective in trying to understand risk factors in the environment such as carcinogens or factors contributing to mental illness.

Definitions [See Appendix D for sources]

Case control study – ... a retrospective epidemiological study in which subjects who have contracted a particular disease (the cases) are compared with similar subjects who did not catch the disease (the controls)

Cross-sectional study – a study that examines the relationship between diseases (or other health-related characteristics) and other variables of interest, as they exist in a defined population at one particular time. [The temporal sequence of cause and effect cannot necessarily be determined in a cross-sectional study]

Epidemiological research – a strategy for trying to determine the causes, both necessary and sufficient, for the distribution and rates of occurrence of disease phenomena in human populations

Epidemiology – the study and distribution and determinants of health-related states or events in specified populations

Retrospective study – a study in which the outcomes have occurred to the participants before the study commenced.

Example

Kritz-Silverstein, D., Barrett-Connor, E. & Corbeau, C. (2001) Cross-sectional and prospective study of exercise and depressed mood in the elderly: the Rancho Bernado study. *American Journal of Epidemiology* 153 (6) 596–603 52 References

This study examined cross-sectional and prospective associations of exercise with depressed mood in a community-based sample of men and women between the ages of 50 and 89. Results showed that exercisers have less depressed mood, but it does not protect against future problems for those not clinically depressed at baseline.

Annotations

2.41.1 Bhopal, R. (2002) *Concepts of epidemiology: an integrated introduction to the ideas, theories, principles and methods of epidemiology.* Oxford: Oxford University Press ISBN 0192631551 References

Book explains and illustrates the language, principles and methods underlying the science of epidemiology, and its application to policy-making, health service planning and promotion (CR 2.2, 3.11).

2.41.2 Brownson, R.C. & Petitti, D.B. (eds) (1998) *Applied epidemiology: theory to practice.* New York: Oxford University Press ISBN 0195111907 References

Textbook is intended for students, practitioners and public health care personnel. It applies traditional epidemiologic methods for determining disease aetiology to the 'real-life' situations of public health and health services research.

2.41.3 Coughlin, S.S. & Beauchamp, T.L. (eds) (1998) *Ethics and epidemiology.* Oxford: Oxford University Press ISBN 0195102428 References

This text of theoretical and practical moral challenges in epidemiology, intended for students and health professionals, highlights the difficulties of keeping subjects informed and protected from unnecessary risks while performing relevant and important research (CR 2.17).

2.41.4 *Dictionary of epidemiology* (2001) 4th edition. Edited by Last, J.M. New York: Oxford University Press ISBN 0195141695

This is the standard English-language dictionary of epidemiology. It covers the common terms in epidemiology and those from many related fields, such as biostatics, infectious disease control, health promotion, genetics, clinical epidemiology, health economics and medical ethics. Epidemiologists from all over the world have made contributions to this book (CR 2.2, 2.17, 2.84).

2.41.5 Grimshaw, J., Wilson, B., Campbell, M., Eccles, M. & Ramsay, C. (2001) Epidemiological methods. In Fulop, N., Allen, P., Clarke, A. & Black, N. (eds) *Studying the organization and delivery of health services: research methods.* London: Routledge ISBN 0415257638 Chapter 4 56–72 26 References

Describes epidemiological approaches, focusing on methods for estimating the magnitude of the benefits of interventions to improve the delivery and organization of health services (CR 3.12.3).

2.41.6 Hulley, S.B., Cummings, S.R., Browner, W.S., Grady, D., Hearst, N. & Newman, T.B. (2001) *Designing clinical research: an epidemiologic approach.* Philadelphia, PA: Lippincott Williams & Wilkins ISBN 0781722187 References

Analyses various methodologies and discusses each step used in the process of epidemiological research.

2.41.7 Keyserling, W.M. (2000) Workplace risk factors and occupational musculoskeletal disorders, Part 2: a review of biomechanical and psychophysical research on risk factors associated with upper extremity disorders. *Aihaj* 61 (2) 231–43 59 References

Epidemiological and laboratory-based research methods have been used to evaluate the significance of various risk factors associated with overuse injuries and disorders. Although epidemiological studies provide important insights to understanding the causes of work-related overuse disorders, they are sometimes criticized for their inability to measure precisely how people respond to specific risk factors in the workplace. The article presents a review of recent laboratory and biomedical models of work factors believed to be associated with increased risk of injury, and although these approaches do not replace epidemiological studies, they do provide complementary information.

2.41.8 Moon, G., Gould, M., Brown, T., Jones, K., Duncan, C., Twigg, L., Subramanian, S.V., Litva, A. & Iggulden, P. (2000) *Epidemiology: an introduction.* Buckingham: Open University Press ISBN 0335200125 References

Book offers insight into the methods and principles of epidemiological study alongside an analysis of the broad context in which this type of research is undertaken. The design and analysis of epidemiological studies is discussed, together with how it may be assessed and applied.

2.41.9   Page, R.M., Cole, G.E. & Timmreck, T.C. (1995) *Basic epidemiological methods and bio-statistics: a practical guidebook.* Sudbury, MA: Jones & Bartlett   ISBN 0867208694   References

This application-oriented text will enable students to learn the basic principles of epidemiologic investigation. Numerous opportunities are presented to apply and test learning through problems and application exercises. Answers are provided.

2.41.10   Silman, A.J. & Macfarlane, G.J. (2002) *Epidemiological studies: a practical guide* (2nd edition). Cambridge: Cambridge University Press   ISBN 0521009391   References

Book provides a user-friendly introduction to the field of epidemiology.

2.41.11   University of Texas *Field epidemiology Internet resources* www.sph.uth.tmc.edu:8054/library/ph2615.htm (Accessed 19/02/03)

This website, developed by librarians at the Health Science Center at Houston School of Public Health, gives an example of specific material to be found on the Internet relating to epidemiology. It includes books, online databases, statistics instruction, federal and Texas statistics.

2.41.12   Unwin, N., Carr, S. & Leeson, J. (1997) *An introductory study guide to public health and epidemiology.* Buckingham: Open University Press   ISBN 0335157858   References

Covers some of the key issues in public health and epidemiology. Epidemiological study designs and weighing up the evidence from them are discussed. The chapters are written in a study guide format, each including a series of questions and exercises to encourage active participation.

2.41.13   Weiss, M.G. (2001) Cultural epidemiology: an introduction and overview. *Anthropology and Medicine* 8 (1) 5–29   72 References

Paper describes the EMIC framework for cultural studies of illness that developed from interdisciplinary collaboration between epidemiology and anthropology. The emergence of an interdisciplinary field of research, cultural epidemiology, is described, including its theoretical underpinnings. Five papers in this overview are concerned exclusively with mental health, but there is also discussion of active research on leprosy, tuberculosis, epilepsy, and tropical infections. Study on neurological and medical disorders is ongoing (CR 2.9, 2.15, 2.29, 2.36, 2.42, 3.22).

2.42   ETHNOMETHODS

'The growth of a new cultural movement, based on the anthropological tradition, developed in the USA in the 1960s, focusing on how people know and understand their world. The term ethnomethods is used to describe a group of techniques which seek to explain human care and health attributes which are part of the social structure, world views, language and different environmental contexts.' (Leininger, 1987: 13) [adapted]

Definitions [See Appendix D for sources]

Culture – a set of shared guidelines that helps a group of people make sense of the world, and includes the 'rules' of appropriate behaviour in that world

Emic – ... perspectives that are shared and understood by members of a particular culture, the 'insiders', in contrast to the perspective of the culture that observers, the 'outsiders', may have

Ethnography – ... the systematic process of observing, detailing, describing, documenting and analysing the life-ways or particular patterns of a culture (or subculture) in order to grasp the life ways or patterns of the people in their familiar environment

Ethnology – the historical-geographical and comparative study of peoples or cultures

Ethnomethodology – a family of related approaches concerned with describing and portraying how people construct their own definitions of a social situation or, more broadly, with the social construction of knowledge

Ethnonursing – the study and analysis of the local or indigenous peoples' viewpoints, beliefs and practices about nursing care phenomena and processes of designated cultures

Ethnoscience – a formalized and systematic study of people from their viewpoint in order to obtain an accurate account of how people know, classify and interpret their life ways and the universe

Ethology – a method of systematically observing, analysing and describing behaviours within the context in which they occur

Etic – ... refers to the outsiders' view of the experiences of a cultural group

Idiographic research – a method of investigation which is concerned with the individual, or unique experiences, rather than with generalities

Nomothetic research – a style of research which seeks to develop abstract generalizations about phenomena

Reflexivity – ... the process of critical self-reflection on one's biases, theoretical predispositions and preferences. The inquirer is part of the setting, context and social phenomenon he or she seeks to understand

Example

Denham, S.A. (1999) Part 2: Family health during and after death of a family member. *Journal of Family Nursing* 5 (2) 160–83   70 References

Reports an ethnographic study of families who used hospice services, which aimed to identify how they defined and practised family health during a time of transition.

Annotations

2.42.1   Agar, M.H. (1996) *The professional stranger: an informal introduction to ethnography* (2nd edition). New York: Academic Press   ISBN 0120444704   References

Book explores the nature of ethnographic research and discusses the key issues involved. It is contrasted with hypothesis-testing approaches and examples are given mainly from the author's own experience. Problems relating to ethnographic interviews and observation are discussed (CR 2.68, 2.72).

2.42.2   Atkinson, P., Coffey, A., Delamont, S., Lofland, J. & Lofland, L.H. (eds) (2001) *Handbook of ethnography*. London: Sage   ISBN 076195824X   References

Handbook provides a critical guide to the principles and practice of ethnography. The contents systematically locate ethnography in its relevant historical and intellectual contexts, examine the contribution of ethnography to major fields of substantive research and consider the key debates and issues from the conduct of research through to contemporary arguments.

2.42.3   *Australian   Institute   for   Ethnomethodology and Conversation Analysis* wwwmcc. murdoch.edu.au/aiem/ (Accessed 13/02/03)

Australian delegates at meetings in 2001 of the International Institute for Ethnomethodology and Conversation Analysis held in Manchester, UK, founded this group. It aims to bring together researchers in the fields of EM and CA across Australia. News and events will be shared, and meetings, symposia and conferences organized (CR 2.89).

2.42.4   Bernard, H.R. (1995) *Research methods in anthropology: qualitative and quantitative approaches* (2nd edition). Walnut Creek, CA: Alta Mira Press   ISBN 0803952457   References

Revised edition of a major methods text intended also for social scientists. New sections include ethics, sampling, focus groups and use of methods for theory development. There is increased emphasis on use of computers (CR 2.1, 2.17, 2.29, 2.36, 2.69).

2.42.5   Brewer, J.D. (2000) *Ethnography.* Buckingham: Open University Press   ISBN 0335202683   References

Book asks what is ethnography, and discusses it as a method and methodology. The research process, analysing, interpreting and presenting ethnographic data, the uses of ethnography and its future are all discussed.

2.42.6   Bryman, A. (ed.) (2001) *Ethnography.* London: Sage   ISBN 0761970916   References 4 Volumes

> Volume 1: The Nature of Ethnography
> Volume 2: Ethnographic Fieldwork Practice
> Volume 3: Issues in Ethnography
> Volume 4: Analysis and Writing in Ethnography

This collection brings together some landmark contributions by key figures such as Geertz, Denzin, Whyte, Emerson and Atkinson, and Delamont, and a wide variety of issues in the field. It provides a complete guide to the methods, significance and contribution of ethnography and will be a resource for scholars and students.

2.42.7   Coffey, A. (1999) *The ethnographic self: fieldwork and the representation of identity.* London: Sage   ISBN 0761952675   References

Book attempts to synthesize accounts of the personal experience of ethnography. The author makes sense of the process of fieldwork research as a set of practical, intellectual and emotional accomplishments. A wide range of material is used for illustration. (CR 2.16).

2.42.8   Couldry, N. (2000) *Inside culture: re-imagining the method of cultural studies.* London: Sage   ISBN 0761963863   References

Offers a reassessment of the direction of cultural studies and argues for a discipline centred on the interrelations of culture and power. There should be a clear focus on empirical research which is accountable and that deals with the real complexities of contemporary lives.

2.42.9   Coulon, A. (1995) *Ethnomethodology.* Thousand Oaks, CA: Sage   ISBN 0803947771 References

Author demystifies the ethnomethodological tradition and the often arcane nomenclature. Its history, major features and the main criticisms levelled at it are discussed. Covering both theory and practices, examples of key work in the area are given.

2.42.10 Denzin, N.K. (1997) *Interpretive ethnography: ethnographic practices for the 21st century.* London: Sage ISBN 0803972997 References

Examines the changes, prospects, problems and forms of ethnographic interpretative writing in the twenty-first century. The author believes that postmodern ethnography is the moral discourse of the contemporary world, and that ethnographers should explore new types of experimental text to form a new ethics of inquiry.

2.42.11 Erikson, K. & Stull, D. (1997) *Doing team ethnography: warnings and advice.* Thousand Oaks, CA: Sage ISBN 0761906673 References

Examines the challenges and opportunities when doing team ethnography, including setting goals, creating a team, observing, sharing and collaborating on a finished product (CR 2.15).

2.42.12 Fetterman, D.M. (1998) *Ethnography: step by step* (2nd edition). Thousand Oaks, CA: Sage ISBN 0761913858 References

This new edition takes readers into the resources of the Internet, including conducting research, collecting census data, conducting interviews by 'chatting' and videoconferencing, sharing notes and pictures about research sites, debating issues with colleagues on listservers and in online journals, and downloading useful data collection and analysis software (CR 2.85).

2.42.13 Foley, D.E. (2002) Critical ethnography: the reflexive turn. *International Journal of Qualitative Studies in Education* 15 (4) 469–90 References

Paper explores the recent debates on ethnographic writing by explicating four types of reflexivity: confessional, theoretical, textual and deconstructive. The author then illustrates how such reflexive practices have been incorporated into his work. The paper advocates blending autobiography and ethnography into a 'cultural Marxist' standpoint perspective that also draws upon multiple epistemologies and feminist notions of science. He also highlights the importance of writing in ordinary language and believes that reflexive epistemological and narrative practices will make ethnography a more engaging, useful, public story-telling genre (CR 2.6, 2.10, 2.78).

2.42.14 Forsythe, D.E. (1998) Using ethnography to investigate life scientists' information needs. *Bulletin of the Medical Library Association* 86 (3) 402–9 35 References

Describes a particular use of ethnographic methods to establish the information needs of life scientists.

2.42.15 Gray, A. (2002) *Research practice for cultural studies: ethnographic methods and lived cultures.* London: Sage ISBN 076195175X References

Book starts from the epistemological and methodological background of a number of key studies in the Birmingham tradition, and explores how to make use of these experiences and how to deploy 'experience' as a tool for research (CR 2.6, 2.16).

2.42.16 Gunaratnam, Y. (2003) *Researching 'race' and ethnicity.* London: Sage ISBN 0761972862 References

Discusses the methodological, epistemological and ethical challenges of doing qualitative research on questions of 'race' and ethnicity. The author explores the construction and use of the categories of 'race' and ethnicity, inter-racial research and ethnic matching, and empirical and ethical concerns about research relations, analysis, representation and activism. Case study examples with white and minoritized research participants are used for illustration (CR 2.6, 2.16, 2.17, 2.22, 2.39, 2.42).

2.42.17 Hammersley, M. & Atkinson, P. (1995) *Ethnography: principles in practice* (2nd edition). London: Routledge ISBN 0415086647 References

Book provides an introduction to the principles and practice of ethnographic research, and is intended for students and experienced researchers. The principle of reflexivity is thoroughly explored, as the authors believe this is the key to development of both theory and methodology in social science generally, and in ethnographic work in particular. Ethnographic research is put in the context of other qualitative methods, and each step in the process is examined using a wide range of examples. Book includes an annotated bibliography.

2.42.18 Hammersley, M. (1998) *Reading ethnographic research: a critical guide* (2nd edition). London: Longman ISBN 0582311047 References

Book provides an overview of ethnography and recent methodological developments. The process of undertaking and assessing ethnographic accounts is explored and illustrated by the author's own work.

2.42.19 Hammersley, M. (2002) Ethnography and realism. In Huberman, A.M. & Miles, M.B. (eds) *The qualitative researcher's companion.* Thousand Oaks, CA: Sage. ISBN 076191191X Chapter 3 65–80 40 References

Author discusses some of the philosophical underpinnings of ethnographic research (CR 2.5, 2.36.62).

2.42.20 Hine, C. (2000) *Virtual ethnography.* London: Sage ISBN 0761917179 References

Author produces a distinctive understanding of the significance of the Internet and shows that it is both a site for cultural formations and a cultural artefact that is shaped by people's understandings and expectations, thus requiring a new form of ethnography. The shape of this ethnography is considered and the book guides readers through its applications in multiple settings (CR 2.85).

2.42.21 Hodgson, I. (2001) Engaging with cultures: reflections on entering the ethnographic field. *Nurse Researcher: The International Journal of Research Methodology in Nursing and Health Care* 9 (1) 41–51 16 References

Paper offers reflections on the experience of starting an ethnographic study. It provides an overview of the study, addresses key elements in entering the field and suggests questions that require further investigation, while identifying those elements that are crucial to effective observation (CR 2.16).

2.42.22 International Institute for Ethnomethodology and Conversation Analysis www.iiemca.mrl.nott.ac.uk (Accessed 13/02/03)

This institute is dedicated to the advancement of theory and method in ethnomethodological and conversation analysis studies, and to the development of research, instructional and other programmes, as well as conferences, symposia and lectures. Its website gives information on current activities, history, publications, web links and future events (CR 2.89).

2.42.23 Katz, J. (2001) From how to why: on luminous description and causal inference in ethnography (Part 1). *Ethnography* 2 (4) 443–73 References

AND

2.42.24 Katz, J. (2002) From how to why: on luminous description and causal inference in ethnography (Part 2). *Ethnography* 3 (1) 63–90 References

Papers illustrate three of seven forms for characterizing the effectiveness of ethnographic data, and the distinctive resources they offer are analysed.

2.42.25 Krumeich, A., Weijts, W., Reddy, P. & Meijer-Weitz, A. (2001) The benefits of anthropological approaches for health promotion research and practice. *Health Education and Research* 16 (2) 121–30 54 References

The value of the 'thick description' is explored together with the anthropological philosophy of improving cultures as opposed to health education.

2.42.26 Lyon, E. (1999) Reflections on the future of applied ethnography. *Journal of Contemporary Ethnography* 28 (6) December Special Issue 620–7 References

Discusses several circumstances affecting the future of applied ethnography. It has now gained visibility across disciplines and within sociology, and attention is being paid to the funding of applied ethnographic research and methodological expansion.

2.42.27 Maggs-Rapport, F. (2000) Combining methodological approaches in research: ethnography and interpretive phenomenology. *Journal of Advanced Nursing* 31 (1) 219–25 25 References

Paper makes a case for the potential of combining ethnography and interpretative phenomenology. The author argues that through a more multidimensional approach the researcher may come closer to understanding their personal interpretation of the research phenomenon and the experience of research participants (CR 2.26, 2.49).

2.42.28 Pink, S. (2001) *Doing visual ethnography: images, media and representation in research.* London: Sage ISBN 0761960546 References

Explores the use and potential of photography, video and hypermedia in ethnographic and social research. It offers a reflexive approach to theoretical, methodological, practical and ethical issues when using these media in the field and in the academy (CR 2.17, 2.36, 2.72).

2.42.29 Reed-Danahay, D. (2002) Turning points and textual strategies in ethnographic writing. *Qualitative Studies in Education* 15 (4) 421–5 13 References

Describes the use of self-reflexive writing to contextualize data gathered in the field of ethnographic research. Considers 'experimental' writing, that is, writing opposed to accepted ethnographic convention, with a view to humanizing the ethnographic encounter.

2.42.30 Roper, J.M. & Shapira, J. (2000) *Ethnography in nursing research.* Thousand Oaks, CA: Sage ISBN 0761908749 References

This 'how to do it' manual describes the principles and methods of ethnography used by researchers to examine issues related to health and illness. Guidance is given on conducting research in health settings, analysing and interpreting data, making ethical decisions related to the role of the ethnographer and how to write a research proposal (CR 2.17, 2.96).

2.42.31 Rose, D. (1990) *Living the ethnographic life*. Newbury Park, CA: Sage   ISBN 080393999X References

Offers an alternative to the corporate mould of ethnography and reshapes it as a democratic form of thinking and being.

2.42.32 Rudge, T. (2002) (Re)writing ethnography: the unsettling questions for nursing research raised by post-structural approaches to 'the field'. In Rafferty, A.M. & Traynor, M. (eds) *Exemplary research for nursing and midwifery*. London: Routledge   ISBN 0415241634   Chapter 8 153–65   12 References

Paper outlines the researcher/researched positioning evidenced within observational records in research into nurse/patient interactions focused on one nursing procedure. What it exposes is that the researcher's position is not static, neither is the position of informant or participant. Researching in the clinical context as a nurse means that it is difficult to remove oneself from the research, even when nurses locate you as outside of the event (CR 2.16, 3.16, 3.21.5).

2.42.33 Saukko, P. (2003) *Doing research in cultural studies: an introduction to classical and new methodological approaches*. London: Sage   ISBN 076196505X   References

Book outlines the key methodological approaches to the study of lived experience, texts and social contexts within the field of cultural studies. It discusses classical methodologies and contemporary debates that have argued for new ethnographic, post-structuralist and multi-scope research methods. Real-life examples and case studies are included, together with practical exercises.

2.42.34 Savage, J. (2000) Ethnography and health care. *British Medical Journal* 321 (7273) 2 December 1400–2   23 References

Author believes that ethnography has been overlooked as a qualitative methodology for the in-depth study of health care issues in the context in which they occur. This article gives a broad indication of the nature of ethnography, and some relevant studies to show how it was used. Its limitations are also briefly outlined (CR 2.6).

2.42.35 Schwartzman, H.B. (1993) *Ethnography in organizations*. Newbury Park, CA: Sage.   ISBN 0803943792   References

Book provides a methodological history of ethnography in organizations and guidelines for its conduct. The Hawthorne study is described as well as the role that anthropologists played in research arising from this work. Recent studies are included to give pointers for other researchers.

2.42.36 Smith, W.N. (2002) Ethno-poetry notes. *Qualitative Studies in Education* 15 (4) 461–7

Offers a personalized view of experimentation with field notes using a free verse poem format (included in the text) and compares this with the accepted form of data collection used in PhD acceptable field notes.

2.42.37 State University of New York, Institute of Technology *Ethnography and research methods in nursing* www.sunyit.edu/library/html/culturedmed/ bib/ethnography/ (Accessed 22/01/03)

Provides an example of a list of texts and journal articles on research methods in ethnography.

2.42.38 Stewart, A. (1998) *The ethnographer's method*. Thousand Oaks, CA: Sage   ISBN 0761903941   References

Author helps ethnographers devise a clearly articulated explanation of their methods. The book also considers what ought to be normative in methods discussions within ethnography from research design to end product.

2.42.39 Taylor, S. (ed.) (2001) *Ethnographic research: a reader*. London: Sage/Open University ISBN 0761973931   References

Reader presents a selection of 10 recently published studies, intended to show the variety of social research that is currently being conducted within the ethnographic tradition. Sections include at society's margins; gendered identities; workplace practices; the consumption of cultural products; and working to improve medical services.

2.42.40 Thomas, J. (1993) *Doing critical ethnography*. Newbury Park, CA: Sage   ISBN 080393923X   References

Book offers a direct style of thinking about relationships between knowledge, society and political action. This type of ethnography can be scientific and critical and offers ways of going beyond conventional studies, without standing in opposition to it.

2.42.41 Van Maanen, J. (2002) The fact of fiction in organizational ethnography. In Huberman, A.M. & Miles, M.B. (eds) *The qualitative researcher's companion*. Thousand Oaks, CA: Sage   ISBN 076191191X   Chapter 5 101–17   27 References

Paper aims to reduce some of the confusion tying empirical discovery and conceptual development in ethnographic work to the specific experience of the researcher (CR 2.36.62).

2.42.42 Wakefield, A. (2000) Ethnomethodology: the problem of unique adequacy ... including commentary by Meerabeau, L. *NT Research* 5 (1) 46–54   23 References

Paper explores the extent to which ethnomethodology can be employed to extrapolate data from the investigative domain. The concept of 'unique adequacy' is examined in detail as this element created significant problems when analysing the data. The debate focuses on the difficulties encountered when attempting to achieve 'ethnomethodological indifference', that is, the researcher's ability to remain non-judgemental when reporting on the findings.

2.42.43   Warren, C.A.B. & Hackney, J.K. (2000) *Gender issues in ethnography* (2nd edition). Thousand Oaks, CA: Sage   ISBN 0761917179   References

Summarizes the state of the art of gender issues in fieldwork both in anthropology and sociology. Authors show how the gender of researchers can affect both the fieldwork relationships and the production of ethnography. Using their own experience, they focus on ways in which researchers represent these expectations through narrative (CR 2.16).

2.43   EVALUATION/OUTCOMES RESEARCH

'[Recently] an important scientific methodology [outcomes research] has been developed to examine the end results of patient care. The strategies used in it are a departure from the traditional scientific endeavours. These include the incorporation of evaluation methods, epidemiology and economic theory perspectives.' (Burns & Grove, 1997: 569–611) [adapted]

'The past two decades have seen a growing emphasis on basing healthcare decisions on the best available evidence. This evidence encompasses all facets of healthcare and includes decisions related to the care of an individual, an organization or at a policy level.' (Evans, 2003: 77)

Evaluating this evidence includes ranking it in the form of a hierarchy to provide means by which a range of methodologically different types of research can be graded. This requires an understanding of the fundamentals of study design and outcomes research and its clinical significance.

Definitions [See Appendix D for sources]

Benchmark – a reference point serving as a standard for comparing or judging other things

Evaluation research – research that investigates how well a programme, practice or policy is working

Evidence-based medicine/nursing – ... the conscientious, explicit and judicious use of current best evidence in making decisions about the care of individual patients

Gold standard – the method, procedure or measurement that is widely accepted as being the best available against which new interventions should be compared. [It is particularly important in studies of the accuracy of diagnostic tests. For example, hand searching is sometimes used as the gold standard for identifying trials against which electronic searches of databases such as MEDLINE are compared]

Hierarchy of evidence – a table that ranks the value of evidence

Intervention research – new methodology for investigating the effectiveness of a nursing intervention in achieving the desired outcome or outcomes in a natural setting

Outcomes research – ... any research that attempts to link either structure or process, or both, to the outcomes of medical care in the community, system, institution or patient level

Example

Manias, E., Bullock, S. & Bennett, R. (2000) Formative evaluation of a computer-assisted learning program in pharmacology for nursing students. *Computers in Nursing* 18 (6) 265–71   20 References

Aim of this study was to demonstrate the benefits of using a combination of objective and naturalistic models when undertaking a formative evaluation of a computer-assisted learning programme. It confirmed the importance and value of collecting a variety of data in order to improve this programme.

Annotations

2.43.1   Aday, L.A., Begley, C., Lairson, D.A. & Slater, C.H. (1998) *Evaluating the healthcare system: effectiveness, efficiency and equity* (2nd edition). Chicago, IL: Health Administration Press   ISBN 1567930794

Presents the fundamentals of health services research. This revised edition includes prevention-oriented and long-term medical care, the influence of environmental and population factors on the design and impact of health services and the use of data systems to evaluate health services delivery (CR 3.11).

2.43.2 Andrews, G.J. (2002) Towards a more place sensitive nursing research: an invitation to medical and health geography. *Nursing Inquiry* 9 (4) 221–38   218 References

Investigates the use of medical and health geography in nursing research. Argues that there is a dynamic relationship between people, health and place and a range of places where health care is provided. Suggests that as nursing research has adopted a range of theoretical frameworks from various disciplines, health geography might be a useful addition to that range.

2.43.3 Bailey, D. & Littlechild, R. (2001) Devising the evaluation strategy for a mental health training programme. *Evaluation* 7 (3) 351–68 References

Authors evaluate the definitions and methods of evaluation that can be developed into an evaluation strategy. This has been derived from the use of case-study research methodology applied to a UK postgraduate multidisciplinary programme in community health. The chosen model is coupled with another adapted from the training literature and it is critically reviewed to see how it may be applied in practice (CR 2.39).

2.43.4 Berk, R.A. & Rossi, P.H. (1998) *Thinking about program evaluation* (2nd edition). Thousand Oaks, CA: Sage   ISBN 0761917659   References

Through the use of specific examples to illustrate evaluation research goals and methods, this book provides readers with an overview of the science and politics of this type of research.

2.43.5 Boruch, R.F. (1997) *Randomized experiments for planning and evaluation: a practical guide*. Thousand Oaks, CA: Sage ISBN 0803935102 . References

Book disentangles the complexities of randomized field experiments to enable researchers to evaluate better the impact of new programmes (CR 2.29).

2.43.6 Borum, F. & Hansen, H.F. (2000) The local construction and enactment of standards for research evaluation: the case of the Copenhagen business school. *Evaluation* 6 (3) 281–99 References

The local adaptation of research at faculty and department level is analysed as well as the processes through which a standard was stipulated and enacted. Three elements are discussed: the interplay of the standard with the local context, conflict resolution and co-ordination and the processing of local problems and issues (CR 3.3).

2.43.7 Boyne, G., Farrell, C., Law, J. & Powell, M. (2003) *Evaluating public management reforms:*

principles and practice. Buckingham: Open University Press   ISBN 0335202462   References

This book develops a framework for a theory-based evaluation of reforms, and then uses this to assess the impact of new arrangements for public service delivery in the UK.

2.43.8 Briggs, A.H. & Gray, A.M. (1999) Handling uncertainty in economic evaluations of health care interventions. *British Medical Journal* 319 (7210) 4 September 635–8   16 References

Explains that economic evaluations help to determine which interventions offer maximum health gain, but points out that there are uncertainties and disagreement regarding the methodologies employed to assess this. The article examines the evidence in respect of cost data and makes recommendations regarding analysis and presentation of findings.

2.43.9 Brown, S.J. (2002) Nursing intervention studies: a descriptive analysis of issues important to clinicians. *Research in Nursing and Health* 25 (4) 317–27   References

Study that aimed to estimate the frequency with which recommendations made in the literature on how to conduct and report intervention studies were actually being reported.

2.43.10 Burns, N. & Grove, S.K. (2001) Intervention research. In Authors *The practice of nursing research: conduct, critique and utilization* (4th edition). Philadelphia, PA: W.B. Saunders ISBN 0721691773   Chapter 13   331–64   91 References

Chapter describes a revolutionary new approach to intervention research that holds great promise for designing and testing nursing interventions. Nursing intervention is defined, the problems of true experiments are discussed, an overview of its use is given, together with the processes required when conducting this type of research (CR 2.1.13, 2.2, 2.29).

2.43.11 Callon, M., Larédo, P. & Mustar, P. (1997) *The strategic management of research and technology: evaluation of programmes*. Paris: Economic International   ISBN 1902282027

Book takes stock of the methods and tools that are being used in Europe to evaluate all types of programme in order to ensure genuine strategic management of all research and technology.

2.43.12 Chelimsky, E. & Shadish, W.R. (eds) (1997) *Evaluation for the 21st century: a handbook*. London: Sage   ISBN 0761906118   References

A group of evaluators explain how evaluation has become what it is today and its future. Topics discussed include what makes evaluation different from other disciplines, the links between evaluation and the auditing professions, which activities have priority in evaluation, new methodological approaches, the issues of advocacy versus truth, and evaluating programmes versus empowering people to evaluate their own.

2.43.13   Clarke, A. (1999) *Evaluation research: an introduction to principles, methods and practice.* London: Sage   ISBN 0761950958   References

Provides a comprehensive introduction to valuation research and shows how social research methods and methodologies can be applied in a variety of evaluation contexts.

2.43.14   Clarke, A. (2001) Evaluation research in nursing and health care. *Nurse Researcher: The International Journal of Research Methodology in Nursing and Health Care* 8 (3) 4–14   38 References

Identifies the broad dimensions of health care evaluation and outlines the role evaluation plays in the context of nursing research.

2.43.15   Closs, S.J. & Cheater, F.M. (1999) Evidence for nursing practice: a clarification of the issues. *Journal of Advanced Nursing* 30 (1) 10–17   33 References

Discusses the confusion and unease within nursing about the emphatic push for all health care to be 'evidence-based' and an anxiety that the emphasis on evidence ignores practitioners' skills and individual patient preferences. The paper attempts to clarify the issues and aims to debunk the misconception that randomized controlled trials are synonymous with evidence, and to increase critical awareness of the nature of evidence in nursing.

2.43.16   Cole, N., Tucker, L.J. & Foxcroft, D.R. (2000) Benchmarking evidence-based nursing … including commentary by Thompson, C. *NT Research* 5 (5) September–October 336–45   22 References

Reports a study that aimed to develop and apply a set of criteria for benchmarking evidence-based nursing. As no previous work was found on benchmarking or assessing evidence-based nursing, the authors developed 14 criteria, organized around four key themes for achieving effective practice: selecting a particular aspect of practice to question and examine; finding out from the literature, professional networks and other sources what is current best practice, and critically appraising the available literature and sources of information; implementing and/or learning how to provide best-known clinical practice; and confirming that you are providing best practice. The authors believe that the benchmarking tool developed in this study may be helpful to other organizations considering how to take forward evidence-based nursing practice (CR 2.37, 2.102).

2.43.17   Daly, W.M. & Carnwell, R. (2001) The case for a multi-method approach. *Nurse Researcher: The International Journal of Research Methodology in Nursing and Health Care* 8 (3) 30–44   57 References

Authors believe that a multimethod approach can be of value when faced with the complexity of evaluating clinical competency. The methodological and practical issues are discussed (CR 2.17, 2.51, 2.66, 2.69, 2.72).

2.43.18   Drummond, M.F., O'Brien, B., Stoddart, S.L. & Torrance, G.W. (1997) *Methods for the economic evaluation of health care programmes* (2nd edition). Oxford: Oxford University Press   ISBN 0192627732   References

The key methodological principles of economic evaluation are outlined using a critical appraisal checklist that can be applied to any study. The features of the basic forms of analysis – cost, cost-effective, cost-utility and cost-benefit – are explained in detail. Chapters are also included on collecting and analysing data, and presenting and using economic and evaluation results (CR 2.64, 2.79).

2.43.19   Estabrooks, C.A. (1998) Will evidence-based nursing make practice perfect? *Canadian Journal of Nursing Research* 30 (1) 15–36   68 References

Before we adopt evidence-based nursing (EBN) as a mantra for the twenty-first century, its origins and consequences should be examined. Related concepts, two of which are the nature and structure of practice-based knowledge and the nature and structure of evidence generally, are discussed. Findings of a recent survey of nurses in western Canada are used to show that nurses use a broad range of practice knowledge, much of which is experientially-based rather than research-based.

2.43.20   *Evaluation thesaurus* (1991) 4th edition. Edited by Scriven, M.C. Newbury Park, CA: Sage ISBN 0803943644   References

Covers major concepts, positions, acronyms, processes, techniques and checklists in the field of evaluation.

2.43.21   Evans, D. (2003) Hierarchy of evidence: a framework for ranking evidence evaluating healthcare interventions. *Journal of Clinical Nursing* 12 (1) 77–84   36 References

Proposes a hierarchy of evidence for grading methodologically different types of research and provides a framework for the development of systematic review protocols.

2.43.22   Ferlie, E., Wood, M. & Fitzgerald, L. (1999) Some limits to evidence-based medicine: a case study from elective orthopaedics. *Quality in Health Care* 8 (2) 99–107   26 References

Case study qualitative data are presented which illuminate the scientific, organizational and behavioural factors that combine to shape clinical behaviour. It is suggested that there are alternative models of what constitutes 'evidence' in use, scientific knowledge is in part socially constructed and clinical professionals retain a monopoly of technical knowledge. The implication is that there may be severe obstacles to the rapid or broad implementation of evidence-based practice (CR 2.36, 2.39).

2.43.23   Fetterman, D.M., Kaftarian, S.J. & Wandersman, A. (eds) (1995) *Empowerment evaluation: knowledge and tools for self-assessment and accountability.* Thousand Oaks, CA: Sage ISBN 076190025X   References

The focus of this book, empowerment evaluation (a method for using evaluation concepts, techniques and findings to foster improvement and self-determination), is to examine the method as it has been adopted in academic and foundation settings.

2.43.24   Fetterman, D.M. (2000) *Foundations of empowerment evaluation.* Thousand Oaks, CA: Sage   ISBN 080395669X   References

Employing both qualitative and quantitative methodologies, empowerment evaluation is the use of evaluation concepts, techniques and findings to foster improvement and self-determination. The background and theory are explored and the three steps of empowerment are discussed (CR 2.9, 2.39).

2.43.25   Fink, A. (1995) *Evaluation for education and psychology.* Thousand Oaks, CA: Sage   ISBN 0803958544   References

Book provides information for those undertaking a programme evaluation within the context of a quantitative approach. Examples and exercises are given, as well as dos and don'ts and advantages and disadvantages (CR 2.29).

2.43.26   Fitz-Gibbon, C.T. & Morris, L.L. (1988) *How to design a program evaluation* (2nd edition). Newbury Park, CA: Sage ISBN 080393128X   References

Book covers evaluation designs in educational settings.

2.43.27   Gomm, R. & Davies, C. (eds) (2000) *Using evidence in health and social care.* London: Sage/Open University Press   ISBN 0761964959 References

Text introduces readers to different kinds of evidence and will enable them to evaluate the unique contributions of each. It acknowledges the variety of contexts in which practitioners work and the challenges of putting research into practice.

2.43.28   Greene, J., Lehn, B. & Goodyear, L. (2001) The merits of mixing methods in evaluation. *Evaluation* 7 (1) 25–44   References

Discusses the complexities of understanding human behaviour and suggests that we need to frame our understanding in a way that honours diversity and respects differences. Case examples from the United States are given.

2.43.29   Grembowski, D. (2001) *Health program evaluation.* Thousand Oaks, CA: Sage   ISBN 0761918477   References

Provides a thorough guide for undertaking an evaluation of a health programme.

2.43.30   Hanney, S., Packwood, T. & Buxton, M. (2000) Evaluating the benefits from health research and development centres: a categorization, a model and examples of application. *Evaluation* 6 (2) 137–160   References

Article describes the development and multidimensional categorization of benefits, or payback, from research and development centre models for conducting evaluations of impact. Two R & D centres were assessed and the acceptability of this approach is discussed (CR 2.6, 3.11).

2.43.31   Hek, G. (2000) Evidence-based practice: finding the evidence. *Journal of Community Nursing* 14 (11) 19–20, 22   14 References

Outlines the three types of evidence needed to provide the foundations for care. These are patients' and carers' views, the expertise of clinical practitioners and the best available evidence. The article concentrates on how to find appropriate literature (CR 1.2).

2.43.32   House, E.R. & Howe, K.R. (1999) *Values in evaluation and social research.* Thousand Oaks, CA: Sage   ISBN 0761911553   References

Book examines the concept of values in programme evaluation. The authors analyse four views of facts and values in evaluation: those rooted in a fact–value dichotomy; radical constructivists; post-modernists; and deliberative democrats.

2.43.33 Jenkinson, C. (ed.) (1997) *Assessment and evaluation of health and medical care: a methods text.* Buckingham: Open University Press ISBN 0335197051 References

Text describes the variety of approaches available in the assessment and evaluation of health care. The principles of randomized controlled trials, case control studies, cohort studies and social surveys are described, together with qualitative methods which may be used (CR 2.12, 2.29, 2.36, 2.41, 2.48, 2.52, 2.92).

2.43.34 Jennings, B.M. & Staggers, N. (1998) The language of outcomes. *Advances in Nursing Science* 20 (4) 72–80   33 References

The potential of outcomes is considerable as a mechanism to evaluate quality, improve effectiveness and link practice to accountability. This article identifies the current confusion in outcomes terminology, begins an outcomes lexicon and issues a call to action for further clarification in the language of outcomes (CR 2.2).

2.43.35 Johnson, M., Maas, M.L. & Moorhead, S. (2000) *Nursing outcomes classification* (2nd edition). St Louis, MO: Mosby   ISBN 0323017509 References

This classification system standardizes the terminology and criteria for measurable or desirable outcomes as a result of interventions performed by nurses.

2.43.36 Kazdin, A.E. (1999) The meanings and measurement of clinical significance. *Journal of Consulting and Clinical Psychology* 67 (3) June 332–9   References

Among the issues raised by the concept of clinical significance are ambiguities regarding the meaning of current measures available, the importance of relating assessment to the goals of therapy and evaluation of the construct(s) that clinical significance reflects. Research directions discussed include developing a typology of therapy goals, evaluating cut-off scores and thresholds for clinical significance, and attending to social as well as clinical impact of treatment.

2.43.37 Koch, T. (2000) 'Having a say': negotiation in fourth-generation evaluation. *Journal of Advanced Nursing* 31 (1) 117–25   20 References

Research, guided by the principles of fourth-generation evaluation, which has negotiation at its centre, is scrutinized. Three case studies are discussed to illustrate its potential applications.

2.43.38 Kushner, S. (2000) *Personalizing evaluation.* London: Sage   ISBN 0761963626 References

Challenges the mainstream approach to programme evaluation and inverts the traditional relationship between programme and person. The three principle concerns discussed are: how to learn about evaluation in ways that are related to the often confusing experience of doing it; how to understand the role of evaluation as a form of personal expression and, even, political action; and how to use it to reveal something about people's lives as well as the programmes and institutions in which they are involved.

2.43.39 Lawrenz, F. & Huffman, D. (2002) The archipeligo approach to mixed method evaluation. *American Journal of Evaluation* 23 (3) Autumn 331–8   References

Authors propose a new metaphorical framework for understanding and using mixed-methods evaluation. Mixed methods can create philosophical and practical dilemmas in the ways data are collected, analysed, interpreted and reported. Using the metaphor of an archipelago helped to clarify and reconceptualize the evaluation approach and its findings by allowing simultaneous consideration of different mixed methods and stances. The results have implications for others who may wish to use a mixed-method approach.

2.43.40 Levin, H.M. & McEwan, P.J. (2000) *Cost-effectiveness analysis: methods and applications* (2nd edition). Thousand Oaks, CA: Sage ISBN 0761919341   References

Book gives advice on planning and implementing a cost analysis study.

2.43.41 Maloney, K. & Chaiken, B.P. (1999) An overview of outcomes research and measurement. *Journal of Health Care Quality* 21 (6) 4–10   23 References

Describes the three outcome domains (clinical, economic and humanistic) and characterizes the activities involved in outcomes research and measurement (CR 2.54).

2.43.42 McKee, M., Britton, A., Black, N., McPherson, K., Sanderson, C. & Bain, C. (1999) Interpreting the evidence: choosing between randomised and non-randomised studies. *British Medical Journal* 319 (7205) 31 July 312–15   22 References

Compares the potential differences in research outcomes between randomized and non-randomized studies. Differences in the characteristics of subjects, potential threats to validity and limits to generalizability are discussed (CR 2.22, 2.25, 2.28, 2.29).

2.43.43 Newman, D.L. & Brown, R.D. (1996) *Applied ethics for program evaluation.* Thousand Oaks, CA: Sage   ISBN 0803951868 References

Book explores a set of principles that can serve as a guide to making ethical decisions in evaluation research. Using vignettes, the authors provide ethical dilemmas and questions to encourage discussion about the positive and negative consequences of each option. Suggestions are made about how evaluators can make informed ethical decisions (CR 2.17).

2.43.44 Nixon, C.T. & Northrup, D.A. (eds) (1997) *Evaluating mental health services: how do programs for children 'work' in the real world?* Thousand Oaks, CA: Sage ISBN 0761907955 References

Book addresses evaluation issues relating to community-based mental health services for children and young people with emotional and behavioural problems. Contributors discuss recent evaluations of the effectiveness of systems of care and specific intervention strategies. Their own research is described and issues facing researchers, limitations and the future are all discussed (CR 2.16).

2.43.45 Orr, L.L. (1998) *Social experiments: evaluating public programmes with experimental methods.* Thousand Oaks, CA: Sage ISBN 0761912959 References

Provides a basic understanding of how to design and implement social experiments and how to interpret their results (CR 2.29, 2.87, 2.93).

2.43.46 Ovretveit, J. (1998) *Evaluating health interventions: an introduction to evaluation of health treatments, services, policies and organizational interventions.* Buckingham: Open University Press ISBN 033519964X References

Book describes the strengths and weaknesses of different approaches to evaluation, together with some of the practical pitfalls and politics associated with it.

2.43.47 Owen, J.M. & Rogers, P. (1999) *Program evaluation: forms and approaches.* London: Sage ISBN 076196178X References

This introductory text on evaluation for beginners and practitioners shows how to identify appropriate forms and approaches, using an original framework.

2.43.48 Patton, M.Q. (1990) *Qualitative evaluation and research methods* (2nd edition). Beverly Hills, CA: Sage ISBN 0803937792 References

Book aims to encourage expansion of the evaluation skills of social scientists. It recognizes that quantitative research is not 'better' than qualitative research, but different methods are appropriate for diverse situations. The emphasis is on developing strategies for using qualitative evaluation methods.

2.43.49 Patton, M.Q. (1997) *Utilization-focused evaluation: the new century text* (3rd edition). Thousand Oaks, CA: Sage ISBN 0803952651 References

Book provides a comprehensive review of the literature on evaluation use and practice. Both theoretical and practical, the book gives advice on conducting programme evaluations (CR 2.12).

2.43.50 Patton, M.Q. (2002) *Utilization-focused evaluation (u-fe) checklist* www.wmich.edu/evalctr/checklists (Accessed 13/02/03)

Utilization-focused evaluation is a process for helping users to select the most appropriate content, model, methods, theory and uses for their particular situation. The checklist on this website enables the tasks to be identified and their related challenges pinpointed.

2.43.51 Pawson, R. & Tilley, N. (1997) *Realistic evaluation.* London: Sage ISBN 0761950095 References

Book shows how programme evaluation needs to be and can be improved. It describes a new paradigm, called realistic evaluation, which promises greater validity and utility from the findings of evaluation studies. A complete blueprint for evaluation activities goes from design to data collection and analysis, the accumulation of findings across programmes and its development into policy (CR 2.25, 3.11).

2.43.52 Perrin, B. (2002) How to – how not to – evaluate innovation. *Evaluation* 8 (1) 13–28 References

Article discusses the nature of innovation and the limitations of traditional evaluation approaches for assessing it. An alternative model, consistent with the nature of innovation, is proposed.

2.43.53 Preskill, H. & Torres, R.T. (1998) *Evaluative inquiry for learning in organizations.* Thousand Oaks, CA: Sage ISBN 0761904549 References

Book provides a databased approach to organizational learning and change, and focuses on the use of the evaluative inquiry processes with organizations rather than across large-scale, multi-site programmes. Illustrative case studies, interview extracts, strategy plans, diagrams and advice boxes are also included.

2.43.54 Ray, L. (1999) Evidence and outcomes: agendas, presuppositions and power. *Journal of Advanced Nursing* 30 (5) 1017–26   92 References

Paper explores philosophical and methodological issues involved in determining 'What counts as making a meaningful difference?' – the fundamental question in health outcomes research and evidence-based practice. It examines how clinical researchers must negotiate the agendas of diverse stakeholders, while maintaining a programme of research that is true to the needs of the clinical population. Presuppositions and power bases that shape the generation and utilization of evidence in health care are described. A discussion follows of the consequences of these agendas, using for illustration research issues with families who are raising chronically ill children (CR 2.102).

2.43.55   Resnick, B. (2000) Incorporating outcomes research into clinical practice: the four-step approach. *AACN Clinical Issues* 11 (3) 453–62   23 References

Describes a four-step approach to demonstrating effectiveness in advanced practice, identifying and describing current practice, collecting data, analysing data, and putting the research into practice (CR 2.18, 2.64, 2.79, 2.102).

2.43.56   Roberts, K.L. (1998) Evidence-based practice: an idea whose time has come. *Collegian: Journal of the Royal College of Nursing, Australia* 5 (3) 24–7   21 References

Paper defines evidence-based practice (EBP), gives a brief history, addresses nurses' current usage of research, examines the need for EBP and addresses what it will mean to the profession. The author believes that Australian nursing is in a stage of pre-evidence-based practice, in which most nurses neither read nor apply research findings to practice. A demand for EBP will encourage nurses to use research in practice.

2.43.57   Roberts, P., Priest, H. & Bromage, C. (2001) Selecting and utilizing data sources to evaluate health care education. *Nurse Researcher: The International Journal of Research Methodology in Nursing and Health Care* 8 (3) 15–29   45 References

Discusses the purposes of educational evaluation and the selection and use of research data to promote improvements in nursing and health care education (CR 2.64, 2.69, 2.75).

2.43.58   Robertson, S.C. & Colborn, A.P. (2000) The issue is: Can we improve outcomes research by expanding research methods? *American Journal of Occupational Therapy* 54 (5) 541–3   18 References

Suggests that occupational therapy outcomes necessitate culling functional performances of individuals to describe the overall outcomes of a treatment programme. The challenge in reporting outcomes is to find ways to demonstrate clearer links between individual treatment and function. The suggestion is made that individual session outcomes become a formal part of the reporting procedure, thus combining both group and individual data.

2.43.59   Robson, C. (1999) *Small-scale evaluation: principles and practice*. London: Sage ISBN 0761955100   References

Book examines the strengths and weaknesses of the various methods of evaluation. The issues of collaboration are examined; stakeholder models are compared with participatory evaluation; ethical considerations are placed in context; and the best ways of communicating findings are discussed. Exercises are included in each chapter (CR 2.15, 2.17, 2.98).

2.43.60   Rolfe, G. (1999) Network. Insufficient evidence: the problems of evidence-based nursing. *Nurse Education Today* 19 (6) 433–42   30 References

Evidence-based practice has gained a foothold in nursing, where, despite calls for a broad and nurse-oriented definition of what should count as evidence, it appears to be propounding the randomized controlled trial as the gold standard. The paper challenges the wisdom of basing nursing practice on the findings of large-scale statistical studies, and offers a number of logical objections to the underpinning philosophy of evidence-based nursing and the randomized controlled trial. The author argues for a rethinking of what should count as evidence and suggests a quasi-legal model based on reflection rather than research, in which evidence is employed to understand and justify practice after the event rather than it being used to plan practice in advance (CR 2.29).

2.43.61   Rossi, P.H., Freeman, H.E. & Lipsey, M.W. (1999) *Evaluation: a systematic approach* (6th edition). Thousand Oaks, CA: Sage ISBN 0761908935   References

This comprehensive text covers the role of evaluation research in the planning, design and implementation of programmes and projects. The latest techniques and approaches are included, and guidelines are given on how to tailor evaluations in particular circumstances.

2.43.62   Rothman, J., Thomas, E.J. & Fauri, F.F. (eds) (1994) *Intervention research: design and development for human service*. Binghampton, NY: Haworth Press Inc. ISBN 1560244216 References

This interdisciplinary book presents a comprehensive, conceptual and methodological treatment of intervention research, and a developing area of empirical inquiry that aims to make research more directly relevant and applicable to practice. Chapters by highly regarded scholars in the field explain how to distinguish intervention research from other modalities, demonstrate a new model of research for the design and development of interventions, and provide guidelines for conducting this type of research in practice.

2.43.63   Sackett, D.L., Straus, S.E., Richardson, W.S., Rosenberg, W. & Haynes, R.B. (2000) *Evidence-based medicine: how to practice and teach EBM* (2nd edition). Edinburgh: Churchill Livingstone   ISBN 0443062404   References

Book, written jointly by British, Canadian and American physicians, discusses the areas to be considered in the development of evidence-based medicine. The authors give advice on questions that can be answered, searching for the best evidence, how it may best be evaluated and its validity for patient care. New chapters are included on screening and guidelines, and those on evaluation and teaching have been updated. A CD-ROM containing parallel cases from other specialities and EBM sources is included (CR 2.25).

2.43.64   Shaw, I.F. (1999) *Qualitative evaluation.* London: Sage   ISBN 0761956905   References

Author shows how evaluation practice can utilize qualitative approaches to gain an understanding that more traditional quantitative research may fail to do. The foundations, recent trends, evaluation and action programmes and policies, and the practice of evaluation are all discussed. Chapters include exercises to assist in application of the ideas (CR 2.36).

2.43.65   Shaw, I.F. & Lishman, J. (eds) (1999) *Evaluation and social work practice.* London: Sage ISBN 0761957936   References

Covers the central issues confronting evaluation in social work that links theory and method to practical application.

2.43.66   Sidani, S. & Braden, C.J. (1998) *Evaluating nursing interventions: a theory-driven approach.* Thousand Oaks, CA: Sage   ISBN 0761903151   References

Book offers a comprehensive perspective on nursing intervention together with theory-driven guidelines for future study. The problems encountered in outcomes and intervention research are explained and the authors then show, via the Intervention Theory, how such studies can be undertaken.

2.43.67   Sonnichsen, R.C. (1999) *High impact internal evaluation: a practitioner's guide to evaluating and consulting inside organizations.* Thousand Oaks, CA: Sage   ISBN 0761911537 References.

Book is intended for all those wishing to undertake evaluation studies within their own organization.

2.43.68   Spath, P.L. (1996) *Medical effectiveness and outcomes management: issues, methods and case studies.* San Francisco, CA: Jossey-Bass   ISBN 1556481500

Book introduces nursing leaders, health care administrators and quality managers to outcomes research. Case studies included come from a wide variety of organizations and illustrate which practices best enhance patient outcomes and decrease cost (CR 2.39).

2.43.69   Stevens, A., Abrams, K., Brazier, J., Fitzpatrick, R. & Lilford, R. (eds) (2001) *The advanced handbook of methods in evidence-based healthcare.* London: Sage   ISBN 0761961445 References

Book covers a spectrum of issues, from primary evidence (clinical trials) through reviews and meta-analysis to identifying and filling gaps in the evidence. It provides the most advanced thinking and the most authoritative resource for a state-of-the-art review of methods of evaluating health care (CR 2.29, 2.92).

2.43.70   Stufflebeam, D.L. (2001a) Evaluation checklists: practical tools for guiding and judging evaluations. *American Journal of Evaluation* 22 (1) Winter 71–9   References

Article provides evaluators, their clients and other stakeholders with checklists for guiding and assessing formative and summative evaluations. The checklists pertain to programme, personnel and product evaluations, and reflect different conceptualizations of evaluation. They are constructed for use in planning, contracting, conducting, reporting and judging evaluations. They are available on Western Michigan University Evaluation Center's website (www.wmich.edu/evalctr/checklists/)

2.43.71   Stufflebeam, D.L. (2001b) The meta-evaluation imperative. *American Journal of Evaluation* 22 (2) Summer 183–209   References

Author defines meta-evaluation, and believes that because the evaluation field has advanced sufficiently in its methodology and public service that evaluators can and should subject their evaluations to systematic meta-evaluations. The advantages of both formative and summative meta-evaluations are discussed. Some tools that have been developed are available.

2.43.72   Sussman, S. (ed.) (2000) *Handbook of program development for health behaviour research and practice.* Thousand Oaks: CA: Sage   ISBN 0761916733   References

Handbook takes the reader from programme development theory, through programme activity analysis and selection, to immediate impact studies, and intermediate and long-term programme outcome measurement.

2.43.73 Torres, R.T., Preskill, H.S. & Piontek, M.E. (1996) *Evaluation strategies for communicating and reporting.* Thousand Oaks, CA: Sage ISBN 0803959273 References

Book provides a model for doing evaluation in a way that helps individuals and organizations to develop.

2.43.74 Trinder, L. & Reynolds, S. (eds) (2000) *Evidence-based practice: a critical appraisal.* Oxford: Blackwell Science ISBN 0632050586 References

Book provides a critical appraisal of the strengths and weaknesses of evidence-based practice, and weighs up the arguments for and against. Its spread as a cross-disciplinary phenomeno is discussed, together with the relevance for disciplines other than medicine. A list of websites is included.

2.43.75 van Eyk, H., Baum, F. & Blandford, J. (2001) Evaluating health care reform: the challenge of evaluating changing policy environments. *Evaluation* 7 (4) 487–503 References

Evaluating health care programmes is difficult because they frequently become entangled in complex, inherently political processes and often shift away from their original objectives when policies are changed. Evaluators in South Australia describe how they attempted to address these challenges through a flexible and dynamic action research approach (CR 2.37, 3.2, 3.11).

2.43.76 *www.nettingtheevidence.org.uk A ScHARR Introduction to Evidence-Based Practice on the Internet* www.shef.ac.uk/~scharr/ir/netting/first. html (Accessed 01/05/03)

Netting the evidence is intended to facilitate evidence-based health care by providing support and access to helpful organizations and useful learning resources, such as an evidence-based virtual library, software and journals.

2.44 EX-POST FACTO RESEARCH

In this type of research attempts are made to explain or describe events that have already occurred, and this has value when research problems cannot be studied by experimentation. Studies investigate cases where variables have been manipulated by life events (for example environmental pollution or the effects of thalidomide) and those that have taken place in natural settings rather than in a laboratory.

Definition [See Appendix D for source]

Ex-post facto research – an after-only evaluation research design where pre-testing is not possible

Example

Dunn, S.A., Lewis, S.L., Bonner, P.N. & Meize-Grochowski, R. (1994) Quality of life for spouses of CAPD patients. *ANNA Journal* 21 (5) 237–46, 257 34 References

Study describes the quality of life for spouses of Continuous Ambulatory Peritoneal Dialysis (CAPD) patients. Authors believe that nurses caring for the whole family can make a difference to the stability and well-being of the patient's spouse.

Annotation

2.44.1 Giuffre, M. (1997) Designing research: ex-post facto designs. *Journal of Perianesthesia Nursing* 12 (3) 191–5 4 References

Article discusses ex-post facto research.

2.45 GROUNDED THEORY RESEARCH

Grounded theory is a highly systematic research approach for the collection and analysis of qualitative data. Its purpose is to generate explanatory theory that furthers the understanding of social and psychological phenomena. It represents an advance in the technology for handling qualitative data gathered in the natural, everyday world. It has its roots in the social sciences, specifically in the symbolic interaction tradition of social psychology and sociology.

Definitions [See Appendix D for sources]

Dimensional analysis – ... an alternative method of generating grounded theory conceived for the purpose of improving the articulation and communication of the discovery process in qualitative research

Grounded theory – an approach to collecting and analysing qualitative data with the aim of developing theories and theoretical propositions grounded in real-world observations

Heuristic research – a style of qualitative analysis ... in which research participants remain visible in the examination of data and continue to be portrayed as whole persons

Symbolic interaction – the study of how the self and the social environment mutually define and shape each other through symbolic communication

Example

Guthrie, C. (1999) Nurses' perceptions of sexuality relating to patient care. *Journal of Clinical Nursing* 8 (3) 313–21   49 References

Using grounded theory, this study explores the perceptions of nurses regarding sexuality related to patient care. Several negative issues were identified which were complex and interrelated, and nurses dealt with questions relating to patient sexuality by adopting various coping strategies.

Original text

Glaser, B.G. & Strauss, A.L. (1967) *The discovery of grounded theory: strategies for qualitative research*. Hawthorne, NY: Walter de Gruyter   ISBN 0202302601

Annotations

2.45.1   Atkinson, P. & Housley, W. (2003) *Interactionism*. London: Sage   ISBN 0761962700 References

Provides a guide to the essential thinking, research and concepts in interactionism, demonstrates the use of this approach and explains why the interactionist influence has not been fully acknowledged in Britain.

2.45.2   Backman, K. & Kyngäs, H.A. (1999) Challenges of the grounded theory approach to a novice researcher. *Nursing and Health Sciences* 1 (3) 147–53   37 References

Discusses the methodological decisions that a researcher has to make in order to undertake a research study using grounded theory and discusses the problems encountered by a researcher using the approach for the first time (CR 2.16).

2.45.3   Berger, K.M. & Allen, M.N. (2001) Symbolic interactionism as a theoretical perspective for multiple-method research. *Journal of Advanced Nursing* 33 (4) 541–7   17 References

Paper presents symbolic interactionism as a theoretical perspective for multiple-method designs with the aim of expanding the dialogue about new methodologies (CR 2.7, 2.29, 2.36).

2.45.4   Cutcliffe, J.R. (2000) Methodological issues in grounded theory. *Journal of Advanced Nursing* 31 (6) 1476–84   34 References

Paper gives a brief overview of grounded theory in order to identify the rudiments of the method. Four key issues are then discussed: sampling, creativity, reflexivity and the use of literature and precision within grounded theory.

2.45.5   Dey, I. (1999) *Grounding grounded theory: guidelines for qualitative inquiry*. London: Academic Press   ISBN 0122146409   References

Discusses the methodological principles on which grounded theory is based, together with its main features. This is not another 'how to' book but aims to show what this theory has to offer qualitative research (CR 2.36).

2.45.6   Eaves, Y.D. (2001) A synthesis technique for grounded theory data analysis. *Journal of Advanced Nursing* 35 (5) 654–63   32 References

Paper examines the issues surrounding current changes in grounded theory methods and describes an innovative synthesis technique that lends clarity to the process.

2.45.7   Glaser, B.G. & Strauss, A.L. (1967) *The discovery of grounded theory: strategies for qualitative research*. Hawthorne, NY: Walter de Gruyter ISBN 0202302601

A seminal work in the field of qualitative research (CR 2.36).

2.45.8   Goulding, C. (2002) *Grounded theory: a practical guide for management, business and market researchers*. London: Sage   ISBN 076196682X   References

Book aims to properly contextualize grounded theory by looking at its background, characteristics and the different sides of the argument of its potential for the researcher, but also outlines how the approach may be used within a research context.

2.45.9   Hall, W.A. & Callery, P. (2001) Enhancing the rigor of grounded theory: incorporating reflexivity and relationality. *Qualitative Health Research* 11 (2) March 257–72   35 References

Authors claim that the principal texts on grounded theory do not attend to the effects of interactions between researcher and participant in interview and participant observation contexts. Descriptions of these interactions are necessary to add to the rigour of grounded theory findings. Reflexivity and relationality should be incorporated into grounded theory.

2.45.10   Happ, M.B. & Kagan, S.H. (2001) Methodological considerations for grounded theory research in critical care settings. *Nursing Research* 50 (3) 188–92   41 References

Article presents methodological considerations for conducting grounded theory research in fast-paced physiologically and technologically complex critical care settings. Barriers to this, strategies and opportunities are all discussed.

2.45.11 Kearney, M.H. (1998) Ready-to-wear: discovering grounded formal theory. *Research in Nursing and Health* 21 (2) 179–86   32 References

Discusses grounded formal theory analysis that can yield high-level, broadly applicable theory from analysis of situation specific substantive theories. Although they may lack the cultural detail and context of similar smaller analyses, they have the potential to serve as 'ready-to-wear' models that fit the experiences of individuals in a variety of settings.

2.45.12 Kushner, K.E. & Morrow, R. (2003) Grounded theory, feminist theory, critical theory: toward theoretical triangulation. *Advances in Nursing Science* 26 (1) 30–43   56 References

Examines variants of grounded theory and proposes a critical feminist grounded theory methodology deriving from theoretical triangulation (CR 2.10, 2.26).

2.45.13 Locke, K.D. (2001) *Grounded theory in management research.* Thousand Oaks, CA: Sage ISBN 0761964282   References

Describes the grounded theory approach and brings together the broadly dispersed discussions of its logic and practices. This book discusses the possibilities and challenges of the method for graduate students and academics teaching research methods courses in management and organization studies.

2.45.14 Melia, K.M. (1997) Producing 'plausible stories': interviewing student nurses. In Miller, G. & Dingwall, R. (eds) *Context and method in qualitative research.* London: Sage ISBN 0803976321 Part 1 Chapter 2 26–36   References

Reviews the recent disagreements between Glaser and Strauss about the nature of the research strategy they promoted in the 1960s. The author tries to establish where this leaves the followers of grounded theory. Interviews as text and as data are discussed, which raises questions about their appropriateness and limits (CR 2.36.88, 2.68).

2.45.15 Norton, L. (1999) The philosophical bases of grounded theory and their implications for nursing practice. *Nurse Researcher* 7 (1) 31–43   36 References

Article considers the philosophical bases of grounded theory and discusses the relevance of these in relation to the generation and writing of a

grounded theory. The links between ontology, epistemology, methodology and method are important and need to be observed when generating a grounded theory in order that research rigour is maintained (CR 2.5).

2.45.16 Schreiber, R. & Stern, P.M. (eds) (2002) *Using grounded theory in nursing.* New York: Springer ISBN 0826114067   References

Book details the expanding knowledge about the use of this qualitative research method in health care. Contributions are included from internationally known qualitative researchers and include a combination of theoretical and practical information (CR 2.36).

2.45.17 Strauss, A.L. & Corbin, J. (eds) (1997) *Grounded theory in practice.* London: Sage ISBN 0761907483   References

Volume presents a series of readings that emphasize different aspects of grounded theory and methodology. Selections are written by some of Strauss's former students and have been chosen for their accessibility and range. Commentaries by the editors are included for each paper.

2.45.18 Strauss, A. & Corbin, J. (1998) *Basics of qualitative research: techniques and procedures for developing grounded theory* (2nd edition). Thousand Oaks, CA: Sage ISBN 0803959397   References

This book offers practical advice and technical expertise that will aid researchers in analysing and interpreting their collected data and ultimately to develop theory from it. A step-by-step guide to undertaking research is given. Many definitions and examples are included, as well as criteria for evaluating a study and responses to frequently asked questions about qualitative research (CR 2.2, 2.7, 2.36, 2.86, 2.93, 2.95, 2.97, 2.100).

2.46 HISTORICAL RESEARCH – DOCUMENTARY

'Historiography provides one important route for researchers from nursing, midwifery and health visiting to interrogate "quality" in research practice and keep an evaluative eagle eye on intellectual standards more generally. We ignore the "lessons" of history … at our peril.' (Rafferty, 1997/98: 15)

Definitions [See Appendix D for sources]

External criticism (appraisal, examination) – a type of examination of historical data that is concerned with the authenticity or genuineness of the data. [External criticism might be used to determine if a letter was actually written by the person whose signature was contained on the letter]

Historical research – the critical investigation of events, developments and experiences of the past, the careful weighing of evidence of past sources of information and the interpretation of this evidence

Historicism – [has two meanings] ... encompasses the idea that history can be explained in terms of fixed laws or principles that explain social change/ ... a perspective that argues that any aspect of social life can be understood only in the context of the historical period in which it exists

Historiography – the writing of history

History – a recorded narrative of past events, especially those concerning a particular period, nation, individual

Internal criticism – a type of examination of historical data that is concerned with the accuracy of the data. [Internal criticism might be used to determine if a document contained an accurate recording of events as they actually happened]

Example

Matilainen, D. (1999) Patterns of ideas in the professional life and writings of Karin Neuman-Rahn: a biographical study of the ideas of psychiatric care in Finland in the early twentieth century. *Advances in Nursing Science* 22 (1) 78–88   50 References

Study aims to increase the understanding of ideas in Finnish psychiatric care, based primarily on texts produced by Neuman-Rahn (1867–1962) and anchored in the history of ideas at that time. Her works reflect a profound ethical stance, an understanding of mental life, mental suffering, the power of human will, and the idea of the possible. The research indicates that history offers much valuable wisdom that we can incorporate into our care today.

Annotations

2.46.1   American Association for the History of Nursing Inc. *Historical methodology* www.aahn. org/methodology.html (Accessed 15/02/03)

Provides a bibliography on historical methodology, nursing library collection issues, using archives – *Using Archives: A Practical Guide for Researchers,* that is a set of guidelines from the National

Archives of Canada – and links to information on oral history (CR 2.47).

2.46.2   Berridge, V. (2001) Historical research. In Fulop, N., Allen, P., Clarke, A. & Black, N. (eds) *Studying the organization and delivery of health services: research methods.* London: Routledge   ISBN 0415257638   Chapter 9 140–53   30 References

Examines historical research methods, their theoretical bases and uses, and shows how historians construct their accounts and find appropriate sources (CR 2.47, 3.12.3).

2.46.3   Black, J. & MacRaild, D.M. (2000) *Studying history* (2nd edition). Basingstoke: Macmillan   ISBN 0333801830   References

Book examines the multifaceted nature of history and offers a comprehensive view of the discipline. The sources and methods that historians use are discussed and students are advised about practical details in conducting studies and writing up results. A section on quantitative history is also included (CR 2.97).

2.46.4   Carr, E.H. (1986) *What is history?* London: Macmillan   ISBN 0333389565   References

A classic text that explores historical theory, the origins of history, its relationship to science and morality, causation and how it expands the horizon of learning.

2.46.5   Church, O.M. (1990) New knowledge from old truths: problems and promises of historical enquiry in nursing. In McCloskey, J.C. & Grace, H.K. (eds) *Current issues in nursing* (3rd edition). St Louis, MO: Mosby   ISBN 0801655250   Chapter 13 94–8   20 References

Discusses the value of historical inquiry to the practice of nursing.

2.46.6   Cushing, A. (1996) Method and theory in the practice of nursing history ... including commentary by Maggs, C. *International History of Nursing Journal* 2 (2) 5–32   35 References

Paper examines two main issues connected to the writing of history: difficulties in writing an account of past events and the role of social theory in historical writing. The contributions of other historians, the diversity of views and underlying assumptions in methodological approaches are all discussed in relation to written documents.

2.46.7   D'Antonio, P. *Rethinking the rewriting of nursing history* www.nursing.upenn.edu/history/ chronicle/s98/antonio.htm (Accessed 14/05/03)

Author suggests that thinking about nursing history in such a way as to reposition identity rather than work as the centre of analysis will enable greater understanding of nurses' roles over time.

2.46.8 Fealy, G.M. (1999) Historical research: a legitimate methodology for nursing research in Ireland. *Nursing Review (Ireland)* 17 (1/2) 24–9 26 References

Identifies the principal philosophical positions related to this type of research. Outlines the principles of conducting historical research and potential sources of material. Suggests that historical research could be of great value in tracing the history of nursing in Ireland (CR 2.47).

2.46.9 Fitzpatrick, M.L. (2001) Historical research: the method. In Munhall, P.L. *Nursing research: a qualitative perspective* (3rd edition). Sudbury, MA: Jones & Bartlett and National League for Nursing ISBN 0763711357 Chapter 13 403–15 8 References

Chapter introduces nurse scholars to the field of historical research in nursing – its objectives, methods, approaches, procedures, analysis and interpretation (CR 2.36.98).

2.46.10 Hill, M.R. (1993) *Archival strategies and techniques.* Newbury Park, CA: Sage ISBN 0803948255 References

Much more than a 'how to' book, the author interprets the archives and their use from a Goffmanian sociological perspective. Readers are guided through the archival process by drawing on a sociological/historical project. The 'rules of the game' on conducting and preparing to work in archives, the protocol of using them and ways of referencing the data obtained are all discussed.

2.46.11 Lusk, B. (1997) Historical methodology for nursing research. *Image: Journal of Nursing Scholarship* 29 (4) 355–9 36 References

Describes the basic tenets of historical research methodology with an emphasis on researching nursing history.

2.46.12 Mansell, D. (1995) Sources in nursing historical research: a thorny methodological problem. *Canadian Journal of Nursing Research* 27 (3) 83–86 9 Endnotes

Discusses some of the difficulties facing nurses when researching any historical subject. Limitations exist in available records that may give a skewed picture of particular groups of nurses and their activities. However, when these are combined with oral data, personal diaries and correspondence, a fuller picture may be gained (CR 2.28, 2.67, 2.71).

2.46.13 Marwick, A. (2001) *The new nature of history: knowledge, evidence, language.* Chicago, IL: Lyceum Books Inc. ISBN 0925065617 References

This updated version of the classic *The Nature of History* offers answers to questions essential to the student of history – What is history? Why do it? And how does one do it? Using the categories in the subtitle, the author presents the first clear and comprehensive expression of the case against post-modernism. He argues that the substance of history is evidence, not speculation, and explicates the production of history as a body of knowledge. He outlines the actual activities of a working historian in discussing the necessity of precise language, the analysis and interpretation of primary and secondary sources, and the vital distinctions between the 'witting' and 'unwitting' testimony of primary sources.

2.46.14 McCulloch, G. & Richardson, W. (2000) *Historical research in educational settings.* Buckingham: Open University Press ISBN 0335202543 References

Book explores how to set about historical research in education. It offers a theoretical guide to the rationales and problems of the field as well as to current opportunities for research. Practical advice is given for getting started and suitable research methods in different projects and detailed case studies are also included.

2.46.15 Morris, R.J. (1991) History and computing: expansion and achievements. *Social Science Computer Review* 9 (2) 215–30 References

Reports on developments in historical research using computers from 1980 to 1990. It includes information on large databases, developments in text analysis, information on associations, journals and data archives (CR 2.76, 2.89).

2.46.16 Rafferty, A.M. (1997/98) Writing, researching and reflexivity in nursing history. *Nurse Researcher* 5 (2) 5–16 34 References

Author considers some of the questions which have 'exercised the minds and hearts of historians' since the nineteenth century. She believes that nurse researchers can learn from history, and particularly from that of other disciplines, to create building blocks for the development of further research in nursing.

2.46.17 Rafferty, A.M. (2000) Historical research. In Cormack, D.F.S. (ed.) *The research process in nursing* (4th edition). Oxford: Blackwell Science ISBN 0632051582 Chapter 17 199–212 30 References

Chapter briefly outlines some signposts to historical research in nursing (CR 2.1.23).

2.46.18 Sarnecky, M.T. (1990) Historiography: a legitimate research methodology for nursing.

Advances in Nursing Science 12 (4) 1–10   36 References

Examines the historical approach, discusses its relevance to nursing and contrasts it with other epistemologies and ontologies (CR 2.5, 2.6).

2.46.19   Sheeley, V.L. *Historical research methods* ericcass.uncg.edu/research/sheeley.html (Accessed 01/05/03)

Discusses historiography, when historical research may be useful and the contribution it can make to gaining knowledge.

2.46.20   Sorenson, E.S. (1988) Archives as sources of treasure in historical research. *Western Journal of Nursing Research* 10 (5) 666–70   11 References

Discusses the use of historical archives and gives some of the sources available for the study of nursing history.

2.46.21   Speziale, H.J.S. & Carpenter, D.R. (2003) Historical research in practice. In Authors *Qualitative research in nursing: advancing the humanistic imperative* (3rd edition). Philadelphia, PA: Lippincott Williams & Wilkins   ISBN 0781734835 Chapter 12 225–43   41 References

Chapter highlights how researchers in nursing practice, education and administration apply historical methodology to understand patterns of our past. Guidelines are given for critiquing historical studies (CR 2.36.132, 2.95).

2.46.22   Speziale, H.J.S. & Carpenter, D.R. (2003) Historical research methods. In Authors *Qualitative research in nursing: advancing the humanistic imperative* (3rd edition). Philadelphia, PA: Lippincott Williams & Wilkins   ISBN 0781734835   Chapter 11 207–23   37 References

Chapter discusses historical research methods (CR 2.36.132).

2.46.23   Stinson, S.M., Johnson, J.L. & Zilm, G. (1992) *History of nursing beginning bibliography: a proemial list with special reference to Canadian sources.* Edmonton, Alberta, Canada: Faculty of Nursing, University of Alberta   ISBN 0888647727

4.4 Nursing research entry nos 828–867
5.2 Historical research methods entry nos 895–963

This bibliography is the first published list of references pertaining to the history of nursing with special reference to Canada. Sections cover the history of nursing research and historical research methods. The latter covers literature from 1952 to 1991 and includes both documentary and oral history (CR 1.3, 2.47).

2.46.24   West Yorkshire History of Nursing (WHYON) University of Huddersfield School of Human & Health Sciences *Historical research methods* www.hud.ac.uk/hhs/departments/hswcs/ nursing_history/historical_research_methods (Accessed 05/03/03)

Gives sources for historical research methods, general sites, resources related to the work of Michel Foucault, post-modernity, qualitative research and oral history (CR 2.47).

2.46.25   Yuginovich, T. (2000) More than time and place: using historical comparative research as a tool for nursing. *International Journal of Nursing Practice* 6 (2) 70–5   15 references

Identifies the contribution that a comparative method of historical research can make to the understanding of past and present political systems and appreciation of health care practice. Makes particular reference to nursing in remote areas of Australia (CR 3.2).

2.47   HISTORICAL RESEARCH – ORAL

'Oral history in some ways is "coming of age", and growing in popularity. It is offering a voice to the unheard and unseen.' (Howarth, 1998: v)

Definition [See Appendix D for source]

Oral history – the interviewing of eyewitness participants in the events of the past for the purposes of historical reconstruction

Example

Fairman, J. & Kagan, S. (1999) Creating critical care: the case of the Hospital of the university of Pennsylvania, 1950–1965. *Advances in Nursing Science* 22 (1) 63–77   57 References

Article examines the development of critical care nursing through the lens of a local story. The methodology used is social history and the data were derived from oral history interviews, archival material and secondary sources. Conclusions are reported and it provides parallels to contemporary nurse workforce issues (CR 2.68, 2.76, 2.91).

Annotations

2.47.1   Bornat, J., Perks, R., Thompson, P. & Walmsley, J. (eds) (1999) *Oral history, health and welfare.* London: Routledge   ISBN 0415191564

Book comprises a collection of papers from the 1996 Oral History Society Conference – Cradle to Grave: Oral History, Health and Welfare. Seventeen contributors show the vigour of the topic and the breadth and depth of scholarship in the field. Sections include the testimonies and lives of health professionals, the experiences of those socially marginalized and the impact of health care during birth and old age.

2.47.2 Caunce, S. (1994) *Oral history and the local historian.* South Melbourne, Victoria: Longman ISBN 0582072948

This book is 'a menu you can choose from, not an instruction manual'. The author sets out to demystify and broaden the basis of oral history.

2.47.3 Davis, C., Back, K. & Maclean, K. (1977) *Oral history: from tape to type.* Chicago, IL: American Library Association ISBN 0838902308 References

An instructional and operating manual designed to guide those beginning an oral history programme and a textbook for instructors. Illustrations and exercises are included to enable the novice to practise certain skills. Sample forms show how to do the paperwork that accompanies oral history interviewing and processing. A glossary and a list of additional sources are included (CR 2.2).

2.47.4 Dunaway, D.K. & Baum, W.K. (eds) (1997) *Oral history: an interdisciplinary anthology* (2nd edition). Thousand Oaks, CA: Alta Mira Press ISBN 0761991891 References

Book explains the basis of oral history and how to make use of it in research. It also includes a significant collection of classic readings by oral historians.

2.47.5 Finnegan, R. (1992) *Oral traditions and the verbal arts: a guide to research practices.* London: Routledge ISBN 0415028419 References

Book is a guide to the practicalities of fieldwork and the range of methods by which oral texts and performances can be observed, collected and analysed (CR 2.86).

2.47.6 Grele, R.J. (1998) Movement without aim: methodological and theoretical problems in oral history. In Perks, R. & Thomson, A. (eds) *The oral history reader.* London: Routledge ISBN 0415133521 Part 1 Chapter 4 38–52 52 Notes and References

Discusses some of the problems in the rapidly developing field of oral history – interviewing, research standards and historical methodology (CR 2.47.18).

2.47.7 Hackmann, M. (1999) Interviews in historical nursing research (German). *Pflege* 12 (1) 28–33 42 References

Interviewing methods in historical nursing research and the concept of oral history are described. Examples are given to illustrate the method (CR 2.68).

2.47.8 Howarth, K. (1998) *Oral history.* Stroud: Sutton Publishing Company ISBN 0750917571 References

This introduction for amateurs and professionals fully explains oral history recording and all its uses. Detailed sections are included on planning and conducting interviews, storage, cataloguing and retrieval. The applications of oral history and ethical issues are discussed and several case studies included (CR 2.17, 2.68).

2.47.9 Humphries, S. (1984) *The handbook of oral history: recording life stories.* London: Inter-Action Inprint ISBN 0904571467 References

Book shows how a more accurate and authentic picture of the past may be created by talking to the people who were actually there. It includes sections on organizing a project, working with different groups and all aspects of presentation and publication.

2.47.10 Hunter, B. (1999a) Oral history and research. Part 1: Uses and implications. *British Journal of Midwifery* 7 (7) 426–9 15 References

AND

2.47.11 Hunter, B. (1999b) Oral history and research. Part 2: Current practice. *British Journal of Midwifery* 7 (8) 481–4 8 References

These two articles discuss the use of oral history research in midwifery and explore its relevance for contemporary and future practice. The author describes how oral history research may be done, and considers its advantages and disadvantages.

2.47.12 Hutching, M. (1993) *Talking history: a short guide to oral history.* Wellington, NZ: Williams, Bridget Books/Historical Department Branch, Department of Internal Affairs ISBN 0908912463

Book is intended for those undertaking oral history for the first time. Oral history is defined and the processes involved, from preparation to interview and processing, are discussed. A list of questions and a short bibliography are included.

2.47.13 Jones, D.W. (1998) Distressing histories and unhappy interviewing. *Oral History* Autumn 49–56 20 Notes and References

Discusses the parallels between therapeutic and research interviewing, handling distress and probing when gathering evidence. Also considered are the impact of interviewing on the interviewer and interviewee, and protecting the interests of both (CR 2.68).

2.47.14   McKenzie, D. & Pifalo, V. (1998) The oral history program: III. Personal views of health sciences librarianship and the Medical Association Library. *Bulletin of the Medical Library Association* 86 (4) 464–74

The Medical Library Association Oral History Programme stores original taped interviews and transcripts that can be accessed for research purposes. Although the subject matter relates to health sciences librarianship, this archive may be of value to others working in the health field (CR 2.68).

2.47.15   Oral History Research Office *Oral history Internet resources* www.columbia.edu/cu/lweb/indiv/oral/offsite.html (Accessed 15/02/03)

Website provides links to oral history organizations in colleges, universities and government programmes. It also gives information on private programmes and projects.

2.47.16   Oral History Society *Oral History Society* www.oralhistory.org.uk/ (Accessed 15/02/03)

Website gives information about oral history and how it can be used. Links are given to the Oral History Society and its journal.

2.47.17   Perks, R. (ed.) (1990) *Oral history: an annotated bibliography.* London: British Library National Sound Archive   ISBN 071230505X

This annotated bibliography identifies a wide range of health topics in over 2,100 entries. Sources of information on the processes involved in oral history are also included (CR 1.3).

2.47.18   Perks, R. & Thomson, A. (eds) (1998) *The oral history reader.* London: Routledge   ISBN 0415133521   References

This reader is an international anthology of key writings about the theory, method and use of oral history. Mainly using previously published papers, it covers key debates, including interviewing methods, ethical questions, the politics of empowerment, analytical strategies for interpreting memories and concerns of archiving and public history. It illustrates similarities and differences in oral history work around the world and details the many subjects to which it has made a contribution. It also includes addresses of useful contacts.

2.47.19   Perks, R. (1999) Oral history websites. *Oral History* 27 (2) Autumn 87–9

Lists websites of key oral history organizations from Australia, Brazil, Israel, New Zealand, Singapore, South Africa, the UK and the USA. Other key and link/search sites give international coverage.
www.essex.ac.uk/sociology/oralhis.htm (UK)
www.baylor.edu/~OHA/ (USA)

2.47.20   Portelli, A. (1998) What makes oral history different? In Perks, R. & Thomson, A. (eds) *The oral history reader.* London: Routledge   ISBN 0415133521   Part I Chapter 6 63–74   11 Notes and References

Chapter discusses the orality of oral sources, oral history as narrative, events and meaning, whether we should believe oral sources, objectivity and who speaks on oral history (CR 2.47.18).

2.47.21   Rickard, W. (1998) Oral history – 'more dangerous than therapy'?: interviewees' reflections on recording traumatic or taboo issues. *Oral History* Autumn 34–48   20 Notes and References

Following a seminar on issues of ethics, methodology and copyright, the author reports and analyses the key points emerging from life history interviews with four people on 'difficult subjects'. These included: coping with an AIDS diagnosis, suicide of a family member, domestic violence, drug addiction, 'coming out', self-identity, prostitution, family friction and sexual abuse (CR 2.17).

2.47.22   Rolph, S. (1998) Ethical dilemmas: oral history work with people with learning difficulties. *Oral History* Autumn 65–72   53 Notes

Introduces some ethical dilemmas that may be encountered in working with people with learning difficulties. Issues of access, anonymity and privacy, information and consent, power and participation, sensitive matters and the use of archival sources are all discussed. It is not simply the research techniques that are being questioned, but the role of the oral historian and researcher without learning difficulties (CR 2.17, 2.76).

2.47.23   Sangster, J. (1998) Telling our stories: feminist debates and the use of oral history. In Perks, R. & Thomson, A. (eds) *The oral history reader.* London: Routledge   ISBN 0415133521 Part 1 Chapter 8 87–100   52 Notes and References

Author examines current theoretical dilemmas encountered by feminist historians, including ethical issues in interpreting other women's lives through oral history and which approaches are the most effective in conceptualizing this methodology (CR 2.10, 2.17, 2.47.18).

2.47.24   Seldon, A. & Pappworth, J. (1983) *By word of mouth: 'elite oral history'*. London: Methuen   ISBN 0416367402   References

This guide gives the history of elite figures, i.e. from or about people eminent in their field. It analyses the advantages of using oral history, offers advice on aspects of interviewing and gives information on the establishment and maintenance of an oral archive. A series of case studies showing the use of oral evidence by contemporary authors is included (CR 2.39, 2.68).

2.47.25   Thompson, P. (2000) *The voice of the past* (3rd edition). Oxford: Oxford University Press ISBN 0192893173   References

The new edition of this major text combines the theory and practice of oral history methodology and puts this in a wider context. The history, development and practice of oral history are discussed and many examples are given (CR 2.68).

2.47.26 Thurgood, G. (2002) Legal, ethical and human rights issues related to the storage of oral history interviews in archives. *International History of Nursing Journal* 7 (2) 38–49   96 References

Provides personal reflections that explore the legal, ethical and human rights issues of conducting oral history interviews with elderly retired nurses. Two methodological approaches were used: analysis of primary and secondary documentary archival sources and oral history interviews. The advantage of oral history to historians is discussed, together with maintaining anonymity, overcoming difficulties, libellous action, tape and transcript, to edit or not to edit and 'there is no rule' (CR 2.90, 2.91).

2.47.27   Vaz, K.M. (ed.) (1997) *Oral narrative research with black women: collecting treasures.* Thousand Oaks, CA: Sage   ISBN 0803974299 References

Oral narrative researchers from a variety of disciplines present strategies they have used to examine the experiences of African and African-American women. The book explores in detail the strengths of oral narrative research for expanding and transforming knowledge and how carrying out this type of research has affected the researchers' personal and professional lives (CR 2.16, 2.78).

2.47.28   Wallot, J.P. & Fortier, N. (1998) Archival science and oral sources. In Perks, R. & Thomson, A. (eds) *The oral history reader.* London: Routledge   ISBN 0415133521   Part V Chapter 30 365–78   58 Notes and References

Chapter discusses the growth of oral testimony and how this has 'challenged' the nature of archival science where material was previously all in written form. Suggestions are made as to how oral sources may be preserved, documented and made readily accessible to scholars (CR 2.47.18).

2.47.29   Ward, A. & Jenkins, A. (1999) Collecting the life stories of graduates: evaluating students' educational experiences. *Oral History* 27 (2) Autumn 77–86   28 Notes and References

Article outlines the methodology used for a long-term follow-up study of graduates in a British university. It shows how oral historians can help to shift the emphasis of course evaluation from short-term questionnaire studies to a long-term perspective that focuses on the individual's development (CR 2.43, 2.75).

2.47.30   Yow, V.R. (1994) *Recording oral history: a practical guide for social scientists*. Thousand Oaks, CA: Sage   ISBN 0803955790   References

Gives advice on all aspects of in-depth interviewing, handling tape recorders and asking probing questions. Ethical and legal issues are also covered (CR 2.17, 2.68).

2.48   LONGITUDINAL/DEVELOPMENTAL RESEARCH

This research strategy is useful for detecting change in individuals or groups over time, for example examining health maintenance or illness recovery.

Definitions [See Appendix D for sources]

Cohort – ... a group that is defined by a specific characteristic, such as a diagnosis or treatment

Cohort study – an observational study in which a defined group of people (the cohort) is followed over time

Developmental research – research focusing on those aspects of human behaviour that changes over time

Longitudinal designs – studies based on longitudinal data include *trend studies*, in which data are compared across time points on different subjects; *cohort studies* in which data from the same age cohort are compared at different points in time; and *panel studies*, in which the same subjects are compared across time points

Example

Hanrahan, P., Raymond, M., McGowan, E. & Luchins, D.J. (1999) Criteria for enrolling dementia patients in hospice: a replication. *American Journal of Hospice and Palliative Care* 16 (1) 395–400   7 References

This longitudinal study, involving 45 dementia patients, examined the value of the National Hospice Organization Guidelines when identifying those for whom hospice care may be appropriate, their limitations and the importance of the actual care plans used. Results are reported (CR 2.13).

Annotations

2.48.1   Boyington, A.R., Tomlinson, B.U. & Dougherty, M.C. (2000) Using a relational database to support nursing research. *Computers in Nursing* 18 (4) July – August. 155–6   References

Designing, implementing and maintaining a relational database for a complex longitudinal clinical research project can be the key to its success. Related issues of data entry, accuracy, confidentiality, security, data analysis and evaluation of research activity are among the considerations that must be addressed. The authors' experience of designing a system that was effective and user-friendly to manage the data collected during a six–year National Institutes of Health-funded nursing research project is highlighted.

2.48.2   Goldstein, H. (1979) *The design and analysis of longitudinal studies: their role in the measurement of change.* London: Academic Press   ISBN 0122895800   References

Provides comprehensive coverage of the theoretical background to this type of design together with a practical approach to the problems encountered in human field studies. Statistical aspects of longitudinal studies are thoroughly explored.

2.48.3   Huber, G.P. & Van De Ven, A.H. (eds) (1995) *Longitudinal field research methods: studying processes of organizational change.* Thousand Oaks, CA: Sage   ISBN 0803970919   References

Book describes procedures on tabulating, coding and interpreting both qualitative and quantitative data collected in the field (CR 2.86, 2.87).

2.48.4   King, M.P. (2001) Cross-sectional and longitudinal research design issues in the studies of human development. *Graduate Research in Nursing Online* June   5 References www.graduate research.com/King.htm (Accessed 29/01/03)

The purposes, advantages and disadvantages of cross-sectional and longitudinal designs are discussed, together with prospective versus retrospective issues. A study of maternal role transition is used to illustrate the use of prospective longitudinal design.

2.48.5   Magnusson, D. & Bergman, L. (eds) (1990) *Data quality in longitudinal research.* Cambridge: Cambridge University Press   ISBN 052138091X   References

Book discusses data quality issues in different areas, drop-out and attrition, design and methods. The importance of ensuring reliability, validity and representativeness is stressed (CR 2.24, 2.25).

2.48.6   Magnusson, D., Bergman, L.R., Rudinger, G. & Torestad, B. (eds) (1991) *Problems and methods in longitudinal research: stability and change.* Cambridge: Cambridge University Press   ISBN 052140195X   References

Covers many of the problems and difficulties that may be encountered in this type of research.

2.48.7   Menard, S. (2002) *Longitudinal research* (2nd edition). London: Sage   ISBN 0761922091   References

Written in non-technical language, this volume brings readers the latest advice on major issues involved in longitudinal research. It covers research design strategies, methods of data collection, and how longitudinal and cross-sectional research compares in terms of consistency and accuracy of results.

2.48.8   Ruspini, E. (2002) *Introduction to longitudinal research.* London: Routledge   ISBN 0415260086   References

Book provides an introduction to the kinds of issues involved in using longitudinal data. It covers the advantages, how to use longitudinal datasets in the European Union, United States and Canada, the implications of integrating micro-level empirical research with macro-level theories of social change, and the choices that need to be made between using trend, panel and duration data.

2.48.9   Smith, C.S., Sayler, J., Geddes, N. & Mark, B.A. (1998) Strategies to enhance internal validity in multi-centre longitudinal research. *Outcomes Management Nursing Practice* 2 (4) 174–9   References

Article addresses several key issues in data collection in multi-centre longitudinal research that may affect the results. Specific strategies used in a particular study are described, and the authors believe that these may also be useful to enhance the internal consistency of experimental and non-experimental cross-sectional research (CR 2.25).

2.48.10   Taris, T.W. (2000) *A primer in longitudinal analysis.* London: Sage ISBN 0761960279 References

Provides an introduction to the theory and practice of longitudinal research and points out its strengths and weaknesses. Designing, collecting data, using statistical techniques and interpretation of results are all included (CR 2.87).

2.48.11   Watson, R. (1998) Longitudinal quantitative research designs. *Nurse Researcher* 5 (4) 41–54   12 References

Author discusses some of the designs, benefits and problems of longitudinal quantitative research (CR 2.29).

2.48.12   Whitney, J.D. (2000) Comparative, observational designs: case-control and cohort studies. *Journal of the Wound, Ostomy and Continence Nurses Society* 27 May 191–3   12 References

Author discusses cross-sectional case-control designs and cohort studies (CR 2.21, 2.41).

2.48.13   Wolfe, F. (1999) Critical issues in longitudinal and observational studies: short-versus long-term selection of study instruments, methodological outcomes, and biases. *Journal of Rheumatology* 26 (2) February 469–72   References

Although longitudinal observational studies (LOS) are easy to perform, they are difficult to perform correctly. Major problems include recruitment, retention and relevance, but the central problems are biases, understanding their nature and reporting them. The author makes suggestions for resolving these problems (CR 2.22, 2.27).

2.48.14   Yarnold, P.R., Feinglass, J., McCarthy, W. & Martin, G.J. (1999) Comparing three preprocessing strategies for longitudinal data: an example in functional outcomes research. *Evaluation and the Health Professions* 22 (2) 254–77 26 References

Study compares three different methods for evaluating clinical outcomes for individual patients: raw change score analysis versus normative and ipsative statistical analysis. Results are reported (CR 2.43).

2.48.15   Young, C.H., Savola, K.L. & Phelps, E. (1991) *Inventory of longitudinal studies in the social sciences.* Newbury Park, CA: Sage ISBN 0803943156   References

Inventory contains information on longitudinal studies conducted over the last 60 years in the United States and Canada. Each one is described in detail, including its purpose, names and addresses of principal investigators, how it was conducted, its current status and a list of related references.

2.49   PHENOMENOLOGICAL RESEARCH

'Phenomenology is a 20th century philosophical movement dedicated to describing structures of experience as they present themselves to consciousness, without recourse to theory, deduction, or assumptions from other disciplines such as the natural science.' (Centre for Advanced Research in Phenomenology – www.phenomenologycenter.org/)

Definitions [See Appendix D for sources]

Bracketing – a process in which qualitative researchers put aside their own feelings or beliefs about a phenomenon that is being studied to keep from biasing their observations

Phenomenography – ... a qualitative, nondualist research approach that identifies and retains the discourse of research participants

Phenomenology – a method of study that attempts to understand human experience through analysis of the participant's description of that experience

---

Example

2.49   Ramritu, P.L. & Barnard, A. (2001) New nurse graduates understanding of competence. *International Nursing Review* 48 (1) 45–57   37 References

Describes the findings of a phenomenological research study used to understand the experiences of competence of new nurse graduates. Eight conceptions of competence were described: safe practice, limited independence, utilization of resources, management of time and workload, ethical practice, performance of clinical skills, knowledge and evolvement of competence. The research highlighted areas for improving undergraduate education programmes as well as clarification of entry-level competency standards.

Annotations

2.49.1   Ahern, K.J. (1999) Pearls, pith and provocation: ten tips for reflexive bracketing. *Qualitative Health Research* 9 (3) 407–11   12 References

Acknowledges that total objectivity is not possible or necessarily desirable in qualitative research but highlights the lack of guidance on how assumptions are put aside. Provides guidance on using reflexivity to identify areas of bias and to bracket them to minimize their influence on the research.

2.49.2 Annells, M. (1999) Evaluating phenomenology: usefulness, quality and philosophical foundations. *Nurse Researcher* 6 (3) 5–19   44 References

Author defines and explains the purpose of phenomenological nursing research and discusses the choices available when seeking to evaluate a report using this method (CR 2.5, 2.95).

2.49.3 Barkway, P. (2001) Michael Crotty and nursing phenomenology: criticism or critique? *Nursing Inquiry* 8 (3) 191–5   21 References

Debates whether Michael Crotty's writings on the nursing approach to phenomenology is a valid scholarly critique or a criticism of nursing research (CR 2.49.14).

2.49.4 Barnard, A., McCosker, H. & Gerber, R. (1999) Phenomenography: a qualitative research approach for exploring understanding in health care. *Qualitative Health Research* 9 (2) 212–26 46 References

Article presents the major assumptions associated with phenomenographic research. An example is included to emphasize its distinctiveness from phenomenological research.

2.49.5 Beech, I. (1999) Bracketing in phenomenological research. *Nurse Researcher* 6 (3) 35–51 22 References

Author discusses the use of bracketing as a methodological principle and considers its effects in conducting phenomenological research (CR 2.5).

2.49.6 Benner, P. (ed.) (1994) *Interpretive phenomenology: embodiment, caring and ethics in health and illness.* Thousand Oaks, CA: Sage ISBN 0803957238 References

Book comprises a collection of theoretical materials offering an introduction to the subject, followed by chapters that illustrate interpretative phenomenology in research.

2.49.7 Caelli, K. (2000) The changing face of phenomenological research: traditional and American phenomenology in nursing. *Qualitative Health Research* 10 (3) 366–77 46 References

Article explores the differences between traditional European and American phenomenology and argues that the latter approach extends the phenomenological project in valuable and meaningful ways that are particularly appropriate for the health sciences.

2.49.8 Center for Advanced Research in Phenomenology www.phenomenologycenter.org/index.html (Accessed 20/02/03)

Index gives access to all aspects of the Center's work.

2.49.9 Center for Advanced Research in Phenomenology *Collective multidisciplinary bibliography of phenomenology* www.phenomenolog center.org/biblio.htm (Accessed 02/05/03)

This resource is a complete list of all works by phenomenologists, both living and deceased, beginning in the 1880s. Entries will be added as they appear.

2.49.10 Center for Advanced Research in Phenomenology *What is phenomenology?* www.phenomenologycenter.org/phenom.htm (Accessed 19/02/03)

This paper outlines seven widely accepted features of the phenomenological approach; its 100-year spread by nation and discipline; tendencies and stages within philosophical phenomenology so far and how it may develop in the twenty-first century.

2.49.11 Centre for Philosophy and Phenomenological Studies *Aims and activities* www.csudh.edu/phenomstudies/ (Accessed 07/05/03)

Organization aims to promote, through electronic media, philosophical inquiries, exchange of findings and interaction with students. A bi-annual electronic journal is published and teleconferences are held (CR 2.5).

2.49.12 Cohen, M.Z., Kahn, D.L. & Steeves, R.H. (2000) *Hermeneutic phenomenological research: a practical guide for nurse researchers.* Thousand Oaks, CA: Sage ISBN 0761917209 References

Volume introduces this methodology and includes site-access, preparation, proposal writing, ethical issues, data collection, bias reduction, data analysis and research publication (CR 2.5, 2.14, 2.17, 2.22, 2.27, 2.86, 2.99).

2.49.13 Corben, V. (1999) Misusing phenomenology in nursing research: identifying the issues. *Nurse Researcher* 6 (3) 52–66   33 References

Explores some of the problems of the phenomenological method and issues surrounding its potential misuse in nursing research. Elements discussed are philosophical, methodological, researcher role, issues of validity and sampling, data analysis and discussion of results (CR 2.5, 2.16, 2.22, 2.25, 2.86, 3.16).

2.49.14 Crotty, M.C. (2000) *Phenomenology and nursing research* (2nd edition). South Melbourne, Australia: Churchill Livingstone ISBN 0443054320 References

Author describes and discusses two phenomenologies and urges a return to 'the unadulterated phenomena'. Ways forward for nurse researchers are considered.

2.49.15   Crowell, S., Embree, L. & Julian, S.J. (eds) *The reach of reflection: issues for phenomenology's second century* www.electronpress.com/ (Accessed 20/02/03)

This electronic book was developed by the Center for Advanced Research in Phenomenology (www.phenomenologycenter.org) to mark the transition from the second to the third millennium. While some chapters take up traditional philosophical themes or phenomenological problem areas, others discuss new subjects, including constructive phenomenology, cognitive science, ecology, ethnicity, gender, genetic phenomenology, horizontality, medicine and non-human animal life. A final chapter relates phenomenology to analytic philosophy.

2.49.16   Draucher, C.B. (1999) The critique of Heideggerian hermeneutical nursing research. *Journal of Advanced Nursing* 30 (2) 360–73   62 References

Article reviews research, focusing on two critical issues: do the reports reflect a convergence of researcher understanding and participant narratives as called for by the Heideggerian tradition? And do these ideas inform and enrich the studies' findings? The review reveals wide variations in how these two issues are reflected in published reports (CR 2.12).

2.49.17   Drew, N. (2001) Meaningfulness as an epistemologic concept for explicating the researcher's constitutive part in phenomenologic research. *Advances in Nursing Science* 23 (4) 16–31 17 References

When phenomenological data are the transcripts of interviews, our connections to the phenomena under study stand out as personally meaningful. Tracing back through past experiences to the origins of that meaningfulness provides a picture of the pre-understanding, assumptions and beliefs that contribute to our unique perception of the phenomena under study. Concrete guidelines are given for initiating the process of discovering one's constitutive part in phenomenologic studies (CR 2.6, 2.68).

2.49.18   Giorgi, A. (2000) Concerning the application of phenomenology to caring research … Crotty, M. Phenomenology and nursing research. Melbourne: Churchill Livingstone (1996). *Scandinavian Journal of Caring Sciences* 14 (1) 11–15   14 References

This article sharpens the distinction between philosophical and scientific phenomenology and demonstrates the confusion that can ensue when philosophical phenomenology is uncritically used as the model for scientific research. It does so by examining the work of Crotty (CR 2.49.14).

2.49.19   Johnson, M.E. (2000) Heidegger and meaning: implications for phenomenological

research. *Nursing Philosophy* 1 (2) 134–46   70 References

Provides a critique of Heideggerian phenomenology, including comparison with Husserl. Describes how Heidegger was introduced into nursing and, using an example, how his philosophy might inform the phenomenological researcher.

2.49.20   Jones, A. (2001) A condensed history of the phenomenology: the first and second phases from Franz Bretano to Hans-Georg Gadamer. *Nurse Researcher: The International Journal of Research Methodology in Nursing and Health Care* 8 (4) 65–75   24 References

Article examines the roots of the phenomenological movement and discusses the potential application to nursing research.

2.49.21   Koch, T. (1999) An interpretive research process: revisiting phenomenological and hermeneutical approaches. *Nurse Researcher* 6 (3) 20–34 26 References

Author examines how researchers move from the research question to the study itself in phenomenological research (CR 2.5, 2.6, 2.86).

2.49.22   Le Vasseur, J.J. (2003) The problem of bracketing in phenomenology. *Qualitative Health Research* 13 (3) March 408–20   27 References

Reviews the philosophical roots of phenomenology and discusses the issue of bracketing within hermeneutic frameworks. A fresh interpretation is offered to resolve the incongruity of employing the technique within essentially hermeneutic research (CR 2.5).

2.49.23   Lowes, L. & Prowse, M.A. (2001) Standing outside the interview process? The illusion of objectivity in phenomenological data generation. *International Journal of Nursing Studies* 38 (4) August. 471–80   References

This paper challenges the idea of researcher objectivity as a necessary feature of phenomenological interviewing by contrasting the philosophies of Husserl and Heidegger in relation to the way they influence the interview process, the generation of data and the role of the researcher in the interview. A failure to distinguish between the two results in methodological confusion. The interviewing process is analysed, and interviewer bias, the pursuit of objectivity and the relevance of subjectivity are all discussed. Quality indicators are also discussed and illustrated with examples from the authors' doctoral studies (CR 2.27, 2.68).

2.49.24   Moustakas, C. (1994) *Phenomenological research methods*. Thousand Oaks, CA: Sage   ISBN 0803957998   References

Author discusses the theoretical underpinnings of phenomenology and takes the reader step by step through the process of conducting a study. Numerous examples are given, together with form letters and other tools used in designing and conducting a study.

2.49.25 Munhall, P.L. (1994) *Revisioning phenomenology: nursing and health science research.* Sudbury, MA: Jones & Bartlett ISBN 0887375979

This book offers a unique approach to finding meaning in human experiences through a post-modern interpretation of the study of being.

2.49.26 Pope, E., Nel, E. & Poggenpoel, M. (1998) The experience of registered nurses nursing in the general adult intensive care unit: a phenomenological qualitative research study. *Curationis: South African Journal of Nursing* 21 (2) 32–38 31 References

The objectives of this study were to explore and describe the experience of registered nurses in an intensive care unit and develop guidelines, based on the information received, to support these nurses in their work. Authors discuss the following aspects of research methodology: data gathering (ethical considerations and informed consent), purposive selection, phenomenological interviews and field notes and data analysis using Tesch's method. This included ways of ensuring trustworthiness, organization of raw data and integration of findings supported by literature (CR 2.36).

2.49.27 Porter, E.J. (1998) On 'being inspired' by Husserl's phenomenology: reflections on Omery's exposition of phenomenology as a method of nursing research. *Advances in Nursing Science* 21 (1) 16–28 53 References

Reflects upon the philosophical origins and methods of phenomenology and its position in nursing research, explaining the basic tenets of Husserl and Omery.

2.49.28 Sadala, M.L.A. & Adorno, R.de C.F. (2002) Phenomenology as a method to investigate the experience lived: a perspective from Husserl and Merleau Ponty's thought. *Journal of Advanced Nursing* 37 (3) 282–93 12 References

By taking nursing as a human relationships activity, in spite of its strong technical-scientific features, this article reflects on the phenomenological method as one of the ways to develop an investigation and acquire knowledge of the topic.

2.49.29 Schoppmann, S. & Pohlmann, M. (2000) Some epistemological reflections on phenomenological research in nursing (German). *Pflege* 13 (6) 361–6 27 References

Paper is concerned with the question of which philosophical traditions underpin the phenomenological perspective in nursing research. Because there is some confusion over the use of some terms and methods, it is difficult to differentiate between the various accounts and use them for a concrete inquiry in nursing. The differences and consequences for phenomenological research methods are described, taking the ideas of Husserl and Heidegger into account (CR 2.6).

2.49.30 Stubblefield, C. & Murray, R.L. (2002) A phenomenological framework for psychiatric nursing research. *Archives of Psychiatric Nursing* 16 (4) August. 149–55 References

Article describes a framework developed to support phenomenological research within the context of psychiatric nursing. It integrates phenomenology as a philosophy and methodology with a method for analysing the experience of living with a mental illness.

2.49.31 Todres, L. & Wheeler, S. (2001) The complementarity of phenomenology, hermeneutics and existentialism as a philosophical perspective for nursing research. *International Journal of Nursing Studies* 38 (1) 1–8 42 References

Paper draws on the thinking of Husserl, Dilthey and Heidegger to identify elements of the phenomenological movement that can provide focus and direction for qualitative research in nursing.

2.49.32 van Manen, M. (2001) *Phenomenology online* www.phenomenologyonline.com/main.cfm (Accessed 11/02/03)

This site provides public access to articles, monographs and other materials discussing and exemplifying phenomenological research.

2.49.33 Whiting, L.S. (2001) Analysis of phenomenological data: personal reflections on Giorgi's method. *Nurse Researcher: The International Journal of Research Methodology in Nursing and Health Care* 9 (2) 60–74 40 References

Author offers some personal insights into using Giorgi's phenomenological method in a small-scale research study that considered the meaning of health promotion as perceived by a group of children's nurses.

2.49.34 Yegdich, T. (2000) In the name of Husserl: nursing in pursuit of things-in-themselves. *Nursing Inquiry* 7 (1) 29–40 71 References

Explores the notion that nurse phenomenologists' pursuit of humanistic inquiry have led them to combine humanism and Husserlian phenomenology. Through an examination of Husserl and Kant's philosophies, it is argued that there are inconsistencies between Husserl's thinking and nursing interpretations of his thought (CR 2.49).

2.50 PRESCRIPTIVE THEORY

Empirical validation of prescriptive theory has lagged behind other methodologies, as multiple studies over a long period of time are essential for this process.

Definition [See Appendix D for source]

Prescriptive theory – ... gives directions or rules as to how something should work or be carried out

---

Example

Kogan, H. & Betrus, P. (1984) Self-management: a nursing mode of therapeutic influence. *Advances in Nursing Science* 6 (4) 55–73   12 References

Study aimed to assess the reduction in stress following self-management training sessions. Results showed that it was successful in reducing symptoms.

Annotations

2.50.1 Huth, M.M. & Moore, S.M. (1998) Prescriptive theory of acute pain management in infants and children. *Journal of the Society of Pediatric Nurses* 3 (1) 23–32   55 References

Explains the concepts of theory, practice and research and how these form middle-range theory. Applies this to pain management in infants and children, in the form of prescriptive theory.

2.50.2 Knudtzon, K. *Prescriptive theories* www.cs.umd.edu/class/fall2002/cmsc838s/tichi/prescriptive.html (Accessed 01/05/03)

Provides an overview, the scope, applications and limitations of prescriptive theories. Gives an example of how it has been used in designing human/computer interaction tools. Reference is made to some seminal works in this field.

2.50.3 Thomas, C. (2002) *HCI introduction* www.cs.umd.edu/class/fall2002/cmsc838s/tichi/ (Accessed 01/05/03)

Discusses several theories, including prescriptive theory, as they are used in the domain of Human Computer Interaction. Their role is briefly discussed.

2.50.4 Zhou, Y. *Some important concepts* www.personal.psu.edu/faculty/y/x/yxz132/INSYS%20525/knowledge%20base/con ... (Accessed 14/11/03)

A table outlines the differences between descriptive and prescriptive theories.

2.51 SIMULATION AND GAMING

Role-playing has been used as a technique in educational research and the social sciences for assessing personality, in business training, and in psychotherapy. Its value is in the possibility of using it for assessment, teaching, and as a therapeutic procedure.

Definitions [See Appendix D for sources]

Monte Carlo Simulation – any generating of random values (most often with a computer) to study statistical models

Role-play – a function performed in a particular situation, process or operation

Simulation – to imitate, represent or feign

Example

Carlisle, C. (1998) A conceptual model described how adults responded to a simulated literacy assessment. [Commentary on Brez, S.M. & Taylor, M. Assessing literacy for patient teaching: perspectives of adults with low literacy skills. *Journal of Advanced Nursing* 1997 25 (5) 1040–7.] *Evidence-Based Nursing* 1 (1) January 29

This study aimed to understand how adults with low literacy skills experienced an assessment of their reading ability. A simulated literary screening experience that used a nurse-administered tool – The Rapid Estimate of Adult Literacy in Medicine – formed part of the data collection process. Results of the study are reported (CR 2.26, 2.39, 2.68, 2.72).

Annotations

2.51.1 Cohen, L., Manion, L. & Morrison, K. (2000) Recent developments: simulations. In Authors (eds) *Research methods in education* (5th edition). London: Routledge/Falmer   ISBN 0415195411   Chapter 22 385–9   References

Discusses the applications, key features, advantages and disadvantages of using simulations in educational research. Several relevant websites are included:

www/santafe.edu
www.brint.com/systems.htm
journals.wiley.com/1076-2787/tocs
life.csu.edu.au/v1_complex/all.html (All accessed
29/01/03) (CR 2.1.20).

2.51.2   Cohen, L., Manion, L. & Morrison, K.
(2000) Role-playing. In Authors (eds) *Research
methods in education* (5th edition). London:
Routledge/Falmer   ISBN 0415195411 Chapter 21
370-9   References

Chapter outlines the history of role-play and discusses its strengths and weaknesses, including the
problem of deception. Evaluating role-play and
simulations is discussed and authors describe how it
may be used in educational settings (CR 2.1.20).

2.51.3   Crookall, D.A. & Arai, K. (eds) (1995)
*Simulations and gaming across disciplines and
cultures: ISAGA at a watershed.* Thousand Oaks,
CA: Sage   ISBN 0803971028   References

Discusses the 'state of play' in simulation and gaming techniques. Abstracts of all papers presented at
the 25th ISAGA conference are also included.

2.51.4   Gates, D.M., Fitzwater, E. & Telintelo, S.
(2001) Using simulations and standardized patients
in intervention research. *Clinical Nursing Research*
10 (4) 387-400   35 References

Article describes the development and use of simulated exercises and standardized patients as an evaluation methodology for intervention research. The
aim of the work was to decrease the incidence of
assaults on caregivers.

2.51.5   Gilbert, N. & Troitzsch, K.G. (1999)
Simulation for the social scientist. Buckingham: Open
University Press   ISBN 0335197442   References

This text gives practical advice on the techniques of
building computer simulations to assist understanding of social and economic issues and problems.

2.51.6   Gredler, M. (1992) *Designing and evalu-
ating games and simulations: a process approach.*
London: Kogan   Page   ISBN   0749404787
References

Book contains a historical survey of games and simulations as learning tools and analyses of well-
known simulations. It identifies a group of key
categories and includes examples from both British
and American sources.

**2.51.7   Miller, A.M., Wilbur, J., Montgomery,
A.C. & Talashek, M.L.** (1998) Standardizing faculty evaluation of nurse practitioner students by
using simulated patients. *Clinical Excellence for
Nurse Practitioners* 2 (2) 102-9   20 References

Biases related to variations among patients and
having faculty evaluate the clinical skills of students
as they interact with simulated patients are discussed. The Student Clinical Performance Scale
was developed to standardize assessment of videotaped simulated patient encounters with family
nurse practitioner students. Findings demonstrated
the importance of a rigorous approach to developing
and testing instruments that guide measurement of
clinical competence. The use of simulated patients
provides opportunities to assess a wide range of
attributes and holds promise for assessing advanced
clinical skills in controlled educational environments
(CR 2.24, 2.27, 2.55).

2.51.8   Mooney, C.Z. (1997) *Monte Carlo simulation.* Thousand   Oaks,   CA: Sage   ISBN
0803959435   References

Monte Carlo simulation is a method of evaluating
substantive hypotheses and statistical estimators by
developing a computer algorithm to simulate a population, drawing multiple samples from this pseudo-
population and evaluating estimates from these
samples. The author explains the rationale behind
the method and demonstrates its uses for social and
behavioural research (CR 2.22).

**2.51.9   North   American   Simulation   and
Gaming Association** *About NASGA* www.nasga.
org/about.htm (Accessed 19/02/03)

This association comprises a group of professionals
working on the design, implementation and evaluation
of games and simulations to improve learning results
in all types of organization. Its primary mission is to
facilitate the use of simulation and gaming principles
and procedures of interactive, experiential approaches
to educational management, problem-solving and
decision-making.

2.51.10   Smith, H.W. (1981) Simulation and
gaming. In Author *Strategies of social research: the
methodological imagination* (3rd revised edition).
Austin, TX: Holt   ISBN 0030230772   References

Discusses the use of simulation as a research technique with its dimensions and properties outlined.
Man, machine and man-machine simulation are discussed (CR 2.95.40).

**2.51.11   *Society for the Advancement of Games
and Simulations in Education and Training
(SAGSET)*** www.ms.ic.ac.uk/sagset/sagset2.htm
(Accessed 19/02/03)

SAGSET is a voluntary professional society dedicated to improving the effectiveness and quality of
learning through the use of interactive learning,
role-play, simulation and gaming. It offers *The
International Simulation and Gaming Yearbook*,
annual conferences, a newsletter, advice for users,

sources of information and interactive learning materials, research topics and contact information.

2.51.12 Trochim, W. & Davis, S. (1996) *Computer simulations for research design* trochim. human.cornell.edu/simul/ (Accessed 12/01/03)

This online workbook introduces the use of computer simulation in applied social research designs. There are two versions of each simulation, one accomplished manually (by rolling dice), the other using MINITAB statistical package. Applications in social research are discussed (CR 2.14).

2.51.13 Whicker, M.L. & Sigelman, L. (1991) *Computer simulation and applications: an introduction.* Newbury Park, CA: Sage   ISBN 0803932464 References

Provides comprehensive coverage of computer simulations, discussing their strengths and weaknesses as a research method. The steps involved are identified, as well as the purposes for which they may be used.

2.51.14 Yardley- Matwiejczuk, K.M. (1997) *Role play: theory and practice.* London: Sage   ISBN 0803984510   References

This book, amply illustrated with helpful and practical vignettes, provides an explanation of role-play theory and practice. Readers are shown how role-play differs from other experimental or therapeutic techniques, and are introduced to the key requirements of good technique.

2.52   SURVEY RESEARCH

Surveys are a commonly used research design where information is sought from a group of people, usually by means of interviews or questionnaires. It is a flexible method, broad in scope and may be used in both quantitative and qualitative studies. There are several types and forms of survey, depending on semantics. Writers and researchers may interchange the names of similar types of study and this can lead to confusion.

Definitions [See Appendix D for sources]

Comparative survey – results from two groups or techniques are compared

Cross-cultural survey – study of more than one culture

Cross-sectional survey – several groups in various stages of development are studied simultaneously

Evaluation survey – researcher looks back at previous activities with a critical eye and evaluates results

Field survey – study conducted in the real world as opposed to in a laboratory

Long-term/longitudinal survey * – a sequence of events is observed over more than five years but there is no control over the outcome

[*Long-term/longitudinal surveys are given different names in the following disciplines: in psychology and education – longitudinal; in anthropology and sociology – historical; and in economics – time-series]

Short-term survey – sequence of events observed over less than five years

Survey – type of research plan undertaken to study a large population by systematically selecting samples from the group to discover the incidence, distribution, inter relationships and behaviour of variables

Example

Thoroddsen, A. (1999) Pressure sore prevalence. *Journal of Clinical Nursing* 8 (2) 170–9   41 References

A cross-sectional nationwide sample was used to determine the point prevalence and grading of pressure sores in patients in all hospitals in Iceland. Results are reported and will be valuable when making international comparisons.

Annotations

2.52.1   Abramson, J.H. (1999) *Survey methods in community medicine: epidemiological research, programme evaluation, clinical trials* (5th edition). Edinburgh: Churchill Livingstone   ISBN 0443061637   References

This book is a guide to the planning and performance of studies such as therapeutic trials and health surveys among groups and populations. It covers the basics of the subject, formulating objectives, methods of data collection, constructing a questionnaire, rather than looking at detailed statistical methods (CR 2.20, 2.41, 2.64, 2.75).

2.52.2 Aday, L.A. (1996) *Designing and conducting health surveys* (2nd edition). San Francisco, CA: Jossey-Bass.   ISBN 0787902942

Book discusses all aspects of designing and conducting surveys in health care.

2.52.3 Aldridge, A. & Levine, K. (2001) *Surveying the social world: principles and practice in survey research.* Buckingham: Open University Press ISBN 0335202403 References

Book discusses the strengths and limitations of social surveys, shows how the principles can be put into practice and how findings are analysed and presented.

2.52.4 Bell, D.S., Mangione, C.M. & Kahn, C.E. Jr (2001) Randomized testing of alternative survey formats using volunteers on the World Wide Web. *Journal of the American Medical Informatics Association* 8 (6) 616–20 13 References

Consenting visitors to a health survey website were randomly assigned to a 'matrix' presentation or an 'expanded' presentation of survey response options. Results are reported, and authors believe that presenting options in a matrix format may not substantially speed survey completion. The study demonstrates a method for rapidly evaluating interface design alternatives using anonymous web volunteers who have provided informed consent (CR 2.17, 2.85).

2.52.5 *CASS* www.scpr.ac.uk/cass/ (Accessed 02/02/03)

CASS is an ESRC (Economic and Social Research Council) Centre that provides short courses in survey methods and operates a Survey Question Bank for use by social scientists and researchers in the academic world, government, market research, and the independent and voluntary sectors. It also provides a reference source for question formats in major social surveys, including the Census and family expenditure.

2.52.6 Coomber, R. (1997) Using the Internet for survey research. *Sociological Research Online* 2 (2) 21 References www.socresonline.org.uk/socresonline/2/2/2.html (Accessed 09/11/03)

Paper outlines some recent Internet survey research using a group of illicit 'drug dealers' who are normally difficult to access. A discussion of sampling issues concludes that the Internet can be a source of indicative as opposed to easily generalizable data. A practical guide to undertaking research on the Internet is included (CR 1.6, 2.22, 2.28, 2.85).

2.52.7 Czaja, R. & Blair, J. (1996) *Designing surveys: a guide to decisions and procedures.* Thousand Oaks, CA: Pine Forge Press ISBN 0803990561 References

Describes how modern survey research is conducted with the novice in mind. Its emphasis is on the initial stages, through to completion of data collection.

2.52.8 de Vaus, D. (ed.) (2002) *Social surveys.* London: Sage ISBN 0761973389 References 4 Volumes

This is the methods 'bible' for social scientists using survey methods. It provides an unparalleled guide to the state of knowledge in the field and is a key asset in practical survey 'know-how'.

2.52.9 Fink, A. & Kosecoff, J. (1998) *How to conduct surveys: a step by step guide* (2nd edition). Thousand, Oaks, CA : Sage ISBN 0761914099 References

Text outlines the basic essentials required to organize a rigorous survey or evaluate the credibility of others using a step-by-step approach. This new edition covers computer and interactive surveys and gives advice on informed consent procedures, sample size, ways to ask questions about ethnicity, reading computer printouts of survey results, preparing an abstract, new data analysis techniques and guidelines for presenting results (CR 2.17, 2.22, 2.86, 2.87, 2.94, 2.99).

2.52.10 Fink, A. (ed.) (2003) *The survey kit* (2nd edition). Thousand Oaks, CA: Sage ISBN 0761925104

This 10-volume survey kit has been completely revised and updated. In addition to separate volumes on in-person and telephone interviews, the new edition contains sections on: data management; literacy and language issues; qualitative survey research techniques, including focus group interviewing and content analysis; survey ethics, including the ethical principles to use in survey development and the characteristics of survey research misconduct; factorial design and conjoint analysis; cultural considerations; translation of interviews into other languages; CAPI interviews; sample size and power; creating a complete codebook; the use of data management and statistical programmes; Internet surveys; and the characteristics of good web reporting. Each of the 10 volumes contains checklists, warnings of things to avoid, examples of what does and does not work, and, new to this edition, exercises with answers and a glossary at the end of each volume.
[Each volume is cross-referenced to the appropriate section within this book.]

2.52.11 Fink, A. (2003) *The survey handbook* (2nd edition). Volume 1 ISBN 0761925805 (CR 2.2, 2.16, 2.22, 2.24, 2.25).

2.52.12 Fink, A. (2003) *How to ask survey questions* (2nd edition). Volume 2 ISBN 0761925791 (CR 2.2, 2.20).

2.52.13 Bourque, L. & Fielder, E.P. (2003) *How to conduct self-administered and mail surveys* (2nd edition). Volume 3 ISBN 0761925627 (CR 2.2, 2.75).

2.52.14   Bourque, L. & Fielder, E.P. (2003) *How to conduct telephone surveys* (2nd edition). Volume 4 ISBN 0761925910 (CR 2.2, 2.70).

2.52.15   Oishi, S.M. (2003) *How to conduct in-person interviews for surveys* (2nd edition). Volume 5   ISBN 0761925708 (CR 2.2, 2.68).

2.52.16   Fink, A. (2003) *How to design survey studies* (2nd edition). Volume 6   ISBN 0761925783 (CR 2.2).

2.52.17   Fink, A. (2003) *How to sample in surveys* (2nd edition). Volume 7   ISBN 0761925775 (CR 2.2, 2.22).

2.52.18   Litwin, M.S. (2003) *How to access and interpret survey psychometrics* (2nd edition). Volume 8   ISBN 0761925619 (CR 2.2).

2.52.19 Fink, A. (2003) *How to manage, analyze and interpret survey data* (2nd edition). Volume 9 ISBN 0761925767 (CR 2.2, 2.81, 2.82, 2.86, 2.87).

2.52.20 Fink, A. (2003) *How to report on surveys* (2nd edition). Volume 10   ISBN 0761925759 (CR 2.2, 2.94, 2.97, 2.100).

2.52.21   Foddy, W. (1994) *Constructing questions for interviews and questionnaires: theory and practice in social research.* Cambridge: Cambridge University Press   ISBN 0521467330   References

Book provides a theoretical basis for the construction of valid and reliable questions for interviews and questionnaires. Chapters address past problems of survey research, defining topics properly, formulating requests, providing response frameworks and using filters. Research literature is practically applied and each chapter summarized (CR 2.24, 2.25, 2.56, 2.68, 2.75).

2.52.22   Folz, D.H. (1996) *Survey research for public administration.* Thousand Oaks, CA: Sage ISBN 0761901531   References

Book helps to clarify the basics of survey research as they apply to public administration. The fundamentals of the research process are covered, together with practical illustrations. Data analysis using computers is covered and illustrations of SPSS screens are given (CR 2.84, Appendix A).

2.52.23   Fowler, F.J. Jr (2002) *Survey research methods* (3rd edition). Thousand Oaks, CA: Sage ISBN 0761921915   References

Book is intended for researchers who are not primarily statisticians or methodologists and differs from previous editions in that options for the researcher, made possible by computers and the Internet, are discussed. New methodological material has been integrated and improved techniques for evaluating survey questions are included.

2.52.24   Gore-Felton, C., Koopman, C., Bridges, E., Thoresen, C. & Spiegel, D. (2002) An example of maximising survey return rates. *Evaluation and the Health Professions* 25 (2) 152–68   20 References

Describes a mail survey that was designed to achieve a high response rate. While this was achieved, the best method was not assessed and further research is recommended to identify the relative effectiveness of each principle.

2.52.25   Jackson, C.J. & Furnham, A. (2000) *Designing and analyzing questionnaires and surveys: a manual for health professionals and administrators.* London: Whurr Publications Ltd   ISBN 1861560729   References

Book aims to provide accessible, detailed good practice guidelines that also address the political and ethical problems of conducting surveys within the health professions (CR 2.17, 2.75).

2.52.26   Kelly, B. & Long, A. (2000) The design and execution of social surveys. *Nurse Researcher: International Journal of Research Methodology in Nursing and Health Care* 8 (2) 69–83   21 References

Examines the use of the social survey design and discusses the various approaches available to social researchers. The strengths and weaknesses of the survey design are highlighted, together with the importance of careful planning (CR 2.22, 2.24, 2.25, 2.27, 2.75).

2.52.27   Leaver, D. (2000) Survey research techniques. *Radiologic Technology* 71 (4) 364–77   38 References

Provides an introduction to survey research, its strengths and weaknesses and basic statistical concepts. It also provides guidance on preparing a research article for publication (CR 2.99).

2.52.28   Lensing, S.Y., Gillaspy, S.R., Simpson, P.M., Jones, S.M. & James, J.M. (2000) Encouraging physicians to respond to surveys through use of fax technology. *Evaluation and the Health Professions* 23 (3) 349–60   18 References

Study describes the success of the option of receiving papers and returning data by fax. This may be an added tool to increase response rates.

2.52.29   Mandal, A., Eaden, J., Mayberry, M.K. & Mayberry, J.F. (2000) Questionnaire surveys in medical research. *Journal of Evaluation In Clinical Practice* 6 (4) 395–408   27 References

Provides an overview of survey methods, including questionnaires, face-to-face and telephone interviews, giving an indication of how to design and phrase questions. It also addresses the growing use of the Internet to conduct surveys (CR 2.68, 2.70, 2.75).

2.52.30 Mangione, T.W. (1995) *Mail surveys: improving the quality.* London: Sage ISBN 0803946627 References

Discusses ways in which data collection can be improved by careful question construction, sampling procedures and use of incentives. Management and processing of data are also considered.

2.52.31 Playle, J. (2000) Research designs: the survey. *Journal of Community Nursing* 14 (6) 17–18, 20, 24 16 References

Provides a general comparison of quantitative and qualitative designs and illustrates where survey research fits into these paradigms. Explains the terminology associated with surveys and the different types, including descriptive/exploratory, crosssectional, prospective/retrospective and correlational. Briefly addresses validity and reliability in respect of survey design (CR 2.9, 2.24, 2.25).

2.52.32 Puleo, E., Zapka, J., White, M.J., Mouchawar, J., Somkin, C. & Taplin, S. (2002) Caffeine, cajoling, and other strategies to maximize clinical survey response rates. *Evaluation and the Health Professions* 25 (2) 169–84 25 References

Reports a four-stage data collection strategy that aimed to better understand organizational factors affecting the adoption and implementation of breast and cervical cancer screening guidelines.

2.52.33 Punch, K.F. (2003) *Survey research: the basics.* London: Sage ISBN 0761947043 References

Book is a short, practical, 'how to' book on a central methodological technique, aimed at the novice researcher. It focuses on small-scale quantitative surveys, studying the relationships between variables. The elements of the survey process are described and guidelines are given (CR 2.29).

2.52.34 Rea, L.M. & Parker, R.A. (1992) *Designing and conducting survey research: a comprehensive guide.* San Francisco, CA: Jossey-Bass ISBN 155542404X References

Covers all aspects of survey research, including developing and administering questionnaires, ensuring scientific accuracy, and analysing and reporting results. Exercises are included in each chapter (CR 2.75).

2.52.35 Sapsford, R. (1999) *Survey research.* London: Sage ISBN 0761955283 References

Book guides both beginners and experienced researchers through the main theoretical and practical

issues of survey research. It covers the technical questions that need to be considered, the ethics and politics of research projects and is illustrated with examples (CR 2.17).

2.52.36 Schuman, H. & Presser, S. (1996) *Questions and answers in attitude surveys: experiments on question form, wording and context.* Thousand Oaks, CA: Sage ISBN 0761903593 References

Covers all aspects of developing questions and analysing answers in attitude surveys (CR 2.56).

2.52.37 Shreffler, M.J. (1999) Culturally sensitive research methods of surveying rural/frontier residents. *Western Journal of Nursing Research* 21 (3) 426–35 13 References

Article describes adaptations to conventional survey research methods, based on knowledge of and respect for characteristics and qualities of rural communities and their culture. Few guidelines are published about appropriate modifications for culturally sensitive research and the author hopes these suggestions may be of value to other researchers.

2.52.38 Thomas, S.J. (1999) *Designing surveys that work.* London: Corwin Press ISBN 0803968523 References

Guide provides detailed instructions for every step of the survey process from choosing the right topic, to designing the survey, selecting and working with the respondents, and making sense of all the data.

2.52.39 University of Michigan Institute for Social Research *Mission and organization* www.isr.umich.edu/about/default.html (Accessed 20/02/03)

The University of Michigan Institute for Social Research is the largest and oldest academic survey and social research organization in the world and its members have conducted empirical research in the disciplines of psychology, political science, economics, anthropology and public health. The website lists some major studies and gives access to its main centres, including The Survey Research Center. (www.isr.umich.edu/src/).

2.52.40 Weisberg, H.F., Krosnick, J.A. & Bowen, B.D. (1996) *An introduction to survey research, polling and data analysis* (3rd edition). Thousand Oaks, CA: Sage ISBN 0803974027 References

Book covers the design of surveys, steps for sampling and question writing, interviewing, coding strategies, and analysing the data. Examples are given from large contemporary surveys and polls. The ethics of survey research are discussed and details given on how to read and write reports (CR 2.17, 2.22, 2.75, 2.86, 2.87).

2.53   TRANSCULTURAL/ CROSS-CULTURAL RESEARCH

'Cross-cultural research seeks to investigate variables which exist in one or more communities. These include age, sexual division of labour, habits of cleanliness, religious ceremonies, courtship patterns, kinship terminology, birth and death rites and the prevention and cure of disease. The major difficulties associated with it are cost, communication difficulties and the maintenance of cultural meanings in an instruments language.' (Treece & Treece, 1986: 208)

[The terms transcultural and cross-cultural are sometimes used interchangeably in the literature.]

Definitions [See Appendix D for sources]

Cross-cultural analysis – ... involves exploring and evaluating concepts and practices from a culture other than one's own, using tolls from one's culture

Cross-cultural method – ... an experimental method used ... for evaluating cultures on several different cultural dimensions

Example

Chesney, M. (1998) Dilemmas of interviewing women who have given birth in Pakistan. *Nurse Researcher* 5 (4) 57–70   23 References

Author discusses the dilemmas that arose when interviewing women from another culture about their birth experiences. These included the researcher's background, research stance and the methodology used. Of prime importance was the responsibility of interpreting the women's words accurately and leaving them unharmed by the experience of being interviewed (CR 2.16, 2.68, 3.16).

Annotations

2.53.1   Alasuutari, P. (1995) *Researching culture: qualitative method and cultural studies.* Thousand Oaks, CA: Sage   ISBN 0803978316   References

Book gives the range of approaches and methodological tools available for undertaking critical research, and shows how cultural studies transcend traditional divisions between qualitative and quantitative method and between social sciences and

humanities. Ethnography, symbolic interactionism, semiotics, narrative analysis, conversation and discourse analysis and quantitative analysis in terms of its relevance to data produced by research on culture are discussed (CR 2.42, 2.45, 2.88, 2.89).

2.53.2   Bradby, H. (2002) Translating culture and language: a research note on multilingual settings. *Sociology of Health and Illness* 24 (6) 842–55   37 References

Identifies that people from multilingual settings often have a hybrid language and suggests that a limited mixing of minority language and English can facilitate communication during the research process (CR 2.42).

2.53.3   Chapple, A. (1998) Interviewing women from an ethnic minority group: finding the sample, negotiating access and conducting semi-structured interviews. *Nurse Researcher* 6 (1) 85–92   18 References

Article discusses issues relating to obtaining the sample, interviewing women from a different culture and the use of a link worker who was able to speak the respondents' languages. Findings and general points are discussed (CR 2.68).

2.53.4   Donnelly, T.T. (2002) Representing 'others': avoiding the reproduction of unequal social relations in research. *Nurse Researcher: The International Journal of Research Methodology in Nursing and Health Care* 9 (3) 57–67   13 References

Author argues that some researchers have represented 'others' in ways that tend to reproduce unequal social relations. Researchers undertaking cross-cultural studies must recognize how meanings are constructed in and through systems of representation.

2.53.5   Grant, C.A. (ed.) (1999) *Multi-cultural research: a reflective engagement with race, class, gender and sexual orientation.* London: Falmer ISBN 075070880   References

Written by a group of American academics, this book gives accounts of their studies in the field of multicultural research. Five themes provide the scaffolding for a collection of papers: systems of reasoning; power in relationships; ideology in response to ethnicity and issues of social justice, involvement in struggles and forming alliances; and methods and procedures.

2.53.6   Leininger, M.M. (1984) *Reference sources for trans-cultural health and nursing.* Thorofare, NJ: Slack Inc.   ISBN 0913590932 Part II D 33–8

Contains selected references on many aspects of transcultural nursing, including theory and research methods.

2.53.7 Lindenberg, C.S., Solorzano, R.M., Vilaro, F.M. & Westbrook, L.O. (2001) Challenges and strategies for conducting intervention research with culturally diverse populations. *Journal of Transcultural Nursing* 12 (2) 132–9 32 References

Article identifies four challenges requiring special consideration when conducting intervention research with culturally diverse, underserved and hard-to-reach populations. These are: building community partnerships, developing acceptable and relevant interventions, promoting successful recruitment, active participation in the intervention and retention of participants, and building a diverse, cohesive and committed team and effective managerial information support systems (CR 2.22).

2.53.8 Lynam, M.J. & Young, R.A. (2000) Towards the creation of a culturally safe research environment. *Health – Interdisciplinary Journal for the Study of Health, Illness and Medicine* 4 (1) 5–23 References

Article examines whether theory, and the research methods associated with it, have the potential for creating a culturally safe environment for the conduct of research. An example is given from adolescent dyads of Indo-Canadian and Euro-Canadian background to illustrate how the methods employed created a safe environment.

2.53.9 McGuigan, J. (ed.) (1997) *Cultural methodologies*. London: Sage ISBN 0803974841 References

Book illustrates the distinctiveness and coherence of cultural studies as a site of interaction between the humanities and social sciences. Major sections cover methodologies, research and reflections on the processes (CR 2.9, 2.10, 2.17, 2.42, 2.86, 2.89, 2.97).

2.53.10 Morse, J. (ed.) (1989) *Cross-cultural nursing: anthropological approaches to nursing research*. Philadelphia, PA: Gordon & Breach Science Publications ISBN 1881243835 References

Comprises a series of studies illustrating anthropological approaches to nursing research.

2.53.11 Ovretveit, J. (1998) *Comparative and cross-cultural health research: a practical guide*. Oxford: Radcliffe Medical Press ISBN 1857752740 References

Book describes concepts and methods for comparing health treatments, organizations, health systems, policies and health reforms. Author believes that our abilities to make valid and useful comparisons by learning methods and principles that are common to research will be enhanced by taking a multidisciplinary perspective (CR 2.15, 3.22).

2.53.12 Strickland, C.J. (1999) Conducting focus groups cross-culturally: experiences with pacific northwest Indian people. *Public Health Nursing* 16 (3) 190–7 29 References

Paper focuses attention on the impact of culture in conducting focus groups. Experiences from 15 focus groups conducted in two qualitative research studies with two Washington State Indian tribes over a five-year period are presented and illustrate the importance of culture. Communication patterns, roles, relationships and traditions were found to be the most important elements that must be considered. While some strategies discovered were helpful, further research still needs to be done (CR 2.25, 2.69).

2.53.13 Temple, B. (2002) Crossed wires: interpreters, translators, and bi-lingual workers in cross-language research. *Qualitative Health Research* 12 (6) 844–54 22 References

Discusses employing interpreters/translators and cultural brokers in research, as it raises methodological issues around the meaning of concepts and how to convey the difference.

2.53.14 Tobin, M. (2000) Developing mental health rehabilitation services in a culturally appropriate context: an action research project involving Arabic-speaking clients. *Australian Health Review* 23 (2) 177–84 12 References

When developing services for the Arab-speaking population it was discovered that the principles of mental health rehabilitation theory were inherently Anglo-Australian and therefore unsuitable. Two new culturally relevant programmes were developed, staff attitudes to rehabilitation were changed and assertive strategies were introduced to alter clients' attitudes and perceptions about mental health rehabilitation (CR 2.37).

2.53.15 van de Vijver, F. & Leung, K. (1997) *Methods and data analysis for cross-cultural research*. London: Sage ISBN 076190106X References

Book covers methodological concepts in cross-cultural research, the theoretical background, methods, design and analysis. The analysis and design of four common kinds of cross-cultural study are discussed.

2.53.16   Warwick, D.P. & Osherson, S. (eds) (1973) *Comparative research methods*. Englewood Cliffs, NJ: Prentice-Hall   ISBN 013153940X References

Papers seek to show how the same problem may be studied in different societies and cultures using a combination of methods. The problems that may occur are included, together with some successful outcomes. The five parts of the book cover an overview of comparative research methods, conceptual equivalence and cultural bias, equivalence of measurement and linguistics, translation and illustrative methods, survey research and participant observation (CR 2.52, 2.72).

Measurement

2.54 MEASUREMENT – GENERAL

The process of measurement involves the delineation of what needs to be measured in terms of the research problem, the development of an instrument to measure it and then analysis of the resulting data. Outcome measures are of particular importance in the current climate of health service development and some references to this literature are included here. Other material may be found in section 2.43.

Definitions [See Appendix D for sources]

Criterion-referenced measures – techniques appropriate for determining whether or not an individual has acquired a set of behaviour or mastered a specific task

Measurement – the assignment of some numerical value to objects or events to represent the kind or amount of some characteristic of those objects or events [Measurement as used in this context, includes qualitative data, in which objects are assigned to categories that represent the kinds of characteristic they possess and that are mutually exclusive and exhaustive]

Norm-referenced measures – techniques appropriate for evaluating the performance of an individual relative to some other individuals in a group

Outcome measures – ... evaluate the efficacy of intervention: the extent to which a medication, procedure or program produced a desired effect

---

Annotations

2.54.1 Addington-Hall, J. & Kalra, L. (2001) Who should measure quality of life? *British Medical Journal* 322 (7299) 9 June 1417–20 28 References

Paper discusses the use of proxies to measure the quality of life of cancer patients, and the advantages and disadvantages of collecting data in this way. Reasons are debated as to why a proxy's view and a patient's view may differ, and suggested directions for further research are given (CR 3.16).

2.54.2 Anderson, K.L. & Burckhardt, C.S. (1999) Conceptualization and measurement of quality of life as an outcome variable for health care intervention and research. *Journal of Advanced Nursing* 29 (2) 298–306 58 References

Presents the historical and conceptual arguments regarding quality of life as an outcome measure for health intervention. Dismisses the traditional approaches to this measurement in favour of a more client-centred approach (CR 2.43).

2.54.3 Ciliska, D., Cullum, N. & DiCenso, A. (1999) The fundamentals of quantitative measurement. *Evidence-based Nursing* 2 (4) 100–1 4 References

Provides an introduction to the measurement of health outcomes assessed in studies of causation, treatment, prognosis, diagnosis and economic evaluation.

2.54.4 Encyclopedia of social measurement (2004) London: Academic Press ISBN 0124438903 3 Volumes www.academicpress.com/measure (Accessed 18/06/03)

Covering all core social science disciplines, the 300+ articles of this encyclopedia will present not only a comprehensive summary of observational frameworks and mathematical models, but it will also offer tools, background information, qualitative methods and guidelines for structuring the research process. The encyclopedia is divided into 15 major subject areas, each containing coherent articles on discreet topics and it will serve as the field's standard reference for audiences worldwide.

2.54.5 ISBN.nu *Health status indicators* www.isbn.nu/sisbn/health%20status%20indicators (Accessed 19/02/03)

Lists books and compendia relating to various aspects of health status indicators.

2.54.6 Jacoby, W.G. (1991) *Data theory and dimensional analysis*. Newbury Park, CA: Sage ISBN 0803941781 References

Examines basic scaling questions and discusses strategies for different research situations. Data theory and the study of how real-world observations can be transformed into data that can be analysed are discussed.

2.54.7 Kelley, D.L. (1999) *Measurement made accessible: a research approach using qualitative, quantitative and quality improvement methods.* Thousand Oaks, CA: Sage ISBN 0761910247 References

Through the use of examples and exercises this student guide teaches methods for sampling, data gathering, developing questionnaires, reliability and validity, and quantitative and qualitative measurement. It also explains the use of quality improvement tools and techniques (CR 2.9, 2.22, 2.24, 2.25, 2.29, 2.36, 2.75, 2.84).

2.54.8 Lange, J.W. (2002) Methodological concerns for non-Hispanic investigators conducting research with Hispanic Americans. *Research in Nursing and Health* 25 (5) October 411–19 51 References

Article discusses methodological concerns for non-Hispanic researchers, including instrument response format, translation issues, population-related extraneous variables and response tendencies that may influence the research results (CR 2.16).

2.54.9 Roland, M. & Torgerson, D. (1998) What outcomes should be measured? *British Medical Journal* 317 (7165) 17 October 1075–80 10 References

Explains the range of outcomes that can be measured in clinical trials, including clinical, economic and patient-related outcomes. The article discusses how these should relate to the nature of the study and the research question that is posed (CR 2.29, 2.43).

2.54.10 Sidani, S. (1998) Measuring the intervention in effectiveness research. *Western Journal of Nursing Research* 20 (5) 621–35 26 References

Identifies the problem of inconsistent implementation of interventions in the field setting, which might result in type II errors. Proposes a strategy using an empirical example to overcome this difficulty (CR 2.43, 2.87).

2.54.11 Taubman Medical Library Guide to tests and measurement instruments www.lib.umich. edu/taubman/info/testsandmeasurement.htm (Accessed 02/05/03)

Lists Internet resources, reference books and additional resources available on tests and measurement instruments. It includes descriptions and websites (CR 2.56, 2.57, 2.58, 2.59, 2.60, 2.61, 2.63).

2.54.12 Waltz, C.F., Strickland, O.L. & Lenz, E.R. (1991) *Measurement in nursing research* (2nd edition). Philadelphia, PA: F.C. Davis Co. ISBN 0803690479 References

This text is for students and experienced researchers who are consumers or developers of nursing measures. The theories and principles of sound measurement practices are discussed, together with the processes involved in designing, selecting and testing instruments. The appendix contains information on compilations of existing tools, a selection of nursing theories and their measurement implications and guidance on resources useful for locating suitable tools (CR 2.17, 2.55, 2.65, 2.66, 2.68, 2.72. 2.73, 2.74, 2.75, 2.88).

2.54.13 Wright State University Libraries *Research guides: tests and measurements* www. libraries.wright.edu/libnet/subj/psy/tandm.html (Accessed 03/05/03)

Guide lists information resources that may be used to locate and evaluate tests and measurements in psychology, education and the health sciences (CR 2.58, 2.60).

2.55 FINDING, DEVELOPING AND USING INSTRUMENTS

An issue that frequently faces nurses undertaking research is whether to use instruments developed by others or to develop new ones. It is generally less costly and time-consuming to use existing ones and this is beneficial from the knowledge-building perspective. Use of existing tools provides an increasing database for evaluating the properties of the instruments themselves.

Definitions [See Appendix D for sources]

Instrument – the device or technique that a researcher uses to collect data (e.g. questionnaires, tests, observation schedules)

Methodological studies – research studies that are concerned with the development, testing, and evaluation of research instruments and methods

Annotations

2.55.1 Achterberg, W.P., Holtkamp, C.C.M., Kerkstra, A., Pot, A.M., Ooms, M.E. & Ribbe, M.W. (2001) Improvements in the quality of co-ordination of nursing care following implementation of the Resident Assessment Instrument (RAI) in nursing homes. *Journal of Advanced Nursing* 35 (2) 268–75   14 References

Study tested an existing tool to determine the quality of co-ordination of nursing care in Dutch nursing homes. Authors believe that its use has led to better case history and care plans that could mean residents are better assessed, but there may still be problems in the standards of care that require further work.

2.55.2 Antonakos, C.L. & Colling, K.B. (2001) Focus on research methods. Using measures of agreement to develop a taxonomy of passivity in dementia. *Research in Nursing and Health* 24 (4) 336–43   26 References

The Passivity in Dementia Scale was developed and revised using six nurse scientists. This article describes the taxonomy, provides details about the statistics applied, and explains the method used to collect and apply expert ratings.

2.55.3 Bakas, T. & Champion, V. (1999) Development and psychometric testing of the Bakas Care-giving Outcomes Scale. *Nursing Research* 48 (5) 250–9   42 References

Reports the development of an instrument to measure changes in family caregiving outcomes in the stroke population. Results are reported and authors conclude that this instrument will be a valuable measure in research, as well as an assessment tool to identify family caregivers in need of intervention (CR 2.24, 2.25).

2.55.4 Brown, V., Sitzia, J., Richardson, A., Hughes, J., Hannon, H. & Oakley, C. (2001) The development of the Chemotherapy Symptom Assessment Scale (C-SAS): a scale for the routine clinical assessment of the symptom experiences of patients receiving cytotoxic chemotherapy. *International Journal of Nursing Studies* 38 (5) October 497–510   27 References

Paper describes the development of a 24-item scale for the routine assessment of symptoms by patients receiving chemotherapy. The process focuses both on the psychometric properties and clinical usefulness of the scale. Patients and health professionals played a significant role in item selection and scale design in order to maximize its clinical utility.

2.55.5 Chalmers, K.I., Luker, K.A., Leinster, S.J., Ellis, I. & Booth, K. (2001) Information and support needs of women with primary relatives with breast cancer: development of the information and support needs questionnaire. *Journal of Advanced Nursing* 35 (4) 497–507   72 References

Study aimed to develop and pilot a newly developed measure – the Information and Support Needs Questionnaire – for use with women whose primary relatives had breast cancer. Its development and properties are described, together with the way in which it was administered. The questionnaire showed promise as a measurement tool but further testing and development is indicated (CR 2.75).

2.55.6 Chen, K.-M., Snyder, M. & Krichbaum, K. (2002) Translation and equivalence: the Profile of Mood States Short Form in English and Chinese. *International Journal of Nursing Studies* 39 (6) 619–24   28 References

Describes the processes used to translate the Profile of Mood States Short Form from English to Chinese and assesses the equivalence in the two languages. The Chinese version was found to be as reliable as the original English version.

2.55.7 Chen, M.-L. & Hu, L.-C. (2002) The generalizability of Caregiver Strain Index in family caregivers of cancer patients. *International Journal of Nursing Studies* 39 (8) November 823–9   12 References

Study aimed to estimate the variance components associated with individual differences and various sources of measurement error of the Caregiver Strain Index. A two-facet (item and occasion) crossed design generalizability study was conducted with 14 caregivers. Based on the findings, alternative decision studies were designed to search for optimal generalizability (CR 2.28).

2.55.8 DeVellis, R.F. (2003) *Scale development: theory and applications* (2nd edition). Thousand Oaks, CA: Sage   ISBN 0761926054

Book guides the reader towards an identification of the latent variable, the generation of an item pool, the format for measurement and optimization of the scale length. This Second edition contains practical tips for students, new sections on face validity, factor analysis, item response theory and qualitative procedures and issues related to differential item functioning (CR 2.25).

2.55.9 Eeva, T. & Katri, V.-J. (1998) The content validity of Humane Caring Scale. In: *Knowledge development: clinicians and researchers in partnership*. Helsinki: The Finnish Federation of Nurses   ISSN 0251–4753   Proceedings of the Workgroup of European Nurse Researchers (9th Biennial Conference 5–8 July 1998 Helsinki, Finland) Volume 2 944–52   27 References

Study describes the development of an instrument for the measurement of humane caring through its seven different stages, and by that means to assess its content validity (CR 2.25).

2.55.10 Eiser, C. (2000) The measurement of quality of life in young children. *Child: Care, Health and Development* 26 (5) 401–14   30 References

Argues the need for a quality of life measure for children between 4 and 8 years, including the problems in developing such instruments. Summarizes and critiques available measures.

2.55.11 Fisher, M. & Parolin, M. (2000) The reliability of measuring nursing clinical performance using a competency-based assessment tool: a pilot study. *Collegian: Journal of the Royal College of Nursing, Australia* 7 (3) July 21–7   28 References

Describes the development of a tool based on the Australian Nursing Council Inc. competency statements that aimed to assess new graduates' clinical competence. The pilot study is described and the problems encountered are discussed (CR 2.23, 2.25).

2.55.12 Fuller, B.F., Neu, M., Smith, M. & Vojir, C.P. (1999) Testing a model of the nursing assessment of infant pain. *Clinical Nursing Research* 8 (1) 69–83   15 References

Study tested whether elements of an infant pain assessment model interacted as postulated. Findings supported its use.

2.55.13 Fulton, T.R. & Wilden, B.M. (1998) Patient requirements for nursing care: the development of an instrument. *Canadian Journal of Nursing Administration* 11 (1) 31–51   12 References

Paper describes the development of an instrument that considers patients' nursing care needs as a determinant of nursing staff mix. Recommendations for the use of the tool are identified (CR 2.61).

2.55.14 Halfens, R.J.G., Van Achterberg, T. & Bal, R.M. (2000) Validity and reliability of the Braden scale and the influence of other risk factors: a multi-centre prospective study. *International Journal of Nursing Studies* 37 (4) August 313–19   26 References

This scale, which predicts the risks of developing pressure sores, was re-examined to see whether adding new risk factors could enhance its sensitivity. The existing instrument was reused and results showed that it was a reliable instrument and that its sensitivity and specificity was sufficient. However, reformulating the factors 'moisture' and 'nutrition' and adding the risk factor 'age' enhanced its value. Suggestions are made on how to use risk assessment scales in practice.

2.55.15 Hall, E.O.C., Wilson, M.E. & Frankenfield, J.A. (2003) Translation and re-standardization of an instrument: the Early Infant

Temperament Questionnaire. *Journal of Advanced Nursing* 42 (2) 159–68   50 References

Reports the testing of the psychometric properties of a Danish translation of the Early Infant Temperament Questionnaire to establish standards for scoring. The processes of translation are described (CR 2.75).

2.55.16 Hambleton, R.K., Swaminathan, H. & Rogers, H.J. (eds) (1991) *Fundamentals of item response theory*. Newbury Park, CA: Sage   ISBN 0803936478   References

Using concepts from classical measurement methods and basic statistics, the book introduces the elements of item response theory. Its application to problems in test construction, identification of biased items, test-equating and computer-adaptation testing are all discussed. New directions are also explored.

2.55.17 Hilton, A. & Skrutkowski, M. (2002) Translating instruments into other languages: development and testing process. *Cancer Nursing* 25 (1) 1–7   References

Discusses the problems that may occur when trying to develop culturally-sensitive instruments. A temptation may be to translate an English version of a questionnaire word-for-word, but this is not adequate to account for linguistic and cultural differences. Strategies adopted by the authors to overcome the various difficulties are described (CR 2.53, 2.75).

2.55.18 Hofmeyer, A. & Cecchin, M. (2001) Enactment of virtue ethics: collaboration between nurse academics and international students in questionnaire design … study to be reported in full elsewhere. *Australian Journal of Advanced Nursing* 18 (3) 8–13   33 References

Study explores issues impacting on the ability of international nursing students to achieve their goals at an Australian university. This paper describes the design of an instrument by lecturers and students in a collaborative process, characterized by a pluralistic worldview and the enactment of virtue ethics. The myth of the term 'ESL' is critiqued and challenged. In designing the instrument it was important to be aware of the conceptual attributes and embedded meanings of language for the unique study population, to ensure face and content validity (CR 2.15, 2.25).

2.55.19 Judkins, S.K., Barr, W.J., Clark, D. & Okimi, P (2000) Consumer perception of the professional nursing role: development and testing of a scale. *Nurse Researcher* 7 (3) 32–9   16 References

Describes the development of a 50-item questionnaire that aimed to measure the gap between consumer perceptions and the role of the professional nurse.

2.55.20   Kalfoss, M.H. & Ringel, K.S. (1998) The World Health Organization's Quality of Life Instruments (The WHOØOL – 100 and WHOØOL Bref). In: *Knowledge development: clinicians and researchers in partnerships.* Helsinki: The Finnish Federation of Nurses   ISSN 0251–4753   Proceedings of the Workgroup of European Nurse Researchers (9th Biennial Conference 5–8 July 1998 Helsinki, Finland) Volume 1 376–87   12 References

Paper describes the background and development of the WHOØOL instruments and the present reliability properties of their use in an outpatient sample of 66 people with diffuse muscle-skeletal problems. A tried-and-tested translation method is also reported.

2.55.21   Kim, S.C., Boren, D. & Solem, S.L. (2001) The Kim Alliance Scale: development and preliminary testing. *Clinical Nursing Research* 10 (3) 314–31   32 References

Paper describes the development and preliminary testing of the Kim Alliance Scale (KAS), which was developed to measure the quality of the therapeutic alliance from the patient's perspective, including patient empowerment. Results are reported and the authors believe it may be a useful tool.

2.55.22   Leinonen, T., Leino-Kilpi, H., Ståhlberg, M.-R. & Lertola, K. (2001) The quality of perioperative care: development of a tool for the perceptions of patients. *Journal of Advanced Nursing* 35 (2) 294–306   45 References

Study aimed to examine patients' views of the quality of perioperative care received in the operating theatre and recovery room. The Good Nursing Care Scale was modified and suggestions made for further improvements.

2.55.23   Little, P., Glew, C., Kelly, J., Griffin, S., Dickson, N. & Sadler, C. (1998) Contraceptive knowledge: development of a valid measure and survey of pill users and general practitioners. *British Journal of Family Planning* 24 (3) 98–100 13 References

Paper discusses the design, piloting and validation of a questionnaire to test contraceptive knowledge in combined oral contraceptive pill users. The method and results are given and the authors conclude that this questionnaire is suitable for use in audit or research, is reliable and has face, content and construct validity. (CR 2.24, 2.25).

2.55.24   Long, A.F., Mercer, G. & Hughes, K. (2000) Developing a tool to measure holistic practice: a missing dimension in outcomes measurement within complementary therapies. *Complementary Therapies in Medicine* 8 (1) 26–31   24 References

Paper reports on an exploratory, qualitative study aimed at developing a measure of holism and holistic

practice. It draws out some key features requiring measurement and provides insights into the emerging measure. Further development work is needed before it can be used within research or routine practice (CR 2.58).

2.55.25   Lopopolo, R.B. (2001) Development of the Professional Role Behaviours Survey (PROBES). *Physical Therapy* 81 (7) 1317–27   33 References

This study examined the content validity, internal consistency and underlying dimensions of the Professional Role Behaviours Survey. Results are reported and the author believes it will be a useful tool for studying the changing roles of professional practitioners, and a link in the study of the effect of organizational change on organizational outcomes such as job satisfaction and commitment (CR 2.25).

2.55.26   Meek, P.M., Nail, L.M., Barsevick, A., Schwartz, A.L., Stephen, S., Whitmer, K., Beck, S.L., Jones, L.S. & Walker, B.L. (2000) Psychometric testing of fatigue instruments for use with cancer patients. *Nursing Research* 49 (4) 181–90   47 References

Article reports the results of psychometric testing of several fatigue instruments in patients undergoing cancer treatment. Results are reported and all the instruments showed responsiveness to changes in cancer treatment-related fatigue. Researchers and clinicians are provided with detailed comparisons of the performance of established measures which can be used when selecting an instrument.

2.55.27   Miles, K., Penny, N., Power, R. & Mercey, D. (2003) Comparing doctor and nurse-led care in a sexual health clinic: patient satisfaction questionnaire. *Journal of Advanced Nursing* 42 (1) 64–72   50 References

Describes the development of a patient satisfaction questionnaire to compare the satisfaction of women attending either a nurse or doctor-led clinic (CR 2.75).

2.55.28   Millward, L.J. & Jeffries, N. (2001) The team survey: a tool for health care team development. *Journal of Advanced Nursing* 35 (2) 276–87   33 References

Reports the validation of a psychometric tool, the team survey, in a health care setting with a range of teams from a large National Health Service Trust. The results suggest that this tool is psychometrically robust within a health care setting (CR 2.63).

2.55.29   Morris, L.L., Fitz-Gibbon, C.T. & Lindheim, E. (1988) *How to measure performance and use tests* (2nd edition). Newbury Park, CA: Sage   ISBN 0803931328   References

Book includes many aspects of the development and use of performance tests: preliminary considerations, locating existing measures, its appropriateness for each programme, constructing tests, assessing validity and reliability and using the data (CR 2.24, 2.25).

2.55.30 Morse, J.M., Hutchinson, S.A. & Penrod, J. (1998) From theory to practice: the development of assessment guides from qualitatively derived theory. *Qualitative Health Research* 8 (3) 329–40   22 References

A method of using qualitative research findings to develop a patient assessment guide is described. Qualitatively derived theory is deconstructed to form the theoretical components of the guide. Nursing assessment questions and behavioural signs are then elicited from the theory. Intervention strategies are extrapolated both from theory and from clinical nursing knowledge. The assessment guide is implemented and evaluated using techniques of qualitative outcome analysis to modify the guide and expand the repertoire of intervention strategies. The process is illustrated using two projects: hope (from concept analysis) and living with bipolar disorders (from grounded theory). Assessment guides provide a method for directly applying qualitative research to practice and constitute a valid and useful means of patient assessment and intervention (CR 2.7, 2.36).

2.55.31 National Council on Measurement in Education Washington, DC. www.ncme.org/ (Acccessed 18/11/03)

Purposes of this organization are to encourage scholarly efforts to advance the science of measurement in education and to improve instruments procedures and applications. It also aims to disseminate knowledge about educational measurement.

2.55.32 Netemeyer, R.G., Bearden, W.O. & Sharma, S. (2003) *Scaling procedures: issues and applications.* Thousand Oaks, CA: Sage   ISBN 0761920277   References

Book examines the issues involved in developing and validating multi-item self-report scales of latent constructs. A four-step approach is discussed, examples are included and the concepts of dimensionality, reliability and validity are reviewed (CR 2.24, 2.25).

2.55.33 Olson, L.L. (1998) Hospital nurses' perceptions of the ethical climate of their work setting. *Image – The Journal of Nursing Scholarship* 30 (4) 345–9   62 References

Reports the development of an instrument to measure how hospital nurses perceive the ethical climate of their work setting and its psychometric

properties. The instrument developed was the Hospital Ethical Climate Survey (HECS) and nurses employed in two acute care hospitals in one US Midwestern city assisted in this process. Results showed that the survey had acceptable initial reliability and validity (CR 2.17, 2.24, 2,25).

2.55.34 PsychInfo *Tests and measurements* www.pub.alleg.edu/dept/psych/Tests.html (Accessed 07/05/03)

Web site provides a general guide to finding tests and measures.

2.55.35 Rhodes, V.A., McDaniel, R.W., Homan, S.S., Johnson, M. & Madsen, R. (2000) An instrument to measure symptom experience: symptom occurrence and symptom distress. *Cancer Nursing* 23 (1) 49–54   28 References

Describes the development of an instrument that measures symptom experience in cancer patients (CR 2.24, 2.25).

2.55.36 Roberts, P. (1998) The service quality approach to developing user satisfaction tools. *Nurse Researcher* 5 (3) 43–50   31 References

Author describes a step-by-step process for creating a user satisfaction tool and suggests there may be some value in health professionals considering adapting established generic instruments or developing contextual tools to measure the satisfaction of specific users.

2.55.37 Roberts, P. (1999) Tester user satisfaction tools. *Nurse Researcher* 6 (3) 67–76   18 References

Author takes readers through the sequential steps of reliability testing for developed instruments (CR 2.24, 2.25).

2.55.38 Rose, D. & Pevalin, D. (2002) *A researcher's guide to the national statistics socio-economic classification.* London: Sage   ISBN 0761973222   References

Introduces researchers to all aspects of the new National Statistics Socio-economic Classification (NS-SEC). It fully describes the NS-SEC and elucidates its conceptual basis, shows how it has been validated as a measure, evaluates how well it works in describing and explaining the relationships between social class and key health and employment variables, and demonstrates its applications in research. Because of its inherent methodological interest, the book will be relevant to undergraduate and graduate courses that discuss how social scientists construct and validate basic measures (CR 2.25).

2.55.39 Söderhamn, U. & Söderhamn, O. (2002) Reliability and validity of the Nutritional Form for the Elderly (NUFFE). *Journal of Advanced Nursing* 37 (1) 28–34 15 References

Reports the testing of the Nutritional Form for the Elderly. It is a tool for nurses to use to assess older patients with the aim of detecting undernourished individuals and those at risk. It has been developed in Scandinavia and should primarily be used there until further testing is done (CR 2.24, 2.25).

2.55.40 Spector, P.E. (1992) *Summated rating scale construction.* Newbury Park, CA: Sage ISBN 0803943415 References

Aims to help researchers construct more effective scales. Information is given on how to estimate the number of items, choose good from bad, and how scales can be validated (CR 2.25).

2.55.41 Stewart, M., Tudiver, F., Bass, M.J., Dunn, E.V. & Norton, P.G. (1992) *Tools for primary care research.* Newbury Park, CA: Sage ISBN 0803944047 References

Covers basic concepts and tools for measurement and data collection.

2.55.42 Templeton, H.R.M. & Coates, V.E. (2001) Adaptation of an instrument to measure the informational needs of men with prostate cancer. *Journal of Advanced Nursing* 35 (3) 357–64 47 References

Reports the adaptation of the Toronto Informational Needs Questionnaire that was then applied to a sample of 90 men from centres in Northern Ireland. The construct and content validity were established so it was felt to be suitable for this group, and also has potential for cross-cultural application (CR 2.53).

2.55.43 Voutilainen, P. (1998) Development of an instrument to measure accountability in nursing. In: *Knowledge development: clinicians and researchers in partnership.* Helsinki: The Finnish Federation of Nurses ISSN 0251–4753 Proceedings of the Workgroup of European Nurse Researchers (9th Biennial Conference 5–8 July 1998 Helsinki, Finland) Volume 2 969–77 16 References

Reports a study that analysed the concept of accountability in order to develop an instrument to measure this attribute in nursing personnel. The first phase of instrument development – concept analysis – is discussed.

SOURCES OF INSTRUMENTS

Sections 2.56 to 2.63 include compendia, books or articles that list or describe instruments of possible relevance to nursing. They are grouped under the following headings: 2.56 Attitudinal; 2.57 Behavioural; 2.58 Health related; 2.59 Medical; 2.60 Mental measures; 2.61 Nursing; 2.62 Physiological; 2.63 Sociological/occupational.

The listing is not exhaustive and there is some overlap between compilations, but it illustrates the wide variety of tools already available. Before developing new tools, existing ones should be carefully examined to see if their validity for nursing practice could be further strengthened by repeated use. Please note that many compilations are 'old' but have not been superseded.

2.56 INSTRUMENTS – ATTITUDINAL

Annotations

2.56.1 Adams, A. (1998) Attitude scales: building a composite picture. *Nurse Researcher* 5 (3) 51–62 11 References

Article explains what attitude scales are and why they are useful. Issues relating to their development and testing are discussed and guidelines are given for using published scales (CR 2.24, 2.25).

2.56.2 Attitude Measurement Corporation *Healthcare research* www.attitudemeasurement. com/healthcare.html (Accessed 19/02/03)

This corporation operates a broad range of market research activities, including several related to health care. It mainly conducts research on behalf of national and international health care organizations and many have involved the evaluation of drugs, instruments and devices and managed care.

2.56.3 Henerson, M.E., Morris, L.L. & Fitz-Gibbon, C.T. (1987) *How to measure attitudes* (2nd edition). Beverly Hills, CA: Sage ISBN 080393131X References

Book covers topics commonly confronted by evaluators of educational programmes. Its use should enable the development of basic skills in designing and using instruments for the assessment of attitudes. Included are preliminary questions, selecting from alternative approaches, finding and developing measures, validity and reliability of attitudinal instruments, analysing the data and its presentation (CR 2.24, 2.25, 2.86, 2.87, 2.94).

2.56.4 Robinson, J.P. & Shaver, P.R. (1973) *Measures of social psychological attitudes.* Ann Arbor, MI: Institute for Social Research, University of Michigan ISBN 0879440694

This compilation of 126 instruments measuring attitudes is organized under the general headings of self-esteem and related constructs, locus of control, alienation, authoritarianism, socio-political attitudes, values, attitudes towards people, religious attitudes and social desirability scales. Bibliographical information is included for 30 additional self-concept measures. For each tool the following are described: variables, format, samples to whom it has been given, reliability and validity, bibliographical sources in which it has been described or used and the method of administration. An evaluation is also made.

2.56.5 Shaw, M.E. & Wright, J.M. (1967) *Scales for the measurement of attitudes*. New York: McGraw-Hill   No ISBN number

A compilation of 176 attitude scales which fall into the general categories of social practices, social issues and problems, international issues, abstract concepts, political and religious attitudes, ethnic and national groups, significant others and social institutions. Each tool is described as well as subjects used for testing, measurement properties of the response mode, reliability and validity data and an evaluation.

2.57   INSTRUMENTS – BEHAVIOURAL

Annotations

2.57.1   Andrulis, R.S. (1977) *A source book of tests and measures of human behaviour*. Springfield, IL: Charles Thomas   ISBN 0398036039   References

Volume contains descriptions of 155 commercially available tests to assess adult behaviour. Tests are categorized under intelligence and aptitude, achievement, cognitive style, general measures of personality, personality adjustment, vocational and interest inventories, attitude devices, personality performance, managerial and creativity tests. Each description includes variables measured, type of measure, where to obtain it, psychometric properties, its purpose, scoring and groups used for testing. Some reliability and validity data are available for about 90 per cent of the tools.

2.57.2   Ciminero, A.R., Calhoun, K.S. & Adams, H.E. (eds) (1986) *Handbook of behavioural measurement* (2nd edition). New York: Wiley   ISBN 0471888494

This book is a comprehensive review of general and specific issues in behavioural measurement. It discusses issues in assessment and a system to classify psychological responses that could be used as a framework for research. General approaches to behavioural assessment, with chapters on interviews, self-report tools, direct observation and psycho-physiologic techniques, are included and descriptions are given on how these approaches may

be used. A number of sources are included and some instruments are described (CR 2.68, 2.71, 2.72).

2.57.3   Lake, D.G., Miles, M.B. & Earle, R.B. Jr (1973) *Measuring human behaviour: tools for the assessment of social functioning*. New York: Teachers College Press   ISBN 0807716480

Eighty-four behavioural instruments are described and critiqued, including personal, interpersonal, group or organizational variables. Each tool is described, variables are tested and its scoring, administration, development, critique and evaluation are discussed. Most have been tested for reliability and validity (CR 2.19, 2.24, 2.25).

2.57.4   Pfeiffer, W.J., Heslen, R. & Jones, J.E. (1976) *Instrumentation in human relations training* (2nd edition). LaJolk, CA: California University Associates Inc.   ISBN 0883901161

Part 1 of this book deals with instrumentation issues such as administration, validity, reliability, instrument development and problems of instrumentation. Part 2 contains a guide to 92 instruments for use in the behavioural sciences. These are categorized as personal, interpersonal and organizational in focus. Although a variable amount of information is included for each instrument, length and time to complete are given, as well as descriptions of scales and sub-scales and purchase information (CR 2.24, 2.25, 2.55).

2.57.5   Sommer, B. & Sommer, R. (1997) *A practical guide to behavioural research: tools and techniques*. (4th edition). New Delhi, India: Oxford University Press   ISBN 0195104188   References

Covers many of the tools and techniques required to conduct behavioural research.

2.57.6   Wilmoth, M.C. & Tingle, L.R. (2001) Development and psychometric testing of the Wilmoth Sexual Bahavoirs Questionnaire–Female. *Canadian Journal of Nursing Research* 32 (4) 135–51   27 References

Article describes the development and testing of a tool to examine the sexual behaviours of women. Initial results suggested that it is a reliable and valid measure (CR 2.24, 2.25).

2.58   INSTRUMENTS – HEALTH RELATED

Annotations

2.58.1   Bowling, A. (1999) *Measuring health: a review of quality of life measurement scales* (2nd edition). Buckingham: Open University Press   ISBN 033519754X   References

This revised and updated edition offers a comprehensive guide to measures of health and functioning, including psychological well-being, emotional well-being, social networks and support. A number of recently developed scales are included. New edition contains an index and a list of scale distributors.

2.58.2 Bowling, A. (2001) *Measuring disease: a review of disease-specific quality of life measurement scales* (2nd edition). Buckingham: Open University Press   ISBN 0335206417   References

Book provides reviews of specific measures of the quality of life. Other scales are also included.

2.58.3 Carr, A.J. & Higginson, I.J. (2001) Are quality of life measures patient centred? *British Medical Journal* 322 (7298) 22 June 1357–60   32 References

Identifies the limitations of quality of life measures in respect of their accuracy and usefulness. Argues for more consideration regarding the individual nature of quality of life and the need for further research into patient-centred measures.

2.58.4 De Leo, D., Diekstra, R.F.W., Lonnqvist, J., Trabucchi, M., Cleiren, M.H.P.D., Frisoni, G.B., Dello Buono, M., Haltunen, A., Zuchetto, M., Rozzini, R., Grigoletto, F. & Sampaio-Faria, J. (1998) LEIPAD, an internationally applicable instrument to assess quality of life in the elderly. *Behavioral Medicine* 24 (1) 17–28   30 References

Describes the multinational collaborative development of a quality of life instrument for the elderly, through the World Health Organization. The instrument uses 49 self-assessment items covering a range of concepts (CR 2.15).

2.58.5 Frank-Stromborg, M. & Olsen, S.J. (eds) (1997) *Instruments for clinical health care research* (2nd edition). Sudbury, MA: Jones & Bartlett   ISBN 0763703168   References

The goals of this Second edition, as with the First (*Instruments for Clinical Nursing Research*) are to provide reviews of clinical research instruments to measure selected clinical phenomena, describe their psychometric properties, review particular studies where they have been used, identify their strengths and weaknesses and discuss the relevance to nursing practice. The new title reflects the present emphasis on a team approach to health care. Major sections are an overview, including evaluating instruments for use in clinical research, instruments for assessing health and function, health promotion activities and clinical problems (CR 2.61.4).

2.58.6 Johnson, O.G. (1976) *Tests and measurements in child development: handbooks* I & II San Francisco, CA: Jossey-Bass   No ISBN

2.58.7 Karoly, P. (ed.) (1991) *Measurement strategies in health psychology*. New York: Wiley ISBN 0471554812   References

Book describes the current state of health psychology assessment and potential new directions. The applications of many tests are discussed and references are given. In most instances the tests themselves are not included but research based on them is reported. Assessments given include quality of life, lifestyles, risk factors, medical compliance, pain, illness cognition and life stress events. Methodological considerations are discussed.

2.58.8 Lorig, K., Stewart, A., Ritter, P., Gonzalez, V., Laurent, D. & Lynch, J. (1996) *Outcome measures for health education and other health care interventions*. Thousand Oaks, CA: Sage ISBN 0761900675   References

Book provides a compilation of more than 50 self-administered scales for measuring health behaviours, health status, self-efficacy and health care utilization (CR 2.43).

2.58.9 McDowell, I. & Newell, C. (1996) *Measuring health: a guide to rating scales and questionnaires* (2nd edition). New York and Oxford: Oxford University Press   ISBN 0195103718

Book brings together scattered information on several types of health measurement technique and aims to provide data necessary to choose, apply and score the chosen method. Fifty measures are reviewed and topics include physical disability and handicap, psychological well-being, depression, mental status testing social health, pain, quality of life and general health. Descriptions cover the purpose of each test, its conceptual basis, reliability and validity and a copy of each is included. Alternative forms, a discussion of the method and the test developer's address are also given (CR 2.24, 2.25, 2.75).

2.58.10 Mukherjee, R. (1989) *The quality of life: valuation in social research*. Newbury Park, CA: Sage   ISBN 08039958873   References

Examines the all-inclusive notion of the quality of life by using two perspectives, that is others' valuation of what people need and what the people involved actually want.

2.58.11 Press, I. (2002) *Patient satisfaction: defining measuring, and improving the experience of care*. Chicago, IL: Health Administration Press ISBN 1567931898   References

Book provides readers with tools to measure, monitor and improve patient satisfaction.

2.58.12 Raina, P., Bonnett, B., Waltner-Toews, D., Woodward, C. & Abernathy, T. (1999) How reliable are selected scales from population-based health surveys? *Canadian Journal of Public Health* 90 (1) 60–4   19 References

Study assessed the internal consistency and test–retest reliability of selected scales from four national and provincial surveys used to examine the health status of community-dwelling seniors. Specific items were selected and administered to a group of 1,054 seniors living in Ontario. Results are reported (CR 2.24).

2.58.13 Reeder, L.G., Ramacher, L. & Gorelnik, S. (1976) *Handbook of scales and indices of health behaviour.* Pacific Palisades, CA: Goodyear   ISBN 0876203799

Seventy-eight studies are included and grouped under health behaviour, status, orientation, illness behaviour and use of health services. Information is presented using the steps of the research process. Approximately 85 per cent of studies used the survey method of data collection, and for about 25 per cent the tools, or sections of them, are included.

2.58.14 Streiner, D.L. & Norman, G.R. (1995) *Health measurement scales: a practical guide to their development and use.* Oxford: Oxford University Press   ISBN 0192626701   References

An explanatory text intended for medical researchers. It covers reliability, validity, response bias, telephone interviewing and other relevant topics (CR 2.24, 2.25, 2.27, 2.70).

2.58.15 Walker, S.R. & Rosser, R.M. (eds) (1992) *Quality of life assessment: key issues in the 1990s.* Dordrecht: Kluwer Academic Publishers ISBN 0792389913   References

Based on presentations given at a workshop, this book comprises sections covering philosophies, concept and key instruments involved in assessing the quality of life and in major disease areas. Viewpoints and perspectives from industry, regulatory authorities and health care purchasers, ethics, policy decisions and cost-effectiveness are all discussed. Appendices include shortened versions of some instruments (CR 2.17, 3.11).

2.59   INSTRUMENTS – MEDICAL

Annotations

2.59.1 Fitzpatrick, R., Davey, C., Buxton, M.J. & Jones, D.R. (1998) Evaluating Patient-based outcome measures for use in clinical trials. *Health Technology Assessment* 2 (14) 74 pages

Reviews the literature regarding patient-based outcome measures. Describes and provides a rationale for the diversity of measures and determines the criteria for selection of measures for use in clinical trials. (CR 2.29).

2.59.2 Fitzpatrick, R. & Hopkins, A. (eds) (1993) *Measurement of patients' satisfaction with their care.* London: Royal College of Physicians ISBN 1873240538

Patient satisfaction is itself an outcome of health care, and so requires measurement. This book explores ways in which this may be done.

2.59.3 Gunning, K. & Rowan, K. (1999) Outcomes data and scoring systems. *British Medical Journal* 319 (7204) 24 July 241–4

Describes the use of scoring systems to enable comparative audit and evaluative research, including APACHE II, Glasgow Coma Scale and the Therapeutic Intervention Scoring System.

2.59.4 Hopkins, A. (ed.) (1992) *Measures of the quality of life, and the uses to which such measures may be put.* London: Royal College of Physicians ISBN 1873240457.

Book explores the various measures of the quality of life and also the uses to which they may be put in terms of resource allocation. Particular stress is laid upon the ethical aspects of such measurements and how they might be used as instruments of social policy.

2.59.5 to 2.59.26 *Medical Care Supplement* (1989) Advances in health status assessment: conference proceedings. *Medical Care* 27 (3) March

The following entry differs in format as it documents a special issue of the journal *Medical Care*. These articles have not been annotated.

2.59.5 Bergner, M. Quality of life, health status, and clinical research. S148–S156   37 References

2.59.6 Breslow, L. Health status measurement in the evaluation of health promotion. S205–S216 20 References

2.59.7 Connelly, J.E., Philbrick, J.T., Smith, G.R. Jr, Kaiser, D.L. & Wymer, A. Health perceptions of primary care patients and the influence on health care utilization. S99–S109   18 References   .

2.59.8 Deyo, R.A. & Patrick, D.L. Barriers to the use of health status measures in clinical investigation, patient care and policy research. S254–S268   63 References

2.59.9 Epstein, A.M., Hall, J.A., Tognetti, J., Son, L.H. & Conant, L. Jr Using proxies to evaluate quality of life: can they provide valid information about patients' health status and satisfaction with medical care? S91–S98   25 References

2.59.10   Erikson, P., Kendall, E.A., Anderson, J. & Kaplan, R.M. Using composite health status measures to assess the nation's health. S66–S76   36 References

2.59.11   Feeny, D.H. & Torrance, G.W. Incorporating utility-based quality-of-life assessment measures in clinical trials: two examples. S190–S204   73 References

2.59.12   Hall, J.A., Epstein, A.M. & McNeil, B.J. Multi-dimensionality of health status in an elderly population: construct validity of a measurement battery. S168–S177   23 References

2.59.13   Kaplan, R.M., Anderson, J.P., Wu, A.W., Matthews, C., Kozin, F. & Orenstein, D. The quality of well-being scale: applications in AIDS, cystic fibrosis and arthritis. S27-S43   36 References

2.59.14   Kaplan, S.H., Greenfield, S. & Ware, J.E. Assessing the effects of physician–patient interactions on the outcomes of chronic disease. S110–S127   69 References

2.59.15   Kazis, L.E., Anderson, J.J. & Meenan, R.F. Effect sizes for interpreting changes in health status. S178–S189   15 References

2.59.16   Lewis, C.C., Pantell, R.H. & Kieckhefer, G.M. Assessment of children's health status: field test of new approaches. S54–S65   14 References

2.59.17   Lipscomb, J. Time preference for health in cost-effectiveness analysis. S233–S253   39 References

2.59.18   Lohr, K.M. Advances in health status assessment: overview of the conference. S1–S11   47 References

2.59.19   Mosteller, F., Ware, J.E. Jr & Levine, S. Finale panel: comments on the conference on advances in health status assessment. S282–S294 34 References

2.59.20   Mulley, A.G. Jr Assessing patient's utilities: can the ends justify the means? S269–S281 56 References

2.59.21   Nelson, E.C. & Berwick, D.M. The measurement of health status in clinical practice. S77–S90   58 References

2.59.22   Patrick, D.L. & Deyo, R.A. Generic and disease-specific measures in assessing health Status and Quality of life. S127–S232   95 References

2.59.23   Rothman, M.L., Hedrick, S. & Inui, T. The Sickness Impact Profile as a measure of the health status of non-cognitively impaired nursing home residents. S157–S267   24 References

2.59.24   Steinwachs, D.M. Application of health status assessment measures in policy research. S12–S26   54 References

2.59.25   Temkin, N.R., Dikmen, S., Machamer, J. & McLean, A. General versus disease-specific measures: further work on the Sickness Impact Profile for head injury. S44–S53   18 References

2.59.26   Verbrugge, L.M. & Balaban, D.J. Patterns of change in disability and well-being. S128–S147   37 References

2.60   INSTRUMENTS – MENTAL MEASURES

Annotations

2.60.1   Buros Institute of Mental Measurements www.unl.edu/buros/catalog.html (Accessed 16/11/03)

The Buros Institute has published series of educational, psychological, personality, English, foreign language, intelligence, mathematics, reading, science, social studies and vocational tests since 1933. In particular it publishes series of mental measurements yearbooks – online from the 9th–15th with monthly updates from the latest review database. Further information may be found in Appendix E and on their website (CR 2.60.16).

2.60.2   Chun, K.T., Cobb, S. & French, J.R.P. Jr (1975) *Measures for psychological assessment: a guide to 3,000 original sources and their applications*. Michigan, IN: University of Michigan, Institute for Social Research   ISBN 0879441682 References

A compilation of annotated references to measures of mental health and related variables, and their uses. A bibliography of all quantitative research that used these measures between 1960 and 1970 is included. Volume consists of two major sections, primary references, applications and two indexes. The section on primary sources lists approximately 3,000 references to articles or other publications in which the measures were first described. The section on application provides over 6,000 instances in which the measures are described. Details relating to each test are not included.

2.60.3   Comrey, A.L., Backer, T.E. & Glaser, E.M. (1973) *A sourcebook for mental health measures*. Los Angeles, CA: Human Interaction Research Institute

Contains abstracts of approximately 1,100 psychological and mental health-related tools. Topics of interest to nurses are alcoholism, drugs, family interaction, geriatrics, mental handicap and evaluation of professional service delivery. Abstracts include title, source, authors' names and addresses, purpose of the tool, a description, major applications and how the test may be obtained. It also indicates for most tools where information on reliability and validity may be obtained (CR 2.61, 2.63).

2.60.4   Follette, W.C. & Houts, A.C. (1996) Models of scientific progress and the role of theory in taxonomy development. *Journal of Consulting and Clinical Psychology* 64 (6) 1120–32

In recent editions of the *Diagnostic and Statistical Manual of Mental Disorders*, the proliferation of categories is an indication that the underlying classification scheme is inadequate and unlikely to produce the scientific progress originally envisioned. It has also put itself in an awkward position by claiming to be atheoretical, which now limits the progression of science. The problems that this poses are discussed, together with possible solutions (CR 2.38).

2.60.5   Frank, S.H. (1992) Inventory of psychological measurement instruments useful in primary care. In Stewart, M., Tudiver, F., Bass, M.J., Dunn, E.V. & Norton, P.G. (eds) *Tools for primary research*. Newbury Park, CA: Sage ISBN 0803944047   References   Appendix 229–70

This inventory contains 179 tests under 30 topic headings. Information on each one includes the number of items, item format, original references and notes. Also, when available, a reference describing its use in the family practice setting is included (CR 2.55.41).

2.60.6   Goldman, B.A. & Mitchell, D.F. (eds) (1995) *Directory of unpublished experimental mental measures.* Volume 6 Washington, DC: American Psychological Association   ISBN 1557982899

This series of eight volumes identifies non-standard and non-commercial experimental test instruments taken from 36 top journals in the fields of psychology, sociology and education and dating from 1970 to 2000. The instruments are not evaluated, but the information given about each test should make it possible for researchers to make a preliminary judgement of its usefulness. Each entry includes test name, purpose, description, statistics, validity, author and source. Indexes allow searching by both author and subject.

AND

2.60.7   Goldman, B.A., Saunders, J.L. & Busch, J.C. (eds) (1996) *Directory of unpublished experimental mental measures.* Volumes 1, 2 & 3 Washington, DC: American Psychological Association ISBN 1557983364

AND

2.60.8   Goldman, B.A., Osbourne, W.L. & Mitchell, D.F. (eds) (1996) *Directory of unpublished experimental mental measures.* Volumes 4 & 5 Washington, DC: American Psychological Association   ISBN 1557983518

AND

2.60.9   Goldman, B.A., Mitchell, D.F. & Egelson, P. (eds) (1997) *Directory of unpublished experimental mental measures.* Volume 7 Washington, DC: American Psychological Association ISBN 1557984492   References

AND

2.60.10   Goldman, B.A. & Mitchell, D.F. (eds) (2002) *Directory of unpublished experimental mental measures.* Volume 8 Washington, DC: American Psychological Association   ISBN 1557989516 References

2.60.11   Halling, S. & Goldfarb, M. (1996) The new generation of diagnostic manuals (DSM-III, DSM-III–R and DSM-IV). An overview and a phenomenologically-based critique. *Journal of Phenomenological Psychology* 27 (1) 49–71

Given the extraordinary influence of the Diagnostic and Statistical Manual of Mental Disorders-III and its successors, the DSM-III–R and the DSM-IV, practitioners are urged to examine these carefully. The article discusses the goals that have guided their development and provides an overview of their basic structure. This is followed by a phenomenologically-based critique, evaluating the claim that these manuals are 'descriptive' and 'atheoretical'. Five guiding principles for phenomenological diagnosis and assessment are discussed (CR 2.38, 2.49).

2.60.12   Kline, P. (2000) *Handbook of psychological testing* (2nd edition). London: Routledge   ISBN 0415211581   References

Book covers psychoanalytic theory and method, types of psychological test, their use and interpretation. It also includes psychological tests, lists, descriptions and evaluations.

2.60.13   Loewenthal, K.M. (2001) *An introduction to psychological tests and scales.* (2nd edition). Hove, East Sussex: Psychology Press Ltd   ISBN 1841691399   References

Provides a jargon-free primer for all those embarking on fieldwork or research analysis. All stages of finding, choosing and developing tests and scales are discussed in detail. A list of websites is also included.

2.60.14   Lyerly, S. (1973) *Handbook of psychiatric rating scales* (2nd edition). Rockville, MD: National Institute of Mental Health   No ISBN found

Describes 61 rating scales that have been used in psychiatric settings, of which 38 include detailed descriptions. A table gives information on the population, type of rater, source of data, reliability and validity.

2.60.15   Mittler, P.J. (ed.) (1974) *The psychological assessment of mental and physical handicaps.* London: Tavistock   ISBN 0422756008   References

Text is designed to assist those who are concerned with systematic assessment of the handicapped. It does not cover the psychometric aspects of testing which may be found in other standard texts but covers comprehensively the diagnostic and assessment aspects. Individual tests are commented upon and extensive references given. Principles of psychological assessment, assessment of children and adults and experimental advances are included.

2.60.16   Murphy, L.L., Impara, J.C. & Plake, B.S. (2001) *Mental measurements yearbook. 14th XY/N1.* Lincoln, NB: Buros Institute of Mental Measurements, University of Nebrasca-Lincoln ISBN 0910674558   References www.unl.edu/buros

The 14th *Mental Measurements Yearbook* (*MMY*) contains reviews of tests that are new, or significantly revised, since publication of the 13th *MMY* in 1998. Review, descriptions and references associated with many older tests can be located in other Buros publications: previous *MMYs* and *Tests in Print V.* The content includes: bibliography of 430 commercially available tests, new or revised, published as separates for use with English-speaking subjects; 802 critical test reviews by qualified professional people; and the following indexes – test titles, classified subject, publishers directory and index, name index, acronyms and a score index. A list of earlier publications in the series is included (CR 2.60.1, Appendix E).

2.60.17   nfer-Nelson *Health and social care assessments* www.nfer-nelson.co.uk (Accessed 02/02/03)

nfer-Nelson publish a wide range of assessments for education and caring professionals who work with children outside the classroom to enable difficult decisions to be made about health, psychological and physical well-being, jobs, careers and lifestyle. Details are available on the website.

2.60.18   Pichot, P.J. (1997) DSM-III and its reception: A European view. *American Journal of Psychiatry* 154 (6) Supplement 470–54

Discusses the reception of the Diagnostic and Statistical Manual of Mental Disorders-III in Europe. Criticisms of this included the atheoretical

syndrome approach, the introduction of quantification and its adherence to alleged American values. These criticisms contrast sharply with its general acceptance, and that of its successors, which rest on their objective merits (CR 2.38).

2.60.19   Sugerman, A. & Kanner, K. (2000) The contribution of psychoanalytic theory to psychological testing. *Psychoanalytic Psychology* 17 (1) 1–21

Article examines the impact of psychoanalytic theory on the clinical practice of psychological testing. Three major thinkers allowed testing to expand far beyond the psychometric and atheoretical approach so prevalent before the 1940s, as well as the descriptive emphasis that is so popular today. The contributions and functions of psychoanalytic theory in testing are discussed.

2.60.20   Sweetland, R. & Keyser, D. (eds) (1987) *Test Critiques compendium: review of major tests from the test critiques series.* Kansas City, MO: Test Corporation of America   ISBN 0933701098 References

Book contains evaluations of psychological, neurophysical and educational tests and measurements.

2.60.21   Sweetland, R. & Keyser, D. (eds) (1991) *Tests: a comprehensive reference for assessments in pyschology, education and business* (3rd edition). Austin, TX: Pro-Ed   ISBN 0890792550

Book contains psychological, educational and occupational aptitude tests.

2.61   INSTRUMENTS – NURSING

Annotations

2.61.1   Beck, C.T. (1999) Quantitative measurement of caring. *Journal of Advanced Nursing* 30 (1) 24–32   50 References

Eleven different quantitative instruments designed to measure caring are reviewed. For each the following information is provided: description of the tool, such as number of items and length of time to administer; conceptual definition of caring upon which it is based; reported reliability and validity; and the instrument's use in research studies. Comparisons between them showed that multiple factors need to be taken into consideration by nurse researchers in deciding which instrument to use to measure caring (CR 2.24, 2.25).

2.61.2   Clayton, G.M. & Broome, M. (1989) *Instruments for use in nursing education research.*

New York: National League for Nursing ISBN 088737424

Monograph categorizes, describes and evaluates instruments used in nursing education research during the 1980s. A wide range of topics is covered which shows a fragmented body of knowledge. The categories are: prediction of success, student attitudes, student roles and socialization, curricula and methods of instruction and faculty roles. The following are given for each instrument: an introduction, description and administrative details, psychometric properties and research using the test. Qualitative studies are not included.

2.61.3 Conner-Spady, B.L., Slaughter, S. & MacLean, S.L. (1999) Assessing the usefulness of the assessment of living skills and resources (ALSAR) in a geriatric day hospital. *Canadian Journal of Rehabilitation* 12 (4) 265–72 19 References

Paper examines the Assessment of Living Skills and Resources as a clinical assessment tool and outcome measure for instrumental activities of daily living in 63 patients attending a geriatric assessment and treatment programme. Some of the problems experienced when using this tool are discussed.

2.61.4 Frank-Stromborg, M. (ed.) (1992) *Instruments for clinical nursing research* (2nd edition). Boston, MA: Jones & Bartlett ISBN 0867203404 References

Book developed from a project undertaken by the Oncology Nursing Society that aimed to describe available instruments. It reviews the tools currently obtainable to measure a selected phenomenon. Their psychometric properties are described, details of the sample or studies that have utilized the tool are given and their strengths and weaknesses are identified. Their use in all areas of nursing is outlined. The evaluation of research instruments is discussed, together with ways of identifying those assessing health, function and commonly occurring clinical problems. Most chapters are summarized and have extensive reference lists (CR 2.58.5).

2.61.5 Holzemer, W.L. (1992) Measurement: a foundation of nursing science. In *Communicating nursing research – silver threads – 25 years of nursing excellence.* Volume 25 Boulder, CO: Western Institute of Nursing No ISBN 45–54 46 References

Paper addresses the contribution made by compilations of instruments to the practice of nursing, centres of excellence, linking measurement and nursing research at the national level. Issues for the future are identified.

2.61.6 Kitson, A. & Harvey, G. (1991) *Bibliography of nursing quality assurance and standards of care 1932–1987.* Harrow, Middlesex: Scutari ISBN 1871364469

An annotated bibliography that cites literature on general theory, principles and methodological background issues related to quality and standards of care. It also includes philosophical aspects, a range of quality assurance measures available to nurses and articles relating quality of care to manpower studies.

2.61.7 Krowinski, W.J. & Steiber, S.R. (1996) *Measuring and managing patient satisfaction* (2nd edition). San Francisco, CA: Jossey-Bass ISBN 1556481578

Book shows how to plan and conduct each step of patient satisfaction studies within the context of today's regulatory environment.

2.61.8 Redman, B.K. (1998) *Measurement tools in patient education.* New York: Springer ISBN 0826198600

Draws together instruments for measuring outcomes in patient education from a wide variety of sources. Fifty-two tools are included and each is accompanied by a descriptive review, critique, information on administration, scoring and psychometric properties.

2.61.9 Rinke, L.T. & Wilson, A.A. (eds) (1987) *Outcome measures in home care.* New York: National League for Nursing ISBN 088737378X References Volume 1 Publication No. 21–2194

Anthology provides a single reference to the classic and current literature addressing outcomes in home care. Part 1 includes: basic issues in evaluating the quality of health care; the relationship of nursing process to nursing outcomes; criterion measures of nursing care quality and status of quality assurance in public health nursing. Parts 2, 3, 4 & 5 include two studies on maternal and child health; using records as a data source; a community-based demonstration project and instrument development.

2.61.10 Rinke, L.T. & Wilson. A.A. (eds) (1987) *Outcome measures in home care service.* New York: National League for Nursing ISBN 0887373798 References Volume 2 Publication No. 21–2195

Volume covers a sample of both published and unpublished measurement outcome indicators for community-based nursing services. The six parts give a historical overview; examples of promulgated outcome standards; programmatic approaches; medical diagnosis approach; discipline specific indicators and a functional approach.

2.61.11 SDSU Library *Sources for nursing research instruments* infodome.sdsu.edu/research/guides/science/nursinstruments.shtml (Accessed 01/05/03)

Gives an example of sources of instruments available at the San Diego University Library (CR 2.56, 2.57, 2.58, 2.60, 2.63).

2.61.12 Strickland, O.L. & Waltz, C.F. (eds) (1988) *Measurement of nursing outcomes.* Volume 1: *Measuring nursing performance, practice education and research.* New York: Springer ISBN 0826152724

Book is a collection of tools focusing on provider-centred outcomes. Some of the major topic areas include measuring professionalism, clinical performance, educational outcomes, research and measurement and future directions. Measurement protocol for each tool includes: critical review and analysis of the literature; review and analysis of existing tools and procedures for measuring the variable; conceptual basis of the measure; purpose and/or objective of the measure; procedures for construction, revision or future development of the tool; procedures for administration and scoring; methodology for testing the reliability and validity of the measure, including approach to data collection, protection of human subjects and statistical analysis procedures (CR 2.43).

2.61.13 Strickland, O.L. & DiIorio, C. (eds) (2002) *Measurement of nursing outcomes. Volume 2: Client outcomes and quality of care* (2nd edition). New York: Springer ISBN 082611427X References

Book presents nearly 80 actual, tested instruments for assessing nursing outcomes in a multitude of settings. A descriptive essay that includes information on purpose, administration, scoring, reliability and validity accompanies each test. They may be used to measure patient outcomes, evaluating patient learning, or assessing the effectiveness of teaching and learning in a nursing school.

2.61.14 Strickland, O.L. & DiIorio, C. (eds) (2002) *Measurement of nursing outcomes. Volume 3: Self caring and coping.* (2nd edition). New York: Springer ISBN 0826117953 References

Book presents nearly 80 actual, tested instruments for assessing nursing outcomes in a multitude of settings. A descriptive essay that includes information on purpose, administration, scoring, reliability and validity accompanies each test. They may be used to measure patient outcomes, evaluating patient learning, or assessing the effectiveness of teaching and learning in a nursing school.

2.61.15 Voge, S. & Beaton, S. (1998) *Measurements for long-term care: a guidebook for nurses.* Thousand Oaks, CA: Sage ISBN 0803953887 References

Book brings together more than 100 of the most frequently used (and some of the most difficult to find) measurement tools for long-term care research. It includes abbreviations, acronyms, an index of instrument authors' names, an index of nursing diagnoses and related instruments, an index of subjects (client disorders and problems), and an index of instrument titles.

2.61.16 Waltz, C.F. & Jenkins, L.S. (eds) (2001) *Measurement of nursing outcomes. Volume 1: Measuring nursing performance in practice, education and research* (2nd edition). New York: Springer ISBN 0826114172

This is a compendium of over 30 tools for the measurement of professional and education outcomes in nursing. The collection of tools and methods is presented, with attention given to purpose and utility, conceptual basis, development, testing, and the results of reliability and validity assessments. Major topic areas focus around clinical decision-making and performance in education and practice, student outcomes, professionalism and research. In most cases the complete instrument is included in the book.

2.61.17 Ward, M.J. & Fetler, M.E. (1979) *Instruments for use in nursing education research.* Boulder, CO: Western Interstate Commission for Higher Education No ISBN References

A major barrier to conducting research is the lack of appropriate data collecting instruments, so this compilation aims to provide a collection relating specifically to nursing education research. It contains descriptions, critiques and reproductions of 78 instruments; brief descriptions and references to another 40; an annotated bibliography of other published compilations; a glossary and appendices. Each tool is described with key concepts, title, author, variables measured, nature and content of the instrument, administration and scoring, rationale for development and sources of items. Data on reliability and validity are included, together with studies where it has been used, selected comments, references, name and address of a contact person and name of the copyright owner.

2.61.18 Ward, M.J. & Lindeman, C.A. (1979) *Instruments for measuring nursing practice and other health care variables.* Hyattsville, MD: Department of Health and Welfare Publication Nos Volume 1 HRA 78–53 and Volume 2 HRA 78–54 No ISBN

Volumes contain descriptions, critiques and reproductions of 138 psychosocial research instruments, descriptions of 19 instruments which measure physiological parameters, an annotated bibliography of other selected compilations, and a glossary of physiological instrument terms (CR 2.62).

2.61.19 Werley, H.H. & Lang, N.M. (eds) (1988) *Identification of the nursing minimum data set.* New York: Springer ISBN 0826153402 References

Book describes development of the nursing minimum data set. This information is unique to nursing practice and represents essential data. It enables nurses to use computers to assemble comparable nursing data across clinical populations, geographical areas and time through the use of consensually derived categories, variables and uniform definitions. Conceptual considerations, existing information about the data set, perspectives on data requirements across settings, multiple perspectives, effectiveness of nursing care, control of practice standards, quality assessment, health policy, work of the task force which generated the data set and future directions are all discussed.

2.62 INSTRUMENTS – PHYSIOLOGICAL

Annotations

2.62.1 Cavanaugh, B.M. (1999) *Nurses manual of laboratory and diagnostic tests* (3rd edition). Philadelphia, PA: F.A. Davis ISBN 0803603630 References

Book will assist students and practitioners of nursing in caring for patients undergoing laboratory tests and diagnostic procedures. The purpose of and indications for each procedure is followed by clinical applications data. For each test reference and critical values, contra-indications, interfering factors and nursing care before and after are included. Case studies and critical thinking exercises are also included, together with references and bibliographies.

2.62.2 Chernecky, C.C. & Berger, B.J. (2001) *Laboratory tests and diagnostic procedures* (3rd edition). Philadelphia, PA: W.B. Saunders ISBN 0721686095 References

This reference book features over 900 laboratory tests and diagnostic procedures. Part 1 lists diseases, conditions and symptoms with the tests most commonly used to confirm them; Part 2 alphabetically lists virtually every test available today so that information can be quickly located. This new edition includes 45 new tests, together with vital information on herbal remedies and natural treatments.

2.62.3 Fulbrook, P. (2000) Physiological measurement. In Cormack, D.F.S. *The research process in nursing* (4th edition). Oxford: Blackwell Science ISBN 0632051582 Chapter 28 337–51 15 References

Chapter discusses measurement, measurement procedures and instruments, data collection and ethical issues (CR 2.1.23, 2.17).

2.62.4 Harris, R., Wilson-Barnett, J., Griffiths, P. & Evans, A. (1998) Patient assessment: validation of a nursing instrument. *International Journal of Nursing Studies* 35 (6) 303–13 40 References

Study evaluated the reliability and validity of the Byron Physical Assessment Framework. This is a systems-based checklist of physiological measurements, signs and symptoms, designed to structure and document the assessment of a patient's physical condition by nursing staff. The processes used are described and results reported (CR 2.24, 2.25).

2.62.5 Malarkey, L.M. & McMorrow, M.E. (2000) *Nurse's manual of laboratory tests and diagnostic procedures* (2nd edition). Philadelphia, PA: W.B. Saunders ISBN 0721678122 References

Book provides essential guidance on over 700 laboratory tests and diagnostic procedures used in nursing. It provides background information on each test, explains normal and abnormal results and emphasizes nursing care for the patient undergoing the test.

2.62.6 McGhee, M. (2000) *A guide to laboratory investigations* (3rd edition). Oxford: Radcliffe Medical Press ISBN 0857753577

Although primarily intended for doctors, this book would also prove useful to nurses. Material is organized under the categories of haematology, microbiology, fertility and pregnancy testing, rheumatology, biochemistry and miscellaneous. Information is given on which tests to carry out, those which are essential and who must be informed in certain circumstances.

2.62.7 McMorrow, M.E. & Malarkey, L.M. (1998) *Laboratory and diagnostic tests: a pocket guide.* Philadelphia, PA: W.B. Saunders ISBN 0721673031 References

This portable resource presents 400 of the most commonly used laboratory tests and diagnostic procedures, together with their nursing implications.

2.62.8 Pagana, K.D. & Pagana, T.J. (1999) *Diagnostic testing and nursing implications: a case study approach* (5th edition). St Louis, MO: Mosby ISBN 0323002897 References

Book teaches nursing students how to use diagnostic tests in patient assessment and emphasizes their special role in this process. The book's organization, case studies with critical thinking questions, review questions and a comprehensive practice test will help nurses apply their knowledge to clinical circumstances.

2.62.9   Pagana, K.D. & Pagana, T.J. (2001) *Mosby's manual of diagnostic and laboratory tests* (2nd edition). St Louis, MO: Mosby ISBN 032301609X   References

Manual is a complete resource for nurses and other health professionals covering virtually every clinically significant test. Priorities for patient teaching are included, as well as and home care information to support the increasing emphasis on early discharge and outpatient testing.

2.62.10   Pagana, K.D. & Pagana, T.J. (2002) *Mosby's diagnostic and laboratory test reference* (6th edition). St Louis, MO: Mosby ISBN 0323020496   References

This clinical handbook features clinically relevant laboratory and diagnostic tests. Over 850 test entries, presented in a consistent format, provide complete coverage.

2.62.11   Tilkian, S.M., Conover, M.B. & Tilkian, A.G. (1996) *Clinical nursing implications of laboratory tests* (5th edition). St Louis, MO: Mosby ISBN 0815188072   References

This comprehensive reference book approaches laboratory tests in the same way as a clinical evaluation. Each test is explained, its value and limitations are defined, and clinical implications, nursing responsibilities and patient preparation are all discussed.

2.63   INSTRUMENTS – SOCIOLOGICAL/ OCCUPATIONAL

Annotations

2.63.1   Beere, C.A. (1979) *Women and women's issues: a handbook of tests and measurements.* San Francisco, CA: Jossey-Bass ISBN 0835748154 References

Volume contains 235 instruments obtained from literature published in 1977. They are divided into the following categories: sex roles, stereotypes, role prescriptions, children's sex roles, gender knowledge, marital, parental, employee and multiple roles, attitudes towards women's issues, somatic and sexual issues. Each category constitutes a chapter and included for many of the instruments is the title, author, date, variables, type of instrument, item content, length, group for whom it is intended, sample items, scoring method, theoretical basis, reliability, validity, possible modifications, source and bibliographical information.

2.63.2   Bonjean, C.M., Hill, R.J. & McLemore, S.D. (1967) *Sociological measurement: an inventory of scales and indices.* San Francisco, CA: Chandler   No ISBN

Contains bibliographical information for 2,080 sociologic scales and indices. Seventy-eight conceptual categories were used to classify the instruments and some of these were authoritarianism, family cohesion and attitudes towards medicine and health. The extent of the discussion varies but generally includes information on its development, use, administration, scoring and the sample used.

2.63.3   Mangen, D. & Peterson, W. (eds) (1982) *Research instruments in social gerontology. Volume 1: Clinical and social psychology.* Minneapolis, MN: University of Minnesota Press ISBN 0816609918

AND

2.63.4   Mangen, D. & Peterson, W. (eds) (1982) *Research instruments in social gerontology. Volume 2: Social roles and social participation.* Minneapolis, MN: University of Minnesota Press ISBN 0816610967

AND

2.63.5   Mangen, D. & Peterson, W. (eds.) (1984) *Research instruments in social gerontology. Volume 3: Health, program evaluation and demography.* Minneapolis, MN: University of Minnesota Press ISBN 0816611122

2.63.6   Murray, A., Strauss, M.A. & Brown, B.W. (1978) *Family measurement techniques: abstracts of published instruments 1935–1974* (revised edition). Minneapolis, MN: University of Minnesota Press ISBN 0816607990

Includes abstracts of 813 instruments to measure the properties of the family or the behaviour of people in family roles. Four broad categories are husband/wife relationships, parent/child and sibling-to-sibling relationships, husband/wife and parent/child variables and sex and pre-marital relationships. Abstract includes author, test name, variables, test description, sample item, length, availability and references. Psychometric properties of the instruments are not included.

2.63.7   Price, J.L. (1986) *Handbook of organizational measurement.* London: Harper Business ISBN 0685104966

Book is structured under 22 organizational concepts, some of which are absenteeism, autonomy, centralization communication, effectiveness, satisfaction and span of control. Each chapter contains a general discussion and definition of the concept, issues pertaining to its measurement and descriptions of relevant instruments. Other information includes: a definition, data collecting information, computation methods, reliability and validity of some instruments, evaluative comments and bibliographical sources.

2.63.8   Raynes, N.V. (1988) *Annotated directory of measures of environmental quality for use in residential services for people with a mental handicap.* Manchester: Department of Social Policy and Social Work, University of Manchester

Contains summaries of 62 instruments that can be used to evaluate aspects of the environment provided for mentally handicapped people, although some may be of relevance to other client groups. Each instrument is described using a standard format which includes title, authors, date of most recent edition, purpose, content, administration, scientific credibility focusing on standardization, reliability, validity and references. An appendix gives names and addresses of people to contact for further information.

2.63.9   Robinson, J.P., Athanasiou, R. & Head, K.B. (1969) *Measures of occupational attitudes and occupational characteristics.* Ann Arbor, MI: Institute for Social Research, University of Michigan   No ISBN

Seventy-seven scales used to measure occupational-related variables are cited. Eight general headings are used: job attitudes for particular occupations, satisfaction with specific job features, concepts related to job satisfaction, occupational values, leadership styles, other work-related attitudes, vocational interests and occupational status. Information provided for most tests includes variables, description, sample, reliability, validity, source, results and comments. There is a wide variation in details of reliability and validity. Several chapters discuss topics such as status inconsistency, occupational similarity and social mobility. An overview of research and survey of literature related to job attitudes and performance is also included (CR 2.56).

2.63.10   Sawin, K.J., Harrigan, M. & Woog, P. (1994) *Measures of family functioning for research and practice.* New York: Springer ISBN 0826176305

Book examines nearly 20 instruments for measuring family functioning. Information on each includes: a history of the instrument; an overview of the model and its conceptual framework; a description of the tool; information on scoring, reliability and validity; sample items; and a description of its sensitivity to cross-cultural issues, gender and variant family structures. Also included is a summary of studies using the instruments.

2.63.11   Touliatos, J., Perlmutter, B.F., Strauss, M.A. & Holden, G.W. (2000) *Handbook of family measurement.* Volumes 1–3 Thousand Oaks, CA: Sage   ISBN 0803972504   References

This text is intended for researchers, clinicians and students in the family and related fields. Volume 1 includes abstracts of 976 family measurement instruments cited in published literature 1929–86. Volume 2 includes 367 instruments from 1987–96. Volumes 1 and 2 are preceded by overviews, written by authorities in family studies, that organize and review the instruments in each chapter. Volume 3 contains 168 of the instruments abstracted in Volume 2, reproducing them in full, along with their scoring instructions. Volume 3 also provides author, instrument titles and subject indexes for all three volumes. An attempt has been made to include instruments that are representative of all areas in family studies, that are conceptually and psychometrically sound and that have been used to evaluate diverse populations.

Data Collection

2.64 DATA COLLECTION – GENERAL

Data collection refers to ways in which information can be obtained from the real world, recorded in a systematic way, quantified and/or explained. There are many data collection methods and sections 2.65 to 2.78 will guide the reader towards appropriate sources.

High-quality data will increase the value of research. Choices therefore need to be made in terms of the degree of structure that is possible or desirable, whether or how the data can be quantified, the obtrusiveness of the researcher that may lead to ethical problems, and how objective or subjective the data are or need to be.

Definitions [See Appendix D for sources]

Data – pieces of information obtained in the course of a study

Data cleaning – ... the checking of data from clinical trials or clinical practice in terms of inconsistent or erroneous codes and entries

Data collection – the gathering of information needed to address a research problem

Data set – a collection of related items

Database – a collection of data organized for rapid research and retrieval, usually by a computer; often a consolidation of many records previously stored separately

Multiple imputation – ... a predictive approach to handling missing data in multivariate analysis

---

Annotations

2.64.1 Ackroyd, S. & Hughes, J. (1992) *Data collection in context* (2nd edition). London: Longman ISBN 0582053110 References

Book, which has been extensively revised and updated, covers many aspects of data collection.

2.64.2 Aitken, L.M. & Mardegan, K.J. (2000) 'Thinking aloud': data collection in the natural setting. *Western Journal of Nursing Research* 22 (7) 841–53 26 References

Authors present two variations of decision-making research conducted in the natural clinical setting, using 'thinking aloud' as the primary means of data collection. The procedures are described and a conclusion reached that this technique is valid and useful, although relatively new and controversial.

2.64.3 Coxon, A.P.M. (1999) *Sorting data: collection and analysis*. London: Sage ISBN 0803973377 References

Book gives advice on collecting, describing, comparing and analysing data. Information is also included on setting the criterion, the pre-test, administration and recording results (CR 2.79).

2.64.4 Dashiff, C. (2001) Data collection with adolescents. *Journal of Advanced Nursing* 33 (3) 343–9 40 References

Defines adolescence, identifies settings where research with adolescents may take place and discusses the potential cultural and ethnic issues that might arise (CR 2.53).

2.64.5 Economic and Social Research Council (1996) Qualitative Data Archival Resource Centre (QUALIDATA). *Sociological Research Online* www.socresonline.org.uk/socresonline/1/3/qualidata. html#top (Accessed 02/02/03)

Describes the QUALIDATA Resource Centre located in the Department of Sociology at the University of Essex. Its aims are: locating, assessing and documenting qualitative data and arranging for their deposit in suitable public archives; disseminating information about these data; and raising archival consciousness among the social science research community. The QUALIDATA database is available on the Internet (www.essex.ac.uk/qualidata (Accessed 02/02/03)) (CR 2.64.9).

2.64.6 Epstein, J. & Klinkenberg, W.D. (2002) Collecting data via the Internet: the development and deployment of a web-based survey. *Journal of*

Technology in Human Services 19 (2/3) 33–47   15
References

Discusses a study designed to replicate a survey originally administered in a traditional manner. Presents data on the characteristics of respondents, hit and completion rates and the effectiveness of different methods of advertising the survey among a gay and lesbian population of Internet users (CR 2.85).

2.64.7 Holcomb, E.L. (1999) *Getting excited about data: how to combine people, passion and proof.* Thousand Oaks, CA: Corwin Press   ISBN 0803967381   References

This 'how to' manual discusses what and how much data should be collected and how it should be analysed and reported, and what should be done with the findings that will improve the next round of results.

2.64.8 Patrician, P.A. (2002) Multiple imputation for missing data. *Research in Nursing and Health* 25 (1) February 76–84   24 References

Reviews the problems associated with missing data, options for handling this situation and recent multiple imputation methods.

2.64.9 Qualitative Data Service *Introduction to Qualitative Data Service* www.qualidata.essex.ac.uk/about/introduction.asp (Accessed 20/02/03)

QUALIDATA provides a national service for the acquisition, dissemination and re-use of social sciences qualitative research data. It can offer specialist advice on research project management, issues of confidentiality and consent, and documentation of data with regard to their archiving. It also offers a resource discovery hub via both the UK Data Archive and its own online catalogue, QUALICAT. Training and seminars are offered to encourage professional researchers and research students to make full use of these rich resources (CR 2.64.5).

2.64.10 Roberts, P. & Woods, L. (2000) Alternative methods of gathering and handling data: maximizing the use of modern technology. *Nurse Researcher: The International Journal of Research Methodology in Nursing and Health Care* 8 (2) 84–95   19 References

Authors describe the principles behind a number of emerging techniques, including computer-assisted and electronic mail interviewing (CR 2.17, 2.68, 2.70, 2.84).

2.64.11 Roberts, P., Priest, H. & Bromage, C. (2001) Selecting and utilizing data sources to evaluate health care education. *Nurse Researcher: The International Journal of Research Methodology in Nursing and Health Care* 8 (3) 15–29   45 References

Authors discuss the purposes of educational evaluation and the selection and use of research data to promote improvements in nursing and health care education (CR 2.43, 2.68, 2.75).

2.64.12 Sapsford, R. & Jupp, V. (eds) (1996) *Data collection and analysis.* London: Sage   ISBN 076195046X   References

Text covers both quantitative and qualitative approaches to data collection and analysis in social research. A wide range of academic and applied research studies illustrate the text and exercises are included to aid understanding (CR 2.79).

2.64.13 Sieber, J.E. (ed.) (1991) *Sharing social science data: advantages and challenges.* Newbury Park, CA: Sage   ISBN 0803940831   References

Book highlights the advantages of data sharing in the social sciences. The reasons for sharing practices in various disciplines, factors affecting the value of these data and concerns that may arise are discussed.

2.64.14 Smith, C.E., Cha, J.J., Kleinbeck, S.V.M., Clements, F.A., Cook, D. & Koehler, J. (2002) Feasibility of in-home telehealth for conducting nursing research. *Clinical Nursing Research* 11 (2) 220–33   49 References

Describes a feasibility study that aimed to determine the reliability of using audio/video telehealth equipment for collecting research data at patients' homes, and administering nursing interventions to families. Findings showed that the use of telehealth visits were just as reliable and less expensive that traditional home visits (CR 2.24, 2.72).

Methods of Data Collection

2.65 CRITICAL INCIDENT TECHNIQUE

The critical incident technique employs a set of principles for collecting data on observable human activities. It provides a flexible way of examining interpersonal communication skills and has been used in many nursing studies. Incidents are of particular value because it is reality that is being described rather than hypothetical situations.

Definitions [See Appendix D for sources]

Critical incident – an observable type of human activity which is sufficiently complete in itself to permit inferences and predictions to be made about the person performing the act. To be critical it must be performed in a situation where the purpose or intent of the act seems fairly clear to the observer, and its consequences are sufficiently definite so there is little doubt concerning its effects

Critical incident technique – a set of procedures for collecting direct observations of human behaviour which have special significance and meet systematically defined criteria

---

Example

Narayanasamy, A. & Owens, J. (2001) A critical incident study of nurses' responses to the spiritual needs of their patients. *Journal of Advanced Nursing* 33 (4) 446–55   35 References

Reports a study which aimed to describe what nurses consider to be spiritual needs; explore how nurses responded to these needs; typify nurses' involvement in spiritual dimensions of care and describe the effects of their interventions. The authors believe that the findings of the study offer prospects for developing the Personal and Cultural Approaches of care as models of spiritual care.

Original articles

Flanagan, J.C. (1947) *The aviation psychology programme in the army air forces. AAF psychology programme research report no. 1.* Washington, DC: Government Printing Office

Flanagan, J.C. (1954) The critical incident technique. *Psychological Bulletin* 51 (4) 327–58   74 References

Annotations

2.65.1   Bermosk, L.S. & Corsini, R.J. (1973) *Critical incidents in nursing.* Philadelphia, PA: W.B. Saunders   ISBN 0721616968

Book concentrates on 38 controversial issues documented in the form of critical incidents under the headings of: nurse and the patient, peers, doctors, the family, supervision and the system. The background to each incident is described. Opinions, reactions and some suggestions for resolution from experienced nurses who examined them are described. Critical incidents enable the complex world in which nurses work to be portrayed.

2.65.2   Busse, D.K. & Wright, D.J. (2000) Classification and analysis of incidents in complex medical environments. *Topics in Health Information Management* 20 (4) 1–11   29 References

Incident analysis theory and methodology from fields other than medicine are applied to an incident reporting scheme in an Edinburgh intensive care unit. The model used emphasizes the importance of latent organizational factors and complex multi-layered incident causation. It also takes the role of cognitive performance-shaping factors into account. This provides an analytical framework that integrates the identification of distal causal factors and a mechanism for comparing alternative causal hypotheses.

2.65.3   Chell, E. (1998) Critical incident technique. In Symon, G. & Cassell, C. (eds) *Qualitative methods and analysis in organizational research: a practical guide.* London: Sage   ISBN 0761953515 Chapter 4 51–72   18 References

The critical incident technique was originally used as a scientific tool whereas now it tends to be used as an investigative tool in organizational analysis from within an interpretative or phenomenological paradigm. Because the technique may be used in both qualitative and quantitative studies, researchers need to carefully consider the nature of the research problem to be investigated, and how it may be applied in a particular case. Author discusses these background assumptions, relates them to three different approaches and illustrates it with a detailed case example (CR 2.36.135).

2.65.4   Clamp, C.G.L. (1984) Learning through incidents: studies in the development and use of critical incidents in the teaching of attitudes in nursing. MPhil thesis (unpublished) University of London, Institute of Education

Study aimed to develop a teaching method that could increase attitude awareness and develop interpersonal communication skills in nursing education. Critical incidents were used as triggers for in-depth discussions on the behaviour, attitudes and feelings reported by nurses. Many aspects of learning and areas of personal growth were highlighted.

2.65.5   Cormack, D.F.S. (ed.) (2000) The critical incident technique. In Author *The research process in nursing* (4th edition). Oxford: Blackwell Science ISBN 0632051582   Chapter 27 327–35   12 References

Describes the origins and applications of critical incidents in nursing (CR 2.1.23).

2.65.6   Cortazzi, D. & Roote, S. (1975) *Illuminative incident analysis*. London: McGraw Hill ISBN 0070844526

Using critical incidents as the focal point, describes the process of learning through illuminative incident analysis. The aim of the book is to encourage constructive team development by drawing the incident, rather than discussing it. This method has been shown to develop understanding of attitudes, role perceptions and motivation. Solutions emerge which can become a 'health care plan' for the team.

2.65.7   Flanagan, J.C. (1954) The critical incident technique. *Psychological Bulletin* 51 (4) 327–58   74 References

Article describes the development of critical incident methodology, its fundamental principles and status. Studies using this technique are reviewed and possible future use identified.

2.65.8   Ghaye, T. & Lillyman, S. (1997) Critical incident analysis. In Authors *Learning journals and critical incidents: reflective practice for health care professionals*. Dinton, Nr. Salisbury: Quay Books ISBN 1856421538   References Section B 5: Critical incident analysis 77–87 and Section B 6: Examples of critical incidents 89–99

Explores the use and value of critical incident analysis and the identification of learning through

experience. It also shows when and how critical incidents can be applied to practice.

2.65.9   Kemppainen, J.K. (2000) The critical incident technique and nursing care quality research. *Journal of Advanced Nursing* 32 (5) 1264–71   34 References

Article describes critical incident methodology, reviews previous applications of the technique to the study of health care quality and provides illustrations from research.

2.65.10   Koponen, P., Perala, M. & Riakkonen, O. (2000) Critical incident technique as a research method (Finland). *Hoitotiede* 12 (4) 164–72   51 References

Describes the application of the critical incident technique (CIT) in previous research. The feasibility and usefulness of the technique is also evaluated. Authors discuss what critical incidents have been used for, appropriate data collection methods and how they may be analysed.

2.65.11   Meurier, C.V. (2000) Understanding the nature of errors in nursing: using a model to analyze critical incident reports of errors which had resulted in an adverse or potentially adverse event. *Journal of Advanced Nursing* 32 (1) 202–7   15 References

Author used Reason's Organizational Accident Model to analyse critical incidents of errors in nursing. Twenty registered nurses produced a report of an error and five were subsequently interviewed to gain more information. The detailed analysis of one incident is discussed, demonstrating the effectiveness of this approach in providing insights into the chain of events that may lead to an adverse event, whether they are organizational, local circumstances or active failures.

2.65.12   O'Connor, J. & Jeavons, S. (2003) Nurses' perceptions of critical incidents. *Journal of Advanced Nursing* 41 (1) 53–62   30 References

Reports a study that aimed to determine the types of clinical event nurses perceived as critical and whether their experiences of critical incidents were associated with any demographic variables such as qualifications and current area of work.

2.66   DELPHI TECHNIQUE/APPROACH

'The Delphi concept may be seen as a spin off from defence research. Project Delphi was the name given to an Air Force-sponsored, Rand Corporation study in the early 1950s, concerning the use of expert opinion. The aim of this study was to select an optimal American industrial target system and estimate the number of atom bombs required to reduce the munitions output by a prescribed amount. The study set out to obtain the most reliable consensus of opinion from a group of experts ... by a series of intensive questionnaires interspersed with controlled opinion feedback.' (Linstone & Turoff, 1975: 10)

[Apollo became master of Delphi upon slaying the dragon Pythos, and he was renowned not only for his youth and perfect beauty but even more for his ability to see the future.]

Definitions [See Appendix D for sources]

Consensus methods – provide a means of synthesizing information ... [using] a wider range of [material] than is common in statistical methods, and when published information is inadequate or non-existent

Delphi technique – ... a method for obtaining expert opinion on a topic ... it employs multiple rounds or waves of questionnaires, with each round utilizing information gathered during previous rounds, in an attempt to converge towards group consensus

---

Example

Sharkey, S.B. & Sharples, A.Y. (2001) An approach to consensus building using a Delphi technique: developing a learning resource in mental health. *Nurse Education Today* 21 (5) 398–408 41 References

Study utilizes a multimethod approach in developing a learning resource in clinical risk management in mental health. Phase I of the project is reported and the Delphi technique was used to facilitate consensus from a range of perspectives. The group views elicited enabled a learning resource to be developed.

Major text

Linstone, H.A. & Turoff, M. (eds) (1975) *The Delphi method: techniques and applications.* Reading, MA: Addison-Wesley ISBN 0201042940 References

Annotations

2.66.1 Beech, B. (2001) The Delphi approach: recent applications in health care. *Nurse Researcher: The International Journal of Research Methodology in Nursing and Health Care* 8 (4) 38–48 22 References

Article examines the range of applications of the Delphi technique, as reported in present-day nursing literature, and discusses a representative cross-section of these studies in greater detail (CR 2.12).

2.66.2 Crisp, J., Pelletier, D., Duffield, C., Nagy, S. & Adams, A. (1999) It's all in a name. When is a 'Delphi study' not a Delphi study? *Australian Journal of Advanced Nursing* 16 (3) 32–7 39 References

Paper discusses some of the complexities encountered while exploring the literature on the Delphi technique, a research method believed to be straightforward. Authors' explorations showed that, rather than being a simple means of obtaining the judgements of experts, modifications and adaptations over the years have dramatically changed the 'Delphi'. Those wishing to use this method need to have a sound knowledge of complex theoretical issues associated with its implementation.

2.66.3 de Meyrick, J. (2003) The Delphi method and health research. *Health Education* 103 (1) 7–16 37 References

Reviews the literature pertaining to the history and use of the Delphi technique, outlining the benefits to policy research and health education. Determines the potential weaknesses of the method and steps to overcome them (CR 2.12, 3.11).

2.66.4 Endacott, R., Clifford, C.M. & Tripp, J.H. (1999) Can the needs of a critically ill child be identified using scenarios? Experiences of a modified Delphi study. *Journal of Advanced Nursing* 30 (3) 665–76 34 References

The abstract and evaluative nature of need was a key issue to arise in the pilot phase of this study. The defining attributes arising from the concept analysis were used to construct two hypothetical case studies for the modified Delphi, and these were used as part of the questionnaire for all three rounds. Authors evaluate the use of this technique to identify needs and discuss key features arising from the results (CR 2.75).

2.66.5 Greatorex, J. & Dexter, T. (2000) An accessible analytical approach for investigating what happens between the rounds of a Delphi. *Journal of Advanced Nursing* 32 (4) 1016–24 20 References

In this paper an accessible analytical approach is outlined, using graphical presentations of means and standard deviations to identify what happens between rounds. An example is given to illustrate the methodology.

2.66.6 Hasson, F., Keeney, S. & McKenna, H. (2000) Research guidelines for the Delphi survey technique. *Journal of Advanced Nursing* 32 (4) 1008–15   39 References

Paper aims to provide an understanding of the preparation, action steps and difficulties inherent in using the Delphi technique. A checklist of points is included (CR 2.17, 2.18, 2.22, 2.24, 2.25, 2.64, 2.86, 2.87).

2.66.7   Linstone, H.A. & Turoff, M. (eds) (1975) *The Delphi method: techniques and applications*. Reading, MA: Addison-Wesley   ISBN 0201042940   References

This major text describes the Delphi technique and its applications. It has been used in technological forecasting and in many other contexts. These include normative forecasts, the ascertainment of values and preferences, estimates concerning the quality of life, simulated and real decision-making and planning. Despite many uses, this technique lacks a completely sound theoretical basis. The book includes philosophy, general applications, evaluation, cross-impact analysis, specialized techniques, computers and the future of Delphi, a checklist of pitfalls and an extensive bibliography.

2.66.8   McPhail, A. (2001) Nominal group technique: a useful method for working with young people. *British Educational Research Journal* 27 (2) 161–70   39 References

Reviews focus groups, brainstorming and the Delphi technique before explaining the process of nominal group technique and how it can overcome some of the problems encountered with the first three. Using findings from an educational study, the value of this technique is illustrated (CR 2.69).

2.66.9   Mead, D. & Mosely, L. (2001) The use of the Delphi as a research approach. *Nurse Researcher: The International Journal of Research Methodology in Nursing and Health Care* 8 (4) 4–23   20 References

Article outlines alternative approaches of collecting data from a group of individuals before describing the processes necessary when conducting a Delphi study and the methodological issues involved.

2.66.10   Mosely, L. & Mead, D. (2001) Considerations in using the Delphi approach: design, questions and answers. *Nurse Researcher: The International Journal of Research Methodology in Nursing and Health Care* 8 (4) 24–37   25 References

Discusses issues around the types of question asked in a Delphi study. The authors offer advice from their personal experience to assist others in avoiding some of the many pitfalls.

2.66.11   Murphy, M.K., Black, N.A., Lamping, D.L., McKee, C.M., Sanderson, C.F.B., Askham, J. & Marteau, T. (1998) Consensus development methods, and their use in clinical guideline development. *Health Technology Assessment* 2 (3) 88 pages   References

Reviews the factors that affect decisions that emerge from consensus development methods and recommends methodological research for improving the use of consensus development as a basis for clinical guideline production.

2.66.12   Powell, C. (2003) The Delphi technique: myths and realities. *Journal of Advanced Nursing* 41 (4) 376–82   49 References

Drawing on seminal texts, recent methodological reviews and a selective range of Delphi studies, the paper aims to demystify Delphi methodology and update knowledge to inform future debate. Emphasis is given to the question of scientific merit and the means by which Delphi studies can be evaluated.

2.67   DIARIES

Diaries can provide information that it is not possible to obtain in any other way. However skilful the questionnaire or interview schedule, inevitably the researcher imposes some structure. A diary may also be structured to a certain extent in that people can be asked to record particular things, but additional insights may be gained.

Definition [See Appendix D for source]

Diaries – a source of data that can provide an intimate descriptive comment on everyday life for an individual

Example

Jones, M.L., Walters, S. & Akehurst, R. (2001) The implications of contact with the mentor for pre-registration nursing and midwifery students. *Journal of Advanced Nursing* 35 (2) 151–160   22 References

Reports a study that examined the extent to which pre-registration nursing and midwifery students had contact with their named mentor, and the implications of this. The main objective of the study was to undertake a cost–benefit analysis of clinical placements and this is reported elsewhere. Both named mentors and students kept an activity diary for one week. Results and implications of the study are reported.

Annotations

2.67.1   Breakwell, G.M. & Wood, P. (2000) In Breakwell, G.M., Hammond, S. & Fife-Schaw, C. (eds) *Research methods in psychology* (2nd edition). London: Sage   ISBN 0761965912   Part III Chapter 21 294–302   References

Chapter identifies the nature of diary techniques, the pros and cons of this approach, getting the best out of them and analysing diary data (CR 2.1.7).

2.67.2   Burman, M.E. (1995) Health diaries in nursing research and practice. *Image: Journal of Nursing Scholarship* 27 (2) 147–52   46 References

Describes current uses of health diaries in nursing research and practice. Types of health diary, factors affecting the quality of data, the costs and analytic issues are all discussed. The implications for nursing research and practice are considered.

2.67.3   Corti, L. *Using diaries in social research. Social Research Update* Issue 2 Guildford: University of Surrey, Department of Sociology www.soc.surrey.ac.uk/sru/SRU2.html (Accessed 20/02/03)

Discusses the use of diaries in social research, including reasons for using diaries, diary design and format, data quality and response rates, coding, editing and processing, relative cost, computer software for processing and analysis, and archiving diary data.

2.67.4   Elliott, H. (1997) The use of diaries in sociological research on health experience. *Sociological Research Online* 2 (2)   34 References www.socresonline.org.uk/socresonline/2/2/7.html (Accessed 14/11/03)

Highlights the value of doing diary research, drawing on the literature of auto/biographies and health service research, together with a qualitative study of need and demand for primary health care (CR 2.36, 2.71).

2.67.5   Gibson, V. (1995) An analysis of the use of diaries as a data collection method. *Nurse Researcher* 3 (1) 66–73   18 References

Provides an overview of the diary as a data collection method and discusses its strengths and weaknesses (CR 2.86).

2.67.6   Jones, R.K. (2000) The unsolicited diary as a qualitative research tool for advanced research capacity in the field of health and illness. *Qualitative Health Research* 10 (4) 555–67   56 References

The place of diary method is examined in the context of qualitative tools. Although it is commissioned or

solicited diaries that are increasingly popular in health research, different kinds of diary usage are examined together with certain possible biases and weaknesses. The analysis of an unsolicited diary account of a patient suffering from cancer of the larynx is explored as a potential data source (CR 2.27).

2.67.7   Keleher, H.M. & Verrinder, G.K. (2003) Health diaries in a rural Australian setting. *Qualitative Health Research* 13 (3) 435–43   14 References

Reports a study that used health diaries to examine use of health services, episodes of illness, actions taken to keep healthy and reflections on services and programmes. A literature review examines the history of the method (CR 2.12).

2.67.8   Malinowski, B. (1982) The diary of an anthropologist. In Burgess, R.G. (ed.) *Field research: a sourcebook and field manual*. London: Allen & Unwin   ISBN 004312013X   Chapter 27 200–205   References

An actual diary extract is reproduced.

2.67.9   Oleske, D.M., Heinze, S. & Otte, D.M. (1990) The diary as a means of understanding the quality of persons with cancer receiving home care. *Cancer Nursing* 13 (3) 158–66   References

Reports a study that discusses the rationale for using diaries as a data collection method with an ill population. Results are reported and the advantages of using diaries are discussed.

2.67.10   Richardson, A. (1994) The health diary: an examination of its use as a data collection method. *Journal of Advanced Nursing* 19 (4) 782–91   53 References

Discusses the advantages and disadvantages associated with use of diaries as a data collection instrument in health care settings. Completion of the diary, respondent co-operation, format and issues surrounding analysis are all considered.

2.67.11   Ruffing-Rahal, M.A. (1986) Personal documents and nursing theory development. *Advances in Nursing Science* 8 (3) 50–7   36 References

Discusses the use of personal documents as a means of providing insights into the nature of health and experiences of illness. Triangulated research strategies are advocated in order to incorporate these experiences into nursing research (CR 2.7, 2.26).

2.67.12   Symon, G. (1998) Qualitative research diaries. In Symon, G. & Cassell, C. (eds) *Qualitative methods and analysis in organizational research: a practical guide*. London: Sage   ISBN 0761953515   Chapter 6 94–117   36 References

Chapter aims to encourage qualitative diary research by offering some practical design and implementation guidelines, as applied to organizational settings (CR 2.36.135).

2.67.13 Verbrugge, L. (1980) Health diaries. *Medical Care* 18 (1) 73–95   52 References

A review and methodological discussion of studies that used health diaries. Evidence is given on the following aspects: levels of reporting compared to retrospective interview, recall error, validity of health reports, value of diary data for a broad view of symptoms and health behaviour. Also considered are individual-level analysis, studies of health dynamics, respondent co-operation, conditioning effects, quality of diary data, survey costs, complexity of data collection, processing and analysis (CR 2.25, 2.68).

2.67.14 Woods, N.F. (1981) The health diary as an instrument for nursing research: problems and promise. *Western Journal of Nursing Research* 3 (1) 76–92   16 References

Discusses use of a health diary as a means of obtaining valid data about symptoms. Its advantages and disadvantages are discussed together with reliability, validity and its purpose. Paper is illustrated by a study where 96 women completed a diary for three weeks. Results were weakly correlated with the Cornell Medical Index Health questionnaire, but the author believes the method should be further explored in nursing research (CR 2.24, 2.25).

2.68 INTERVIEW

'Research interviews require a systematic approach to data collection which maximize the chances of maintaining objectivity and achieving valid and reliable results. … And it is for all practical purposes an infinitely flexible tool for research.' (Breakwell, Hammond & Fife-Schaw, 2000: 239) [Adapted]

Definitions [See Appendix D for sources]

Depth interview – an unstructured interview in which the aim is to probe deeply and obtain an exhaustive account of the subject's views and experiences

Exploratory interview – unstructured, intended to develop ideas and hypotheses, and to explore possible ways of gathering data

Interview – a data collection method employing a verbal questioning technique

Interview schedule – a set of questions with guided instructions for an interviewer to use in carrying out an interview

Pilot interview – mainly intended as an aid to the design of later research

Semi-structured interview – partly standardized but also allows the interviewer greater flexibility at the expense of possibly incurring greater bias

Shadowed data – information that participants give … about the types, characteristics and dimensions of concepts, perceptions, behaviours and opinions of others

Standardized/structured interview – involves each subject being asked the same questions in exactly the same order

Transcript – the written form of a tape recording of an interview

Example

de Veer, A.J.E. & Kerkstra, A. (2001) Feeling at home in nursing homes. *Journal of Advanced Nursing* 35 (3) 427–34   27 References

Discusses a study that examined determinants of feeling at home, and in particular the privacy in nursing homes in The Netherlands. The data were collected from individual interviews with 686 residents and family members in 36 nursing homes. Results are reported and problems are highlighted.

Annotations

2.68.1 Anderson, K. & Jack, D.C. (1998) Learning to listen. In Perks, R. & Thomson, A. (eds) *The oral history reader*. London: Routledge ISBN 041513352   Part 11 Chapter 14 156–71   15 Notes and References

Chapter discusses shedding agendas and listening for meaning during oral history interviews (CR 2.47.18).

2.68.2 Arksey, H. & Knight, P.T. (1999) *Interviewing for social scientists: an introductory resource with examples*. London: Sage ISBN 0761958703   References

Book provides a comprehensive introduction to interviewing for graduates and undergraduates (CR 2.26, 2.97, 2.98).

2.68.3 Åstedt-Kurki, P., Paavilainen, E. & Lehti, K. (2001) Methodological issues in interviewing families in family nursing research. *Journal of Advanced Nursing* 35 (2) July 288–93   28 References

Discusses the methodological problems that can be met when conducting family research. There may be one member or multiple family members, the family as a unit and sometimes children as informants. All of these different groupings need to be considered when planning the research project.

2.68.4   Atkinson, R. (1998) *The life story interview*. Thousand Oaks, CA: Sage   ISBN 076190428X References

This volume provides specific suggestions and guidelines for preparing and carrying out a life-story interview. It also deals with the issues of transcribing and interpreting the interview. A sample life-story interview is provided in an appendix.

2.68.5   Bricher, G. (1999) Children and qualitative research methods: a review of the literature related to interview and interpretive processes. *Nurse Researcher* 6 (4) 65–77   50 References

Reviews North American and British literature from 1988 to 1999 that examines the challenges presented in undertaking interviews with children. Their differing needs, techniques required and differences in interpreting data are all included (CR 2.12, 2.36).

2.68.6   Chapple, A. (1999) Reducing risk when interviewing in threatening areas: a personal view. *Nurse Researcher* 6 (4) 79–88   12 References

Paper deals with measures that can be taken to reduce the risk of harmful events occurring during fieldwork. It is concerned with the risks associated with physical violence rather than psychological abuse (CR 2.16).

2.68.7   Docherty, S. & Sandelowski, M. (1999) Focus on qualitative methods: interviewing children. *Research in Nursing and Health* 22 (2) 177–85   81 References

Authors suggest using recent scholarship on the development of children's narrative competence to clarify the problems that still need to be resolved in eliciting useful and meaningful information from children. This literature suggests the importance of combining the influences of developmental age, the target under investigation, interview structure, multiple interviewers and research design on the nature of the data collected. Evaluating these mutual influences will further the goal of faithfully rendering childhood experience (CR 2.36, 2.78).

2.68.8   Dunne, S. (1995) *Interviewing techniques for writers and researchers*. London: A. & C. Black ISBN 0713641924   References

Book covers methods and types of interview, tools, finding subjects, preparing for and conducting the interview, transcribing and writing-up the findings (CR 2.22).

2.68.9   Edwards, R. (1998) A critical examination of the use of interpreters in the qualitative research process. *Journal of Ethnic and Migration Studies* 24 (1) 197–208   41 References

Explores the need, role and use of interpreters in the qualitative research process and offers an alternative model which poses that researchers should carry out research with, rather than through, interpreters (CR 2.36).

2.68.10   Elliott, E., Watson, A.J. & Harries, U. (2002) Harnessing expertise: involving peer interviewers in qualitative research with hard-to-reach populations. *Health Expectations* 5 (2) 172–8   14 References

Explores the issues, problems and advantages of using peer interviewers in a study of the experiences of parents who use illegal drugs. The challenges included the need to provide support for the interviewers, and the difficulties of gaining from their skills and experiences without exploiting their labour. This should be weighed against the advantages of gaining a greater understanding of their experiences (CR 2.22, 2.36).

2.68.11   Erickson, P.I. & Kaplan, C.P. (2000) Maximizing qualitative responses about smoking in structured interviews. *Qualitative Health Research* 10 (6) 829–40   32 References

Addresses the important methodological issue of whether face-to-face or self-administered interviews elicit better qualitative data on reasons for smoking and quitting.

2.68.12   Fielding, N.G. (ed.) (2002) *Interviewing*. London: Sage   ISBN 0761973397   References   4 Volumes

The aim of this collection is to bring together all of the key articles that have been published in professional journals. It is a comprehensive collection addressing: the philosophy of interview methods and its epistemological foundations, the ethics of interview research and the criteria for assessing interview-based research. It covers both interviewing in quantitative research, such as the survey method, and qualitative research in its many forms. The collection explores the principle types of interview (standardized, semi-standardized and non-standardized) and the different modes of interviewing (e.g. telephone interviewing, life-history interviews and focus groups). There is a section on formulating interview questions, the practicalities of recording, transcribing and managing interview data. Other sections address power relations, the role of gender, interviewing on sensitive topics and special respondents such as elites, children and the vulnerable (CR 2.17, 2.29, 2.36, 2.69, 2.70, 2.71).

2.68.13 Foddy, W. (1993) *Constructing questions for interviews and questionnaires: theory and practice in social research*. Cambridge: Cambridge University Press   ISBN 0521467330   References

Book integrates the empirical findings on question design reported in the literature. The theoretical framework used leads to a set of principles that increases the validity and reliability of verbal data collected for research (CR 2.24, 2.25, 2.75).

2.68.14 Gillham, B. (2000) *The research interview*. London: Continuum   ISBN 082644797X   References

Book provides comprehensive coverage of the basic techniques of interviewing for students and professionals. It includes controlling the interview, preparing a schedule, using techniques of questioning and prompting, and probing and analysing the content (CR 2.88).

2.68.15 Gubrium, J.F. & Holstein, J.A. (eds) (2001) *Handbook of interviewing: context and method*. Thousand Oaks, CA: Sage   ISBN 0761919511   References

Handbook offers a comprehensive examination of the interview at the cutting-edge of information technology. It covers forms of interviewing, distinctive respondents, auspices of interviewing, technical issues, analytical strategies, reflection representation (CR 2.22, 2.42, 2.53, 2.70, 2.72, 2.84, 2.85).

2.68.16 Gubrium, J.F. & Holstein, J.A. (eds) (2003) *Postmodern interviewing*. Thousand Oaks, CA: Sage   ISBN 0761928502   References

Offers readers an exploration of the post-modern interview, a conversation with diverse purposes in which the communication format is constructed as much within the interview conversation as it stems from predesignated research interests. The book discusses new horizons in interviews, featuring reflexivity, poetics and power as new ways of gathering experiential knowledge (CR 2.27, 2.72, 2.85).

2.68.17 Hardin, P. (2003) Constructing experience in individual interviews, autobiographies and on-line accounts: a poststructuralist approach. *Journal of Advanced Nursing* 41 (6) 536–44   26 References

Develops a methodological perspective for the production and analysis of data, with regard to form, context and function, using accounts from individuals with anorexia nervosa (CR 2.89).

2.68.18 Higgins, P.A. & Daly, B.J. (1999) Research methodology issues relating to interviewing the mechanically ventilated patient. *Western Journal of Nursing Research* 21 (6) 773–84   24 References

Article describes issues involved in the process of interviewing chronically critically ill patients who required the continuous support of mechanical ventilation (CR 2.17, 2.22).

2.68.19 Holstein, J.A. & Gubrium, J.F. (eds) (2003) *Inside interviewing: new lenses, new concerns*. Thousand Oaks, CA: Sage   ISBN 0761928510   References

Highlights the fluctuating and diverse moral worlds put into place during interview research when gender, race, culture, the age of respondents and other subject positions are brought narratively to the foreground. It explores the 'facts', thoughts, feelings and perspectives of respondents and how this impacts on the research process. Readers will be enabled to select the most appropriate analytical strategy for explicating data that emerges from related activities in the interview process.

2.68.20 Keats, D. (2000) *Interviewing: a practical guide for students and professionals*. Buckingham: Open University Press   ISBN 0335206670   References

Book is a guide for those wishing to improve their interviewing skills, whether experienced professionals or beginners. Practical ideas and information about such issues as building rapport and interpreting verbal and non-verbal responses are included. There are chapters on interviewing children, adolescents, older people, people with disabilities, and interviewing across cultures and in stressful situations. Case studies, sample interviews, activities for students and chapter summaries also feature.

2.68.21 Kvale, S. (1996) *Interviews: an introduction to qualitative research interviewing*. Thousand Oaks, CA: Sage   ISBN 080395820X   References

Provides theoretical underpinnings and practical aspects of the interviewing process (CR 2.36).

2.68.22 Maple, F.F. (1998) *Goal-focused interviewing*. Thousand Oaks, CA: Sage   ISBN 0761901809

Book presents Maple's model for categorizing information elicited from clients. Techniques for focusing on the competencies of clients rather than their deficiencies are discussed (CR 2.86).

2.68.23 McCracken, G. (1988) *The long interview*. Newbury Park, CA: Sage   ISBN 0803933533   References

Provides a systematic guide to the theory and method of the long qualitative interview. Key theoretical and methodological issues are identified, and research strategies and a simple four-step model of inquiry are described. Its value as a tool in scientific studies is outlined.

2.68.24   McEvoy, P. (2001) Interviewing colleagues: addressing the issues of perspective, inquiry and representation. *Nurse Researcher: The International Journal of Research Methodology in Nursing and Health Care* 9 (2) 49–59   32 References

Discusses some of the issues that may arise when practitioner researchers conduct conversational interviews with colleagues as part of a practice-based project.

2.68.25   Melia, K. (2000) Conducting an interview. *Nurse Researcher* 7 (4) 75–89   27 References

While undertaking interviews with intensive care nurses, the author considered the traditional advice that researchers should say as little as possible to encourage the respondents to talk. The paper reconsiders this idea and her points are illustrated with extracts from some of these interviews.

2.68.26   Mills, J. (2001) Self-construction through conversation and narrative in interviews. *Educational Review* 53 (3) 285–301   40 References

Paper scrutinizes the role of interviewing in educational research, both in terms of product and process. The dialogic nature of interviews is addressed and their role in the performance and construction of self is explored. Subtleties in the interview process, frequently overlooked, are discussed (CR 2.89).

2.68.27   Mishler, E.G. (1991) *Research interviewing: context and narrative.* Cambridge, MA: Harvard University Press   ISBN 0674764617   References

Examines current views and practices of interviewing and concludes that they reflect a restricted conception of the interview process. Author makes the proposition that an interview is a form of discourse that is shaped and organized by asking and answering questions. He advocates using a family of methods as a framework for developing an alternative.

2.68.28   Morse, J.M. (2001) Editorial *Qualitative Health Research* 11 (3) 291–2   1 Reference

Editor discusses the value of shadowed data obtained during unstructured, interactive interviews (CR 2.64).

2.68.29   Moyle, W. (2002) Unstructured interviews: challenges when participants have a major depressive illness. *Journal of Advanced Nursing* 39 (3) 266–73   32 References

Paper gives an overview of the challenges involved in conducting unstructured interviews with patients who have a mental illness. Methodological issues are discussed, and the author believes that more information on this technique should be included in research texts to help novice researchers.

2.68.30   Price, B. (2002) Laddered questions and qualitative data research interviews. *Journal of Advanced Nursing* 37 (3) 273–81   23 References

Paper defines and explains a technique designed to direct the use of probing in interviews. The author believes that its selected use might provide richer data than other *ad hoc* approaches used by neophyte researchers (CR 2.36).

2.68.31   Rubin, H.J. & Rubin, I.S. (1995) *Qualitative interviewing: the art of hearing data.* Thousand Oaks, CA: Sage   ISBN 0803950969   References

Book considers the underlying philosophy of qualitative work and research designs (CR 2.36).

2.68.32   Samuel, R. (1998) Perils of the transcript. In Perks, R. & Thomson, A. (eds) *The oral history reader.* London: Routledge   ISBN 0415133521   Part V Chapter 32 389–92

Chapter discusses some of the difficulties involved in transcribing oral material (CR 2.47.18).

2.68.33   Saris, W.E. (1991) *Computer-assisted interviewing.* Newbury Park, CA: Sage   ISBN 0803940661   References

Book aims to help researchers improve the quality of their data. The possibilities and difficulties of computer-assisted interviewing are identified. Examples are annotated so that comparisons can be made with paper questionnaires. An overview is given of the important features to consider when purchasing a CADAC programme. An appendix lists computer programmes (CR 2.75, 2.84).

2.68.34   Seidman, I. (1998) *Interviewing as qualitative research: a guide for researchers in education and the social sciences* (2nd edition). New York: Teachers College Press   ISBN 080773697X   References

This book covers the purpose of interviewing, a structure for in-depth phenomenological interviewing, proposing research, establishing access to participants, affirming informed consent, research techniques, interviewing as a relationship and analysing, interpreting and sharing interview material (CR 2.36).

2.68.35   Spradley, J.P. (1979) *The ethnographic interview.* New York: Holt, Rinehart & Winston ISBN 0030444969   References

This book, together with its companion volume *Participant Observation*, aims to provide a systematic handbook for doing ethnography and develops techniques initially used mainly by anthropologists. Ethnographic research is set in context and a series of steps designed to develop skills in this type of interviewing are discussed. The text is illustrated by many examples from the author's own and others' research (CR 2.42, 2.72.25).

2.68.36   Sullivan, K. (1998/99) Managing the 'sensitive' research interview: a personal account. *Nurse Researcher* 6 (2) 72–85 16   References

Paper presents an account of the interview process used to collect data for a study that described the experience of bereavement of 14 people. The challenges, problems and realities of undertaking this work are described (CR 2.14, 2.16, 2.17, 3.16).

2.68.37   Wengraf, T. (2001) *Qualitative research interviewing: biographic narrative and semi-structured methods.* London: Sage ISBN 0803975015 References

Book focuses on the minutiae of preparing for interviews, analysing transcripts, comparing of cases, and writing-up the results.

2.68.38   Wilson, K., Roe, B. & Wright, L. (1998) Telephone or face-to-face interviews?: a decision made on the basis of a pilot study. *International Journal of Nursing Studies* 35 (6) December 314–21   16 References

Five key considerations may be key factors in deciding whether to use telephone or face-to-face interviews for survey work. These are response rates, ability to produce representative samples, effects on interview schedule design, quality of responses and implementation problems. These issues were then applied to the experiences of the researchers conducting a study on continence care. Pilot interviews explored both interview modes and the main study used telephone interviews. Ideas in this discussion are supported and challenged by reference to other literature and the success of the decision to use telephone interviews in the main study is evaluated and recommendations are made (CR 2.22, 2.23, 2.52, 2.70).

2.68.39   Wimpenny, P. & Gass, J. (2000) Interviewing in phenomenology and grounded theory: is there a difference? *Journal of Advanced Nursing* 31 (6) 1485–92   48 References

Paper explores the differences and similarities that may exist in respect of using the interview method in phenomenological and grounded theory methodologies. A discussion of the interview is developed from both theoretical perspectives (CR 2.45, 2.49).

2.69   INTERVIEW – FOCUS GROUP

'The focus group is a discussion-based interview that produces a particular type of qualitative data. ... Its roots are in sociology ... [but] its methodological evolution is attributable ... to marketing consultants. In that domain it has largely evolved as a "quick and dirty" means of fulfilling client needs rather than as a sophisticated research tool. ... Focus groups can enhance the ability of researchers to answer specific questions but need to be rigorously conducted.' (Millward, in Breakwell, Hammond & Fife-Schaw, 2000: 304) [Adapted]

Definition [See Appendix D for source]

Focus group – a small group of individuals drawn together to express views on a specific set of questions in a group environment

Example

Ross, M.M., Carswell, A., Hing, M., Hollingworth, G. & Dalziel, W.B. (2001) Seniors' decision making about pain management. *Journal of Advanced Nursing* 35 (3) 442–51   71 References

Study investigated seniors' decision making regarding the management and control of their musculoskeletal pain. Focus groups and a mail-back questionnaire were used for data collection and results are reported (CR 2.75).

Annotations

2.69.1   Barboor, R.S. & Kitzinger, J. (eds) (1999) *Developing focus groups research: politics, theory and practice.* London: Sage ISBN 0761955682   References

Book casts a critical eye over focus group research and suggests ways forward in harnessing this versatile and powerful method. Areas discussed are the input of context of data, combining focus groups and interviews, and their use for sensitive topics – feminist research, social research, minority groups, organizational change and community views. Issues in analysing material, presenting data, ethical issues and the politics involved are all discussed (CR 2.10, 2.17, 2.68, 2.86, 2.94).

2.69.2   Bloor, M., Frankland, J., Thomas, M. & Robson, K. (2000) *Focus groups in social research*. London: Sage ISBN 076195743X References

Book addresses the key issues and practical requirements of the social researcher, namely, the kinds of social research issue for which focus groups are most or least suitable, optimum size group and composition and the designing of focusing exercises, facilitation and appropriate analysis.

2.69.3   Catterall, M. & Maclaren, P. (1997) Focus group data and qualitative analysis programs: coding the moving picture as well as snapshots. *Sociological Research Online* 2 (1)   63 References www.socresonline.org.uk/socresonline/2/1/6.html (Accessed 14/11/03)

Literature on the analysis of focus group data is reviewed. This showed that important communication and learning also takes place during this method of data collection (CR 2.86).

2.69.4   Fern, E.F. (2001) *Advanced focus group research*. Thousand Oaks, CA: Sage ISBN 0761912495   References

Written for researchers and students with a fundamental knowledge of focus group research. Numerous examples of what researchers should and should not do in designing their own research projects are given.

2.69.5   Goldman, K.D. & Schmalz, K.J. (2001) Tools of the trade. Focus on focus groups. *Health Promotion Practice* 2 (1) 14–18   3 References

Provides a definition and the attributes of focus groups and identifies nine steps in conducting focus group research. Indicates further reading.

2.69.6   Greenbaum, T.L. (1998) *The handbook for focus group research* (2nd edition). Thousand Oaks, CA: Sage   ISBN 0761912533   References

Provides the latest information on conducting focus groups. New chapters discuss the technology revolution with particular reference to video-conferencing and the Internet, the need to understand the major differences between focus group research in different countries and how to make comparisons. Its weaknesses are also discussed.

2.69.7   Greenbaum, T.L. (2000) *Moderating focus groups: a practical guide for group facilitation*. Thousand Oaks, CA: Sage   ISBN 0761920447 References

This comprehensive guide covers everything form pre-session participant recruitment to post-session reporting. New and advanced techniques are provided, including those for managing group dynamics, energizing a tired group, projective techniques, personality association and position fixing (CR 2.2, 2.73).

2.69.8   Horner, S.D. (2000) Focus on research methods. Using focus group methods with middle school children. *Research in Nursing & Health* 23 (6) 510–17   29 References

Paper discusses the suitability of using the focus group method with middle school children, and describes application of the method for gaining insight into their perspectives on health and illness. The weaknesses of the method are described when used in this particular context.

2.69.9   Jackson, P. (1998) Focus group interviews as a methodology. *Nurse Researcher* 6 (1) 72–84   27 References

Article identifies the nature of focus groups and the key issues related to their use. The strengths and weaknesses, issues of reliability and validity, factors that influence the degree of disclosure and the diversity of uses for focus groups are all examined. Analysis of data is also discussed.

2.69.10   Kennedy, C., Kools, S. & Krueger, R. (2001) Methodological considerations in children's focus groups. *Nursing Research* 50 (3) 184–7   12 References

Discusses the use of child subjects in focus groups and highlights methodological considerations with particular attention to the integration of developmental principles.

2.69.11   Kidd, P.S. & Parshall, M.B. (2000) Getting the focus and the group: enhancing analytical rigor in focus group research. *Qualitative Health Research* 10 (3) 293–308   67 References

Author describes analytical challenges inherent in the interpretation of focus group data, and suggests approaches for enhancing the rigour of analysis and the reliability and validity of focus group findings (CR 2.24, 2.25).

2.69.12   Krueger, R.A. & Casey, M.A. (2000) *Focus groups: a practical guide for applied research* (3rd edition). Thousand Oaks, CA: Sage ISBN 0761920714   References

Book provides a comprehensive text to the use of focus group techniques. A new chapter compares and contrasts market research, academic, non-profit and participatory approaches to focus group research. Planning, procedures and analysing material are discussed. Also included are examples of questions that ask how to do more than just discuss and suggestions on how to answer questions about the quality of this method.

2.69.13　Lane, P., McKenna, H., Ryan, A.A. & Fleming, P. (2001) Focus group methodology. *Nurse Researcher: The International Journal of Research Methodology in Nursing and Health Care* 8 (3) 45–59　58 References

Authors offer a critique of the practical application of focus group methodology in exploring the needs and experiences of informal carers of older people in Ireland.

2.69.14　McDougall, P. (1999) Focus groups: an overview of their use as a research method. *Community Practitioner* 72 (3) 48–9　17 References

Gives an overview of focus groups as a research method. Its usefulness and application in a research project are considered, together with potential strengths and weaknesses.

2.69.15　Morgan, D.L. (1997) *Focus groups as qualitative research* (2nd edition). Thousand Oaks, CA: Sage　ISBN 0761903437　References

Book gives an updated view of current social science approaches to focus groups. They are compared with interviews and their strengths and weaknesses are described. Suggestions are made for planning, conducting and analysing these data.

2.69.16–2.69.22　Morgan, D.L. & Krueger, R.A. (1997) *Focus group kit*. Thousand Oaks, CA: Sage　ISBN 0761907602　6 Volumes

The following entry differs in format as it documents a series of 6 volumes. The annotation includes the whole series.

2.69.17　Krueger, R.A. (1997) *Developing questions for focus groups*. Volume 3　ISBN 0761908196

2.69.18　Krueger, R.A. (1997) *Moderating focus groups*. Volume 4　ISBN 0761908218

2.69.19　Krueger, R.A. (1997) *Involving community members in focus groups*. Volume 5　ISBN 076190820X

2.69.20　Krueger, R.A. (1997) *Analyzing and reporting focus group results*. Volume 6　ISBN 0761908161

2.69.21　Morgan, D.L. (1997) *The focus group guidebook*. Volume 1　ISBN 0761908188

2.69.22　Morgan, D.L. (1997) *Planning focus groups*. Volume 2　ISBN 076190817X

This kit provides information on running successful focus groups, from the initial planning stages to asking questions, the final analysis of data to the reporting of findings.

2.69.23　Morrison-Beedy, D., Cote-Arsenault, D. & Feinstein, N.F. (2001) Maximizing results with focus groups: moderator and analysis issues. *Applied Nursing Research* 14 (1) February 48–53 References

Advice is given on how to maximize the collection of high-quality data by paying specific attention to the selection and training of the moderator, the development of the interview guide and the analysis that addresses intra-group and inter-group processes.

2.69.24　Suter, E.A. (2000) Focus groups in ethnography of communication: expanding topics of enquiry beyond participant observation. *The Qualitative Report* 5 (1/2) 12 pages　30 References www.nova.edu/ssss/QR/QR5-1/suter.html (Accessed 14/11/03)

Poses the view that participant observation is not always the most productive method for ethnographic research and suggests focus groups as an alternative when observation fails to yield appropriate data (CR 2.42, 2.72).

2.69.25　Vaughn, S., Schumm, J.S. & Sinagub, J.M. (1996) *Focus group interviews in education and psychology*. Thousand Oaks, CA: Sage　ISBN 0803958935　References

Book covers all aspects of conducting focus groups in educational and psychological settings. Areas covered are how to prepare for a focus group, creating a moderator's guide, selecting a setting and analysing results. A chapter is included on focus groups with children.

2.69.26　Vissandjée, B., Abdool, S.N. & Dupéré, S. (2002) Focus groups in rural Gujarat, India: a modified approach. *Qualitative Health Research* 12 (6) 826–43　16 References

Describes the need for culturally competent focus groups and how this might be achieved by awareness of geographic, political, economic and socio-cultural knowledge of the research area. Makes recommendations for future studies, using rural India as an example.

2.69.27　Webb, B. (2002) Using focus groups as a research method: a personal experience. *Journal of Nursing Management* 10 (1) 27–35　33 References

Using an example from personal experience, the benefits of using a qualitative research methodology and focus group methods are outlined. The practicalities of using and facilitating groups are explained, and strengths and challenges of the method are discussed (CR 2.36).

2.69.28　Webb, C. & Kevern, J. (2001) Focus groups as a research method: a critique of some aspects of their use in nursing research. *Journal of Advanced Nursing* 33 (6) 798–805   47 References

Paper evaluates and critiques reports in the nursing literature between 1990 and 1999 of the use of focus groups as a research method. Problems identified in the literature are discussed and the authors believe that there should be more in-depth consideration at the research planning stages of the underlying assumptions of methodological approaches that may be used to underpin focus group research, and methods to be used to analyse and report the data generated (CR 2.12, 2.45, 2.49, 2.86).

2.69.29   Williams, R.D. (1999) Use of focus groups with rural women of lower socio-economic status. *Applied Nursing Research* 12 (1) 45–50   28 References

Describes the use of focus groups in studies of low income, rural populations.

2.70   INTERVIEW – TELEPHONE

Telephone interviews are one of the tools, used particularly in market research, to ascertain people's views on a wide range of topics, for example customer services provided by a particular company, or aspects of health care. New developments in this field include the use of computer-assisted and direct computer interviewing.

Definition [See Appendix D for source]

Telephone interview – questioning by telephone

Example

Chapple, A. (1999) The use of telephone interviewing for qualitative research. *Nurse Researcher* 6 (3) 85–93   12 References

Reports a study that used telephone interviewing as a follow-up method after patients had initially sought advice about the treatment of thrush from community pharmacists. The technical aspects involved are discussed, and the author recommends using this type of data collection if the population is geographically dispersed (CR 2.36).

Annotations

2.70.1   Anderson, J.C., Nelson, D.E. & Wilson, R.W. (1998) Telephone coverage and measurement of health risk indicators: data from the national health interview survey. *American Journal of Public Health* 88 (9) 1392–5   18 References

Study compared health behaviour variables for all US households and those with telephones to measure the potential impact of telephone coverage on estimates from telephone surveys. Telephone non-coverage effects appeared to be small, supporting the use of this type of survey for health risk behaviour surveillance with most population groups (CR 2.52, 2.90).

2.70.2   Barriball, K.L., Christian, S.L., While, A.E. & Bergen, A. (1996) The telephone survey method: a discussion paper. *Journal of Advanced Nursing* 24 (1) 115–21   36 References

Gives an account of strategies employed to recruit a study sample, minimize non-response and bias, and ensure sound practices during data collection. Suggestions are made for further work (CR 2.22, 2.27).

2.70.3   de Bortoli Cassiani, S.H., Zanett, M.L. & Pela, N.T.R. (1992) The telephone survey: a methodological strategy for obtaining information. *Journal of Advanced Nursing* 17 (5) 576–81   7 References

Reports some methodological considerations in a study that aimed to assess the level of knowledge about existing nursing schools in Brazil.

2.70.4   de Leeuw, E.D. (1994) Computer-assisted data collection, data quality and costs: a taxonomy and annotated bibliography. *Bulletin de methodologie Sociologique* 44 60–72   References

Includes a taxonomy on different forms of computerized interviewing. The influence on data quality and costs are discussed (CR 2.84).

2.70.5   Frey, J.H. (1989) *Survey research by telephone* (2nd edition). Beverly Hills, CA: Sage   ISBN 0803929854   References

The history of telephone interviewing is outlined and comparisons are made with mail and face-to-face methods. Sampling procedures and question wording are discussed, and techniques are suggested for administering and implementing this method of data collection. Ethical issues are discussed, together with the future of telephone surveys (CR 2.17, 2.22, 2.52, 2.68).

2.70.6   Groves, R.M., Biemer, P., Lyberg, L.E., Massey, J., Nicholis, W.L. & Waksberg, J. (eds) (2001) *Telephone survey methodology*. New York: Wiley   ISBN 0471209562   References

Noted survey experts present recent developments in telephone survey techniques from around the world, including trends in covering household populations, effects due to mode of data collection, and the state of the art in technology. The use of computer-assisted telephone interviewing is discussed, together with in-depth reviews of the literature (CR 2.12, 2.85).

2.70.7 Korner-Bitensky, N. & Wood-Dauphinee, S. (1995) Barthel Index information elicited over the telephone: is it reliable? *American Journal of Physical Medicine and Rehabilitation* 74 (1) 9–18 20 References

Reports a study that examined the comparability of estimates of functional status elicited through both telephone and face-to-face interviews. The index, a commonly used instrument for assessing the activities of daily living, was administered to 366 individuals over the telephone and at home with both health professionals and trained lay interviewers being used. Results showed that, with the exception of a small sub-group of patients, functional status could be elicited reliably over the telephone by both lay people and health professionals (CR 2.69).

2.70.8 Lavrakas, P.J. (1993) *Telephone survey methods: sampling, selection and supervision* (2nd revised edition). Beverly Hills, CA: Sage   ISBN 0803953062   References

Three major elements of telephone survey techniques are explored in depth: generating and processing telephone survey sampling pools, selecting a respondent and securing co-operation, and structuring the work of interviewers and supervisors. Contains a glossary of terms relevant to this method (CR 2.2).

2.70.9 Minnick, A., Roberts, M.J., Young, W.B., Kleinpell, R.M. & Micek, W. (1995) An analysis of post-hospitalisation telephone survey data. *Nursing Research* 44 (6) 371–5   9 References

Reports on some methodological aspects of a study in which 4,600 adults were interviewed by telephone after hospitalization. Response rate differences and reasons for non-participation by gender, age, ethnicity and race are highlighted. Other issues discussed are understanding and reporting response rates, reducing losses due to ineligibility, dealing with refusals and tailoring approaches to special populations (CR 2.22).

2.71   LIFE HISTORY/BIOGRAPHY

Life histories may provide nurses with valuable 'inside' information about an individual for whom they may be caring, or wish to invite to co-operate in a research programme. Although the information gained will be 'subjective' in nature, it will nevertheless give valuable insights into the views of the patient or client about their experiences. Perhaps too often researchers impose structure upon their data gathering that can 'hide' the realities that respondents need to express.

Definitions [See Appendix D for sources]

Biographical method – that combination of research approaches which draws upon life stories, life histories, case studies, oral histories, personal narrations and self-stories

Biography – a written account of a person's life

Interpretative biography – ... a form of biography that is based on the author being present in the study and open recognition that biographical writing is, in part, autobiographical of the author

Life history – a narrative self-report about a person's life experiences regarding some theme of interest to the researcher

Self-report – an indirect method for assessing health status

Example

Glass, N., Taylor, B., Stirling, K. & McFarlane, J. (1999) Making a difference with dying people: positive nurse–patient interactions. *Contemporary Nurse: A Journal for the Australian Nursing Profession* 8 (4) 159–65   19 References

Paper presents some qualitative findings from a study that examined the nature and effects of palliative nursing care for patients. Data were collected through story-telling with patients relating their own experiences. Results are reported and discussion is included about the potential ethical problems of assessing patients' suitability for research (CR 2.17, 2.22).

Annotations

2.71.1 Atkinson, R. (1998) *The life story interview*. Thousand Oaks, CA: Sage ISBN 076190428X   References

Volume provides guidelines and suggestions for carrying out a life-story interview. In addition to putting it into context, advice is given on planning, conducting the interview, and dealing with issues of transcribing and interpreting the data. A sample life-story interview is included (CR 2.68).

2.71.2 Denzin, N.K. (1989) *Interpretive biography*. Newbury Park, CA: Sage   ISBN 0803933592 References

Book links post-modernism and interpretative social science to re-examine the biographical and autobiographical genres and shows a new way in which biographies can be conceptualized and shaped (CR 2.42).

2.71.3   Dex, S. (ed.) (1991) *Life and work history analyses: qualitative and quantitative developments*. London: Routledge   ISBN 0415053382   2 References

Book examines a growing interest in the collection of life and work histories and discusses methods of analysing these data. Each paper takes a specific research topic and many common questions are answered. New concepts and methods of handling these data are reported (CR 2.9).

2.71.4   Entwhistle, V. & Tritter, J.Q. (2002) Researching experiences of cancer: the importance of methodology. *European Journal of Cancer Care* 11 (3) 232–7   21 References

Focuses on the use of self-report methods to investigate experiences of cancer and cancer care. Highlights the challenges of using this method both pragmatically and contextually.

2.71.5   Gabriel, Y. (1998) The use of stories. In Symon, G. & Cassell, C. (eds) *Qualitative methods and analysis in organizational research: a practical guide*. London: Sage   ISBN 0761953515   Chapter 8 135–60   55 References

Author argues that stories open up valuable windows into the emotional and symbolic lives of organizations, offering researchers a powerful instrument. Chapter describes how field research on stories may be conducted and how the material generated may be classified and analysed (CR 2.36.135).

2.71.6   Giele, J.Z. & Elder, J.H. Jr (eds) (1998) *Methods of life-course research: qualitative and quantitative approaches*. Thousand Oaks, CA: Sage ISBN 0761914374   References

Discusses the most effective methods for doing life-course research, the art and method of appropriate research designs, the collection of data and the search for meaningful patterns within it (CR 2.9, 2.21, 2.64).

2.71.7   Grady, K.E. & Wallston, B.S. (eds) (1988) Self-report and other reports. In Authors *Research in health care settings*. Newbury Park, CA: Sage   ISBN 0803928742 Chapter 7 101–16 References

Chapter explores where self-report may be appropriate, gives examples and discusses possible biases (CR 2.27).

2.71.8   Hayes, D. (2001) Reflections on the meaning of 'non-participation' in research. *Research in Education* 65 20–30   37 References

Discusses some of the problems of non-participation in a study of teacher involvement in decision-making. The concept of non-participation, earning trust, data collection, informal exchanges, influence of the researcher's presence and validity of the study are all considered.

2.71.9   Johnstone, M. (1999) Reflective topical autobiography: an under-utilized interpretive research method in nursing. *Collegian: Journal of the Royal College of Nursing, Australia* 6 (1) 24–9 31 References

Reflective topical autobiography (an autobiographical method) belongs to the genre of testimonial research and is located within the post-positive interpretative research paradigm. It is used by researchers in the human and literary disciplines, but remains largely unknown in nursing research domains. Author believes that it is an important research method in its own right, and could make a major contribution to advancing nursing inquiry and knowledge.

2.71.10   Josselson, R. (ed.) (1996) *Ethics and process in the narrative study of lives*. London: Sage   ISBN 0761902376   References

The emphasis in this book is studying what happens after narratives have been obtained, how experts try to understand the material, re-narrate it for their own ends and assess the impact this may have on those involved. The 18 essays are addressed mainly from a psychological perspective (CR 2.17).

2.71.11   Miller, R.L. (2000) *Researching life stories and family histories*. London: Sage   ISBN 0761960929   References

Book covers methods and issues involved in collecting and analysing family and life histories. Three main approaches are discussed: realist, neo-positivist and narrative. Extensive exercises are also included (CR 2.36).

2.71.12   Musson, G. (1998) Life histories. In Symon, G. & Cassell, C. (eds) *Qualitative methods and analysis in organizational research: a practical guide*. London: Sage   ISBN 0761953515   Chapter 2 10–27   39 References

Chapter gives some background to the development of the life-history technique, followed by an analysis of its relevance to organizational research, and some examples of its application in case studies drawn from doctoral research. The chapter concludes by evaluating the usefulness of the approach and summarizing the circumstances in which it might best be used (CR 2.36.135).

2.71.13 Plummer, K. (2000) *Documents of life 2: an invitation to critical humanism* (2nd edition). London: Sage   ISBN 0761961321   References

This classic text championed the use of life stories and other personal documents in social research. Recent developments are included in this new edition, including the emergence of an auto/biographical society, writing and narrative, memory and truth, and humanism.

2.71.14 Roberts, B. (2002) *Biographical research*. Buckingham: Open University Press   ISBN 0335202861   References

Book examines the methodological and theoretical developments associated with research on lives in sociology, oral history, ethnography, biography and narrative analysis. Numerous examples are included for illustration (CR 2.42, 2.47, 2.89).

2.71.15 Scott, D. (2000) Biography and autobiography. In Author *Realism and educational research*. London: Routledge/Falmer   ISBN 0750709189   Chapter 8 95–111   References

Chapter discusses the complex interactional activity of individuals and groups, all seeking to create and recreate themselves in the context of lives that are continually undergoing transformation (CR 2.6.8).

2.71.16 Slim, H., Thompson, P., Bennett, O. & Cross, N. (1998) Ways of listening. In Perks, R. & Thomson, A. *The oral history reader*. London: Routledge   ISBN 0415133521   Part 2 Chapter 10 114–25   19 Notes and References

Discusses different types of interview, props and mnemonics and visual techniques which may be used during oral history inquiries (CR 2.47.18).

2.72   OBSERVATION

'Observation is one of the major methods by which data are gathered and is particularly appropriate for complex research situations. These may be viewed as complete entities and would be difficult to measure either as a whole or separately.' (Fox, 1982: 197)

Definitions [See Appendix D for sources]

Non-participant observation – observer watches and records but does not participate as a member of the group of study subjects being observed

Observation – a method of collecting data in which the researcher scientifically watches and records pertinent information

Participant observation – observer watches, collects and records data while interacting with the group of study subjects as a member of the group

Structured observation – when using structured observation techniques, the researcher identifies beforehand which behaviours are to be observed and recorded

Unobtrusive measure – ... a method of making observations without the knowledge of those being observed

Unstructured observation – the collection of descriptive information through direct observation, whereby the observer is guided by some general research questions but does not follow a pre-specified plan for observing, enumerating, or recording the information

Vignettes – consist of text, images or other forms of stimuli to which research participants are asked to respond

Example

Gerdtz, M.F. & Bucknall, T.K. (2001) Triage nurses' clinical decision making: an observational study of urgency assessment. *Journal of Advanced Nursing* 35 (4) 550–61   38 References

Paper reports a structured observational study that aimed to describe the data triage nurses collect from patients, using the Australasian Triage Scale, and the duration of their decision-making. It also explored the impact of patient and nurse variables on the duration of this decision-making in a clinical setting. Findings are reported.

Annotations

2.72.1 Andersen, C. & Adamsen, L. (2001) Continuous video recording: a new clinical research tool for studying the nursing care of cancer patients. *Journal of Advanced Nursing* 35 (2) 257–67   47 References

Reports the use of continuous videorecording around the patient–nurse interaction during pulsed dose rate brachytherapy. Authors believe that using videorecording as a research tool can document accurately interaction and behaviour between cancer patients and nursing staff. It discloses examples of both eminent and negligent nursing care and as such can be a useful tool for instruction and future research. The credibility, validity and limitations of using videorecordings are discussed.

2.72.2 Barter, C. & Renold, E. (1999) The use of vignettes in qualitative research. *Social Research Update* Issue 25 Guildford: University of Surrey, Department of Sociology 19 References www.soc.surrey.ac.uk/sru/SRU25.html (Accessed 14/11/03)

Identifies the purposes of vignettes, their use within the qualitative paradigm, methodological challenges and their implementation.

2.72.3 Berman, H., Ford-Gilboe, M., Moutrey, B. & Cekic, S. (2001) Portraits of pain and promise: a photographic study of Bosnian youth. *Canadian Journal of Nursing Research* 32 (4) 21–41 39 References

Paper presents the results of a study with seven Bosnian children, aged 11–14, who went to Canada as refugees in 1990 following the Balkans war. The everyday challenges and struggles faced by this group were explored using an innovative research method called photo novella. A secondary purpose was to evaluate the merits and limitations of photo novella as a method for capturing children's perspectives and feelings. Participants were given disposable cameras and asked to take pictures of important people, places and events. These were then explored through a dialogic process the researchers called phototalk. Results and the implications for nurses are discussed.

2.72.4 Bonner, A. & Tolhurst, G. (2002) Insider-outsider perspectives of participant observation. *Nurse Researcher: The International Journal of Research Methodology in Nursing and Health Care* 9 (4) 7–19 33 References

Authors give personal accounts of their experiences in conducting research involving participant observation. Issues discussed include the advantages and disadvantages of nurse researchers as insiders and outsiders. Strategies are suggested to overcome both researcher effect and participant response to the researcher (CR 2.16, 3.16).

2.72.5 Elder, J.H. (1999) Clinical methods: videotaped behavioural observations: enhancing validity and reliability. *Applied Nursing Research* 12 (4) 206–9 8 References

Author identifies several problems commonly encountered while studying behaviour in natural settings, and suggests methods for enhancing validity and reliability through videotaped observations. Results of a newly developed calibration procedure are discussed with implications for rater training. This information should be useful for evaluating interventions in applied settings (CR 2.24, 2.25).

2.72.6 Emmison, M. & Smith, P. (2000) Researching the visual: images, objects, contexts and interactions in social and cultural inquiry. London: Sage ISBN 0761958460 References

Book provides students with a comprehensive introduction to the field of visual research. This includes photographic images, the analysis of everyday objects, places and forms of social interactions. The relevance of leading theorists, such as Foucault, Bourdieu, Goffman and Hall, are discussed and numerous exercises are provided.

2.72.7 Harrison, B. (2002) Seeing health and illness worlds – using visual methodologies in a sociology of health and illness: a methodological review. *Sociology of Health and Illness* 24 (6) 856–72 72 References

Analyses the potential value of a visual approach to data collection and assesses the advantages and disadvantages. Draws upon studies that have utilized a visual methodology, including examples of painting, drawing, photography and video.

2.72.8 Hayes, D. (2001) Reflections on the meaning of 'non-participation' in research. *Research in Education* 65 May 20–30 37 References

Discusses some lessons learnt during a two-year ethnographic study of teacher involvement in decision-making at a time of rapid change.

2.72.9 Hughes, R. & Huby, M. (2002) The application of vignettes in social and nursing research. *Journal of Advanced Nursing* 37 (4) 382–6 40 References

Paper reviews the potential for, and limitations of, the use of vignettes in research that seeks an understanding of people's attitudes, perceptions and beliefs in health care. The differences between vignettes and real-life processes are addressed, and some of the practical advantages and pitfalls of using vignettes are discussed (CR 2.29, 2.36).

2.72.10 Jorgensen, D.L. (1989) *Participant observation: a methodology for human studies.* Newbury Park, CA: Sage ISBN 0803928777

Book is an introduction to the basic principles and strategies of participant observation for students and the more experienced researcher. Sections cover methodology, the process of defining a problem, gaining entry to a setting, participating in everyday life, and developing and sustaining relationships. Observing and gathering information, keeping notes, records and files, analysing and theorizing, leaving the field and communicating the results are also discussed (CR 2.18).

2.72.11 Kennedy, C. (1999) Participant observation as a research tool in a practice-based profession. *Nurse Researcher* 7 (1) 56–65 19 References

Paper offers a personal account of the use of participant observation for exploring and uncovering the knowledge base of experienced district nurses in relation to first assessment visits. The rationale for using this technique, the issues relating to adopting the role of observer, and its strengths as a method for nursing research are analysed (CR 2.16, 3.16).

2.72.12   Kite, K. (1999) Participant observation, peripheral observation or apart-icipant observation? *Nurse Researcher* 7 (1) 44–55   9 References

Describes some of the many difficulties involved in 'doing' participant observation when studying the intensive care unit as a learning environment for registered nurses (CR 2.16).

2.72.13   Lomax, H. & Casey, N. (1998) Recording social life: reflexivity and video methodology. *Sociological Research Online* 3 (2)   www. socresonline.org.uk/socresonline/3/2/1.html (Accessed 31/01/03)

Explores the academic debate related to the use of video recordings as valid research data. Authors believe that video-generated data is an ideal resource in as far as it can provide a faithful record of the process as an aspect of the naturally occurring interaction which comprises the research topic (CR 2.25, 2.42, 2.72, 2.89).

2.72.14   McGarvey, H.E., Chambers, M.G. & Boore, J. (1999) Collecting data in the operating department: issues in observational methodology. *Intensive and Critical Care Nursing* 15 (5) October 288–97   References

The UK literature contains few references to nursing in the operating department and even fewer for researching nursing in what is a complex and stressful environment. Paper focuses on some of the key issues that occurred during one study where an observational methodology was used. Authors suggest that observation is an important component of contextual investigation and requires careful planning and preparation. Sensitivity and skill are required for this role in stressful environments.

2.72.15   Moore, L. & Savage, J. (2002) Participant observation, informed consent and ethical approval. *Nurse Researcher: The International Journal of Research Methodology in Nursing and Health Care* 9 (4) 58–69   14 References

Paper outlines the specific dilemmas raised by participant observation in one practice setting. The difficulties experienced in complying with a predetermined process designed for gaining fully informed consent are discussed. The authors believe that researchers need to be flexible in responding to circumstances as they arise in the field (CR 2.17).

2.72.16   Mulhall, A. (2003) In the field: notes on observation in qualitative research. *Journal of Advanced Nursing* 41 (3) 306–13   36 References

Paper discusses the importance of unstructured observation as a research method, and critically examines the problems associated with both access and field notes (CR 2.36).

2.72.17   Mwanga, J.R., Mugashe, C.L., Magnussen, P., Gabone, R.M. & Aagaard-Hansen, J. (1998) Pearls, pith and provocation. Experience from video-recorded focus group discussions on schistosomiasis in Magu, Tanzania. *Qualitative Health Research* 8 (5) 707–17   19 References

Video-recorded focus group discussions were conducted to explore common perceived illnesses in a rural community co-endemic for urinary and intestinal schistosomiasis in Magu District, Tanzania. The methodological experience with video is discussed in detail, with recommendations for observing methodological triangulation when conducting qualitative health research to enhance the validity of data (CR 2.69).

2.72.18   Nason, J. & Golding, D. (1998) Approaching observation. In Symon, G. & Cassell, C. (eds) *Qualitative methods and analysis in organizational research: a practical guide*. London: Sage   ISBN 0761953515   Chapter 12 234–49   24 References

Authors challenge some of the assumptions underlying typical approaches to observation. They believe that rather than observation being seen as a separate category among a list of alternative research approaches, it might be conceived as consisting of processes which form part of other 'methods' too – from those as disparate as experimentation and modelling to the administering of postal questionnaires. This chapter reconfigures the problems of what constitutes observation in research through an exploration of alternative conceptions of the processes involved (CR 2.36.135).

2.72.19   Prosser, J. (ed.) (1998) *Image-based research: a source book for qualitative researchers*. London: Falmer Press   ISBN 075070649X References

Book gives a theoretical overview of image-based research, images in the research process and in practice (CR 2.36).

2.72.20   Radford, M.J. & Foody, J.M. (2001) How do observational studies expand the evidence base for therapy? *Journal of the American Medical Association* 286 (10) 1228–9

Explains the use of observation studies where it is not possible to undertake a randomized clinical trial and describes the use of propensity analysis in observational studies in order to eliminate potential methodological problems (CR 2.29).

2.72.21　Richman, J. & Mercer, D. (2002) The vignette revisited: evil and the forensic nurse. *Nurse Researcher: The International Journal of Research Methodology in Nursing and Health Care* 9 (4) 70–82　41 References

Article aims to define the vignette in research terms and briefly classifies the various types, according to the variability in their form and use. The author describes how the vignette was used within a secure psychiatric hospital to access some of the informal rules by which nursing staff constructed accounts of the mentally disordered offender (CR 2.36).

2.72.22　Rodriguez, N.M. & Ryave, A.I. (2002) *Systematic self-observation: a method for researching the hidden and elusive features of everyday social life*. Thousand Oaks, CA: Sage　ISBN 076192308X　References

Book describes this research method used by social scientists to gather information about those social actions that are hidden, restricted or subjective (CR 2.36).

2.72.23　Savage, J. (2000) Participant observation: standing in the shoes of others? *Qualitative Health Research* 10 (3) 324–39　62 References

Article argues that participant observation is more than mere method and is in need of greater theoretical attention. It discusses the nature and varieties of participant observation, participant observation as a methodology and its relationship to nursing, and the non-linguistic nature of knowledge from participation.

2.72.24　Spiers, J.A., Costantino, M. & Faucett, J. (2000) Video technology: use in nursing research. *AAOHN Journal* 48 (3) March 119–24　References

Discusses the uses of video technology as a research tool and the issues related to its credibility as a data collection method.

2.72.25　Spradley, J.P. (1980) *Participant observation*. New York: Holt, Rinehart & Winston　ISBN 003044501　References

Book describes the techniques of participant observation when carrying out ethnographic research. Part 1 defines ethnography, identifies assumptions and distinguishes it from other approaches. Part 2 discusses the 'Developmental Research Sequence', that is a series of 12 tasks designed to guide the reader through each stage of observations in ethnographic research (CR 2.42, 2.68.35).

2.72.26　Stiles, D. (1998) Pictorial representation. In Symon, G. & Cassell, C. (eds) *Qualitative methods and analysis in organizational research: a practical guide*. London: Sage　ISBN 0761953515　Chapter 10 190–210　27 References

Chapter explores the origins and use of pictorial representation as an innovative research technique for the exploration of organizational constructs. A background to the use of image and a note of its philosophical roots are also discussed. Some methods developed by the author are included to give the reader some methodological insight into the use of image in research (CR 2.36.135).

2.72.27　Stockdale, A. (2002) *Tools for digital recording in qualitative research*. Guildford: Department of Sociology, University of Surrey Social Research Update Issue 38　4 References www.soc.surrey.ac.uk/sru/SRU38.html　(Accessed 11/02/03)

The technology needed to make digital recordings of interviews and meetings for the purpose of qualitative research is described. The advantages of using digital audio technology and the technical background needed to make an informed choice of technology are outlined, and brief evaluations are given of the types of audio recorder currently available (CR 2.36, 2.68).

2.73　PROJECTIVE TECHNIQUES

'Projective techniques encompass many different measurement tools, devices, and strategies which may be used to examine fundamental aspects of psychological functioning.' (Waltz, Strickland & Lenz, 1984: 255)

Definition [See Appendix D for source]

Projective techniques – personality tests which are distinctive in that the subject has to respond to an ambiguous stimulus. In doing so the subject is supposed to reveal aspects of his personality such as needs, attitudes and unconscious desires

Example

Catterall, M. & Ibbotson, P. (2000) Using projective techniques in educational research. *British Educational Research Journal* 26 (2) 245–56　36 References

The various types of projective technique are described and their benefits and drawbacks are examined. A project, involving students completing a range of techniques, is used for illustration.

Annotations

2.73.1   Finch, A.J. (1993) Projective techniques. In Finch, A.J. & Belter, R.W. (eds) *Handbook of child and adolescent assessment*. Newton, MA: Allyn & Bacon   ISBN 0205145922   Part II Chapter 15 224–36   References

Describes the processes necessary when undertaking projective techniques.

2.73.2   Rabin, A.I. (1981) *Assessment with projective techniques: a concise introduction*. New York: Springer   ISBN 0826135501

Provides an introductory text to this range of techniques.

2.73.3   Semeonoff, B. (1976) *Projective techniques*. New York: Wiley   No ISBN   References and Bibliography

Describes the history of projective psychology and classifies the techniques.

2.74   Q METHODOLOGY

'Q methodology … is most often associated with quantitative analysis … but it is designed to examine elements which frequently engage the attention of the qualitative researcher interested in more than just life measured by the pound. It combines the strengths of both quantitative and qualitative research traditions.' (Brown, 1996: 561–2)

Definition [See Appendix D for source]

Q sort – a research method comprised of rank ordering objects by sorting, and then assigning numbers to the subsets for statistical purposes

Example

Aldrich, S. & Eccleston, C. (2000) Making sense of everyday pain. *Social Science and Medicine* 50 (11) 1631–41   47 References

A social constructionist analysis is reported of how sense is made of everyday pain. Q factor analysis is used within a critical framework as Q methodology. Eight factors or accounts were derived from 61 participants. Common to all accounts is the theme of how pain relates to self, and, in particular, whether pain can change self. Implications of this study in understanding the experience of 'abnormal' pain are discussed, as are possible new research routes.

Original text

Stephenson, W. (1953) *The study of behaviour: Q technique and its methodology*. Chicago, IL: University of Chicago Press   No ISBN

Annotations

2.74.1   Brown, S.R. *The history and principles of Q methodology in psychology and the social sciences*   facstaff.uww.edu/cottlec/Qarchive/Bps. htm (Accessed 07/03/03)

Restates the principles of Q methodology and contrasts it with earlier understandings in British psychology. The roots of the Q–R controversy, its current status, main principles and the future are all discussed.

2.74.2   Karim, K. (2001) Q methodology – advantages and the disadvantages of this research method. *Journal of Community Nursing* 15 (4) 8, 10   9 References

Describes how nurse researchers may use this technique, what it is and the advantages and disadvantages of the method.

2.74.3   McKeown, B. & Thomas, D. (1988) *Q methodology*. Newbury Park, CA: Sage   ISBN 0803927533   References

Covers the principles, techniques and procedures of the Q method.

2.74.4   qmethod.org   www.qmethod.org/sitemap. htm (Accessed 06/05/03)

The official website of the International Society for the Scientific Study of Subjectivity (ISSSS). It provides information and links to websites on many aspects of Q methodology.

2.74.5   Q Method Page www.rz.unibw-muenchen. de/~p41bsmk/qmethod/ (Accessed 12/02/03)

This website introduces Q methodology, lists software packages for the analysis of Q-sort data, and other Q resources on the World Wide Web.

2.74.6   WebQ   www.rz.unibw-muenchen.de/ ~p41bsmk/qmethod/webq/webdoc.htm (Accessed 20/02/03)

Paper discusses and demonstrates WebQ which is a JavaScript application for Q-sorting questionnaire items online.

2.75   QUESTIONNAIRE

'The humble questionnaire is probably the single most common research tool in the social sciences …

with the principle advantages being its apparent simplicity, versatility and low cost as a method of data gathering. ... Designing the perfect questionnaire is, however, probably impossible ... too many ... produced over the years have contained simple errors that have seriously undermined the value of the data collected.' (Fife-Schaw, in Breakwell, Hammond & Fife-Schaw, 2000: 158–9) [Adapted]

Definition [See Appendix D for source]

Questionnaire – a data collection technique consisting of a set of written items requesting a response from subjects

Example

Henderson, A. & Zernike, W. (2001) A study of the impact of discharge information for surgical patients. *Journal of Advanced Nursing* 35 (3) 435–41   29 References

Using written questionnaires and telephone interviews, this study aimed to establish whether the routine information surgical patients receive about the management of pain and wound care during hospitalization was sufficient for them to care for themselves after discharge. Findings are reported (CR 2.70).

Annotations

2.75.1   Bulmer, M. (ed.) (2003) *Questionnaires.* London: Sage   ISBN 0761971483   References   4 Volumes

This collection presents the ideas of leading authorities in the field to provide the researcher and student with a panoramic view of this area of social science research. It provides a complete guide to the key methodological issues on the collection of social data by means of asking people questions.

2.75.2   Drennan, J. (2003) Cognitive interviewing: verbal data in the design and pretesting of questionnaires. *Journal of Advanced Nursing* 42 (1) 57–63   28 References

Describes the process of cognitive interviewing and discusses its use in the reduction of sampling error and increase in response rates. Its use for validating questions is discussed and the author believes the method is useful where complex, sensitive and intrusive questions are employed (CR 2.22, 2.25, 2.68).

2.75.3   Gillham, B. (2000) *Developing a questionnaire.* London: Continuum   ISBN 0826447953   References

Book provides a guide to the successful design and implementation of questionnaires as a data collection method.

2.75.4   Hague, P. (1993) *Questionnaire design.* London: Kogan Page   ISBN 0749409177 References

Book is a comprehensive and practical guide to questionnaire design. Rules and principles are set out and numerous examples are included. The use of questionnaires, types, framing and examples of questions, layout and interviewer instructions are all discussed (CR 2.68).

2.75.5   Harkness, J.A., Schoua-Glusberg, A. & Pennell, B.-E. (1998) *Questionnaire translation and questionnaire design* www.jpsm.umd.edu/qdet/view.asp?SSN=342 (Accessed 01/04/03)

Paper sets out to illustrate the close connections between translation issues and questionnaire design, and to indicate how improving the design of survey translation procedures can change and improve questionnaire design. It includes the following elements: placing the growing need for translated instruments in a cross-national and within-country perspective; illustrating how current questionnaire design practice affects both the goals and products of questionnaire translation; the need for cross-disciplinary uptake and research; new advances in survey translation procedures and assessment; shifting the focus from how design impacts on translation to how translation can be used to inform and improve questionnaire design. It also outlines initiatives that are underway or needed to secure the place of translation in survey design.

2.75.6   Madu, C.N. (1998) An empirical assessment of quality: research considerations. *International Journal of Quality Science* 3 (4) 348–55   7 References

Paper focuses on the empirical study of quality as a whole and looks at the design of questionnaires, their administration, cross-country studies, questionnaire validation and testing, and interpretation of results.

2.75.7   McColl, E., Jacoby, A., Thomas, L., Soutter, J., Bamford, C., Steen, N., Thomas, R., Harvey, E., Garratt, A. & Bond, J. (2001) Design and use of questionnaires: a review of best practice applicable to surveys of health service staff and patients. *Health Technology Assessment* 5 (31) 256 pages

A selective, narrative review focusing on modes of administration, question wording and sequencing, and choice of response formats. Other themes of the review include questionnaire formatting and presentation and techniques for enhancing response rates.

2.75.8 Oppenheim, A.N. (2001) *Questionnaire design* (2nd edition). London: Continuum ISBN 0826451764 References

This classic text has been considerably expanded and revised and is now a general survey research handbook. New chapters are included on surveys, analytic and descriptive design, sampling, interviewing, questionnaire development, statistical analysis and pilot work (CR 2.22, 2.23, 2.52, 2.56, 2.68, 2.69, 2.70, 2.73).

2.75.9 Peterson, R.A. (2000) *Constructing effective questionnaires*. Thousand Oaks, CA: Sage ISBN 0761916415 References

Asking the right questions is at the heart of survey research. This text will show students and new researchers how to commission, conduct and evaluate research based on these questions (CR 2.52).

2.76 RECORDS/ARCHIVAL DATA

Records are a readily available and valuable source of data and may be found everywhere. Sources include government records and those kept by institutions and individuals.

Definitions [See Appendix D for sources]

Archival research – a method of studying organizations or societies, based on the collected records they have produced

Archives – primary material and results of empirical studies. It encompasses all technical areas in which procedures and historical social research are used

Records – compilations of writing, photographs and figures that individuals have collected

Example

Russell, D. (1997) An oral history project in mental health nursing. *Journal of Advanced Nursing* 26 (3) 489–95 24 References

This study produced material that would support, or challenge, the content of a piece of historical writing based largely on primary archival sources. It confirmed an assumption of the usefulness of oral history as a record (in addition to written documents), which enriches the descriptions of historical processes (CR 2.47, 2.90).

Annotations

2.76.1 Hill, M.R. (1993) *Archival strategies and techniques*. Newbury Park, CA: Sage ISBN 0803948255 References

Book aims to improve and increase the use of historical records in social research, in particular the use of records found in special collections. Practical and detailed advice is given in the form of contextual description and methodological advice.

2.76.2 Hodson, R. (1999) *Analyzing documentary accounts*. Thousand Oaks, CA: Sage ISBN 0761917438 References

Book shows how to use documentary works as data sources and how quantitative and qualitative analysis techniques can be combined. Reliability and validity issues are discussed, together with how to start statistical exploration once the data are assembled (CR 2.22, 2.24, 2.25, 2.42).

2.76.3 Iezzoni, L.I. (2002) Using administrative data to study persons with disabilities. *The Millbank Quarterly* 80 (2) 347–79 120 References

Identifies the types of administrative data that are recorded by health care systems, what they might be used for and the advantages and disadvantages of using this data.

2.76.4 Prior, L. (2002) *Using documents in social research*. London: Sage ISBN 0761957464 References

Provides an introduction to the use of documents as tools within social science research. Key features include: making students aware of the diversity of documents available; outlining the various strategies and debates that need to be considered in order to integrate the study of documents into a research project; and offering examples of where documents have been used within a wide variety of research contexts (CR 2.36).

2.76.5 Scott, J. (1992) *A matter of record: documentary sources in social research*. Cambridge: Polity Press ISBN 0745600700 References

Illustrates the diversity of documentary sources available for social research and discusses ways in which they may be used. Chapters cover social research and documentary sources, assessing sources, the official realm, public and private records, administrative routines and decisions. Explorations in official documents, the public sphere, mass communications and personal documents are all discussed.

2.76.6 Webb, E.J., Campbell, D.T., Schwartz, R.D. & Sechrest, L. (1999) *Unobtrusive measures* (revised edition). Thousand Oaks, CA: Sage ISBN 0761920129 References

Book builds on the previous edition to justify novel techniques of survey and archival research. Using illustrations, it authorizes and motivates ingenuity in obtaining information (CR 2.52).

2.77   REPERTORY GRID AND PERSONAL CONSTRUCT THEORY

Personal construct theory, which forms the basis of the repertory grid technique, stresses the importance of eliciting constructs of the subject rather than those supplied by a researcher. A construct is a way of viewing elements as alike or different, where the researcher provides these objects of study. These elements are then developed into a grid. The construct is examined and scores are generated.

Definitions [See Appendix D for sources]

Personal construct – a cover term for each of the ways in which a person attempts to perceive, understand, predict and control the world

Repertory grid – a series of judgements made by a person, using his or her constructs, on some aspect of the world

Example

Hopper, T.F. (2000) Personal construct psychology for developing reflective teaching in physical education: a story of decentering 'self' as teacher. *Avante* 6 (3) 46–56   24 References

Paper shows how the repertory grid process from personal construct psychology offers a tool to develop reflective thinking in a teacher preparation course.

Original texts

Kelly, G.E. (1955) *The psychology of personal constructs*. New York: Norton   No ISBN 2 Volumes

Kelly, G.E. (1963) *Theory of personality*. New York: Norton & Coy   ISBN 0393001520

Annotations

2.77.1   Bannister, D. (1981) Personal construct theory and research method. In Reason, P. & Rowan, J. (eds) *Human inquiry: a sourcebook of new paradigm research*. Chichester: Wiley ISBN 0471279358   Chapter 16 191–9   References

Outlines the personal construct theory developed by Kelly in the 1950s and discusses the use of the repertory grid technique as a tool in various psychological fields (CR 2.11.7).

2.77.2   Bannister, D. & Fransella, F. (1990) *Inquiring man: theory of personal constructs* (3rd revised edition). London: Routledge ISBN 0415034604   References

Book summarizes personal construct theory and reviews the research it has generated. It examines its value for psychologists and psychotherapists and challenges orthodox thinking.

2.77.3   Beail, N. (ed.) (1985) *Repertory grid technique and personal constructs: applications in clinical settings*. London: Croom Helm ISBN 0709932642   References

This collection of readings explores various applications of the repertory grid technique. Included are a brief introduction to the technique and sections covering construct systems, constructs and disability, evaluation of change, exploring relationships through grids, practical applications in education, constructs of handicap and a caveat on some aspects of validity (CR 2.25).

2.77.4   Brint Institute *Personal construct theory and repertory grid*   www.brint.com/PCT.htm (Accessed 22/02/03)

Website gives an overview of personal construct theory, a list of sites for resources on the theory, together with software programs and Internet links on repertory grids.

2.77.5   Cohen, L., Manion, L. & Morrison, K. (2000) Personal constructs. In Authors (eds) *Research methods in education* (5th edition). London: Routledge/Falmer ISBN 0415195411 Chapter 19 337–48   References

Chapter examines the method suggested by Kelly of eliciting constructs and assessing the mathematical relationships between them, i.e. the repertory grid technique. Its characteristics, 'elicited' versus 'provided' constructs, allocating elements to constructs, grid administration and analysis are all discussed. Its strengths and weaknesses are identified and examples are included (CR 2.1.20).

2.77.6 Fransella, F. & Bannister, D. (1977) *A manual for repertory grid technique*. London: Academic Press   ISBN 0122654560   References

Manual describes a technique developed from George Kelly's personal construct theory which aimed to 'look beyond words'. A variety of commonly used grid formats are discussed and the many difficulties that may be encountered are outlined. It offers advice on designing grids while also becoming aware of their limitations. Appendices contain an example of the use of grids and the first published annotated bibliography on grid usage.

2.77.7 Fransella, F. (ed.) (2003) *International handbook personal construct psychology*. Chichester: John Wiley & Sons   ISBN 0470847271   References

This handbook brings together, for the first time, a wide range of theories, research and practice that have grown out of Kelly's original concept. It provides a reference on what has been done and insights into how further applications can be made within psychology and psychotherapy, and also informs non-psychologists and those unfamiliar with Kelly's techniques of its usefulness and applicability in other disciplines.

2.77.8 Mazhindu, G.N. (1992) Using repertory grid research: methodology in nurse education and practice: a critique. *Journal of Advanced Nursing* 17 (5) 604–8   28 References

Paper defines and describes the repertory grid technique and evaluates its potential as a research tool in nurse education and practice. Its merits and limitations are discussed and suggestions made for developing the technique.

2.77.9 Neimeyer, G.J. & Neimeyer, R.A. (eds) (2002) *Advances in personal construct psychology: new directions and perspectives*. Westport, CT: Greenwood Press   ISBN 0275972941   References

Volume offers an authoritative review of leading scholarship in personal construct theory and related approaches. Critical appraisal of repertory grid measures, as well as new strategies for textual analysis, are discussed (CR 2.89).

2.77.10 O'Connor, K.P. & Blowers, G.H. (1996) *Personal construct psychology in the clinical context*. Ottawa: University of Ottawa Press   ISBN 0776604228

Discusses the resurgence of George Kelly's personal construct psychology (PCP), a unique comprehensive theory of personality and clinical practice. Authors demonstrate how PCP methods can be adapted for both evaluation and treatment purposes, and case examples are given.

2.77.11 Psychology of Personal Constructs Information Centre *Books on PCP* www.pcp-net.de/info/books.html (Accessed 23/02/03)

This list of books/papers in English, with a link to those in German, contains information on Kelly, the history of PCP, comprehensive texts and other edited books, introductions to repertory grid technique, conference reports, clinical psychology and related areas, development and education, and organization and business.

2.77.12 Ravenette, T. (2001) *Personal construct theory in educational psychology: a practitioner's view*. London: Whurr   ISBN 1861561210   References

Comprises a selection of papers by the author, representing the development over some 40 years of a psychological practice based on the relatively unknown personal construct theory of George Kelly.

2.77.13 Winter, D.A. (1992) *Personal construct psychology in clinical practice: theory, research and application*. London: Routledge   ISBN 0415005272   References

Book is intended for psychologists but contains many examples of clinical applications that would be of interest to nurses.

2.78   TALK/CONVERSATION/NARRATIVE

Talk is increasingly being recognized and used as a technique for obtaining information from research participants. Conversations are complex to analyse, but may yield data which can be of considerable value to researchers.

Definitions [See Appendix D for sources]

Conversation – an informal spoken exchange of thoughts and feelings

Discourse – ... written and spoken conversation and the thinking that underlies it

Narrative – an orderly, continuous account of an event or series of events

Storyline graph – ... a data collection technique ... introduced to visually display research participants' location, sequencing and evaluation of events

Talk – to converse by means of spoken language

Example

Svedlund, M., Danielson, E. & Norberg, A. (2001) Women's narratives during the acute phase of their myocardial infarction. *Journal of Advanced Nursing* 35 (2) 197–205   31 References

The study reports the narrated experiences of 10 women during their stay in a coronary care unit following a myocardial infarction. Three major themes are reported and discussed (CR 2.68, 2.71).

Annotations

2.78.1   Adelman, C. (ed.) (1981) *Uttering, muttering: collecting, using and reporting talk for social and educational research*. London: Grant McIntyre   ISBN 0862160421   References

Compilation of studies written by leading researchers that brings together the theory and practice of using talk in research. Details on how to gather, interpret and make use of talk in educational and cultural settings are given (CR 2.89).

2.78.2   Berger, A.A. (1996) *Narratives in popular culture, media, and everyday life*. London: Sage ISBN 0761903453   References

Book explores important narrative theorists and techniques. Key terms and concepts are discussed. Readers will be enabled to interpret narratives and make their analyses accessible (CR 2.2, 2.86, 2.89).

2.78.3   Carson, A. & Fairbairn, G. (2002) The whole story: towards an ethical research methodology. *Nurse Researcher: The International Journal of Research Methodology in Nursing and Health Care* 10 (1) 15–29   15 References

Authors believe that sharing and telling stories is a more professional and valid way of generating and developing new models of nursing practice than either simply qualitative or quantitative approaches. They believe it is both central to research and its dissemination, and can provide a way of helping researchers, educators and practitioners to share and develop together.

2.78.4   Clough, P. (2002) *Narratives and fictions in educational research*. Buckingham: Open University Press   ISBN 033520791X   References

Book sets out to locate narrative and fictional methods within the traditions of education research, exemplify the use of narrative in studies of educational and social settings and to explain the processes of composing narrative and fictional research. Five 'fictional' stories demonstrate the use of narrative in reporting research.

2.78.5   Czarniawska, B. (1998) *A narrative approach to organization*. London: Sage   ISBN 0761906630   References

Book guides the reader through the narrative approach to qualitative research, from setting up the fieldwork to writing up the research. The author demonstrates that narratives are still the main carriers of knowledge in all societies (CR 2.36).

2.78.6   Emden, C. (1998) Theoretical perspectives on narrative inquiry. *Collegian: Journal of the Royal College of Nursing, Australia* 5 (2) 30–5   11 References

Paper addresses the theoretical influences upon a particular narrative inquiry into nursing scholars and scholarship. Perspectives that relate to the notion of stories as 'imaginative constructions' and as 'cultural narratives' highlight the profound importance of stories as being individually and culturally meaningful. Reference is made to narrative inquiry from the nursing literature that lies within the broader context of phenomenology (CR 2.49, 2.89).

2.78.7   Frid, I., Öhlén, J. & Bergbom, I. (2000) On the use of narratives in nursing research. *Journal of Advanced Nursing* 32 (3) 695–703   49 References

Article deals with the narrative and its use in nursing care and research. Paul Ricoeur's narrative theory, with its dimensions of interpretation, time, action and ethics, is presented as a possible methodological basis. This narrative theory is examined and a nursing research approach to the narrative, based on the life-world, is suggested.

2.78.8   Gabriel, Y. (1998) The use of stories. In Symon, G. & Cassell, C. (eds) *Qualitative methods and analysis in organizational research: a practical guide*. London: Sage   ISBN 0761953515   Chapter 8 135–60   55 References

Author argues that stories open up valuable windows into the emotional and symbolic lives of organizations, offering researchers a powerful instrument. Chapter describes how field research on stories may be conducted and how the material generated may be classified and analysed (CR 2.36.135, 2.89).

2.78.9   Gilbert, K.R. (2002) Taking a narrative approach to grief research: finding meaning in stories. *Death Studies* 26 (3) 223–39   40 References

Describes the narrative approach, its implications for grief research and the use of this approach in pursuit of qualitative research. It includes identification of the roles of investigator and participant, selecting and gathering narratives, and strategies for data analysis (CR 2.36, 2.86, 2.89).

2.78.10   Josselson, R., Lieblich, A., Sharabany, R. & Wiseman, H. (1997) *Conversation as method: analyzing the relational world of people*

who were raised communally. Thousand Oaks, CA: Sage   ISBN 0761905138   References

Book explores a methodology evolving from people coming together to talk, listen and learn from one another. Four feminist scholars discuss different ways of knowing from both quantitative and qualitative perspectives (CR 2.6, 2.10, 2.29, 2.36, 2.89).

2.78.11   Josselson, R. & Lieblich, A. (1999) *Making meaning of narratives*. Thousand Oaks, CA: Sage   ISBN 0761903275   References

Volume provides guides for doing qualitative research, analysis of several autobiographies, hints on how to interpret what is *not* said in narrative interviews, discussion on how cultural meanings and values are transmitted across generations, and illustrations on the transformational power of stories (CR 2.36, 2.68, 2.71).

2.78.12   Kralik, D., Koch, T. & Brady, B.M. (2000) Pen-pals: correspondence as a method for data generation in qualitative research. *Journal of Advanced Nursing* 31 (4) 909–17   18 References

Reports a study that aimed to understand the impact of chronic illness on the lives of midlife women and examine the ways in which they adapted to, or tolerated, it. Corresponding with the researcher-generated data and issues relating to this innovative method of data collection are analysed. As the literature to guide this process is scarce, the authors describe the preparation phase in setting up the study, discuss some practical issues, share their experiences in generating narratives from dialogues and hear from the women themselves (CR 2.10).

2.78.13   Lieblich, A. & Josselson, R. (1997) *The narrative study of lives*. Thousand Oaks, CA: Sage   ISBN 0761903259   References

Book explores the challenges of performing narrative work in an academic setting. Specific topics are given for illustration and the use of narrative as an additional approach within a larger quantitative project is discussed (CR 2.29).

2.78.14   Lieblich, A., Tuval-Mashiach, R. & Zilber, T. (1998) *Narrative research: reading, analysis and interpretation*. Thousand Oaks, CA: Sage   ISBN 0761910433   References

Book introduces readers to four models of reading and interpreting a text: holistic-content, holistic-form, categorical-content and categorical-form reading. Two complete narratives are presented so that readers can compare the authors' interpretations against the text as well as analyse the stories on their own. Subsequent chapters provide readings, interpretations and analyses of the narrative data from the models (CR 2.89).

2.78.15   Vaz, K.M. (ed.) (1997) *Oral narrative research with black women: collecting treasures*. Thousand Oaks, CA: Sage   ISBN 0803974280   References

Book is a collection of studies by black women, based on interviews with black women, which give insight into the oral narrative research process. It gives examples of different techniques and approaches, providing a useful pedagogical tool for teachers (CR 2.47).

2.78.16   Wardhaugh, R. (1990) *How conversation works*. Oxford: Blackwell   ISBN 0631139397   References

Book discusses the structure of conversation and describes what happens when people talk to each other.

Data Analysis, Interpretation and Presentation

2.79 DATA MANAGEMENT AND ANALYSIS – GENERAL

'Data analysis consists of examining, categorizing, tabulating or otherwise re-combining the evidence, to address the initial propositions of a study.' (Yin, 1984: 99)

Definitions [See Appendix D for sources]

Analytic induction – ... [involves] the intensive examination of a strategically selected number of cases so as to empirically establish the causes of a specific phenomenon

Clinical significance – a result is said to be clinically significant if it is generally considered on clinical grounds to be important [A clinically significant result may or may not be statistically significant. Conversely, a statistically significant result may not be considered to be clinically significant]

Coding – the process of assigning numbers or categories to data or information

Data analysis – application of one or more techniques to a set of data for the purpose of discovering trends, differences or similarities. The type of technique used is guided by the subject matter of the problem

Non-parametric statistics – a set of statistical procedures that are not based on assumptions about population parameters, or the shape of the underlying population distribution. They are most often used when data are measures on the nominal or ordinal scales

Parametric statistics – statistical procedures for estimating population parameters, with assumptions about the distribution of variables and for use with interval or ratio measures

Raw data – observations as originally recorded, i.e. with no operations, transformations or recategorization performed on the numbers or values

Statistical significance – ... a result is said to be statistically significant at, say, the 5% level, this

means that you are 95% confident that the result did not occur by chance [See *clinical significance*]

Annotations

2.79.1 Birbili, M. (2000) Translating from one language to another. *Social Research Update* Issue 31 Guildford: University of Surrey, Department of Sociology 24 References www.soc.surrey.ac. uk/sru/SRU31.html (Accessed 14/11/03)

Discusses the factors affecting the translation of material from one language to another that include the quality of the translation and potential translation-related problems. Techniques for dealing with problems are discussed and also the need to make translation decisions explicit (CR 2.54, 2.64, 2.86, 2.87).

2.79.2 Bland, J.M. & Altman, D.G. (2000) Statistics notes: the odds ratio. *British Medical Journal* 320 (7247) 27 May 1468   3 References

Explains the purpose of the odds ratio in research reports and demonstrates how to calculate it using data from a cross-sectional study on children with asthma.

2.79.3 Bradley, W.J. & Schaefer, K.C. (1998) *The uses and misuses of data and models.* Thousand Oaks, CA: Sage   ISBN 0761909222   References

Book develops principles that can guide the use of data and models in the human sciences. Influences on information, measurement of human information and its limits in the social sciences, the nature of social science data, causality, models and policy-making are all discussed (CR 3.11).

2.79.4 Chen, P.Y. & Popovich, P.M. (2002) *Correlation: parametric and non-parametric measures.* Thousand Oaks, CA: Sage   ISBN 0761922288

After reading this book, the reader will be able to compare and distinguish the concepts of similarity and relationship, identify the distinction between correlation and causation, and interpret correlations correctly.

2.79.5 Chow, S.L. (1996) *Statistical significance: rationale, validity and utility*. Thousand Oaks, CA: Sage ISBN 0761952055 References

Book gives an overview of the most fundamental methodological issue for empirical researchers – how should statistical significance be interpreted? An introduction to null hypothesis testing and statistical significance is given, together with arguments for and against current interpretations and the use of significance testing in research. The book contributes to the debate on the proper role of significance testing in empirical research (CR 2.20, 2.25, 2.87).

2.79.6 Chu, K. (1999) An introduction to sensitivity, specificity, predictive values and likelihood ratios. *Emergency Medicine* 11 (3) 175–81 10 References

Explains how the accuracy of diagnostic tests can be assessed and demonstrates how to calculate sensitivity and specificity and predictive values. Discusses multiple testing and receiver operating characteristics, and summarizes by demonstrating how to calculate likelihood ratios (CR 2.83, 2.87).

2.79.7 de Vaus, D. (2002) *Analyzing social science data: 50 key problems in data analysis*. London: Sage ISBN 0761959386 References

Directs students to the core of data analysis, providing an authoritative guide to the problems facing beginners in the field.

2.79.8 Earl-Slater, A. (2002) Statistical tests: 10 ways to cheat with statistical tests/statisticians [and] general statistical checklists. In Author *The handbook of clinical trials and other research*. Oxford: Radcliffe Medical Press ISBN 1857754859 317–20

Gives two lists that may be used to check the essential elements of appropriate choice of test, and its use, in any particular research study (CR 2.2.13).

2.79.9 Erickson, B.H. & Nosanchuk, T.A. (1992) *Understanding data* (2nd edition). Buckingham: Open University Press ISBN 033509662X References

Book is intended for professional sociologists and students who have always feared numbers. It utilizes the techniques of exploratory data analysis. Students are fully involved in the data and its analysis, draw on their strengths and are allowed to develop their own ideas. Suggestions for examination questions and homework are included.

2.79.10 Fergusson, D., Aaron, S.D., Guyatt, G. & Herbert, P. (2002) Post randomisation exclusions: the intention to treat principle and excluding patients from analysis. *British Medical Journal* 325 (7365) 21 September 652–5 16 References

Examines the legitimacy of excluding randomized patients from analysis in clinical trials.

2.79.11 Fox, J. & Long, J.S. (eds) (1990) *Modern methods of data analysis*. Newbury Park, CA: Sage ISBN 0803933665 References

Volume aims to raise the standard of statistical analysis and presentation of data in the social sciences. It focuses on four themes: graphical data analysis, use of computers, regression analysis and sampling characteristics of data (CR 2.84, 2.94).

2.79.12 Greenhalgh, T. (1997a) Statistics for the non-statistician. I. Different types of data need different statistical tests. *British Medical Journal* 315 (7104) 9 August 364–6 11 References

Provides a checklist of preliminary questions to help the reader appraise the statistical validity of a paper (CR 2.95).

2.79.13 Greenhalgh, T. (1997b) Statistics for the non-statistician. II. 'Significant' relations and their pitfalls. *British Medical Journal* 315 (7105) 16 August 422–5 12 References

Continues the checklist of questions to appraise the statistical validity of a paper, including correlation, regression and causation (CR 2.25).

2.79.14 Hagen, S. (1998a) 1. Data and data summaries. *Nursing Times Learning Curve* 2 (8) 4–6 1 Reference.

Outlines levels of measurement, the process of summarizing data and the calculation of the standard deviation.

2.79.15 Hagen, S. (1998b) 2. Making inferences from data. *Nursing Times Learning Curve* 2 (9) 6–7 3 References

Describes sampling, the implications of sample size, sampling error and confidence intervals (CR 2.22).

2.79.16 Horn, R.V. (1993) *Statistical indicators for the economic and social sciences*. Cambridge: Cambridge University Press ISBN 0521423996 References

Gives comprehensive coverage of indicators in a wide range of disciplines, explores their limitations and reviews many alternatives.

2.79.17 Jairath, N., Fain, J.A. (1999) Methodology: a strategy for converting clinical data into research databases. *Nursing Research* 48 (6) 340–4 15 References

The process for converting clinical data into research databases is described.

2.79.18   Johnson, P. (1998) Analytic induction. In Symon, G. & Cassell, C. (eds) *Qualitative methods and analysis in organizational research: a practical guide*. London: Sage   ISBN 0761953515 Chapter 3 28–50 59   References

Chapter outlines the rationale and procedures of analytic induction through a brief discussion of its epistemological commitments, a review of its historical development and an illustration of its empirical application in an accountancy/industrial relations context. Some problems that may be encountered are also discussed (CR 2.36.135).

2.79.19   Keren, G. & Lewis, C. (1993) *A handbook for data analysis in the behavioural sciences*: *methodological issues*. Hillsdale, NJ: Erlbaum ISBN 0805810366   References

Covers many methodological issues of data analysis in the social sciences.

2.79.20   MacCluskie, K.C., Welfel, E.R. & Toman, S.M. (2002) *Using test data in clinical practice*. Thousand Oaks, CA: Sage   ISBN 0761921885   References

Few resources exist to assist mental health clinicians with the task of learning to synthesize test data from numerous instruments into a meaningful treatment plan and strategy for a client. This book is a systematic explanation of how to understand and integrate data from multiple sources. It also shows how to interpret test data for clients in language that is understandable.

2.79.21   Maisel, R. & Persell, C.H. (1995) *How sampling works: a guide to decisions and procedures*. Thousand Oaks, CA: Sage   ISBN 0803990618   References

Book explains the principles of statistical sampling and inference. Software included with the book helps to clarify these concepts in a visual and non-mathematical way.

2.79.22   Rose, D. & Pevalin, D. (eds) (2003) *A researcher's guide to the national statistics socio-economic classification*. London: Sage   ISBN 0761973222   References

Introduces researchers to all aspects of the new National Statistics Socio-economic Classification (NS-SEC). It describes and elucidates its conceptual basis, shows how it has been validated as a measure, evaluates how well it works in describing and explaining the relationships between social class and key health and employment variables. It also demonstrates the applications of NS-SEC in

research. The book will be of methodological interest to show how social scientists construct and validate basic measures (CR 2.91).

2.79.23   Sijtsma, K. & Molenaar, I.W. (2002) *Introduction to nonparametric item response theory*. Thousand Oaks, CA: Sage   ISBN 0761908137

Book addresses an important and complex topic in test development and will be accessible to students and practitioners with a modest background in classical test theory.

2.79.24   Thompson, S.G. & Barber, J.A. (2000) How should cost data in pragmatic randomised trials be analysed? *British Medical Journal* 320 (7243) 29 April 1197–200   26 References

Discusses the use of health economic evaluations to inform policy and indicates how to determine the most appropriate cost information from clinical trials (CR 2.43).

2.80   STATISTICAL AND OTHER TEXTS

There are many statistical texts on the market. Some are suitable for any discipline and others have been written with nurses in mind. A selection of books is included here, several of which were written to develop the students' ability to understand complex statistical techniques.

Annotations

2.80.1   Allison, P.D. (1999) *Multiple regression: a primer*. Thousand Oaks, CA: Sage   ISBN 0761985336   References

Book is intended for undergraduates in the social sciences taking their first research methods or statistics module and is designed to supplement other texts. It assumes that readers will be consumers rather than producers of research. Its format comprises a series of questions and answers.

2.80.2   Altman, D.G. (1998) Confidence intervals for the number needed to treat. *British Medical Journal* 317 (7168) 7 November 1309–12   13 References

Suggests that number needed to treat (NNT) is a useful way of reporting randomized clinical trials and that sensible confidence intervals can be constructed for the NNT and should always be quoted where this value is given (CR 2.29, 2.83).

2.80.3   Altman, D.G. & Bland, J.M. (1998) Time to event (survival) data. *British Medical Journal* 317 (7156) 15 August 468–9   7 References

Explains the importance of survival data in research studies and warns how results can be distorted if not analysed properly.

2.80.4   Altman, D., Machin, D., Bryant, T.N. & Gardner, M.J. (eds) (2000) *Statistics with confidence* (2nd edition). London: BMJ Books   ISBN 0727913751

A text and disk for health care professionals and medical researchers who need to understand statistics.

2.80.5   Anthony, D. (1999) *Understanding advanced statistics: a guide for nurses and health care researchers*. Edinburgh: Churchill Livingstone ISBN 0443059330

Book sets out in simple language how advanced statistical methods can be used. Many examples and exercises are included to test and consolidate knowledge (CR 2.2).

2.80.6   Argyrous, G. (2000) *Statistics for social and health research: with a guide to SPSS*. London: Sage   ISBN 0761968172

Aims to help students acquire an understanding of statistical methods for research and the associated SPSS procedures (CR Appendix A).

2.80.7   Campbell, M.J. (2001) *Statistics at square two: understanding modern statistical applications in medicine*. London: BMJ Books   ISBN 0727913948

Illustrated with examples from the *British Medical Journal*, this book clearly explains the more complex statistical methods found in medical journals.

2.80.8   Castle, W.M. & North, P.M. (1995) *Statistics in small doses* (3rd edition). Edinburgh: Churchill Livingstone   ISBN 0443045429

A programmed learning text covering topics in statistics needed by medical students and those in related professions. Learning is progressively assessed by questions (with answers included) and each chapter is illustrated with a practical example and concludes with a short summary.

2.80.9   Caulcott, E. (1992) *Statistics for nurses*. London: Scutari   ISBN 187136471X

Intended as a basic text for nursing degree students and others in the health care field. No assumptions are made about previous knowledge and examples are given from the health care field.

2.80.10   Chatfield, C. (1998) *Problem solving: a statisticians guide* (2nd edition). Dordrecht: Kluwer ISBN 0412286807   References

Written for students and statisticians who feel unsure how to tackle a real problem where the data is 'messy' or the objectives unclear. General principles are given, along with a series of exercises to illustrate the practical problems of analysing real data. A digest of statistical techniques with brief notes on two packages – MINITAB and GLIM – is included, as well as useful addresses and statistical tables. Advice is given on choosing computer software and the role of statisticians (CR 2.83, 2.84, Appendix A).

2.80.11   Coggan, D. (2002) *Statistics in clinical practice* (2nd edition). London: BMJ Books ISBN 0727916092   References

Book explains the principles of statistics using clinical examples.

2.80.12   Cramer, D. (1998) *Fundamental statistics for social research: step-by-step calculations and computer techniques using SPSS for windows*. London: Routledge ISBN 0415172047 References

Describes the role of statistics in the social sciences, dedicating chapters to levels of measurement and specific statistical tests. It aims to provide understanding by providing simple examples to be calculated by hand, which are then translated into exercises to be practised on SPSS (CR Appendix A).

2.80.13   Diamond, I. & Jefferies, J. (2000) *Beginning statistics: an introduction for social scientists*. London: Sage   ISBN 0761960627

With an emphasis on description, examples, graphs and displays rather than statistical formulae, this book provides an introductory guide for students.

2.80.14   Driscoll, P., Leeky, F. & Crosby, M. (1999) An introduction to statistics: an introduction to everyday statistics 1. *Journal of Accident and Emergency Medicine* 17 (3) 205–11   3 References

Provides an overview of statistics, explaining the common terms and looking at their use in everyday practice. Includes a recommended reading section.

2.80.15   Field, A. (2000) *Discovering statistics using SPSS for windows: advanced techniques for beginners*. London: Sage   ISBN 0761957553

Integrating statistical theory and the functions of SPSS, the student is provided with a thorough grounding in statistics through learning to use this software package (CR Appendix A).

2.80.16   Fielding, J.L. & Gilbert, G.N. (2000) *Understanding social statistics*. London: Sage ISBN 0803979835

Assumes that most students will have little or no previous experience in statistics and will not have studied mathematics formally for some years, yet also contains material useful to students at postgraduate level. Covers the nature of qualitative and quantitative data, an introduction to the use of computers in data analysis and the use of SPSS. Includes a glossary and standard tables, chapter summaries and exercises (CR 2.2, 2.9, 2.29, 2.36, 2.84, 2.89, Appendix A).

2.80.17   Frankfort-Nachmias, C. (1999) *Social statistics for a diverse society* (2nd edition). Thousand Oaks, CA: Pine Forge Press ISBN 0761986685   References

This introductory text relates statistics to social science research. The use of graphics, real data, and SPSS (Version 9) are discussed. This revised edition includes clear, precise presentation of topics, revisions to the chapters on testing hypotheses, exercises, and an accompanying disk with data sets from the United States General Survey (CR 2.86, Appendix A).

2.80.18   Gibbons, J.D. (1993) *Nonparametric statistics: an introduction*. Newbury Park, CA: Sage   ISBN 0803939515   References

Book provides the specific methodology and logical rationale for many of the most frequently used non-parametric statistics, applicable for both small and large sample sizes.

2.80.19   Greenfield, M.V., Kuhn, J.E. & Wojtys, E.M. (1998a) A statistics primer: confidence intervals. *The American Journal of Sports Medicine* 26 (1) 145–9   19 References

Explains that, in the search for statistical significance, the clinical significance of studies can be missed. The paper argues that confidence intervals provide considerably more information regarding the magnitude, direction and differences in treatment effects than is provided by estimates of statistical significance using the *p* value.

2.80.20   Greenfield, M.V., Kuhn, J.E. & Wojtys, E.M. (1998b) A statistics primer: correlation and regression analysis. *The American Journal of Sports Medicine* 26 (2) 338–46   7 References

A step-by-step guide to correlation and regression analysis. Definitions are provided using worked examples.

2.80.21   Hinton, P.R. (1995) *Statistics explained: a guide for social science students*. London: Routledge   ISBN 0415102863

Book outlines the major statistical tests used by undergraduates in psychology and the social sciences. Easy-to-understand explanations of how and why they are used are given. Book also helps students to understand the results of statistical analysis by computer.

2.80.22   Hooke, R. (1983) *How to tell the liars from the statisticians*. New York: Marcel Dekker ISBN 0824718178

Without using any mathematical calculations, this guide spotlights the effects of statistical reasoning and its misuse. It highlights the fascination of statistics and their value in decision-making. Seventy-six mini-essays, on a very wide range of topics, point out statistically incorrect arguments and dubious inferences. Illustrations are included which feature key points.

2.80.23   Huff, D. (1991) *How to lie with statistics*. Harmondsworth: Penguin   ISBN 0140136290

Discusses ways in which statistics are used to deceive. Everyday examples are used to expose 'the preposterous religion of our time'.

2.80.24   Jaeger, R.M. (1990) *Statistics* (2nd edition). Beverly Hills, CA: Sage   ISBN 0803934211 References

Designed for those who want to understand rather than compute statistics. No equations, which can sometimes obscure the meaning of the subject, are included. Illustrations are provided from educational research and evaluation studies. Each chapter is summarized and contains example problems (CR 2.2, 2.20, 2.54, 2.81, 2.82).

2.80.25   Kerr, A.W., Hall, H.K. & Kozub, S. (2003) *Doing statistics with SPSS*. London: Sage ISBN 0761973850

Book is suitable for any student undertaking an introductory statistics course as part of a science-based undergraduate programme (CR Appendix A).

2.80.26   Knapp, B.G. (1989) *Basic statistics for nurses* (2nd edition). New York: Delmar   ISBN 0827342713   References

Book is intended for undergraduate nursing students as an introductory statistics text. The emphasis is on teaching students to be consumers of research and not statisticians. Each chapter includes an overview, detailed objectives, worked examples and solutions taken from many nursing settings, exercises and a summary. A new chapter in this edition enables students to select the most appropriate statistical test in relation to the research question being asked.

2.80.27   Knapp, T.R. (1996) *Learning statistics through playing cards*. Thousand Oaks, CA: Sage ISBN 0761901094

Book aims to teach statistics in a non-threatening way using a deck of cards.

2.80.28   Kranzler, J.H. (2002) *Statistics for the terrified* (3rd edition). New York: Prentice-Hall ISBN 0130983403

A user-friendly introduction to elementary statistics, primarily intended for the maths-anxious/avoidant person. Its aim is to enable students to make the leap from apprehension to comprehension when learning about statistical techniques.

2.80.29   Lewis, J.P. (1998) *Statistics explained.* Don Mills, Ontario: Addison-Wesley Longman Inc. ISBN 0201178028

The emphasis in this book is on explanation, which is achieved without the complicated mathematics. A series of examples is also included.

2.80.30   Lindsey, J.K. (1999) *Revealing statistical principles*. London: Arnold   ISBN 0340741201 References

All stages of carrying out a research project requiring statistical analysis are covered, from the initial protocol to giving a presentation. No statistical knowledge is assumed.

2.80.31   Moore, D.S. (2001) *Statistics, concepts and controversies* (5th edition). New York: W.H. Freeman   ISBN 0716740087   References

Book gives insights and ideas rather than statistical techniques. Its aim is to give non-mathematical readers an aid to clear thinking when collecting data, organizing it and drawing conclusions. 150 new exercises are included, together with reviews at the end of each chapter. Examples have been updated and an expanded section on data analysis is included (CR 2.79).

2.80.32   Moroney, M.J. (1990) *Facts from figures*. Harmondsworth: Penguin   ISBN 0140135405 References

Provides a 'tool-kit' of essential statistical techniques. Limitations and dangers of misuse are discussed and examples are given.

2.80.33   Munro, B.H. (2001) *Statistical methods for health care research* (4th edition). Philadelphia, PA: Lippincott-Raven   ISBN 078172175X

Book demonstrates the best way to read, analyse and write up nursing research results. Practical solutions address real challenges and computer printouts are used for illustration. Exercises are given to enhance learning and a free disk with data sets will help with the application of statistical approaches (CR 2.2).

2.80.34   Owen, S.V. & Froman, R.D. (1998) Focus on qualitative methods. Uses and abuses of the analysis of covariance. *Research in Nursing and Health* 21 (6) 557–62   19 References

Explores the assumptions for using ANCOVA, giving examples of how it can increase or reduce statistical power. The paper includes a section on using ANCOVA procedures in statistical packages and a brief synopsis of how it has been used in nursing research.

2.80.35   Pett, M.A. (1997) *Non-parametric statistics in health care research: statistics for small samples and unusual distributions*. Thousand Oaks, CA: Sage   ISBN 0803970390   References

Gives a comprehensive overview of the uses of non-parametric tests, the process of hypothesis testing, the character of data, assumptions and violations of parametric tests. Practical examples are given from the fields of health and social care research and tables enable students to select the most appropriate test.

2.80.36   Pett, M.A., Lackey, N.R. & Sullivan, J.J. (2003) *Making sense of factor analysis: the use of factor analysis for instrument development in health care research*. Thousand Oaks, CA: Sage ISBN 076191949X   References

Book presents a straightforward explanation of the complex statistical procedures involved in factor analysis. A step-by-step approach to analysing data using computer packages like SPSS and SAS is provided. Advice is also given on creating new data collection instruments and examining the reliability and structure of those already in existence (CR 2.24, 2.55, 2.87, Appendix A).

2.80.37   Phillips, J.L. Jr (2000) *How to think about statistics* (6th edition). New York: Freeman ISBN 0716740087   References

Book shows applications of statistics in a wide range of fields, from public policy to the sciences. The approach to data analysis has established this book as a leader in the field. The use of new technology is introduced, together with helpful pedagogical features.

2.80.38   Rowntree, D. (1991) *Statistics without tears: a primer for non-mathematicians*. Harmondsworth: Penguin   ISBN 0140136320   References

Intended for the non-mathematical reader and is a 'tutorial in print'. The basic concepts of statistics are illustrated by means of words and diagrams rather than by figures, formulae and equations. Questions are included at frequent intervals so that students can test understanding of the concepts.

2.80.39   Salkind, N.J. (2000) *Statistics for people who (think they) hate statistics*. Thousand Oaks, CA: Sage   ISBN 0761916229

Book offers a step-by-step introduction to statistics, giving each chapter a 'Difficulty Rating Index'. These include tips for each statistical technique, top tens for the best way of creating graphs or collecting data, SPSS tips, and 'time to practice' exercises followed by worked solutions.

2.80.40   Sim, J. & Reid, N. (1999) Statistical inference by confidence: issues of interpretation and utilization. *Physical Therapy* 79 (2) 186–95 33 References

Examines the role of confidence intervals and its advantages over conventional hypothesis testing in the context of clinical practice. Its usefulness is cited for parametric and non-parametric tests, individual studies and meta-analyses (CR 2.20, 2.84, 2.92, Appendix A).

2.80.41   Sirkin, R.M. (1999) *Statistics for the social sciences*. Thousand Oaks, CA: Sage   ISBN 0761914196   References

Book covers statistical analysis at an elementary level. Topics included are the scientific method, levels of measurement and interpretation of tables. Discusses how statistics relate to the larger field of research methodology (CR 2.8).

2.80.42   Smithson, M.J. (1999) *Statistics with confidence: an introduction for psychologists*. London: Sage   ISBN 0716960317   References

This text is an introduction to statistics for undergraduate psychology and social science students. It covers all the key areas in quantitative methods with exercises and problems, and includes a free CD-ROM with tutorial modules.

2.80.43   StatPages.net *Web pages that perform statistical calculations!* members.aol.com/johnp71/javasta6.html (Accessed 26/02/03)

The Interactive Statistical Pages website project represents an ongoing effort to develop and disseminate statistical analysis software in the form of web pages. Those listed comprise a powerful, convenient, accessible, multi-platform statistical software package. There are also links to online statistics books, tutorials, downloadable software, and related resources. All of these resources are freely available.

2.80.44   StatSoft, Inc. (2002) *Electronic statistics textbook*. Tulsa, OK: StatSoft.WEB: www.stasoft.com/textbook/stathome.html (Accessed 19/02/03)

This electronic textbook offers training in the understanding and application of statistics for different disciplines. It gives an overview of elementary concepts and continues with in-depth exploration of specific areas of statistics. A glossary of

statistical terms and a list of references are also included (CR 2.2).

2.80.45   Swinscow,   T.D.V.   (Revised   by Campbell, M.J.) (2002) *Statistics at square one* (10th   edition).   London: BMJ Books   ISBN 0727915525   References

Provides step-by-step instruction on the basic tools of the statistician. This new edition includes methods adapted for pocket calculators, together with commonly asked questions with answers.

2.80.46   Wright, D.B. (1997) *Understanding statistics: an introduction for the social sciences*. London: Sage   ISBN 0803979185

Book describes the most popular statistical techniques, and explains their principles and use in a wide range of social research. The theoretical relationship between statistics and research is explained, t-tests are described in detail together with the three main families of tests – regression, analysis of variance and two-variable tests. A guide is also given to more advanced techniques.

2.80.47   Wright, D.B. (2002) *First steps in statistics*. London: Sage   ISBN 0761951636

Book is an introduction to the most common statistics taught on first-year research methods courses. Coverage includes: descriptive statistics, t-tests, ANOVAs, correlations, regressions and the chi-squared test. The importance of graphing data is stressed, and carefully chosen examples illustrate each test to convey conceptual aspects.

2.81   DESCRIPTIVE STATISTICS

The aim of descriptive statistics is to summarize in precise, standard ways, the characteristics and measurements of a sample.

Definition [See Appendix D for source]

Descriptive statistics – methods of summarizing large quantities of data so that patterns and relationships within the data may be seen, as distinct from statistical methods of hypothesis tests

Annotations

2.81.1   Clark, E. (1990) Making sense of descriptive statistics. *Nursing Standard* 4 (44) 8 August 36–41   8 References

Discusses the use of descriptive statistics and covers some of the tests which may be used.

2.81.2 Gissane, C. (1998) Understanding and using descriptive statistics. *British Journal of Occupational Therapy* 61 (6) 267–72 26 References

Identifies the correct statistical techniques to be used in particular settings, together with different ways of displaying information graphically and summarizing data numerically. Advises readers to consider their choice of test carefully and be able to justify their choice (CR 2.83).

2.81.3 Greenfield, M.V., Kuhn, J.E. & Wojtys, E.M. (1997) A statistics primer: descriptive measures for continuous data. *The American Journal of Sports Medicine* 25 (5) 720–5 6 References

Describes the properties of continuous data and how this data could be used. Explains measures of central tendency and standard deviation.

2.81.4 Hallett, C. (1997) The use of descriptive statistics in nursing research. *Nurse Researcher* 4 (4) 4–16 18 References

Discusses the value of using descriptive statistics for analysing and presenting large and complex sets of data. They fulfil some purposes of both quantitative and qualitative research, offering techniques for handling figures generated in quantitative studies and means for expressing data in a descriptive, diagrammatic or pictorial manner (CR 2.29, 2.36, 2.94).

2.81.5 Miller, H. (1995) *Descriptive statistics*. Edinburgh: Churchill Livingstone ISBN 0443053413

Book forms part of an open learning series. Each section contains an introduction, objectives, text, activities, commentaries, examples and a summary.

2.81.6 Neely, J.G., Stewart, M.G., Hartman, J.M., Forsen, J.W. & Wallace, M.S. (2002) Tutorials in clinical research, Part VI: Descriptive statistics. *The Laryngoscope* 112 (1) 1249–55 10 References

Organized into five sections from an overview to understanding the dispersion of data, this tutorial provides information on how to assess the validity of clinical studies (CR 2.25).

2.81.7 Trochim, W.M. *Descriptive statistics* trochim.human.cornell.edu/kb/statdesc.htm (Accessed 26/02/03)

Describes the uses and methods of descriptive statistics.

2.82 INFERENTIAL STATISTICS

In many instances in research there is a need to do more than just describe data, and inferential statistics provide a means for drawing conclusions about a sample. Researchers are then able to make judgements or generalize about a large class of individuals based on the information gained from a limited number.

Definition [See Appendix D for source]

Inferential statistics – statistics used for hypothesis testing and prediction

---

Annotation

2.82.1 Brown, J.K., Porter, L.A. & Knapp, T.R. (1993) The applicability of sequential analysis to nursing research. *Nursing Research* 42 (5) 280–2 17 References

Summarizes the basic principles of sequential hypothesis testing, its applications and disadvantages (CR 2.20).

2.82.2 Carlin, J.B. & Doyle, L.W. (2000) Statistics for clinicians. 3: Basic concepts of statistical reasoning: standard error and confidence intervals. *Journal of Paediatric and Child Health* 36 (5) 502–5 3 References

Explains the fundamental role of populations, samples and probability in understanding the concept of sampling variability. This in turn is used to explain standard error and confidence intervals in order to establish the principles of inferential statistics (CR 2.22).

2.82.3 Carlin, J.B. & Doyle, L.W. (2001) Statistics for clinicians. 4: Basic concepts of statistical reasoning: hypothesis tests and the t test. *Journal of Paediatric and Child Health* 37 (1) 72–7 8 References

Explains the basic logic of hypothesis testing, one and two tailed tests and interpretation of the hypothesis test. Discusses the t-test and normal distributions, the paired t-test and when it is appropriate to use the t-test.

2.82.4 Lowry, R. *Concepts and applications of inferential statistics* faculty.vassar.edu/lowry/intro.html (Accessed 26/02/03)

This website is a free, full-length and occasionally interactive statistics textbook. It is a companion site to VassarStats: Website for Statistical Computation.

2.82.5   Trochim, W.M. *Inferential statistics* trochim.human.cornell.edu/kb/statinf.htm (Accessed 26/02/03)

Explains the uses of inferential statistics.

2.83   CHOOSING A STATISTICAL TEST

Many research textbooks listed in section 2.1 include sections on statistics, but few actually give direct guidance on how to select an appropriate test. Because of the increasingly easy access to computer software, students need more advice about which test to use, rather than how to undertake the calculations. Several texts included in section 2.80 also give some guidance.

Annotations

2.83.1   Bohannon, R.W. (1999) Selecting an appropriate statistical test. *Topics in Geriatric Rehabilitation* 14 (3) 61–6   13 References

Gives a general overview of measurement issues fundamental to all statistics and includes a flow chart indicating appropriate tests for different types of data.

2.83.2   Hagen, S. (1998) 3. Statistical tests: continuous data. *Nursing Times Learning Curve* 2 (10) 4–6   5 References

Explains the rationale for using paired and unpaired *t*-tests, using example calculations. It also outlines the use of non-parametric tests where parametric assumptions are not fulfilled.

2.83.3   Hagen, S. (1999a) 4. Tests for categorical data. *Nursing Times Learning Curve* 2 (11) 4–6   2 References

Provides several examples of how a chi-squared test can be used to consider relationships between two categorical variables.

2.83.4   Hagen, S. (1999b) 5. ANOVA and linear regression. *Nursing Times Learning Curve* 2 (12) 8–10   2 References

Describes the concepts of one-way analysis of variance and the method of linear regression.

2.83.5   Jordan, K., Ong, B.N. & Croft, P. (1998) *Mastering statistics: a guide for health service professionals and researchers*. Cheltenham: Stanley Thornes ISBN 0748733256   References

Using real-life examples, this book takes the reader through the most common issues when using statistical tests. It emphasizes the importance of designing good research, including rules for sampling and questionnaire design. The book provides chapters on surveys and randomized controlled trials, and includes a 'navigation map' to help in the choice of statistical tests, explaining the conventions used in making an appropriate choice (CR 2.22, 2.29, 2.52, 2.75).

2.83.6   Knapp, B.G. (1989) Selection of an appropriate statistical test. In Author *Basic statistics for nurses*. (2nd edition). New York: Delmar   ISBN 0827342713   References

Chapter gives advice on choosing suitable statistical tests. Several examples with their solutions are provided, together with a flow chart (CR 2.80.26).

2.83.7   Lehmkuhl, L.D. (1996) Nonparametric statistics: methods for analysing data not meeting assumptions required for the application of parametric tests. *Journal of Prosthetics and Orthotics* 8 (3) 105–13   16 References

Contrasts the basic characteristics of non-parametric and parametric tests and explains how non-parametric statistical methods can yield important data regarding the differences between two groups.

2.83.8   Martin, C.R. & Thompson, D.R. (2000) Choice of statistical tests. In Authors *Design and analysis of clinical nursing research studies*. London: Routledge   ISBN 041522599X   Chapter 5 30–3

Chapter briefly discusses the two main types of statistical test – parametric and non-parametric.

2.83.9   Newton, R.R. & Rudestam, K.E. (1999) *Your statistical consultant: answers to your data analysis questions*. Thousand Oaks, CA: Sage ISBN 0803958234   References

This guide introduces, describes and makes recommendations regarding difficult statistical problems and techniques. Frequently asked questions are answered, a conceptual overview of topics and techniques is given, new topics of debate are highlighted and key terms are explained (CR 2.80).

2.83.10   Riegelman, R.K. (2000) *Studying a study and testing a test: how to read the medical evidence* (4th edition). Philadelphia, PA: Lippincott Williams & Wilkins   ISBN 0781718600 (includes CD-ROM for Windows and Macintosh) Part V Selecting a statistic 275–318

A framework for selecting a statistic is suggested and three questions are used to provide this: what question is being asked by the statistical test being used?; is the method appropriate to the type of data being collected?; and are the conclusions drawn from the statistical procedure appropriate? A summary is included in the form of flow charts.

2.83.11 Schechtman, E. (2002) Odds ratio, relative risk, absolute risk reduction, and the number needed to treat – which of these should we use? *Value in Health* 5 (5) 430–5   19 References

Answers some of the questions posed by practitioners about which method for comparing treatments should be used, how different measures can result in different interpretations and makes recommendations that researchers report relative and absolute measures, together with confidence intervals.

2.83.12 Trochim, W.M. *Selecting statistics: how many variables does the problem involve?* www. trochim.human.cornell.edu/selstat/ssstart.htm (Accessed 03/02/03)

This online statistical adviser will answer the question posed and will lead to an appropriate statistical test for your data (CR 2.19).

2.83.13 Williams, C., Soothill, K. & Barry, J. (1991) Nursing: just a job? Do statistics tell us what we think? *Journal of Advanced Nursing* 16 (8) 910–19   5 References

Article examines a particular statistical technique called latent class analysis, and considers its validity and possible use in classifying elements in the complex world of nursing. Authors believe that it can allow for fluidity and fluctuations that occur in nurses' work and personal lives, and can help explore conceptions and attitudes about work (CR 2.25).

2.84 USING COMPUTERS IN RESEARCH

Now that computer software is readily available researchers have the opportunity to assemble, correlate and present large amounts of both qualitative and quantitative data in sophisticated ways. Some programs are included here and further information may be found in Appendix A.

Example

Darbyshire, P. (2000) The practice politics of computerized information systems: a focus group study. *Nurse Researcher: The International Journal of Research Methodology in Nursing and Health Care* 8 (2) 4–17   34 References

Reports an Australian study that used focus group interviews with nurses and midwives to investigate their use of computerized Patient Information Systems. Their attitudes, the impact on practice, the question of power and ownership of information and participation in the development of new systems are all discussed (CR 2.69).

Annotations

2.84.1 Anthony, D. (2000) Current issues in nursing informatics. *Nurse Researcher: The International Journal of Research Methodology in Nursing and Health Care* 8 (2) 18–28   29 References

Author discusses the clinical use of informatics. The issues covered include the problems of locating relevant information on the Internet, accessing the Internet and human networking.

2.84.2 Babbie, E.R., Halley, F. & Zaino, J. (2003) *Adventures in social research: data analysis using SPSS 11.0/11.5* (5th edition). Thousand Oaks, CA: Pine Forge Press ISBN 076197584 References

Guides students step by step through the process of data analysis using General Social Survey Data and versions 11.0/11.5 of SPSS (CR 2.87, Appendix A).

2.84.3 Brown, R.A. & Beck, J.S. (1996) *Medical statistics on personal computers* (2nd edition). London: BMJ Books ISBN 0727907719 References

Authors show how to get the best out of software available for analysing statistical data. New chapters include survival analysis, statistical power calculations, writing up medical papers and notes on available packages.

2.84.4 Bryman, A. & Cramer, D. (1996) *Quantitative data analysis with Minitab: a guide for social scientists*. London: Routledge ISBN 0415123240   References

Using a non-technical approach, this book explains statistical tests for Minitab users (CR Appendix A).

2.84.5 Burnard, P. (1993) *Personal computing for health professionals*. London: Chapman & Hall ISBN 0412496704   References

This introductory text for health professionals will encourage the development of personal computing skills. Advice is given on selecting and purchasing a computer, the organization of a hard disk, software, word processing, databases and spreadsheets in the health care context. The use of a personal computer for writing essays, projects, reports or books is discussed, together with its value in the organization, analysis and reporting of research. Appendices provide further information (CR 2.2).

2.84.6 Burnard, P. (1995) Tips and traps in using computers for research. In Author *Health care computing: a survival guide for pc users*. London: Chapman & Hall   ISBN 0412605309   Chapter 10 173–97   References

Offers advice on the value and problems inherent in using computers at various stages of the research process. Information is given on using a word processor to content analyse textual data (CR 2.88, 2.89).

2.84.7   Buston, K. (1997) NUD*IST In action: its use and usefulness in a study of chronic illness in young people. *Sociological Research Online* 2 (3) www.socresonline.org.uk/socresonline/2/3/6.html (Accessed 14/11/03)

Paper describes use of NUD*IST when studying the experiences of chronically ill children and assesses the epistemological effect of its use. Practical information is given on some of its functions and issues are raised in the CAQDAS debate (CR 2.86, Appendix A).

2.84.8   Cooper, C., Oldham, J. & Hillier, V. (1998/99) Do computers have value in the data collection process for nurse researchers? *Nurse Researcher* 6 (2) 86–93   4 References

Paper examines the question of whether computers do have value for data collection or is it just the domain of 'computer techies'? It considers the use made of computers during the data collection stage of a study that examined if gender affects nurse teachers' attitudes to IT (CR 2.64).

2.84.9   Cooper, C. (1999) General overview of the use of computers in nursing research. *Nurse Researcher* 7 (1) 5–14

Offers some useful tips on using computer programs to enhance nursing research. A list of websites is included.

2.84.10   Davidson, F. (1996) *Principles of statistical data handling*. Thousand Oaks, CA: Sage ISBN 0761901035   References

Book explores the principles of data handling and how to make better use of computer data in research or study. It shows how to input, manipulate and debug data to make analysis easier and more accurate. Using a series of principles, problems or situations are presented and the author suggests how they might be resolved. The implementation of each principle is demonstrated as it appears in the command language of SAS and SPSS (CR Appendix A).

2.84.11   Durkin, T. (1997) Using computers in strategic qualitative research. In Miller, G. & Dingwall, R. (eds) *Context and method in qualitative research*. London: Sage   ISBN 0803976321 Part II Chapter 7 92–105   References

Considers how qualitative researchers may incorporate computer-based analyses into their studies. The opportunities and pitfalls of using computer software in qualitative research are critically examined

and practical advice is given on how to choose the most appropriate packages (CR 2.36.88, 2.86).

2.84.12   Einspruch, E.L. (1998) *An introductory guide to SPSS for Windows*. Thousand Oaks, CA: Sage   ISBN 0761900012   References

Book aims to enable readers to become proficient in using SPSS (Statistical Package for the Social Sciences). All aspects of creating, running, using, manipulating and analysing data are covered (CR Appendix A).

2.84.13   Fielding, N.G. & Lee, R.M. (eds) (1991) *Using computers in qualitative research*. Newbury Park, CA: Sage   ISBN 0803984251   References

Profiles and compares the principal programs available for analysing qualitative data, identifying their strengths and limitations. Ways are suggested as to how computer-based techniques may be incorporated into research methods training (CR 2.36, 2.42, 3.17).

2.84.14   Fielding, N.G. & Lee, R.M. (1998) *Qualitative research on computers*. Thousand Oaks, CA: Sage   ISBN 0803974833

Provides an accessible text on the nature of the change to handling qualitative data using computer programs. They report on findings from the first systematic field research on the impact of computer-assisted qualitative data analysis (CAQDAS). They examine users' experiences of CAQDAS and the advantages and disadvantages of computer use in analysing these data. They provide a framework for developing the craft and practice of CAQDAS and examine new techniques to meet new challenges (CR 2.36).

2.84.15   Francis, I. (1981) *Statistical software: a comparative review*. New York: North Holland ISBN 0444006583

Book presents a taxonomy of statistical software with broad comparisons being made rather than in-depth evaluations. Packages are grouped under the following program headings: data management, editing, tabulation, survey variance estimation, survey analysis, general statistics, specific purpose interactive batch, multiway contingency table analysis, econometric and time series, and mathematical sub-routine libraries. Each package is introduced and its capabilities listed. Its extensibility, proposed improvements, sample job, developers name and address, computer makes, interfaced language, source language, cost and documentation are all identified.

2.84.16   Gahan, C. & Hannibal, M. (1997) *Doing qualitative research using QSR NUD*IST*. London: Sage   ISBN 0761953906

Book provides a practical guide to the latest version of QSR NUD*IST (Version 4), a software package for development, support and management of qualitative data analysis. Taking the user's perspective, the software is presented as a set of tools for approaching a range of research issues. The key stages in carrying out qualitative data analysis are described, together with how to code, index and search the data. Practical exercises are included (CR 2.86, Appendix A).

2.84.17   Goossen, W. (2000) Nursing informatics research. *Nurse Researcher: The International Journal of Research Methodology in Nursing and Health Care* 8 (2) 42–54   28 References

Nursing informatics needs a scientific base in which a range of research methods can be applied. The author explores the research questions, and the methods available, and discusses why and how they should be applied.

2.84.18   Healey, J.F., Babbie, E.R. & Halley, F. (1997) *Exploring social issues using SPSS for Windows*. Thousand Oaks, CA: Pine Forge Press ISBN 0761985263   References

Book includes information on using SPSS (Statistical Package for the Social Sciences) in its Windows version. A self-contained package guides students step by step through all exercises and research reports follow a standardized, fill-in-the-blank format for presenting and analysing results (CR Appendix A).

2.84.19   Hine, C. (2000) *Virtual ethnography*. London: Sage   ISBN 0761958967   References

Author produces a distinctive understanding of the significance of the Net and shows that it is a site for cultural formations and artefacts that is shaped by people's understandings and expectations. This requires a new form of ethnography, which is explored, and readers are guided through its application in multiple settings (CR 2.42).

2.84.20   Jones, S. (ed.) (1998) *Doing Internet research: critical issues and methods for examining the Net*. Thousand Oaks, CA: Sage   ISBN 0761915958   References

Discusses the methodological issues that arise when one tries to understand the social processes occurring within it. Contributors offer original responses in the search for, and critique of, methods with which to study the Internet and the social, political, economic, artistic and communicative phenomena occurring within and around it.

2.84.21   Kelle, U. (1997) Theory building in qualitative research and computer programs for the management of textual data. *Sociological Research*

Online 2 (2) 46 References www.socresonline. uk/socresonline/2/2/1.html (Accessed 14/11/03)

Outlines recent debates about the potential methodological costs and benefits of computer use in qualitative research, and certain aspects of qualitative theory building are discussed (CR 2.36, 2.86, 2.89).

2.84.22   Kirby, K.N. (1993) *Advanced data analysis with SYSTAT*. New York: Van Nostrand Reinhold   ISBN 0442308604

Bridges the gap between statistics texts and SYSTAT manuals and provides step-by-step instructions for carrying out complete data analysis (CR 2.80).

2.84.23   Mann, C. & Stewart, F. (2000) *Internet communication and qualitative research: a handbook for searching online*. London: Sage   ISBN 0761966277   References

Guide covers basic Internet technology, reviews current online research practice and looks in detail at online researcher skills, ethics, confidentiality, security, legal issues and the implications of the virtual venue for data. Authors show how online researchers can use the new configurations of qualitative methods to collect rich, descriptive, contextually-situated data. Collecting data through in-depth online interviewing, virtual focus groups and participant observation in virtual communities are included (CR 2.17, 2.36, 2.68, 2.69, 2.72).

2.84.24   Ryan, B.F., Joiner, B.L. & Ryan, T.A. Jr (1992) *MINITAB handbook* (3rd edition). Boston, MA: PWS-Kent   ISBN 0534933661   References

Book is designed to be used with MINITAB, a general purpose statistical system. It emphasizes aspects of statistics particularly suitable for computer use, and includes many examples and exercises (CR Appendix A).

2.84.25   Saba, V.K. & McCormick, K.A. (2000) *Essentials of computers for nurses: informatics for the new millennium* (3rd edition). New York: McGraw-Hill   ISBN 0766825167   References

Provides an update of the fundamentals of computer technology as applied to nursing education. It included increased coverage on specialized software within the nursing curriculum, using the Internet as a research tool and the advent of distance leaning.

2.84.26   Stine, R. & Fox, J. (eds) (1996) *Statistical computing environments for social research*. Thousand Oaks, CA: Sage   ISBN 0761902708

Describes seven statistical computing environments – APL2STAT, GAUSS, Lisp-Stat, Mathematica, S, SAS/IML and Stata – which can be used in graphical and exploratory modelling.

2.84.27   Tait, M. & Slater, J. (1999) Using computers in nursing research. *Nurse Researcher* 7 (1) 17–29   4 References

Discusses specific tasks for which computers may be used at all stages of developing nursing research projects. Some software packages are discussed (CR Appendix A).

2.84.28   Walker, B.L. (1993) Computer analysis of qualitative data: a comparison of three packages. *Qualitative Health Research* 3 (1) 91–111   13 References

Describes and compares three computer programs designed to assist in the analysis of narrative text. These are Ethnograph, GATOR and Martin. A particular study is used to describe the links between research purposes and programs capabilities and the influence the latter may have on research methods or analysis (CR 2.86).

2.84.29   Weitzman, E. & Miles, M.B. (1995) *Computer programs for qualitative data analysis.* Thousand Oaks, CA: Sage   ISBN 0803955375

Provides a critical, in-depth look at 24 applications for analysing qualitative data. In addition to describing the special features of each program their strengths and weaknesses are highlighted (CR 2.86).

2.84.30   Woods, L. & Roberts, P. (2000) Generating theory and evidence from qualitative computerized software. *Nurse Researcher: International Journal of Research Methodology in Nursing and Health Care* 8 (2) 29–41   26 References

Discusses the use of QSR NUD*IST in the management and analysis of qualitative data and argues that technology is something to be embraced rather than rejected (CR 2.86, Appendix A).

2.85   RESEARCH AND THE INTERNET

This section includes some of the literature relating to research and the Internet. It includes more general articles, with specific ones included in relevant sections.

Example

Kim, H.S., Kim, E. & Kim, J.W. (2001) Development of a breast self-examination program for the Internet: health information for Korean women. *Cancer Nursing* 24 (2) 156–61   25 References

Describes the processes involved in the development of an accessible multimedia Internet program about breast self-examination. The contents posted on the Internet included general information about breast cancer, the diverse methods of self-examination, the monthly checklist graph and the social network for consultation. Sufficient information is included to enable access using existing search engines.

Annotations

2.85.1   Cooper, C.D. (2000) The use of electronic mail in the research process. *Nurse Researcher* 7 (4) 24–30   18 References

Examines the growing use of email and outlines its uses as found in the nursing literature for sample recruitment, data collection, sample interviews, networking and collaboration (CR 2.15, 2.22, 2.64, 2.68).

2.85.2   Duffy, M.E. (2002) Methodological issues in web-based research. *Journal of Nursing Scholarship* 34 (1) 83–8   24 References

Discusses what constitutes web-based research and methodological issues: nature of the sample, testing environment and environmental factors, privacy and confidentiality, response rates and security. Research potential exists but methodological issues are real and, if not addressed, can seriously affect the validity of findings (CR 2.22, 2.17, 2.25).

2.85.3   Gomez, E.G. & Clark, P.M. (2001) The Internet in oncology nursing. *Seminars in Oncology Nursing* 17 (1) 7–17   37 References

Explores the implications of the Internet for oncology nursing practice, education and research. The authors believe it will give oncology nurses a voice extending to millions of Internet users. Among the greatest challenges for users are the quality of information and privacy of the data transmitted (CR 2.17).

2.85.4   Hewson, C., Yule, P., Laurent, D. & Vogel, C. (2002) *Internet research methods: a practical guide for the social and behavioural sciences.* London: Sage   ISBN 0761959203

Offers a concise, comprehensive guide to conducting research on the Internet, and a detailed explanation of all the main areas of Internet research. It distinguishes between primary research (using the Internet to recruit participants, to administer the research process and to collect results) and secondary research (using the Internet to access available material online).

2.85.5   Hynes-Gay, P.M. & Hagle, L.M. (2000) Nursing and the Net. *Canadian Journal of Nursing Leadership* 13 (2) May–June 5–10   11 References

Paper discusses the advantages of Internet/Intranet functionality for nurses, and describes an Intranet application designed specifically for an adult critical care unit at Mount Sinai Hospital in Toronto.

2.85.6 Im, E. & Chee, W. (2001) A feminist critique on the use of the internet in nursing research. *Advances in Nursing Science* 23 (4) 67–82 45 References

Article analyses the use of the Internet in nursing and critiques it from a feminist viewpoint. Its limitations include selection bias, lack of contextual data on research encounters, women's subjective experiences may not be discovered in marginalized situations, and power issues between researcher and participants may be raised. It also has many advantages and feminist challenges for the future are proposed (CR 2.10, 2.27).

2.85.7 Leaffer, T. & Gonda, B. (2000) The Internet: an under-utilized tool in patient education *Computers in Nursing* 18 (1) January–February 47–52 17 References

Reports a two-stage pilot study involving 100 senior citizens who received instruction on how to conduct health information searches on the Internet. The goal was to enable senior citizens to assume an active role in their health care and share information with family and friends. Positive results are reported and suggestions are made for further improvement. These findings are relevant to patient education in nursing curricula.

2.85.8 Mann, C. & Stewart, F. (2000) *Internet communication and qualitative research: a handbook for researching online.* London: Sage ISBN 0761966277 References

Book is an introduction to data sources that will come to the fore in the new millennium. It discusses techniques, ethics and methods of analysing Internet data (CR 2.17, 2.36, 2.68, 2.69).

2.85.9 Menon, G.M. (ed.) (2002) *Using the Internet as a research tool for social work and human services.* Binghampton, NY: Haworth Press Inc. ISBN 0789014483 References

By introducing various methodologies and insights, this book explains how the World Wide Web can be a valuable and legitimate form of research. It examines the problems associated with studying virtual communities and cyber culture, explores methodologies for data collection, and discusses sampling, psychological testing, and online surveys (CR 2.52).

2.85.10 Nartz, M. & Schoech, D. (2000) Use of the Internet for community practice: a Delphi study. *Journal of Community Practice* 8 (1) 37–59 20 References

Reports research, using the Delphi technique, to elicit the opinions of experts on how the Internet tools of email, newsgroups, text, listservs, search engines and chat rooms are used by the four primary models of community practice found on the Internet: these are information dissemination, organization building, mobilization and community planning. The most useful tools were text presentation and email. Barriers to Internet community practice included quality and currency of information, bandwidth, staff time, agency support, rapid technological change, marketing, browser consistency, user skills and the lack of Internet access by potential users (CR 2.66).

2.85.11 Ó Dochartaigh, N. (2001) *The Internet research handbook: a practical guide for students and researchers in the social sciences.* London: Sage ISBN 0761964401 References

A number of different skills are required for using the Internet as a mainstream research resource. The book covers learning how to access the correct sites and extract information in the shortest possible time; maximizing the possibilities of email contact with other researchers around the world; finding out about the major databases which are devoted to the social sciences; and learning how to do the detective work necessary to evaluate and cite documents whose authorship and origins are often unclear.

2.85.12 Ribbons, R. & Vance, S. (2001) Using e-mail to facilitate nursing scholarship. *Computers in Nursing* 19 (3) May–June 105–113 16 References

Article describes an interdisciplinary curricular project in which email was employed as a vehicle to support the development of students' understanding of scholarship within a cohort of first-year undergraduate nursing students. The project involved the establishment of 'Virtual Colleague' activity, which used email to conduct activities, including critical analysis of electronic journals and websites and peer review. The theoretical underpinning and evaluation of the project are discussed, together with possible future applications (CR 3.17).

2.85.13 Rice, R.E. & Katz, J.E. (eds) (2001) *The Internet and health communication: experiences and expectations.* Thousand Oaks, CA: Sage ISBN 0761922334 References

Book provides an in-depth analysis of the changes in human communication and health care resulting from the Internet revolution. The contributors, representing a wide range of expertise, provide an extensive variety of examples to illustrate their findings and conclusions.

2.85.14 Selwyn, N. & Robson, K. (1998) Using e-mail as research tool. *Social Research Update*

Issue 21 Guildford: University of Surrey, Department of Sociology   28 References   www.soc.surrey.ac.uk/sru/SRU21.html (Accessed 14/11/03)

Discusses uses of email as a research tool, some methodological considerations, electronic questionnaires and electronic interviewing (CR 2.68, 2.75).

2.85.15   Sery-Ble, O.R., Taffe, E.R., Clarke, A. & Dorman, T. (2001) Use of and satisfaction with a browser-based tool in a surgical intensive care unit. *Computers in Nursing* 19 (2) March–April 82–6   8 References

Authors' goal was to determine if a computerized tool was an effective teaching method for nurses in a high-stress intensive care unit. A web-based Microsoft Power Point presentation, located on the Intranet at nursing stations, was designed to provide instruction on the methodology and use of the APACHE III medical system, prior to its implementation. Positive and negative results are reported, but nurses thought this browser-based tool was easily accessible and an effective way of communicating new material to medical staff.

2.85.16   Sixsmith, J. & Murray, C.D. (2001) Ethical issues in the documentary data analysis of Internet posts and archives. *Qualitative Health Research* 11 (3) May 423–32   49 References

Article outlines ethical issues surrounding this form of research, including issues of accessing voices, consent, privacy, anonymity, interpretation, authorship and ownership of research material (CR 2.17, 2.86).

2.85.17   Thomas, B., Stamler, L.L., Lafreniere, K. & Dumala, R. (2000) The Internet: an effective tool for nursing research with women. *Computers in Nursing* 18 (1) January–February 13–18   17 References

Article outlines the methodology of using the Internet to survey an international population of women about their perceptions of breast health education and screening. Issues to consider in planning and implementing the project are discussed, together with its benefits and limitations. It was found to be an appropriate medium for health-related research and it also attracted national and international media interest. The address for the website is included (CR 2.22, 2.52).

2.86   ANALYSING QUALITATIVE DATA

Qualitative data are frequently expressed in words and the researcher must organize this material into groups and patterns in order to understand its meaning. Some qualitative data will also lend itself to description through the use of measures of central tendency, dispersion and correlation coefficients. Several computer programs are now available; some are documented here, others can be found in section 2.84 and Appendix A.

Definitions [See Appendix D for sources]

Concept map – … a special form of a web diagram for exploring knowledge and gathering and sharing information

Concept mapping – the strategy employed to develop a concept map [A concept map consists of nodes or cells that contain a concept, item or question and links. The links are labelled and denote direction with an arrow symbol. The labelled links explain the relationship between the nodes. The arrow describes the direction of the relationship and reads like a sentence]

Constant comparison – a procedure used in qualitative research wherein newly collected data are compared in an ongoing fashion with data collected earlier, to refine theoretically relevant categories

Dramaturgical perspective – … a method that uses the theatrical metaphor of the stage, actors and audiences to observe and analyse the intricacies of social interaction

Matrix analysis – a set of numbers or terms arranged in rows or columns that within which, or within and from which, something originates, takes form or develops

Qualitative analysis – the organization and interpretation of non-numerical information for the purpose of discovering important underlying dimensions and patterns of relationships

Qualitative meta-synthesis – … the theories, grand narratives, generalizations, or interpretative translations produced from the integration or comparison of findings from qualitative studies

---

Example

Hoz, R. & Gonik, N. (2001) The use of concept mapping for knowledge-oriented evaluation in nursing education. *Evaluation and Research in Education* 15 (4) 207–27   References

Reports a study that examined a course in paediatric surgery for integration of the contents of several previously taught courses. Concept mapping and Link Strength Matrices were used to study their learning outcomes. Results are reported, together with subsequent changes to the curriculum.

Annotations

2.86.1   Aneshensel, C.S. (2002) *Theory based data analysis for the social sciences*. Thousand Oaks, CA: Pine Forge Press   ISBN 0761987363

The advent of powerful computer-generated statistical models has greatly eroded the former prominence of social theory in data analysis, replacing it with an emphasis on statistical technique. To correct this trend the author presents a method for bringing data analysis and statistical technique into line with theory.

2.86.2   Averill J.B. (2002) Matrix analysis as a complementary analytic strategy in qualitative inquiry. *Qualitative Health Research* 12 (6) 855–66   25 References

Explains the uses of matrix analysis as a strategy to enhance the development of evidence in qualitative research. Uses an example from a study of rural elders to demonstrate the technique.

2.86.3   Ball, M.S. & Smith, G.W.H. (1992) *Analyzing visual data*. Newbury Park, CA: Sage   ISBN 0803934351   References

The major form of visual presentation addressed by this book is the still photograph. Chapters cover the use of photographs in disciplines of words: anthropology, ethnography and sociology. Analysing the content of visual representations, symbolist and structuralist analyses and the social organization of visual experiences are all discussed (CR 2.42, 2.72, 2.88).

2.86.4   Bates, A.J. (2002) Matrix analysis as a complementary analytic strategy in qualitative inquiry. *Qualitative Health Research* 12 (6) 855–66 References

In the current health care environment, researchers are asked to share meaningful results with interdisciplinary professional audiences. Emphasis is placed on effective care outcomes and evidence so that any strategy that facilitates clear, accurate communication of findings will benefit all. The author proposes matrix analysis as a strategy to enhance the development of evidence in qualitative research (CR 2.36, 2.43).

2.86.5   Bazeley, P. & Richards, L. (2000) *The NVivo qualitative project book*. London: Sage   ISBN 0761970002

In this hands-on text readers follow the basic steps for creating and conducting a real project with real data using the enclosed QSR NUD*IST Vivo (NVivo) demonstration software. Tools are introduced as needed and explained as progress is made. The reader is in control throughout and guided by

the experts, with frequent tips and reflections on what is being done (CR Appendix A).

2.86.6   Boyatzis, R.E. (1998) *Thematic analysis: coding as a process for transforming qualitative information*. Thousand Oaks, CA: Sage   ISBN 0761909613   References

Book discusses thematic analysis, a process for encoding qualitative information. Readers are helped to recognize themes and develop codes through the use of numerous examples.

2.86.7   Bryman, A. & Burgess, R.G. (eds) (1994) *Analyzing qualitative data*. London: Routledge   ISBN 0415060621   References

A group of experienced researchers explore and explain the ways in which they have analysed qualitative data. Examples are given from ethnographers, case study workers, lone researchers and team-based investigators. Specialist approaches, including discourse analysis, are discussed (CR 2.36, 2.39, 2.42, 2.89).

2.86.8   CAQDAS Networking Project *Computer assisted qualitative data analysis software*   caqdas. soc.surrey.ac.uk/ (Accessed 26/02/03)

The Computer Assisted Data Analysis Software project, funded by the Economic and Social Research Council, aims to disseminate an understanding of the practical skills needed to use software that has been designed to assist qualitative data analysis. It provides demonstration versions of various qualitative analysis packages, information on short courses, a bibliography on computer software and information about the qual-software mailing list (CR 2.84).

2.86.9   Clayton, D.K., Rogers, S. & Stuifbergen, A. (1999) Answers to unasked questions: writing in the margins. *Research in Nursing and Health* 22 (6) 512–22   36 References

During a large quantitative study of health promotion and quality of life in multiple sclerosis, a quarter of the respondents added extensive qualitative comments to their 36-page questionnaire booklet. These were analysed to develop an understanding of this unsolicited narrative material. The findings and conclusions are reported (CR 2.29, 2.36, 2.75, 2.91).

2.86.10   Coffey, A. & Atkinson, P. (1996) *Making sense of qualitative data*. Thousand Oaks, CA: Sage   ISBN 0803970536   References

Describes and illustrates a number of approaches to analysing qualitative data.

2.86.11   Dey, I. (1993) *Qualitative data analysis: a user-friendly guide for social scientists*. London: Routledge   ISBN 041505852X   References

Book aims to fill the gap in texts on qualitative data analysis. It is written for undergraduates and post-graduates who need to handle data using computers. A variety of ways in which computers can be used are discussed, providing background knowledge and learning experiences. Hypersoft is used as the medium through which methodological problems can be approached. Appendix 2 provides details of Hypersoft (CR 2.84).

2.86.12   Feldman, M.S. (1994) *Strategies for interpreting qualitative data*. Thousand Oaks, CA: Sage   ISBN 0803959168   References

Book outlines four key strategies for interpreting qualitative data: ethnomethodology, semiotics, dramaturgy and deconstruction. The strengths and weaknesses of each are identified and the author suggests when they may best be used. The techniques of each method are applied to a single data set by way of illustration and the differences highlighted (CR 2.42).

2.86.13   Fielding, N.G. & Fielding, J.L. (1986) *Linking data*. Beverly Hills, CA: Sage   ISBN 0803925182   References

Book concentrates on techniques for linking and analysing data obtained from both qualitative and quantitative research methods (CR 2.29, 2.36, 2.87).

2.86.14   Gahan, C. & Hannibal, M. (1998) *Doing qualitative research using QSR NUD*IST*. London: Sage   ISBN 0761953906

This is the first practical guide to using QSR NUD*IST, the software package for development, support and management of qualitative data analysis projects. Book identifies its intentions and the different types of problem that it can be applied to. The key stages in carrying out a qualitative analysis are discussed and practical exercises are included throughout (CR Appendix A).

2.86.15   Gibbs, G.R. (2002) *Qualitative data analysis: explorations with NVivo*. Buckingham: Open University Press   ISBN 0335200842

Book explores the role of computers in analysing qualitative data. It also shows, in outline, with the use of worked examples, how qualitative researchers analyse their data. Use of one particular piece of software, NVivo, is discussed (CR Appendix A).

2.86.16 Gilbert, L.S. (2002) 'Closeness' in qualitative data analysis software. *International Journal of Social Research Methodology: Theory and Practice* 5 (3) July Special issue: 215–28 Qualitative research and computing: methodological issues and practices in using QSR Nvivo and NUD*IST.

This study about researchers' transitions to using qualitative data analysis (QDA software) identified three stages of 'closeness to the data': the tactile digital divide, the coding trap and the meta-cognitive shift. Each of these transitions is explored. Readers are invited to reflect on the nature of 'cognitive tools' and their own levels of expertise, which have implications for evaluating research and considering trustworthiness.

2.86.17   Hardin, P.K. (2003) Constructing experience in individual interviews, autobiographies and on-line accounts: a post-structuralist approach. *Journal of Advanced Nursing* 41 (6) 536–44   26 References

Presents a methodological perspective addressing the importance of form, context and function in account production and data analysis (CR 2.71, 2.78).

2.86.18   Hayes, N. (ed.) (1997) *Doing qualitative analysis in psychology*. Hove, East Sussex: Psychology Press Ltd   ISBN 0863777414 References

Gives examples of how different psychologists have used qualitative analysis in research. Each chapter is based around a real piece of research and each contributor discusses his/her analytic strategy. A wide range of theoretical and methodological approaches is included (CR 2.45, 2.49, 2.77, 2.89).

2.86.19   Jackson, K.M. & Trochim, W.M.K. (2002) Concept mapping as an alternative approach for the analysis of open-ended survey responses. *Organizational Research Methods* 5 (4) October 307–36   References

Presents concept mapping as an alternative method to existing code-based and word-based text analysis techniques for one type of qualitative text data – open-ended survey questions. A detailed example of concept mapping on such data is presented. Reliability and validity issues associated with this technique are discussed (CR 2.24, 2.25, 2.52).

2.86.20   Kinchin, I.M., Hay, D.B. & Adams, A. (2000) How a qualitative approach to concept map analysis can be used to aid learning by illustrating patterns of conceptual development. *Educational Research* 42 (1) 43–57   References

Paper describes an approach to analysing students' concept maps. Three major patterns emerged and can be seen as progressive levels of understanding. Teachers may then use the results to plan and structure groups more effectively (CR 2.36).

2.86.21   King, N. (1998) Template analysis. In Symon, G. & Cassell, C. (eds) *Qualitative methods and analysis in organizational research: a practical guide*. London: Sage   ISBN 0761953515   Chapter 7 118–34   18 References

Template analysis, often referred to as 'codebook analysis' or 'thematic coding', is an approach that the researcher uses to produce a list of codes (a template) representing themes identified in textual data. It can be seen to occupy a position between content analysis, where codes are all predetermined and their distribution is analysed statistically, and grounded theory, where there is no a priori definition of codes. A study of managing mental health in primary care is used to illustrate this technique (CR 2.36.135).

2.86.22 Kuckartz, U. (2001) *An introduction to the computer analysis of qualitative data*. London: Sage   ISBN 0761969020

Book examines the methodological foundations, including qualitative and classical content analysis, the 'Grounded Theory', and the practical application of these new programmes and computer-based techniques. Using examples from winMAX, the author gives an overview of the latest analytical techniques and the methodological concepts associated with computer analysis of qualitative data (CR 2.36).

2.86.23 Miles, M.B. & Huberman, A.M. (1994) *Qualitative data analysis: an expanded sourcebook* (2nd edition). Thousand Oaks, CA: Sage   ISBN 0803955405   References

This practical sourcebook will assist all researchers who make use of qualitative data. Strong emphasis is put on new types of data display and 49 methods are described and illustrated, with practical suggestions for their use. This new edition includes an appendix giving criteria for choosing from available software (CR 2.83, 2.94).

2.86.24 Morison, M. & Moir, J. (1998) The role of computer software in the analysis of qualitative data: efficient clerk, research assistant or Trojan horse? *Journal of Advanced Nursing* 28 (1) 106–16   39 References

The purpose of this paper is to encourage researchers contemplating the use of computer software to consider carefully the possible consequences of their decision, and to be aware that such programmes can alter the nature of the analytic process in unexpected and perhaps unwanted ways. An example of where the package called NUD*IST was used is cited, together with its advantages and limitations. The role of the Computer Assisted Qualitative Data Analysis Networking Project in providing up-to-date information and support for researchers contemplating the use of software is discussed (CR 2.36, Appendix A).

2.86.25 Patton, M.Q. (1999) Enhancing the quality and credibility of qualitative analysis. *Health Services Research* 34 (5) 1189–208   12 References

Examines the ways of enhancing qualitative data analysis by using rigorous techniques and methods for gathering data, establishing the credibility, competence and trustworthiness of the researcher and by establishing the philosophical beliefs of the evaluation users (CR 2.36).

2.86.26 Pope, C., Ziebland, S. & Mays, N. (2000) Analysing qualitative data. *British Medical Journal* 320 (7227) 8 January 114–16   17 References

Outlines the requirements for the rigorous analysis of qualitative data and how the use of software can assist in the process. Identifies the stages of analysis and a framework for undertaking it (CR Appendix A).

2.86.27 Priest, H., Roberts, P. & Woods, L. (2002) An overview of three different approaches to the interpretation of qualitative data. Part 1: theoretical issues. *Nurse Researcher: The International Journal of Research Methodology* 10 (1) 30–42   52 References

AND

2.86.28 Woods, L., Priest, H. & Roberts, P. (2002) An overview of three different approaches to the interpretation of qualitative data. Part 2: practical illustrations. *Nurse Researcher: The International Journal of Research Methodology* 10 (1) 43–51   12 References

In Part 1 the authors discuss the essential features and methods inherent within three approaches to the interpretation of qualitative data: grounded theory, qualitative content analysis and narrative analysis. The philosophical bases of each method and their inherent principles are considered, and key stages and steps are described. Part 2 goes on to illustrate, with reference to a section of text, how the three approaches can be applied to the practical analysis of interview data (CR 2.36, 2.45, 2.88, 2.89).

2.86.29 Richards, L. (1999) *Using NVivo in qualitative research*. London: Sage   ISBN 0761965254

This book is a practical guide to using the latest qualitative software package. An accompanying CD-ROM carries a demonstration version of the software together with six tutorials to use with personal data. Advice is given with each section, addressing a range of research approaches and priorities (CR Appendix A).

2.86.30 Riley, J. (1996) *Getting the most from your data: a handbook of practical ideas on how to analyze qualitative data*. Bristol: Technical and Educational Services   ISBN 0947885315

This practical text includes many ideas for the analysis of qualitative data.

2.86.31   Rodgers, B.L. (1998) Teaching computer-assisted qualitative data analysis to new users: NUD*IST demonstrations and workshops. *Health Informatics* 4 (2) 63–71   6 References

This paper offers insights into the ways in which demonstrations and workshops can be provided to familiarize users with software for qualitative data analysis, especially the popular programme NUD*IST (CR Appendix A).

2.86.32   Rose, K. & Webb, C. (1998) Analyzing data: maintaining rigor in a qualitative study. *Qualitative Health Research* 8 (4) 556–62   25 References

Taking a reflexive approach, this article considers the process of data analysis adopted by a nurse researcher conducting a study into the experiences of informal carers of terminally ill patients. The particular strategy adopted is discussed and the rigour of the method is defended by defining the stages of the process arguing that there should be room for creativity within data analysis.

2.86.33   Roulston, K. (2001) Data analysis and 'theorizing as ideology'. *Qualitative Research* 1 (3) 279–302   47 References

Author revisits data produced from her first study and discusses how novice researchers might approach qualitative analysis. Provides a detailed account of how two different approaches (thematic and conversation analysis) might produce different readings of data.

2.86.34   Russell, C.K. & Gregory, D.M. (2003) Evaluation of qualitative research studies. *Evidence-based Nursing* 6 (2) April 36–40   35 References

Provides guidance on evaluating qualitative research studies.

2.86.35   Sandelowski, M., Docherty, S. & Emden, C. (1997) Focus on qualitative methods. Qualitative meta-synthesis: issues and techniques. *Research in Nursing and Health* 20 (4) 365–71   47 References

Article considers the appropriateness and feasibility of attempting qualitative meta-synthesis. Several efforts to create such synthesis are discussed, together with methodological issues.

2.86.36   Savage, J. (2000) One voice, different tunes: issues raised by dual analysis of a segment of qualitative data. *Journal of Advanced Nursing* 31 (6) 1493–500   37 References

Explores the relationship between the way in which data are analysed and the nature of findings that emerge.

2.86.37   Sharpe, T. & Koperwas, J. (2003) *Behavior and sequential analysis: principles and practice.* Thousand Oaks, CA: Sage   ISBN 0761925600   References

Book provides a step-by-step approach to the principles and practices of direct observation and behaviour analysis research and evaluation procedures. It contains references to software resources, including the BEST and BESTPCC data collection and evaluation package, highlighting technological innovations in methods for this field (CR 2.43, 2.72, Appendix A).

2.86.38   Silverman, D. (ed.) (1997) *Qualitative research: theory, method and practice.* London: Sage   ISBN 0803976666   References

Contributors to this book reflect on the analysis of observations, texts, talk and interviews. Key themes include the centrality of the relationship between analytic perspectives and methodological issues; the need to broaden our conception of qualitative research beyond issues of subjective 'meaning' towards issues of language; representation and social organization; searching for ways to build links between social science traditions; and having a dialogue between social science and the community (CR 2.68, 2.72, 2.76, 2.78).

2.86.39   Silverman, D. (2001) *Interpreting qualitative data: methods for analyzing talk, text and interaction* (2nd edition). London: Sage   ISBN 0761968652   References

This text, which is based on worked-through examples and student exercises, spans the range of different approaches in the qualitative tradition. It focuses on the strengths of particular methodologies, observation, analysis and validity in qualitative research, ethnography, symbolic interactionism and conversational analysis. Ways in which communication can be studied through the analysis of interviews, texts and transcripts are described (CR 2.9, 2.24, 2.25, 2.36, 2.42, 2.68, 2.72, 2.89).

2.86.40   Silvester, J. (1998) Attributional coding. In Symon, G. & Cassell, C. (eds) *Qualitative methods and analysis in organizational research: a practical guide.* London: Sage   ISBN 0761953515   Chapter 5 73–93   43 References

Chapter discusses the method known as attributional coding which enables the researcher to extract, code and thereby analyse patterns of public attributions, defined here as attributions communicated through either discourse (e.g. conversations, team meetings, speeches) or written material (e.g. company reports, letters, email). It is a method that can be used in both qualitative and quantitative research, depending on the theoretical perspective and objectives of the researcher (CR 2.36.135).

2.86.41 Sofaer, S. (1999) Qualitative methods: what are they and why use them? *Health Services Research* 34 (5) 1101–18   28 References

Gives an overview of the range of qualitative methods, the rationale for use in health services research and provides examples of their application (CR 3.12).

2.86.42 Speer, S.A. (2002) What can conversation analysis contribute to feminist methodology? Putting reflexology into practice. *Discourse and Society* 13 (6) 783–803   41 References

Examines the use of conversation analysis as a respondent-centred approach to data collection. The author uses her own work to illustrate that researchers need to consider their own impact on the data collection process, particularly in the light of feminist perspectives of research design (CR 2.10, 2.89).

2.86.43 Thorne, S. (2000) Data analysis in qualitative research. *Evidence-based Nursing* 3 (3) July 68–70   9 References

Article aims to assist readers to make sense of some of the assertions made about qualitative data analysis in order to develop a critical eye for when an analytical claim is convincing or not.

2.86.44 Trochim, W.M.K. *An introduction to concept mapping for planning and evaluation* trochim.human.cornell.edu/research/epp1/epp1.htm (Accessed 02/02/03)

Concept mapping is a type of structured conceptualization that can be used by groups to develop frameworks to guide evaluation or planning. In a typical case, six steps are involved and these are described. Major methodological issues and problems are discussed together with computer programs that may be used.

2.86.45 Twinn, S. (2000) The analysis of focus group data: a challenge to the rigour of qualitative research. *NT Research* 5 (2) 140–6   27 References

Analysing the data from focus group interviews may be time-consuming and difficult, so close collaboration between researchers is essential to ensure consistency in interpretation of words and meanings. This is particularly important if interviews are conducted in a language other than that of the researchers (CR 2.69).

2.86.46 Van Leeuwen, T. & Jewitt, C. (eds) (2000) *The handbook of visual analysis*. London: Sage   ISBN 0761964770   References

Handbook offers a wide range of methods for visual analysis: content, historical, structuralist, iconography, psychoanalysis, social semiotic, film analyses and ethnomethodology. Using many examples, it shows how each method can be applied to specific research projects (CR 2.88).

2.86.47 Webb, C. (1999) Analyzing qualitative data: computerized and other approaches. *Journal of Advanced Nursing* 29 (2) 323–30   29 References

Article reviews the background to, and advantages and disadvantages of, computerized approaches and compares them with manual techniques used in a number of recent PhD studies. Although a number of computer software packages are now available, the author believes that novice researchers, conducting small-scale studies, would be best recommended to use a manual approach in order to gain insight into the intuitive aspects of analysis (CR Appendix A).

2.86.48 Weitzman, E.A. (1999) Analysing qualitative data with computer software. *Health Services Research* 34 (5) 1241–63   17 References

Describes the process of qualitative data analysis and the role of computer software. Asserts that software can benefit the research in terms of speed, consistency and rigour, but should not replace methodological training (CR 2.84, Appendix A).

2.86.49 Woods, L. & Roberts, P. (2000) Generating theory and evidence from qualitative computerized software. *Nurse Researcher* 8 (2) 29–41   26 References

Paper utilizes the authors' experiences of using QSR NUD*IST 4 to manage, analyse and generate theory from large qualitative data sets. Its strengths and weaknesses are also discussed (CR 2.84, Appendix A).

2.86.50 Yanow, D. (1999) *Conducting interpretive policy analysis*. Thousand Oaks, CA: Sage ISBN 0761908277

Book describes what interpretative approaches are and what they can mean to policy analysis. The frame of reference is then moved from thinking about values as costs and benefits to thinking about them more as a set of meanings. The book concludes with a chapter on how to move from 'fieldwork to textwork' (CR 3.11).

2.87   ANALYSING QUANTITATIVE DATA

Statistical tests enable quantitative data to be made meaningful and intelligible. Having chosen the appropriate test and carried it out, the researcher is then in a position to reduce, organize, evaluate, interpret and communicate the results. Descriptive and/or inferential statistics will be utilized depending on the problem and data obtained.

Definitions [See Appendix D for sources]

Event history analysis – a regression method that is used for explaining or predicting the timing of events

Exploratory data analysis – a type of statistical analysis that uses a special collection of largely graphical descriptive statistics for summary research findings

Quantitative data analysis – the manipulation of numerical data through statistical procedures for the purpose of describing phenomena or assessing the magnitude and reliability of relationships among them

---

Annotations

2.87.1　Aiken, L.S. & West, S.G. (1996) *Multiple regression: testing and interpreting interactions*. Newbury Park, CA: Sage　ISBN 0761907122　References

Book provides a clear set of prescriptions for estimating, testing and probing interactions in regression models. The latest research is also included.

2.87.2　Allen, M.P. (1997) *Understanding regression analysis*. Dordrecht: Kluwer Academic/Plenum Publishers　ISBN 0306456486

This introduction to the widely used statistical techniques is intended for those who only have a rudimentary knowledge of mathematics. It discusses descriptive statistics; the logic of sampling distributions and simple hypothesis testing; the basic operations of matrix algebra; and structural equation models (CR 2.81).

2.87.3　Allison, P.D. (1999) *Multiple regression: a primer*. Thousand Oaks, CA: Pine Forge Press ISBN 0761985336

Book is a complete introduction to multiple regression designed for the first social statistics course taken by undergraduates.

2.87.4　Antonius, R. (2002) *Interpreting quantitative data with SPSS*. London: Sage ISBN 0761973990　References

This book will be an invaluable resource for students learning about descriptive and inferential statistics for the first time. Key features include: 14 SPSS lab sessions demonstrating how it can be used in the practical research context; sets of exercises and 'real-life' examples; a step-by-step guide to enable integration of these examples in a descriptive written report; lists of key terms and further reading (CR 2.81, 2.82).

2.87.5　Banks, S. (1999) Analysis of quantitative research data: Part 1. *Professional Nurse* 14 (9) 634–7　6 References

Provides a brief overview of the types of quantitative data, how to describe them and outlines the different shapes of distributions. Includes suggestions for further reading.

2.87.6　Banks, S. (1999) Analysis of quantitative research data: Part 2. *Professional Nurse* 14 (10) 710–13　4 References

Describes which tests can be used with different types of quantitative data and outlines the process of reporting and interpreting hypothesis tests. Includes suggestions for further reading.

2.87.7　Bernstein, I.A. & Rowe, A. (2001) S*tatistical data analysis using your personal computer*. Thousand Oaks, CA: Sage　ISBN 0761917810　References

Book asks what should you see when analysing real data using one of the major statistical packages, such as SPSS, SAS or Microsoft Excel? It guides the reader through the output from a variety of statistical sources. Using actual demonstrations, the authors supply readers with the computer programs necessary to simulate data sets with the statistical properties (usually multivariate) that are often assumed of real data.

2.87.8　Bijleveld, C.J.H. (1998) *Longitudinal data analysis: designs, models and methods*. Thousand Oaks, CA: Sage　ISBN 0761955380

Examines all the main approaches to longitudinal analysis as well as newer developments (such as structural equation modelling, multilevel modelling and optimal scaling). Readers will gain a thorough understanding and make appropriate decisions about which technique can be applied to the research problem (CR 2.48).

2.87.9　Blaikie, N. (2003) *Analyzing quantitative data: from description to explanation*. London: Sage　ISBN 0761967591　References

Book is designed for social researchers who need to know what procedures to use under what circumstances, in practical research projects. It accomplishes this without requiring an in-depth understanding of statistical theory, but also avoids both trivializing procedures or resorting to 'cookbook' techniques.

2.87.10   Bokbo, P. (2001) *Correlation and regression: applications for industrial organizational psychology and management* (2nd edition). Thousand Oaks, CA: Sage   ISBN 0761923039

Provides statistical theory in correlation and regression in an accessible format using words, equations and a variety of applied examples.

2.87.11   Bryman, A. & Cramer, D. (1994) *Quantitative analysis for social scientists* (revised edition). London: Routledge   ISBN 0415113075 References

Provides social science students with a non-technical introduction to the use of statistical techniques. The most up-to-date version of SPSS is used and no previous knowledge is assumed (CR Appendix A).

2.87.12   Byrne, D. (2002) *Interpreting quantitative data*. London: Sage   ISBN 076196262X

Jargon-free and written with the needs of students in mind, this text offers students a guide on how to interpret the complex reality of the social world.

2.87.13   Chen, P.Y. & Popovich, P.M. (2002) *Correlation: parametric and nonparametric measures*. Thousand Oaks, CA: Sage ISBN 0761922288

Book will enable the reader to compare and distinguish the concepts of similarity and relationship, identify the distinction between correlation and causation, and interpret correlations correctly.

2.87.14   Chu, K. (1999) An introduction to statistics, significance testing and the *p* value. *Emergency Medicine* 11 (1) 28–34   45 References

Explains the *p* value when using statistical tests and discusses how type I and type II errors can occur. Emphasizes the need to look for clinical as well as statistical significance in research findings and that *p* values need to be interpreted along with other issues, such as sample size and the validity of the study.

2.87.15   Cramer, D. (2003) *Advanced quantitative data analysis* Buckingham: Open University Press   ISBN 0335200591   References

Book explains the various statistical techniques used to analyse quantitative data. Commonly used software is introduced and instructions are given for SPSS Release 11, and a version of LISREL which is freely available online.

2.87.16   Diamantopoulos, A. & Schlegelmilch, B.B. (1997) *Taking the fear out of data analysis: a step-by-step approach*. London: The Dryden Press ISBN 0030990068

Book is intended for all students studying quantitative research methods in all disciplines. Its three parts cover understanding data, preparing and carrying out its analysis (CR 2.84).

2.87.17   Diggle, P.J., Liang, K.-Y. & Zeger, S.L. (1994) *The analysis of longitudinal data*. Oxford: Clarendon Press   ISBN 0198522843   References

Describes statistical models and methods for the analysis of longitudinal data (CR 2.48).

2.87.18   Faithfull, S. (1997) Analysis of data over time: a difficult statistical issue. *Journal of Advanced Nursing* 25 (4) 853–8   16 References

Discusses the problems encountered when trying to analyse longitudinal data in a study concerning somnolence and cranial radiotherapy. The paper explores and illustrates the process of time-series analysis and weighs its advantages and disadvantages (CR 2.48).

2.87.19   Firebaugh, G. (1997) *Analyzing repeated surveys*. Thousand Oaks, CA: Sage ISBN 0803973985   References

Author explicates different methods for studying social change through analysing data from repeated surveys. Four basic uses are identified – description, decomposition, explanation of aggregate trends and assessment of changing individual parameters (CR 2.52).

2.87.20   Foster, J.J. (2001) *Data analysis using SPSS for windows versions 8–10: a beginners guide*. London: Sage   ISBN 0761922687

Written in a non-technical style, the author explains the basics of SPSS, including the input of data, data manipulation, descriptive analyses and inferential techniques (CR Appendix A).

2.87.21   Fox, J. (1991) *Regression diagnostics: an introduction*. Newbury Park, CA: Sage   ISBN 080393971X   References

Explains the techniques for exploring problems that compromise a regression analysis, and for deciding whether certain assumptions seem reasonable.

2.87.22   Fox, J. (1997) *Applied regression analysis, linear models, and related methods*. Thousand Oaks, CA: Sage   ISBN 080394540X   References

Using graphs and numerous examples using real data from the social sciences, this book considers the role of statistical data analysis in social research. Many topics are covered which will enable appropriate analysis of data.

2.87.23   Garson, G.D. (1998) *Neural networks: an introductory guide for social scientists.*

Thousand Oaks, CA: Sage   ISBN 0761957316
References

Book provides numerous studies and examples that illustrate the advantages of neural network analysis over other procedures. The methods are presented in an accessible style for the reader who does not have a background in computer science.

2.87.24   Guo, S. & Hussey, D. (1999) Note on research methodology. Analyzing longitudinal rating data: a three-level hierarchical linear model. *Social Work Research* 23 (4) 258–68 18 References

Using generalizability theory as a guide, this study discusses statistical problems and strategies of analysing longitudinal rating data involving multiple raters. To disentangle raters' bias from clients' true change, the authors show the importance of looking into the multifaceted structure of measurement error. Proposals are made for analysis in similar studies (CR 2.27, 2.28, 2.48).

2.87.25   Hagenaars, J.A. (1990) *Categorical longitudinal data: log-linear panel, trend and cohort analysis*. Newbury Park, CA: Sage ISBN 0803929579 References

The problems that may occur with statistical analysis of longitudinal data are covered, together with solutions shown by actual examples. The tools developed over the last decade are discussed (CR 2.48, 2.86).

2.87.26   Hagle, T.M. (1996) *Basic math for social scientists: problems and solutions*. Thousand Oaks, CA: Sage   ISBN 0803972857   References

Provides an introduction to basic mathematical problems in the quantitative analysis of social science data.

2.87.27   Hart, A. (2000) Towards better research: a discussion of some common mistakes in statistical analyses. *Complementary Therapies in Medicine* 8 (1) 37–47   11 References

Using scenarios from complementary medicine research common statistical mistakes are identified and discussed. Suggestions are made to help avoid problems, including the clear identification of research objectives and checking of test assumptions.

2.87.28   Jaccard, J. (2003) *Interaction effects in multiple regression* (2nd edition). Thousand Oaks, CA: Sage   ISBN 0761927425

Provides students and researchers with a readable and practical introduction to conducting analyses of interaction effects in the context of multiple regression. This new edition expands coverage on the analysis of three-way interactions in multiple regression analysis.

2.87.29   Kahane, L.H. (2001) *Regression basics*. Thousand Oaks, CA: Sage   ISBN 0761919589

Book shows readers how to get the most from regression by providing a friendly, non-technical introduction to the subject.

2.87.30   Klein, J.H. (2001) *Critical path analysis*. **Wisniewski, M.** (2001) *Linear programming*. Basingstoke: Palgrave ISBN 0333763556 References

Book is part of a new series focusing on the practical relevance of operational research. Critical path analysis, a method of scheduling projects, is discussed and the author shows how it may be used in the management of projects of all sizes. The use of critical path analysis software is also covered. The linear programming model is developed using a business model and the relevance of its use is discussed (CR 2.84).

2.87.31   LeFort, S.M. (1993) The statistical versus clinical significance debate. *Image: Journal of Nursing Scholarship* 25 (1) 57–62   36 References

Paper compares and contrasts statistical and clinical significance to provide an overview of the issues surrounding their use, as described in methodological literature from a variety of disciplines. Some implications for nursing research are discussed.

2.87.32   Leik, R.K. (1997) *Experimental design and the analysis of variance*. Thousand Oaks, CA: Sage ISBN 0803990065   References

Book provides comprehensive coverage of the concepts behind ANOVA as well as its implementation. It emphasizes the importance of assisting students to understand the principles before embarking on computation.

2.87.33   Lewis-Beck, M. (ed.) (1994) *Factor analysis and related techniques*. London: Sage/ Toppan Company ISBN 080395431X   References

Book covers all aspects of factor analysis together with principal components. Also covered are confirmatory analysis and covariance structure models.

2.87.34   Liebrand, W.B.G., Nowak, A. & Hegselmann, R. (eds) (1998) *Computer modeling of social processes*. London: Sage ISBN 0761954244   References

This edited book is the first coherent collection that surveys the impact that computer-based methods have had on the social and behavioural sciences and illustrates the potential for future research. The authors assume no prior knowledge of computer science.

2.87.35   Maruyama, G.M. (1997) *Basis of structural equation modelling*. Thousand Oaks, CA: Sage   ISBN 0803974094   References

Through the use of narrative explanation, the author describes the logic underlying structural equation modelling (SEM) approaches. Its relationship to techniques like regressions and factor analysis is described, together with its strengths and weaknesses. Carefully constructed exercises are included.

2.87.36   Miles, J. & Shevlin, M. (2000) *Applying regression and correlation: a guide for students and researchers*. London: Sage   ISBN 0761962301

Introduces regression analysis through a simple model-building approach and maintains a conceptual, non-mathematical approach throughout the text.

2.87.37   Pallant, J. (2001) *SPSS survival manual: a step-by-step guide to data analysis using SPSS for windows (version 10)*. Buckingham: Open University Press   ISBN 0335208908   References

This book aims to demystify statistics and data analysis by guiding readers through the research process and choosing the right statistical techniques for any particular project (CR 2.83).

2.87.38   Polit, D.F. (1996) *Application manual to accompany data analysis and statistics for nursing research*. Stamford, CT: Appleton & Lange   ISBN 0838563341

AND

2.87.39   Polit, D.F. (1996) *Data analysis and statistics for nursing research*. Stamford, CT: Appleton & Lange   ISBN 0838563295

Book is intended for nursing students undertaking a course on statistics and data analysis. It is written in a non-technical manner, assumes no prior knowledge and its emphasis is on understanding how to use and interpret statistics, not how to calculate them. Computer printouts are included to help students understand them, with actual and fictitious examples being given. Each chapter is summarized and exercises are included. An application manual is available to accompany this book (CR 2.2, 2.80, 2.87.38).

2.87.40   Ratcliffe, P. (1998) Using the 'new' statistics in nursing research. *Journal of Advanced Nursing* 27 (1) 132–9   36 References

Author argues that quantitative methods are underused in nursing research. Although this is often because the qualitative approach is most appropriate, it may also be that nurse researchers are unfamiliar with modern, sophisticated data analysis techniques. Probability and survival modelling techniques, suitable for use in complex nursing research situations, are discussed. Although mathematically complex, they are easily applied in practice using dedicated computer programs. The paper describes their application using one such program, GLIM 4 (CR 2.9, 2.29, Appendix A).

2.87.41   Raudenbush, S.W. & Bryk, A.S. (2002) *Hierarchical linear models: applications and data analysis methods* (2nd edition). Thousand Oaks, CA: Sage   ISBN 076191904X

Book gives examples and lucid explanations of the theory and use of hierarchical linear models (HLM). This new edition includes an intuitive introductory summary of the basic procedures for estimation and inference used with HLM models; a new section on multivariate growth models; a discussion of research synthesis or meta-analysis applications; analytic advice on the centring of level 1 predictors and new material on plausible value intervals and robust standard estimators.

2.87.42   Rose, D. & Sullivan, O. (1996) *Introducing data analysis for social scientists* (2nd edition). Buckingham: Open University Press   ISBN 0335196179   References

This revised and updated edition assumes no previous knowledge of statistics or computer use and aims to assist students taking a first course in quantitative analysis. The principles of analysing these data are explained and a floppy disc of SPSS is included (CR Appendix A).

2.87.43   Smithson, M.J. (2003) *Confidence intervals*. Thousand Oaks, CA: Sage   ISBN 0761922091

Using easy-to-understand examples from different disciplines, the author introduces the basis of the confidence interval framework and provides the criteria for 'best' confidence intervals, along with trade-offs between confidence and precision.

2.87.44   Snijders, T.A.B. & Bosker, R.J. (1999) *Multilevel analysis: an introduction to basic and advanced multilevel modelling*. London: Sage   ISBN 0761958908

The main methods, techniques and issues for carrying out multi-level modelling and analysis are covered in this introduction to the topic.

2.87.45   Sterne, J.A.C. & Davey Smith, G. (2001) Sifting the evidence: what's wrong with significance tests? *British Medical Journal* 322 (7280) 27 January 226 31   4 References

Article gives a brief history of the p value and significance testing, explaining how researchers have come to misinterpret them. Suggests guidelines for reporting which would provide a more useful indication of whether results are significant or not.

2.87.46 Tacq, J. (1997) *Multivariate analysis techniques in social science research: from problem to analysis*. London: Sage ISBN 076195273X References

Book gives a range of actual research examples in the social sciences to show how to make the most appropriate choice of technique. All classical multivariate techniques are covered. The step-by-step explanation works through each analysis both by calculation and by reproducing the computer output from SPSS for Windows. A summary is also included of all the statistical concepts needed for dealing with more advanced techniques (CR 2.83).

2.87.47 Toothaker, L.E. (1993) *Multiple comparison for researchers*. Newbury Park, CA: Sage ISBN 0803941773 References

Discusses all aspects of multiple comparison procedures. These are: when they may be of value, types of procedure, comparisons between them, violations of assumptions and robustness, multiple comparisons for the two-way ANOVA, and factorial or randomized blocks.

2.87.48 Turner, J.R. & Thayer, J. (2001) *Introduction to analysis of variance: design, analysis and interpretation*. Thousand Oaks, CA: Sage ISBN 0803970757

Moving from the simplest type of design to more complex ones, the authors introduce five different kinds of ANOVA technique and explain which design/analysis is appropriate to answer specific questions.

2.87.49 Vermunt, J.K. (1997) *Log-linear models for event histories*. Thousand Oaks, CA: Sage ISBN 0761909370

Book presents a general approach to missing data problems in event history analysis, where this is based upon the similarities between log-linear, hazard and event history models.

2.87.50 Walsh, M. (1988) Beyond statistical significance. *Applied Nursing Research* 1 (2) 101–3 10 References

Article discusses the question of whether statistical significance is a necessary condition for clinical significance. When caring for people, it is not so much the 'average' difference that is of interest, but rather the individual's difference.

2.87.51 Weisberg, H.F. (1992) *Central tendency and variability*. Newbury Park, CA: Sage ISBN 0803940076 References

Book covers levels of measurement, measures of centre and spread and shows how to generalize sample results to the population. The use of exploratory data analysis is also discussed (CR 2.28).

2.87.52 Yamaguchi, K. (1991) *Event history analysis*. Newbury Park, CA: Sage ISBN 080393324X References

Provides a systematic introduction to models, methods and applications of event history analysis.

2.88 CONTENT ANALYSIS

'Recorded words and sentences provide rich and varied sources of data about people and the contexts in which they live. In order to use these data, objective and systematic procedures need to be employed to render them valid and reliable.' (Waltz, Strickland & Lenz, 1984: 285)

Definition [See Appendix D for source]

Content analysis – a procedure for analysing written or verbal communications in a systematic and objective fashion, typically with the goal of quantitatively measuring variables

Example

Waters, T. (1998) The role of the nurse practitioner in the gastroenterology setting. *Gastroenterology Nursing* 21 (5) 198–206 11 References

Study examined the role of a nurse practitioner working in the specialized field of gastro-enterology. Data collection involved researcher-designed open-ended interview methods and content analysis (CR 2.36).

Annotations

2.88.1 Cavanagh, S. (1997) Content analysis: concepts, methods and applications. *Nurse Researcher* 4 (3) 5–16 29 References

Discusses content analysis as a qualitative methodology, considerations about its use, assessing reliability and validity, and ways in which these data can be analysed (CR 2.24, 2.25, 2.86).

2.88.2 *A concept dictionary of English with computer programs for content analysis* (1990) Edited by Laffal, J. Essex, CT: Gallery ISBN 0913622060

Book is a thesaurus-type dictionary of over 42,000 words, classified into 168 concept categories. The development of the system is described and a number of applications in textual analysis are discussed. Several computer programs on diskette are provided (CR 2.89).

2.88.3 Kelly, A.W. & Sime, A.M. (1990) Language as research data: application of computer content analysis in nursing research. *Advances in Nursing Science* 12 (3) 32–40   27 References

Discusses the use of the Minnesota Contextual Content Analysis Program in categorizing, reducing data and interpreting manifest and latent meaning in linguistic communications (CR 2.84, 2.89).

2.88.4 Krippendorf, K. (1980) *Content analysis: an introduction to its methodology.* Beverly Hills, CA: Sage   ISBN 0803914970   References

Intended for a fairly wide audience, this book can serve as a text and practical guide to content analysis in research contexts. An overview of the technique is given, together with a comprehensive discussion of the key elements that need to be considered when it is used. Chapters on computer-based content analysis techniques, reliability and validity are included (CR 2.24, 2.25, 2.84).

2.88.5 Mackenzie, J. (1994) Analyzing data: alternative methods. *Nurse Researcher* 1 (3) 50–6   11 References

Two approaches to content analysis are described, one from a pragmatic point of view and the other from a more complex discussion of the methodological and philosophical issues involved (CR 2.68).

2.88.6 Morgan, D.L. (1993) Qualitative content analysis: a guide to paths not taken. *Qualitative Health Research* 3 (1) 112–21   8 References

Argues that qualitative content analysis is distinctive in its approach to coding and interpretation of counts from codes. Researchers need to consider carefully whether counting codes is an appropriate method of analysis (CR 2.9, 2.86, 2.89).

2.88.7 Moseley, L.G., Mead, D.M. & Murphy, F. (1997) Applying lexical and semantic analysis to the exploration of free-text data. *Nurse Researcher* 4 (3) 46–68   19 Reference

Discusses the categorization of a large number of free-text responses by using a computer. A study of primary nursing provided the data, part of which was to understand the leadership styles of ward sisters (CR 2.84).

2.88.8 Neuendorf, K.A. (2002) *The content analysis guidebook.* Thousand Oaks, CA: Sage   ISBN 0761919783

Author provides an accessible text for upper-level undergraduate and graduate students on this complex methodology. It comprises step-by-step instructions and practical advice.

2.89   CONTEXTUAL/NARRATIVE/ DISCOURSE ANALYSIS

'Contextual analysis assumes that objects, and mostly words, have more in common, the more the context they are in is alike. Context means the linguistic environment of words or within data surroundings of a recording unit.' (Krippendorf, 1980: 117)

[Both qualitative and quantitative analytical techniques may be used for these data.]

Definitions [See Appendix D for sources]

Categorization analysis – ... a method for the study of situated social action [offers a complementary method to sequential analysis used in the study of naturally occurring talk and text]

Contextual analysis – analysis which focuses on the individual's behaviour or attitudes, with reference to a group context

Contextualization – the placement of data into a larger perspective

Conversation analysis – ... focuses ... on issues of meaning and context in interaction

Dialectical analysis – the process of locating events or actions in a wider social and historical context and involves conceptually moving backwards and forwards between the specific part and contextual whole

Discourse analysis – a general term covering a wide variety of approaches to the analysis of recoded talk (sometimes used interchangeably with conversation analysis) ... it is principally concerned with the analysis of the process of communication itself

Discourse theory – ... defines all social phenomena as structured semiotically by codes and rules and therefore amenable to linguistic analysis using semiotic concepts

Network analysis – an efficient way of contextualizing actors' behaviour, based on description and inductive modelling of a specific aspect of this context: the relational pattern or 'structure' of the social setting in which action is observed

Semiotics – ... the theory of signs or the theory investigating the relationship between knowledge and signs

Example

Baird, C.L. (2000) Living with hurting and difficulty doing: older women with osteoarthritis. *Clinical Excellence for Nurse Practitioners* 4 (4) 231–7　31 References

Reports a study that described the many problems experienced by women with the chronic progressive disease of osteoarthritis. Eighteen women participated in narrative, descriptive research based on naturalistic-framework and qualitative analysis methods. Methods of data collection are described, together with the deconstructions and reconstructions of the narratives. Recommendations are made for improving care (CR 2.36).

Annotations

2.89.1　Allen, D. & Hardin, P.K. (2001) Discourse analysis and the epidemiology of meaning. *Nursing Philosophy* 2 (2) 163–76　42 References

Examines a semiotic theory of language and how semiotics relates to discourse and discourse analysis. Discusses the implications for phenomenological research in nursing, where, it is argued, the context of language is often ignored.

2.89.2　Barker, C. & Galasinski, D. (2001) *Cultural studies and discourse analysis: a dialogue on language and identity.* London: Sage　ISBN 0761963847　References

Book demonstrates that critical discourse analysis is able to provide the analytic context, skills and tools to study how language constructs, constitutes and shapes the social world. It demonstrates in detail how this methodological approach can enhance cultural studies.

2.89.3　Boje, D.M. (2001) *Narrative methods for organizational and communication research.* Thousand Oaks, CA: Sage　ISBN 0761965874　References

Book examines alternative discourse analysis strategies. Eight analysis options, which can deal with stories in organization studies, are covered.

2.89.4　Boklund-Lagopoulou, K., Lagopoulos, A. & Gottdiener, M. (eds) (2002) *Semiotics.* London: Sage　ISBN 0761974164　References　4 Volumes

This anthology is a unique research tool for students and scholars alike in all areas of the social sciences and humanities, including linguistics, social and cultural anthropology, sociology, cultural studies, philosophy, psychology, literature, and media and communication studies.

2.89.5　Burnard, P. (1996) Teaching the analysis of textual data: an experimental approach. *Nurse Education Today* 16 (4) 278–81　26 References

Paper offers a group method, based on experimental principles, for teaching the analysis of textual data. Variants of the method are also described and various objections to it are addressed (CR 2.36, 2.87).

2.89.6　Cameron, D. (2001) *Working with spoken discourse.* London: Sage　ISBN 0761957731 References

Book provides a comprehensive account of the expanding field of discourse analysis. Its three sections cover: a definition of discourse and uses of discourse analysis; approaches to this technique and its applications in social research; and designing and writing up projects.

2.89.7　Cortazzi, M. (1993) *Narrative analysis.* London:　Falmer　Press　ISBN　1850009635 References

Book discusses the collection and analysis of narrative material drawing on models within the disciplines of sociology, psychology, literature analysis and anthropology. Quotations and analysis of teachers' narratives are used for illustration.

2.89.8　Coulthard, M. (ed.) (1994) *Advances in written text analysis.* London: Routledge　ISBN 0415095204　References

Provides an overview of approaches to written text analysis. It includes classic and specially commissioned papers containing a variety of foci. Examples used come from pure science, social science, academic journals, weekly magazines, newspapers and literary narrations.

2.89.9　Drew, P., Chatwin, J. & Collins, S. (2001) Conversation analysis: a method for research into interactions between patients and health care professionals. *Health Expectations* 4 (1) 58–70　25 References

Outlines the perspective and method of conversation analysis and reviews studies of doctor–patient interactions in order to identify how it can be applied.

2.89.10　Emden, C. (1998) Conducting a narrative analysis. *Collegian: Journal of the Royal College of Nursing, Australia* 5 (3) July 34–9　9 References

Paper describes the process of narrative analysis as undertaken within a nursing study on scholars and scholarship. Strategies used for analysis are described in sufficient detail for others to use them where appropriate (CR 2.78).

2.89.11 Geanellos, R. (2000) Exploring Ricoeur's hermeneutic theory of interpretation as a method of analyzing research texts. *Nursing Inquiry* 7 (2) June 112–19   24 References

Through exposition of Ricoeur's theory of interpretation, which include distanciation, appropriation, explanation and understanding, guess, and validation, a hermeneutic approach to textual analysis is presented, discussed and critiqued. Examples from nursing research are used to demonstrate points under discussion (CR 2.5, 2.6).

2.89.12 Howarth, D. (2000) *Discourse.* Buckingham: Open University Press ISBN 0335200702   References

This book is an overview of different conceptions and methods of discourse analysis and traditions of thinking in which these conceptions have emerged.

2.89.13 Iverson, G.R. (1991) *Contextual analysis.* Newbury Park, CA: Sage ISBN 0803942729 References

Discusses contextual analysis and guidance is given on selecting the most appropriate statistical model.

2.89.14 Jaworshi, A. & Coupland, N. (eds) (1999) *The discourse reader.* London: Routledge ISBN 0415197341   References

Reader presents a comprehensive collection of important, original writings on discourse analysis. The book covers the foundations of modern discourse analysis and reports all its contemporary methods and traditions. Also included are discussions of research methods and resources, and reflexive commentaries highlighting key differences between sub-traditions. Studies and papers show what it is able to achieve when applied to different social issues and settings.

2.89.15 Jørgenson, M. & Phillips, L. (2002) *Discourse analysis as theory and method.* London: Sage   ISBN 0761971122   References

This systematic introduction to discourse analysis identifies a body of theories and methods for social research. It brings together three central approaches – Laclau and Mouffe's discourse theory, critical discourse analysis and discursive psychology – in order to establish a dialogue between different forms of discourse analysis often kept apart by disciplinary boundaries.

2.89.16 Lepper, G. (2000) *Categories in text and talk: a practical introduction to categorization analysis.* London: Sage ISBN 0761956662 References

Describes the application of 'membership categorization analysis' and introduces the concepts

through an analysis of data samples and exercises. Its application to other disciplines is also discussed.

2.89.17 Lucas, J. (1997) Making sense of interviews: the narrative dimension. *Social Sciences in Health: International Journal of Research and Practice* 3 (2) 113–26   49 References

Article looks at the difficulties of narrative analysis within qualitative research. Illustrated by data from a study of women's experiences of personal crisis, it shows that interview extracts, taken out of context, can be interpreted in many ways (CR 2.36, 2.69).

2.89.18 Masterson, A. (1998) Discourse analysis: a tool for change in nursing, policy, practice and research. In Smith, P. (ed.) *Nursing research: setting new agendas.* London: Arnold   ISBN 0340661941   Chapter 5 81–107   108 References

Discourse analysis is proposed as a powerful tool to assist nurses in influencing health care policies, research agendas and enabling them to become more politically astute. Some methodological issues associated with it are discussed, including its tools, techniques, advantages, disadvantages, validity, reliability and rigour (CR 3.7.7).

2.89.19 McKee, A. (2003) *Textual analysis: a beginner's guide.* London: Sage   ISBN 0761949933 References

This introductory book on the analysis of cultural texts starts from the basic philosophical foundations that underlie the practice, explains the importance of texts and what they tell us about the world they represent. Case studies and exercises are included.

2.89.20 Phillips, D.A. (2001) Methodology for social accountability: multiple methods and feminist, post-structural, psychoanalytic discourse analysis. *Advances in Nursing Science* 23 (4) 49–66   31 References

Bridging the gap between the individual and social context, this methodology aims to explore the regulatory function of discourse on subjectivity production, and moves nursing research beyond the individual level in order to theorize social context and its influence on health and well-being. This article describes the multiple methods used in a recent study that explored links between cultural discourses of masculinity, performativity and practices of male violence (CR 2.10).

2.89.21 Phillips, N. & Hardy, C. (2002) *Discourse analysis: investigating processes of social construction.* Thousand Oaks, CA: Sage ISBN 0761923624   References

Book is a concise, straightforward guide for students and researchers who are interested in understanding and using discourse analysis.

2.89.22 Popping, R. (2000) *Computer-assisted text analysis*. London: Sage   ISBN 0761953795

Book focuses on the methodological and practical issues of coding and handling data, including sampling and reliability and validity issues. An appendix of computer programs for text analysis is included (CR 2.24, 2.25, 2.36, 2.84, 2.88, Appendix A).

2.89.23 Powers, P. (2001) *The methodology of discourse analysis*. Sudbury, MA: Jones & Bartlett   ISBN 0763718041   References

Book presents the theoretical, philosophical and conceptual underpinnings of discourse analysis, including the contribution of feminism to the method. Steps in implementing the method are suggested, and the presentation of a discourse analysis of nursing diagnosis elucidates the method (CR 2.10, 2.36).

2.89.24 Priest, H.M. (2000) The use of narrative in the study of caring: a critique. *NT Research* 5 (4) 245–50 37   References

Author believes that narrative analysis is an appropriate methodology with which to study nurses' perceptions of caring as it enables the researcher to enter their world. It is compatible with other approaches and retains the factual and emotional context in which the data were gathered (CR 2.29, 2.36, 2.64).

2.89.25 Psathas, G. (1995) *Conversation analysis: the study of talk-in-interaction*. Thousand Oaks, CA: Sage   ISBN 0803957475   References

Book provides an introduction to conversation analysis, outlines its procedures and major accomplishments. Also included are discussions on verbal sequence, institutional constraints on interaction and the deep structure of talk.

2.89.26 Samra-Fredericks, D. (1998) Conversation analysis. In Symon, G. & Cassell, C. (eds) *Qualitative methods and analysis in organizational research: a practical guide*. London: Sage   ISBN 0761953515   Chapter 9 161–89   82 References

Chapter discusses some of the complexities of analysing conversation and examines *one* aspect of the 'moment-to-moment existence' of directors and senior managers attending a board meeting (CR 2.36.135).

2.89.27 Scott, J. (2000) *Social network analysis: a handbook* (2nd edition). London: Sage   ISBN 0761963391   References

Text provides an introduction to the theory and practice of network analysis in the social sciences. It is a guide to the general framework of network analysis, the basic concepts and technical measures

required, and available computer programs are reviewed.

2.86.28 Silverman, D. (ed.) (1997) *Qualitative research: theory, method and practice*. London: Sage   ISBN 0803976666   References

Contributors to this book reflect on the analysis of observations, texts, talk and interviews. Key themes include the centrality of the relationship between analytic perspectives and methodological issues; the need to broaden our conception of qualitative research beyond issues of subjective 'meaning' towards issues of language; representation and social organization; searching for ways to build links between social science traditions; and having a dialogue between social science and the community (CR 2.68, 2.72, 2.76, 2.78).

2.89.29 Stillar, G.F. (1998) *Analyzing everyday texts: discoursal, rhetorical, and social perspectives*. Thousand Oaks, CA: Sage   ISBN 0761900616   References

By outlining and integrating three different perspectives – discourse, rhetoric and social theory – this volume provides a comprehensive and well-illustrated framework for the analysis of everyday texts. The book describes the tools and resources which can be drawn from these perspectives, and these are then brought together in an extensive analysis. The last chapter reflects on the principles and consequences of conducting theoretically informed critical textual analysis.

2.89.30 ten Have, P. (1998) *Doing conversational analysis: a practical guide*. London: Sage   ISBN 0761955860   References

Provides hands-on experience in training to use conversation analysis. Sections include an introduction, specific methodology, making and transcribing recordings, analytic strategies, applying conversation analysis and writing up and publishing results (CR 2.97, 2.99).

2.89.31 Titscher, S., Meyer, M., Wodak, R. & Vetter, E. (2000) *Methods of text and discourse analysis: in search of meaning*. London: Sage   ISBN 0761964835   References

Book provides a comprehensive overview of linguistic and sociological approaches to text and discourse analysis. Ten models are surveyed which will enable readers to compare, contrast and apply a range of methods (CR 2.45, 2.88).

2.89.32 Wetherell, M., Taylor, S. & Yates, S. (eds) (2001) *Discourse as data: a guide for analysis*. London: Sage/Open University   ISBN 0761971580   References

Book explains how to do discourse research. Step-by-step examples are given to illustrate a typical analysis. The role of the researcher, transcription, ethics, formulating research questions, the process of writing up research, evaluating, validating and the application of research are all discussed (CR 2.17, 2.20, 2.25, 2.95, 2.97, 2.102, 3.16).

2.89.33 Wetherell, M., Taylor, S. & Yates, S. (eds) (2001) *Discourse theory and practice: a reader*. London: Sage/Open University press   ISBN 0761971564   References

The aim of this reader is to introduce students to the major figures in the field, and to some of their writings. These, combined with editorial commentaries, should allow the key epistemological and theoretical issues to be put into context.

2.89.34 Wiklund, L., Lindholm, L. & Lindström, A. (2002) Hermeneutics and narration: a way to deal with qualitative data. *Nursing Inquiry* 9 (2) 114–25   42 References

Presents an account of the hermeneutic philosophy and narration. Exemplifies this with a case from a larger study about suffering using Ricoeur's theory of interpretation which is modified to encompass a caring science paradigm.

2.89.35 Wodak, R. & Meyer, M. (2001) *Methods of critical discourse analysis*. London: Sage   ISBN 0761961542   References

Designed as an introduction to discourse analysis, the book gives an overview of the various theories and methods associated with this socio-linguistic approach. Students are also introduced to the leading experts in this field and the methods with which they are particularly associated.

2.89.36 Wood, L.A. & Kroger, R.O. (2000) *Doing discourse analysis: methods for studying action in talk and text*. London: Sage   ISBN 0803973519   References

Providing the theoretical justification and practical steps for doing discourse analysis, the book shows how the social world revolves around talk and text. Authors draw on conversation analysis, critical discourse analysis, pragmatics and the discursive approach developed in social psychology.

2.90 LEVELS OF DATA ANALYSIS – PRIMARY

There are three levels of data analysis: primary, secondary and meta-analysis. Primary analysis in the health field usually involves examining archives such as personal or public health records.

Definition [See Appendix D for source]
Primary data analysis – the initial analysis of data, whether those data were collated originally for research or other purposes

Example

Jowell, R., Curtice, J., Park, A., Thomson, K., Jarvis, L., Bromley, C. & Stratford, N. (eds) (2000) *British social attitudes: focusing on diversity: the 17th report*. London: Sage/The National Centre for Social Research   ISBN 0761970452

This book is a compilation, description and commentary upon a range of social attitudes and values in Britain. The National Centre for Social Research conducts annual surveys from a nationwide sample of around 3,500 people and this report summarizes and interprets the most recent data and makes comparisons with findings from previous years.

Annotations

2.90.1 Black, C., Roos, L.L., Rosser, W. & Dunn, E.V. (1992) Analyzing large data sets. In Tudiver, F., Bass, M.J., Dunn, E.V., Norton, P.G. & Stewart, M. (eds) *Assessing interventions: traditional and innovative methods*. Newbury Park, CA: Sage   ISBN 0803947704   Chapter 17 169–81   27 References

Chapter defines large data sets, identifies different types and describes their relevance for primary research. Some important issues in their analysis are discussed.

2.90.2 Kapborg, I. & Berterö, C. (2002) Critiquing bachelor candidates' theses: are the criteria useful? *International Nursing Review* 49 (2) June 122–8   16 References

Reports a study that analysed 13 theses using particular criteria. An evaluation of these criteria in the primary analysis of the theses is reported (CR 3.18).

2.91 LEVELS OF DATA ANALYSIS – SECONDARY

The next level of data analysis is called secondary analysis. The data used may be raw data, statistical databases or archival material.

Definitions [See Appendix D for sources]

Meta-matrix construction – a second level analysis when used for triangulation and occurs following traditional qualitative and quantitative data analyses

Secondary data analysis – a form of research in which data collected by one researcher are re-analysed by another investigator, usually to test new research hypotheses

Example

Hinchcliffe, R. (1999) Noise hazards to the general population: hearing surveys reassessed. *Journal of Audiological Medicine* 8 (2) 113–21   19 References

Author reports the results of an extended analysis of data collected in a Medical Research Council hearing survey 40 years ago (CR 2.46, 2.52, 2.91).

Annotations

2.91.1   Barrett, R.E. (1994) *Using the 1990 US census for research.* Thousand Oaks, CA: Sage   ISBN 0803953909   References

This book explains the 'ins' and 'outs' of using American Census data for research. It covers the history of the Census, its design, procedures and problems, and preparing data for analysis (CR 2.79).

2.91.2   Clarke, S.P. & Cossette, S. (2000) Secondary analysis: theoretical, methodological and practical considerations. *Canadian Journal of Nursing Research* 32 (3) 109–29   44 References

Article highlights difficulties that may arise when researchers use data from previous clinical research projects, including theoretical issues and problems involving sampling, measurement and external and ecological validity. Practical suggestions are made for undertaking secondary analysis together with criteria for their evaluation.

2.91.3   Gorard, S. (2002) The role of secondary data in combining methodological approaches. *Educational Review* 54 (3) 231–7   15 References

Author urges greater use of numerical secondary data as a routine part of all studies, whatever their primary method. The current poor public image of UK educational research and some possible reasons for this are discussed. It is believed that particularly poor quality research, allied to the potential of

secondary data, might empower novice researchers, enabling them to critique established work and conduct powerful and informative analysis of their own.

2.91.4   Heaton, J. (1998) Secondary analysis of qualitative data. *Social Research Update* Issue 22 Guildford: University of Surrey, Department of Sociology   16 References www.soc.surrey.ac.uk/sru/SRU22.html (Accessed 14/11/03)

Describes secondary analysis, suggests why it is useful, explores methodological and ethical considerations, and discusses how the approach may be developed (CR 2.17).

2.91.5   Hilton, T.L. (1992) *Using national databases in educational research.* Hillsdale, NJ: Laurence Erlbaum Associates   ISBN 080580840X

Book is designed to enable educational researchers make better use of the many large, longitudinal and cross-sectional data files now readily available in the USA. It is not a 'how to' book, but should facilitate research at the planning and design stage. Studies show what can and cannot be done with large national databases (CR 2.14, 2.92).

2.91.6   Kneipp, S.M. & Yarandi, H.N. (2002) Complex sampling designs and statistical issues in secondary analysis. *Western Journal of Nursing Research* 24 (5) 552–66   15 References

Addresses the issues that rise from conducting secondary analysis on large, national survey data sets. Defines the terms and procedures for different types of sampling, what difficulties this might pose for analysis and strategies (including the types of statistical package available) that may assist in dealing with these difficulties (CR 2.22, Appendix A).

2.91.7   Orsi, A.J., Grey, M., Mahon, M.M., Moriarty, H.J., Shepard, M.P. & Carroll, R.M. (1999) Conceptual and technical considerations when combining large data sets. *Western Journal of Nursing Research* 21 (2) 130–42   14 References

Explains the necessity of a standardized method for combining large data sets and outlines the process of doing so using the authors' previous work.

2.91.8   Riedel, M. (2000) *Research strategies for secondary data: a perspective for criminology and criminal justice.* Thousand Oaks, CA: Sage   ISBN 0803958382   References

Book describes approaches to the evaluation and analysis of secondary data in criminological research. It focuses on secondary data originating in surveys, information collected by organizations, and data sets available from archives (CR 2.52, 2.76).

2.91.9 Stewart, D.W. (1993) *Secondary research: information sources and methods* (2nd edition). Beverly Hills, CA: Sage ISBN 0803950373 References

This monograph is designed as an introduction to locating, using, evaluating and integrating information that is available from printed materials and computer databases. It includes issues in evaluating research, information sources, including computer-assisted information searches, and integrating data from multiple sources. Exercises are included and more relevant topic areas could easily be substituted for any particular discipline.

2.92 LEVELS OF DATA ANALYSIS – META-ANALYSIS

'The third level of data analysis is meta-analysis which enables the researcher to summarize and integrate findings from several studies. It can be performed using either raw data from original studies or summary measures to generate effect sizes.' (Woods & Catanzaro, 1988: 335)

Definitions [See Appendix D for sources]

Cumulative meta-analysis – ... studies are added one at a time in a specified order (e.g. according to date of publication or quality) and the results are summarized as each new study is added

Meta-analysis – ... a quantitative method of combining the results of independent studies (usually drawn from published literature) and synthesizing summaries and conclusions which may be used to evaluate therapeutic effectiveness [and] plan new studies

Meta-data-analysis – ... the study of the findings of reported research in a particular substantive area of inquiry by means of processing the 'processed data'

Meta-method – ... the study of the rigour and epistemological soundness of the research methods used in research studies

Meta-study – ... a research approach involving analysis of the theory, methods and findings of qualitative research and the synthesis of these insights into new ways of thinking about phenomena

Meta-synthesis – a method of synthesizing qualitative accounts to construct adequate interpretive explanations from multiple studies

Meta-theory – ... analysis of the underlying structures on which the research is grounded

QUOROM – ... an acronym for quality of reporting of meta-analyses of randomized controlled trials

Example

Burke, S.O., Kaufmann, E., Costello, E., Wiskin, N. & Harrison, M.B. (1998) Stressors in families with a child with a chronic condition: an analysis of qualitative studies and a framework. *Canadian Journal of Nursing Research* 30 (1) 71–95 50 References

Article presents a comprehensive, research-based, clinically usable framework of stressors and tasks for families with a chronically ill child. The steps in the early development of the framework and its uses are briefly described and more detail is given of its final stages. This was a meta-analysis of qualitative research findings that confirmed the components of the framework. Conclusions are drawn for subsequent research steps and its potential clinical uses (CR 2.36, 2.55).

Annotations

2.92.1 Barroso, J. & Powell-Cope, G.M. (2000) Meta-synthesis of qualitative research on living with HIV infection. *Qualitative Health Research* 10 (3) 340–53 34 References

Purpose of this meta-synthesis was to understand the experience of adults living with HIV infection as described in published research. Findings are reported (CR 2.26).

2.92.2 Beck, C.T. (1999) Focus on research methods. Facilitating the work of a meta-analyst. *Research in Nursing and Health* 22 (6) 523–30 24 References

After briefly identifying the benefits and criticisms of meta-analysis, specific problems a meta-analyst may encounter in conducting a quantitative review of the literature are discussed. Pointers for removing some of these roadblocks are addressed, along with recommendations to authors, editors and manuscript reviewers for publishing research reports that are more usable for meta-analysis studies.

2.92.3 Britten, N., Campbell, R., Pope, C., Donovan, J. & Morgan, M. (2002) Using meta-ethnography to synthesize qualitative example: a worked example. *Journal of Health Service Research and Policy* 7 (4) October 209–15 23 References

Four papers about lay meanings of medicines were chosen at random. A seven-step process for conducting a meta-ethnography was employed: getting started, deciding what is relevant, reading the studies, determining how they were related, translating the studies into one another, synthesizing translations and expressing the synthesis. Results are reported and authors believe it is possible to synthesize the results of qualitative research. The worked example has produced middle-range theories in the form of hypotheses that could be tested by other researchers (CR 2.36, 2.42).

2.92.4   Brown, S.A., Upchurch, S.L. & Acton, G.J. (2003) A framework for developing a coding scheme for meta-analysis. *Western Journal of Nursing Research* 25 (2) 205–22   18 References

Emphasizes the importance of a formal process of data extraction for systematic reviews and offers a framework for a coding instrument (CR 2.12, 2.24, 2.25).

2.92.5   Byers, J.F. & Stullenbarger, E. (2003) Meta-analysis and decision analysis research and practice. *Western Journal of Nursing Research* 25 (2) 193–204   35 References

Compares the respective elements of meta-analysis and decision analysis and describes the usefulness of the latter for the implementation of research findings into practice (CR 3.8).

2.92.6–2.92.18 *Evaluation and the Health Professions* (1995) Special issue 18 (3) The meta-analytic revolution in health research. Part I

The following entry differs in format as it documents two special issues of the journal *Evaluation and the Health Professions*. These articles have not been annotated.

2.92.6   Bangert-Drowns, R.L. Misunderstanding meta-analysis. 304–14   12 References

2.92.7   Bausell, R.B. Introduction 235–7   4 References

2.92.8   Bausell, R.B., Li, Y.-F., Gau, M.-L. & Soeken, K.L. The growth of meta-analytic literature from 1980 to 1993. 238–51   11 References

2.92.9   Preiss, R.W. & Allen, M. Understanding and using meta-analysis. 315–35   55 References

2.92.10   Soeken, K.L., Bausell, R.B. & Li, Y.-F. Realizing the meta-analytic potential. 336–44   3 References

2.92.11   Wieland, D., Stuck, A.E., Siu, A.L., Adams, J. & Rubenstein, L.Z. Meta-analytic methods for health services research: an example from geriatrics. 252–82   57 References

2.92.12   Yeaton, W.H., Langenbrunner, J.C., Smyth, J.M. & Wortman, P.M. Exploratory research synthesis: methodological considerations for addressing limitations in data quality. 283–303   40 References

Evaluation and the Health Professions (1995) Special issue 18 (4) The meta-analytic revolution in health research. Part II

2.92.13   Bausell, R.B. Introduction 347–8   3 References

2.92.14   Hall, J.A. & Rosenthal, R. Interpreting and evaluating meta-analysis. 393–407   40 References

2.92.15   Kavale, K.A. Meta-analysis at 20: retrospect and prospect. 349–69   88 References

2.92.16   Miller, N. & Pollock, V.E. Use of meta-analysis for testing theory. 370–92   62 References

2.92.17   Sakala, C. & Hunter, J.E. The Cochrane pregnancy and childbirth database: implications for peri-natal care policy and practice in the US. 428–66   91 References

2.92.18   Schmidt, F. & Hunter, J.E. The impact of data-analysis methods on cumulative research knowledge: statistical significance testing, confidence intervals and meta-analysis. 408–27   39 References

2.92.19   Eysenck, H.J. (1995) Problems with meta-analysis. In Chalmers, I. & Altman, D.G. *Systematic reviews.* London: British Medical Journal Publishing Group   ISBN 0727909045   Chapter 6 64–74   20 References

Discusses some problems which occur in meta-analysis: regressions are often not linear, effects are often multivariate rather than univariate, coverage can be restricted, bad studies may be included, the data summarized may not be homogeneous, grouping different causal factors may lead to meaningless estimated effect sizes, and the failure to relate data to theories may obscure discrepancies (CR 2.12.3).

2.92.20   Greener, J. & Grimshaw, J. (1996) Using meta-analysis to summarize evidence within systematic reviews. *Nurse Researcher* 4 (1) 27–38   30 References

Authors discuss the relationship between meta-analysis and systematic review (CR 2.12).

2.92.21   Hunt, M. (1999) *How science takes stock: the story of meta-analysis.* New York: Russell Sage Foundation   ISBN 0871543982   References

Book includes accounts by key practitioners of strategies used to resolve practical and theoretical problems and discusses the impact of meta-analysis on the science and policy communities. It shows how the statistical techniques produce more accurate data than from the standard literature review, and the issue of quality control is addressed. The future of meta-analysis, its potential for further refinements, its growth in the scientific literature and exciting possibilities for the future are all discussed. An appendix offers some finer points of the mechanics of conducting a meta-analysis investigation.

2.92.22 Hunter, J.E., & Schmidt, F.L. (1989) *Methods of meta-analysis: correcting error and bias in research findings.* Newbury Park, CA: Sage ISBN 0803932227   References

Book reviews all the methods proposed for cumulating knowledge across studies, including the narrative review, counting statistically significant findings, and the averaging of quantitative outcome measures (CR 2.27).

2.92.23 Lipsey, M.W. & Wilson, D.B. (2000) *Practical meta-analysis.* Thousand Oaks, CA: Sage ISBN 0761921680   References

By integrating and translating current methodological and statistical work into a practical guide, the authors provide a state-of-the-art introduction to the various approaches to doing meta-analysis.

2.92.24 Muncer, S., Taylor, S. & Craigie, M. (2002) Power dressing and meta-analysis: incorporating power analysis into meta-analysis. *Journal of Advanced Nursing* 38 (3) 274–80   30 References

It is suggested that by incorporating power analysis into meta-analysis, misleading conclusions could be avoided. Changes to protocol design, which would highlight the importance of power analysis, are advocated.

2.92.25 Oxman, A.D. & Stachenko, S.J. (1992) Meta-analysis in primary care: theory and practice. In Tudiver, F., Bass, M.J., Dunn, E.V., Norton, P.G. & Stewart, M. (eds) *Assessing interventions: traditional and innovative methods.* Newbury Park, CA: Sage   ISBN 0803947704   Chapter 19 191–207   60 References

Chapter highlights the major issues and decisions to be made when undertaking a meta-analysis. Examples are included from recently published literature.

2.92.26 Paterson, B.L., Thorne, S.E., Canam, C. & Jillings, C. (2001) *Meta-study of qualitative health research: a practical guide to meta-analysis and meta-synthesis.* Thousand Oaks, CA: Sage ISBN 0761924159   References

Meta-study is an exciting new opportunity for the analysis and synthesis of qualitative research findings.

This Book provides step-by-step directions on how to conduct a meta-study, as well as making recommendations for tools and standards for the application of this approach. The authors use their own experience to explain the process, including past mistakes and retrospective insights (CR 2.36).

2.92.27 Reynolds, N.R., Timmerman, G., Anderson, J. & Stevenson, J.S. (1992) Meta-analysis for descriptive research. *Research in Nursing and Health* 15 (6) 467–75   52 References

A case is made for the value of meta-analysis as a technique for integrating descriptive research. An overview of different meta-analytic approaches to data analysis using the correlational index with descriptive research is described (CR 2.36, 2.86).

2.92.28 Rosenthal, R. (1991) *Meta-analytic procedures for social research* (revised edition). Newbury Park, CA: Sage   ISBN 080394246X References

Covers the latest techniques in the field, as well as providing a comprehensive text on meta-analytic procedures.

2.92.29 Rosenthal, R. & DiMatteo, M.R. (2001) Meta-analysis: recent developments in quantitative methods and literature reviews. *Annual Review of Psychology* 52 59–82   References

The history and current status of the meta-analytic enterprise, its advantages and historical criticisms are described, as are the basic steps in a meta-analysis. Advantages of these procedures include seeing the 'landscape' of a research domain, keeping statistical significance in perspective, minimizing wasted data, becoming intimate with the data summarized, asking focused research questions and finding moderator variables (CR 2.12, 2.29).

2.92.30 Riegelman, R.K. (2000) *Studying a study and testing a test: how to read the medical literature* (4th edition). Philadelphia, PA: Lippincott Williams & Wilkins   ISBN 0781718600 (includes CD-ROM for Windows and Macintosh) Chapter 11 Meta-Analysis 85–99

Discusses the principles of meta-analysis and examines its strengths and weaknesses. A list of questions to ask is included (CR 2.83.10).

2.92.31 Smith, D.G. & Egger, M. (1998) Meta-analysis: unresolved issues and future developments. *British Medical Journal* 316 17 January 221–5

Article discusses some topics for future examination and appropriate practice in the domain of meta-analysis.

2.92.32   Soeken, K.L. & Sripusanapan, A. (2002) Assessing publication bias in meta-analysis. *Nursing Research* 52 (1) January–February 57–60 13 References

Demonstrates several methods, both graphical and statistical, of assessing publication bias (CR 2.27, 2.99).

2.92.33   Sterne, J.A.C., Egger, M. & Smith, G.D. (2001) Investigating and dealing with publication and other biases in meta-analysis. *British Medical Journal* 323 (7304) 14 July 101–5   37 References

Explains how bias can arise in publications and how it might be detected by graphical and statistical means. Suggests strategies to prevent or remedy bias arising in meta-analyses.

2.93   INTERPRETING THE FINDINGS

The final steps in any research project are to interpret the data, so that it becomes meaningful within the context of a particular piece of research. It may then take its place in the literature.

Annotations

2.93.1   Anderson, A.J.B. (1989) *Interpreting data: a first course in statistics.* London: Chapman Hall   ISBN 0412295709   References

Designed for students undertaking a statistics module, this book clarifies the basic requirements of data collection, examines the reliability of published data and the validation and analysis of data by computer. Examples are included from a wide range of disciplines and exercises conclude each chapter (CR 2.24, 2.25, 2.84).

2.93.2   Denzin, N.K. (1994) The art and politics of interpretation. In Denzin, N.K. & Lincoln, Y.S. (eds) *Handbook of qualitative research.* Thousand Oaks, CA: Sage   ISBN 0803946791   Chapter 31 500–15   68 References

Chapter discusses how the complex art of interpretation and story-telling is practised. The constructivist, grounded theory, feminist, Marxist, cultural studies and post-structural perspectives are explored, and predictions are made for the future (CR 2.10, 2.45, 2.97).

2.93.3   DiCenso, A. (2001) Clinically useful measures of the effects of treatment. *Evidence-based Nursing* 4 (2) 36–9   9 References

Describes the process of determining clinically significant outcome measures, including relative risk reduction and the number needed to treat.

2.93.4   Hunter, A., Lusardi, P., Zucher, D., Jacelon, C. & Chandler, G. (2002) Making meaning: the creative component in qualitative research. *Qualitative Health Research* 12 (3) 388–98   19 References

Authors present complementary contributions on how to reflect on qualitative data in order to find meaning (CR. 2.36).

2.93.5   Manski, C.F. (1999) *Identification problems in the social sciences.* Cambridge, MA and London: Harvard University Press   ISBN 0674442849 References

Book provides a language and set of tools for finding bounds on the predictions that social and behavioural scientists can logically make from non-experimental and experimental data.

2.93.6   Mays, N., Roberts, E. & Popay, J. (2001) Synthesizing research evidence. In Fulop, N., Allen, P., Clarke, A. & Black, N. (eds) *Studying the organization and delivery of health services: research methods.*   London: Routledge   ISBN 0415257638   Chapter 12 188–220   36 References

Chapter focuses on the issues encountered in synthesizing mainly non-experimental evidence, including qualitative data (CR 2.36, 3.12.3).

2.93.7   Williamson, J.W., Weir, C.R., Turner, C.W., Lincoln, M.J. & Cofrin, K.M.W. (2002) *Healthcare informatics and information synthesis: developing and applying clinical knowledge to improve outcomes.* Thousand Oaks, CA: Sage   ISBN 0761908242   References

Book covers the process of research synthesis for the purpose of evidence-based health care improvement. The authors integrate the conceptual and procedural dimensions of research synthesis in each stage of the process to produce step-by-step instructions for clinically applicable research synthesis. It also includes a compendium of Internet sources and useful addresses (CR 2.43, 2.102).

2.94   PRESENTING DATA

Once data has been carefully analysed, the next step is to present it verbally and/or in writing in the most clear and unambiguous way so that others may have no difficulty in its interpretation. Depending on the type of research undertaken, data may be presented in the form of tables, graphs, charts, narrative or various visual means.

Annotations

2.94.1   Curran, C.R. (1999) Clinical methods. Data display techniques. *Applied Nursing Research* 12 (3) 153–8   12 References

The reader's ability to perceive, comprehend and recall information contained within data is affected by how it is presented. Advantages and limitations of different types of data format are presented and techniques for the use of colour are also included.

2.94.2   Her Majesty's Stationery Office (1997) *Plain figures*. London: HMSO   ISBN 0117020397   References

Demonstrates and discusses ways of presenting numbers effectively so that their value can be realized. It also aims to help the reader interpret data more competently and confidently. No statistical tests are discussed and the book concentrates on bringing together advice and research findings on statistical presentation.

2.94.3   Hicks, C. (1994) Using tables and graphs to present research findings. *Nurse Researcher* 2 (1) 54–74   11 References

Discusses the different types of data that may be obtained and suggests how this may be presented graphically to bring it to life.

2.94.4   Jacoby, W.G. (1997) *Statistical graphics for univariate and bivariate data*. Thousand Oaks, CA: Sage   ISBN 0761900837

Providing strategies for examining data more effectively, this volume focuses on displaying univariate and bivariate methods graphically (CR 2.87).

2.94.5   Kosslyn, S.M. (1993) *The elements of graph design*. Oxford: W.H. Freeman   ISBN 071672362X   References

Book gives a step-by-step approach to creating effective displays of quantitative data. Crucial communication between the design, data and the reader are made for those who prepare, use and interpret graphic data.

2.94.6   McKinney, V. & Burns, N. (1993) The effective preparation of graphs. *Nursing Research* 42 (4) 250–2   18 References

Discusses the use and effective preparation of graphs.

2.94.7   Office of Health Economics (1997) *Compendium of health statistics* (10th edition). London: Office of Health Economics   No ISBN

Provides a comprehensive statistical description of the National Health Service in the United Kingdom. Various ways of presenting data are shown.

2.94.8   Pearson, L. (1997) Quantitative analysis: the principles of data presentation. *Nurse Researcher* 4 (4) 41–53   9 References

Paper introduces some of the main principles of data presentation in relation to quantitative analysis. Ways of enhancing the clarity and integrity of the data are suggested (CR 2.87).

2.94.9   Sprent, P. (1988) *Understanding data*. Harmondsworth, Middlesex: Penguin   ISBN 0140772065   References

This practical text aims to develop skills in the selection and presentation of numerical data. Data is discussed and presented in a number of different contexts and exercises to consolidate learning are interspersed throughout the text.

2.94.10   Tufte, E.R. (2001) *The visual display of quantitative information* (2nd edition). Cheshire, CT: Graphics Press   ISBN 0961392142

Using numerous examples, the author shows how to rearrange and simplify tabulated lists, schedules, graphs, diagrams and maps in a way that reveals otherwise hidden relationships and patterns.

2.94.11   Wallgren, A., Wallgren, B., Persson, R., Jorner, U. & Haaland, J.-A. (1996) Graphing statistics and data: creating better charts. Thousand Oaks, CA: Sage   ISBN 0761905995   References

Book covers all aspects of organizing and presenting data, using real examples. Readers are shown step by step how to work from the raw data to a finished chart.

Communicating Nursing Research

2.95 EVALUATING RESEARCH FINDINGS

'A research critique is an objective, systematic attempt to identify, appreciate and weigh the merits and demerits of a particular piece of scientific research.' (Phillips, L.R.F., 1986: 364)

Literature included in this section will help nurses to develop their skills in evaluating published works and in making decisions about relevance to practice.

Definition [See Appendix D for source]

Evaluating research findings – a creative, constructive and positive process conducted for the purpose of identifying the strategies and limitations of a research project

Major text

Phillips, L.R.F. (1986) *A clinician's guide to the critique and utilization of nursing research.* Norwalk, CT: Appleton-Century-Crofts ISBN 0838511627 References

Annotations

2.95.1 Bell, P., Staines, P. & Mitchell, J. (2001) *Evaluating, doing and writing research in psychology.* London: Sage ISBN 0761971750 References

Book will enable students to grasp essential skills needed to think theoretically about arguments, to use methods for data analysis and be able to present their findings so that psychology is seen as an empirical science. It also contains chapter summaries, clarification of terms, problem areas in psychological argument and questions and exercises. A guide to doing a literature review is also included (CR 2,12).

2.95.2 Black, T.R. (2001) *Understanding social science research* (2nd edition). London: Sage ISBN 761973699 References

Text explains clearly how students can evaluate research, with particular emphasis on studies involving some aspect of measurement.

2.95.3 Bowers, D., House, A. & Owens, D. (2001) *Understanding clinical papers.* Chichester: John Wiley ISBN 047148976X References

This book, which focuses on quantitative research, uses a straightforward style to take readers through the sequence of a research report. Published examples, largely from the medical literature, describe research from around the world. A chapter, entitled 'Reading between the lines', shows how authors use text, tables and pictures to tell you what they have done.

2.95.4 Burns, N. & Grove, S.K. (2002) *Understanding nursing research* (3rd edition). Philadelphia, PA: W.B. Saunders ISBN 0721600115 References

This extensively revised edition reflects the most current literature and clinical studies. Each step in the research process is identified to enable students read, summarize and use findings in clinical practice. An introduction to interventions research is included, examples of qualitative research have been expanded, and the concept of evidence-based practice is discussed (CR 2.2).

2.95.5 Crookes, P. & Davies, S. (1998) *Research into practice.* Philadelphia, PA: W.B. Saunders ISBN 0702020680 References

This book introduces the skills of research appreciation and prepares the reader to access, critically evaluate, understand and use research-based literature within the multidisciplinary context of today's health services.

2.95.6 Cutcliffe, J. & Ward, M. (2002) *Critiquing nursing research.* Dinton, Nr. Salisbury: Quay Books ISBN 1856421945 References

Book aims to assist nurses in developing their critiquing skills. It explains the theoretical, substantive, methodological and presentational dimensions of the process.

2.95.7 Dempsey, P.A. & Dempsey, A.D. (2000) *Using nursing research: process, critical evaluation*

and utilization (5th edition). Philadelphia, PA: Lippincott   ISBN 0781717906   References

This new edition discusses the importance of nursing research, both quantitative and qualitative. Chapters show how to read and critique published research and how these findings may be used in practice (CR 2.1, 2.9, 2.102).

2.95.8 Devine, F. & Heath, S. (1999) *Sociological research methods in context.* Basingstoke: Macmillan   ISBN 0333666321

Text offers a detailed critique of eight research studies. Researchers are introduced to 'real-life' challenges in research by discussing how the sociologists actually undertook their work. Issues include politics of the research process; the influence of researchers' personal values; difficulties of sampling hidden populations; the practical and epistemological implications of using multiple methods and questions relating to informed consent in ethnographic fieldwork (CR 2.22, 2.42).

2.95.9 Fain, J.A. (1999) *Reading, understanding and applying nursing research: a text and workbook.* Philadelphia, PA: J.A. Davis   ISBN 0803602278   References

This interactive text introduces readers to research and explains its importance to the profession. Each step of the research process is covered and approaches to evaluating and applying nursing research are discussed. Chapters include objectives, a glossary, summary, learning activities and references (CR 2.2, 2.102, 3.7).

2.95.10 Gehlbach, S.H. (2002) *Interpreting the medical literature* (4th edition). New York: McGraw-Hill   ISBN 0071387625   References

Book demystifies the complex language of research studies and makes reading medical literature more palatable, digestible and profitable.

2.95.11 Girden, E.R. (2001) *Evaluating research articles from start to finish* (2nd edition). Thousand Oaks, CA: Sage   ISBN 0761922148   References

This new edition includes examples of recent good and flawed studies. All chapters but one include two articles, one critiqued by the author with copious notes to highlight potential flaws or good aspects, and the second is for self-critique. New to this edition are lists of 'caution factors', assumptions of/about statistical tests, an expanded introduction to the particular research design featured in each chapter, and expanded coverage of qualitative research techniques (CR 2.2).

2.95.12 Gomm, R. & Davies, C. (eds) (2000) *Using evidence in health and social care.* London:

Sage/Open University Press   ISBN 0761964959   References

Text introduces readers to different kinds of evidence and assists in evaluating the unique contributions of each. It supports evidence-based practice but seeks to ensure that the interpretations and uses of it are broad, thoughtful and informed (CR 2.43).

2.95.13 Gomm, R., Needham, G. & Bullman, A. (eds) (2000) *Evaluating research in health and social care: a reader.* London: Sage Publications/ Open University Press   ISBN 0761964916   References

Book contains examples of a wide range of research techniques and provides a critical commentary for each. The commentary is designed to tackle jargon and demystify the text, highlighting the compromises that need to be made in the real world and the complexity of controlling relevant variables. The book also seeks to underline the challenges of interpreting and generalizing results both for the researcher and those who fund their work (CR 2.19, 2.28, 2.29, 2.36, 2.41, 2.52, 2.95).

2.95.14 Gott, R. & Duggan, S. (2003) *Understanding and using scientific evidence: how to critically evaluate data.* London: Paul Chapman Educational Publishing   ISBN 0761970835   References

Aims to assist teachers to develop an understanding of how evidence is collected, analysed and evaluated.

2.95.15 Greenhalgh, T. (2001) *How to read a paper: the basics of evidence-based medicine* (2nd edition). London: BMJ Books   ISBN 0727915789

Book covers searching the literature and assessing methodological quality. Advice is given on finding papers, assessing scientific validity and, where relevant, puting the findings into practice (CR 2.43, 2.102).

2.95.16 Guyatt, G.H., Sackett, D.L. & Cook, D.J. (1993) Users' guides to the medical literature. II How to use an article about therapy or prevention: (a) are the results of the study valid? *Journal of the American Medical Association* 270 (21) 2598–601 20 References

Utilizes a clinical scenario to demonstrate how to locate and appraise articles that will help in making decisions about patient care. Provides a framework for assessing the validity of research studies related to therapy or prevention (CR 1.2, 2.25, 2.101).

2.95.17 Guyatt, G.H., Sackett, D.L. & Cook, D.J. (1994) Users' guides to the medical literature. II How to use an article about therapy or prevention: (b) what were the results and will they help me in caring for my patients? *Journal of the American Medical Association* 271 (1) 59–63   13 References

Provides a clinical scenario and a suggested search strategy. Addresses the main questions clinicians need to ask in order to determine whether articles on therapy or prevention are useful in decisions regarding care (CR 1.1, 2.101).

2.95.18   Hayward, R.S.A., Wilson, M.C., Tunis, S.R., Bass, E.B. & Guyatt, G. (1995) Users' guides to the medical literature. VIII How to use clinical practice guidelines: (a) are the recommendations valid? *Journal of the American Medical Association* 274 (7) 570–4   30 References

Provides a framework for assessing the value and applicability of clinical guidelines to patient care (CR 2.25, 2.101).

2.95.19   Jacob, R.F. & Carr, A.B. (2000) Hierarchy of research design used to categorize the 'strength of evidence' in answering clinical dental questions. *Journal of Prosthetic Dentistry* 83 (2) 137–52   6 References

Offers a systematic means of categorizing the quality of research reports for clinicians and clinical investigators.

2.95.20   Jaeschke, R., Guyatt, G.H. & Sackett, D.L. (1994a) Users' guides to the medical literature. II How to use an article about a diagnostic test: are the results of the study valid? *Journal of the American Medical Association* 271 (5) 389–91   11 References

Indicates a search strategy to help answer a problem outlined in a clinical scenario, together with a framework for assessing the validity of research studies related to diagnostic tests (CR 2.25, 2.101).

2.95.21   Jaeschke, R., Guyatt, G.H. & Sackett, D.L. (1994b) Users' guides to the medical literature. III How to use an article about a diagnostic test: (b) what are the results and will they help me in caring for my patient? *Journal of the American Medical Association* 271 (9) 703–7   14 References

Uses a clinical scenario to suggest questions that need to be asked in order to determine how useful studies about diagnostic tests are when making decisions about the care of patients (CR 2.101).

2.95.22   Kearney, M.H. (2001) Levels and applications of qualitative research evidence. *Research in Nursing and Health* 24 (2) 145–53   32 References

Article contributes to the continuing dialogue on the role of qualitative research findings in improving nursing care. The role of qualitative research evidence, degrees of complexity and discovery, and applying qualitative findings in all health care encounters are discussed (CR 2.36).

2.95.23   Langford, R.W. (2001) *Navigating the maze of nursing research: an interactive learning adventure*. St Louis, MO: Mosby ISBN 0323009476   References

This hands-on approach to nursing research presents a total learning package, teaching students about research and information application in a unique, activity-based format. Its primary focus is on the ability to read, understand, interpret and apply research results in multiple clinical settings. The package combines traditional text with CD-ROM and a special website. Package includes a Computerized Test Bank (ISBN 0323010121) and an Instructor's Manual (ISBN 0323010156) (CR 2.102).

2.95.24   Lanoë N. (ed.) (2002) *Ogier's reading research: how to make research more approachable* (3rd edition). London: Ballière Tindall ISBN 0702026700   References

Book will enable nurses to get started in finding, reading and understanding research. Changes in locating research using new technologies are discussed. It also highlights the political and professional challenges and pressures for every practising nurse to be accountable for the quality of care delivered.

2.95.25   Laupacis, A., Wells, G., Richardson, S. & Tugwell, P. (1994) Users' guides to the medical literature. II How to use an article about prognosis. *Journal of the American Medical Association* 271 (3) 234–7   19 References

Suggests a framework for assessing articles that deal with prognosis, including asking questions about validity and usefulness to patient care (CR 2.25, 2.101).

2.95.26   Leininger, M. (2001) Founder's focus: theoretical research and clinical critiques to advance transcultural nursing scholarship. *Journal of Transcultural Nursing* 12 (1) 71   1 Reference

Author encourages nurses to renew their commitment to critiques in transcultural nursing and all theoretical, research and clinical studies to ensure scholarship in these endeavours. The processes involved in critiquing literature are briefly discussed, together with the qualities required in those undertaking this task (CR 2.53).

2.95.27   Levine, M., Walter, S., Lee, H., Haines, T., Holbrook, A. & Moyer, V. (1994) Users' guides to the medical literature. II How to use an article about harm. *Journal of the American Medical Association* 271 (20) 1615–19   22 References

Outlines a brief search strategy to address a clinical problem. Suggests questions to ask in order to assess the validity of research studies about harm and their implications for practice (CR 2.25, 2.101).

2.95.28 Light, R.J. & Pillemer, D.B. (1984) *Summing up the science of reviewing research.* Cambridge, MA: Harvard University Press ISBN 0674854314 References

Discusses the art of combining information from several studies in a practical way. General guidelines and step-by-step procedures are included, with examples given from several disciplines. Also included is checklist for evaluating reviews. The book is written in non-technical language and is likely to become a methodological classic (CR 2.12, 2.92).

2.95.29 Locke, L.F., Spirduso, W.W. & Silverman, S.J. (1998) *Reading and understanding research.* Thousand Oaks, CA: Sage ISBN 0761903070 References

Authors introduce and frame the notion of reading research within a wider context. Information is provided on finding, selecting and evaluating reports for trustworthiness. A step-by-step guide to reading reports from both qualitative and quantitative studies is included (CR 2.29, 2.36).

2.95.30 Naylor, C.D. & Guyatt, G.H. (1996) Users' guides to the medical literature. VI How to use an article about a clinical utilization review. *Journal of the American Medical Association* 275 (18) 1435–9 34 References

Advises how to critique an article that measures the quality of the process of care and assists in decision-making if undertaking a utilization review (CR 2.25, 2.101).

2.95.31 Oxman, A.D., Sackett, D.L., Cook, D.J. & Guyatt, G.H. (1994) Users' guides to the medical literature. VI How to use an overview. *Journal of the American Medical Association* 272 (17) 1367–71 39 References

Discusses how to use systematic reviews in order to assess the validity and usefulness of the results in caring for patients (CR 2.25, 2.101).

2.95.32 Phillips, L.R.F. (1986) *A clinician's guide to the critique and utilization of nursing research.* Norwalk, CT: Appleton-Century-Crofts ISBN 0838511627 References

Book is designed to complement existing texts and aims to provide the information needed to conduct an objective research critique and to use this to make decisions about research utilization. Major units in the text focus on the current research–practice gap

in nursing, development of critiquing skills and the utilization of clinical nursing research. Each chapter is summarized and includes additional learning activities and a bibliography. Two examples of published research are used to illustrate each aspect of the critiquing process (CR 2.102, 3.8).

2.95.33 Playle, J. (2000) Critically appraising research reports. *Journal of Community Nursing* 14 (11) 10, 13–16 22 References

Outlines the structure of research reports, the nature of critical appraisal and some of the key issues and questions to be addressed. Suggests that changes in practice should be driven by a critical and systematic evaluation of a body of knowledge.

2.95.34 Polit, D.F., Beck, C.T. & Hungler, B.P. (2000) *Essentials of nursing research: methods, appraisal and utilization* (5th edition). Philadelphia, PA: Lippincott Williams & Wilkins ISBN 0781725577 References

This new edition retains all its previous features and has a more user-friendly presentation. Additional material on qualitative methods and actual research examples are included. An Instructor's Manual, Test Bank, Study Guide for Students and a CD-ROM providing review questions are also available (CR 2.2, 2.95.35, 2.102).

2.95.35 Polit, D.F. & Hungler, B.P. (2000) *Study guide to accompany essentials of nursing research* (4th edition). Lippincott Williams & Wilkins ISBN 0781725585

Book will assist nurses in evaluating research findings in terms of scientific merit and potential utilization. It compares quantitative and qualitative data with regard to each aspect of study. Research examples, both real and fictional will assist students to read and analyse the strengths and weaknesses of the studies presented. Two full research reports, which will facilitate the development of critical reading skills, are included (CR 2.95.34).

2.95.36 Poulson, L. & Wallace, M. (eds) (2003) *Learning to read critically in teaching and learning.* London: Paul Chapman Publishing ISBN 0761947973 References

Book provides students with a framework for the critical analysis of any text, and shows how to incorporate it into a literature review. A further section presents accounts of leading-edge research and invites readers to practise literature review skills. A final section shows how a high-quality literature review can be constructed (CR 2.12).

2.95.37 Riegelman, R.K. (2000) *Studying a study and testing a test: how to read the health science literature* (4th edition). Philadelphia, PA: Lippincott

Williams & Wilkins   ISBN 0781718600 (includes CD-ROM for Windows and Macintosh)

Provides a step-by-step approach to a clinical review of the medical literature. It assumes no prior training in epidemiology, maths or statistics and teaches students, residents and clinicians how to read journal articles more critically and efficiently (CR 2.2, 2.83.10).

2.95.38   Rose, G. (1983) *Deciphering sociological research*. Beverly Hills, CA: Sage ISBN 00803920423   References

This book, which complements existing texts, provides an approach to analysing sociological research. Systematic methods are given for deciphering reports and 12 selected examples, which are edited versions of articles originally published in sociological journals, provide the data for analysis. These illustrate a range of approaches to research and are chosen from three major areas of sociology: deviance, education and stratification. The link between theory and empirical evidence is thoroughly explored in the analyses.

2.95.39   Schiavetti, N. & Metz, D.E. (2002) *Evaluating research in communication disorders* (4th edition). Boston, MA: Allyn & Bacon/ Longman   ISBN 0205337724   References

This new edition explains and discusses how to read, understand and evaluate research published in communicative disorders and sciences journals. Numerous examples are included, together with study questions.

2.95.40   Smith, H.W. (1981) *Strategies of social research: methodological imagination* (3rd revised edition). Austin, TX: Holt ISBN 0030230772 References

This reader comprises four major parts: sociology as a science; the production of data; improving data quality; and the analysis and presentation of data. The emphasis is on evaluating research rather than doing it. Each chapter ends with readings for advanced students and suggested research projects. Case histories are used to illustrate ethical and moral problems in social research (CR 2.17).

2.96   RESEARCH PROPOSALS

'A research proposal is a written document specifying what the investigator proposes to study. Proposals serve to communicate the research problem, its significance, and planned procedures for solving the problem.' (Polit & Hungler, 1991: 535)

Definition [See Appendix D for source]

Research proposal – the written plan and justification for a research project prepared before it begins. It is also used when applying for financial support to do the research

Example

Morse, J.M. (1996) The qualitative proposal. In Morse, J.M. & Field, P.A. *Nursing research: the application of qualitative approaches* (2nd edition). London: Chapman & Hall ISBN 0412605104 Appendix A 161–93 [Appendix B 194–6 Critique of the proposal]

Reproduces a proposal which was submitted to the National Center for Nursing Research, National Institutes of Health (USA), funded as a three-year foreign award in 1989, to conduct a series of studies on comfort and its application within nursing. A critique of the proposal is also included (CR 2.36.89).

Annotations

2.96.1   Bent, K.N. (1999) Seeking the both/and of a research proposal. *Advances in Nursing Science* 21 (3) 76–89   43 References

Article examines the layers of assumptions that circumscribe an ethnographic study of the relationships among health, environment, policy and culture in one Hispanic community. The author seeks to analyse these assumptions as sources of meaning and interpretation by illuminating discourses contained within the text of the proposal. This discourse analysis provides perspectives from which to consider questions of knowledge, power, and relationships in nursing inquiry (CR 2.42, 2.89).

2.96.2   Boyd, C.O. & Munhall, P.L. (2001) Qualitative research proposals and reports. In Munhall, P.L. (ed.) *Nursing research: a qualitative perspective* (3rd edition). Sudbury, MA: Jones & Bartlett and National League for Nursing   ISBN 0763711357   Chapter 24 613–38   14 References

Chapter offers practical guidance on developing qualitative research proposals (CR 2.36.98).

2.96.3   Coley, S.M. & Scheinberg, C.A. (2000) *Proposal writing* (2nd edition). Thousand Oaks, CA: Sage   ISBN 0761919600   References

Covers all aspects of proposal writing for beginners and moderately experienced grant writers. Appendices contain information on estimating time, a sample proposal, critique and funding resource information (CR 3.13).

2.96.4 Connelly, L.M. & Yoder, L.H. (2000) Improving qualitative proposals: common problem areas. *Clinical Nurse Specialist* 14 (2) 69–74 23 References

Outlines the problems that are frequently observed in qualitative proposals, offering advice on how to correct them, and providing examples from the authors' own funded proposals (CR 2.36).

2.96.5 Cutcliffe, J. & Stevenson, C. (2001) The long and winding road: obtaining funding for qualitative research proposals. *Nurse Researcher: The International Journal of Research Methodology in Nursing and Health Care* 9 (1) 52–62 26 References

Paper considers a range of strategies to help aspiring qualitative researchers produce proposals that stand a greater chance of being successful and gaining funding (CR 2.36, 3.13).

2.96.6 Davitz, J.R. & Davitz, L.L. (1996) *Evaluating research proposals: a guide for the behavioural sciences* (3rd edition). Englewood Cliffs, NJ: Prentice-Hall ISBN 0133485668 References

Book designed for students who are planning or critically evaluating research studies. The points to be considered when evaluating research proposals are discussed and a series of questions accompanies each section.

2.96.7 Ezell-Kalish, S.E., McCullum, T., Henry, Y., Schoenthaler, A. & Grady, S. (1981) *The proposal writer's swipe file: 15 winning fundraising proposals ... prototypes of approaches, styles and structures*. Washington, DC: Taft Corporation ISBN 0914756451

Provides a resource book of successful research proposals. Examples, covering a wide range of disciplines, are written by professional proposal writers and give insight into how fund-raising proposals should be constructed, organized, styled and presented.

2.96.8 Gitlin, L.N. & Lyons, K.J. (1996) *Successful grant writing: strategies for health and human service professionals*. New York: Springer ISBN 0826192602 References

Book is specially written for those in academic and practice settings. A range of strategies and work models are presented. Parts cover the perspective of funding agencies and the grantee, writing the proposal, models for their development and life after its submission (CR 3.13).

2.96.9 Heath, A.W. (1997) The proposal in qualitative research. *The Qualitative Report* [Online serial] 3 (1) March (41 paragraphs) www.nova.edu/ssss/QR/QR3-1/heath.html (Accessed 14/11/03)

Gives a generic outline for qualitative research proposals. It applies specifically to the research paradigm and methods that seem most applicable to the study of families and family therapy (e.g. post-positivist, phenomenological clinical observation and long interviews) (CR 2.49, 2.68).

2.96.10 Jacox, A.K. (1980) Nursing's statement: testifying in Washington. In Davis, A.J. & Krueger, J.C. (eds) *Patients, nurses, ethics*. New York: American Journal of Nursing Company ISBN 0937126845 References

[A testimony presented on 3 May 1977 at a public hearing before the National Commission for the Protection of Human Subjects of Biomedical and Behavioural Research, National Institute of Health, Bethesda, Maryland.]

Presenter reports on the difficulties encountered in getting research proposals accepted by research committees. Author contends that committees are composed largely of physicians and representatives of the biomedical sciences. This creates a powerful pressure to encourage research designs that are experimental rather than non-experimental. The place and value of nursing research is explored, and examples where permission has been refused are used to illustrate these points. Physicians, in their role as gatekeepers, are discussed, and the case for nursing representation on committees is outlined (CR 2.17).

2.96.11 Jones, S.P. & Bundy, A. *Writing a good grant proposal* www.dcs.gla.ac.uk/uk-cs-research/proposals.html (Accessed 05/02/03)

Website gives advice on approaching a proposal, criteria for a good proposal and some common shortcomings (CR 3.13).

2.96.12 Locke, L.F., Spirduso, W.W. & Silverman, S.J. (1999) *Proposals that work: a guide for planning dissertations and grant proposals* (4th edition). Thousand Oaks, CA: Sage ISBN 0761917063 References

Book gives practical advice on all aspects of writing research proposals, and the specimens show different designs and paradigms from several disciplines. The book is updated with a discussion of the effects of new technologies and the Internet on the process, a new chapter on funding for student research, a revised chapter on qualitative research, and two new specimen proposals (CR 2.13, 2.17, 2.23, 3.13).

2.96.13   Marshall, C. & Rossman, G.B. (1998) *Designing qualitative research* (3rd edition). Thousand Oaks, CA: Sage   ISBN 0761913394   References

Authors provide clear and direct guidance for writing successful proposals that fit into the framework of qualitative research. There is expanded coverage of focus groups, action research and interviewing, and many vignettes are included that illustrate the methodological challenges facing the researcher (CR 2.37, 2.68, 2.69, 2.72).

2.96.14   Medical Research Council (1994) *Developing high quality proposals in health services research*. London: Medical Research Council   No ISBN

Booklet provides guidance on developing research proposals (CR 3.13).

2.96.15   Miller, D.C. (2002) The art and science of grantsmanship. In Miller, D.C. & Salkind, N.J. *Handbook of research design and social measurement* (6th edition). Thousand Oaks, CA: Sage   ISBN 0761920463   Part 7 B3 596–641   References (extensive)

Section covers all aspects of proposal writing, contract research, pre- and post-doctoral fellowships, funding institutions (both government and private), together with information sources. Advice is also given on costing research projects (CR 2.1.52, 2.99, 3.13).

2.96.16   Munhall, P.L. (2000) *Qualitative research proposals and reports: a guide* (2nd edition). Sudbury, MA: Jones & Bartlett   ISBN 0763711713   References

This 'how to' book provides information on formatting and reporting qualitative research reports and abstracts.

2.96.17   National Science Foundation *A guide for proposal writing* www.nsf.gov/pubs/1998/nsf9891/nsf9891.htm (Accessed 05/02/03)

Discusses the review process for awarding grants, criteria for evaluation, the likely impact of the research and advice to proposal writers (CR 3.13).

2.96.18   Ogden, T.E. (1995) *Research proposals: a guide to success* (2nd edition). New York: Raven Press   ISBN 0781703131   References

Book is a complete guide to the preparation of research proposals written from the perspective of a grant reviewer. Focusing on the National Institute of Health (NIH) system in the USA the book covers basic grantsmanship for the novice and unsuccessful applicant, and advanced grantsmanship for scientists beginning academic and research careers. Appendices include information sources at NIH,

categorical institute programmes and examples of pink sheets, preliminary data and informed consent.

2.96.19   Punch, K.F. (2000) *Developing effective research proposals*. London: Sage   ISBN 0761963561   References

Book shows how to design and prepare a research proposal and present it effectively to a university review committee, funding body or commercial client. It is organized around three themes: what are research proposals?; who reads them and why?; what general strategies and guidelines might be useful and what might a finished proposal look like? The advice given is appropriate for both quantitative and qualitative and mixed-method studies.

2.96.20   Stewart, R.D. & Stewart, A.L. (1992) *Proposal preparation* (2nd edition). New York: Wiley   ISBN 0471552690   References

Although largely aimed at business enterprises, this book shows how to present the information required for successful research applications to funding bodies. It also describes how they are evaluated, which gives clues about the preparation of a winning proposal.

2.96.21   University of Wisconsin-Madison *Proposal writing: Internet resources* www.library.wisc.edu/libraries/Memorial/grants/proposal.htm (Accessed 08/02/03)

Lists Internet sources that give advice to individuals or organizations on planning and writing grant proposal (CR 3.13).

2.96.22   Woods, L.P. (2000) Responding to calls for bids: process and preparation. *Nurse Researcher: The International Journal of Research Methodology in Nursing and Health Care* 8 (1) 19–27   5 References

Article focuses on how individuals and groups might respond to invitations to tender for specific research contracts. The issues that need to be addressed are highlighted, together with some of the potential problems likely to be encountered.

2.97   WRITING ABOUT RESEARCH

'To write is to convey to others the facts, and the relationships between facts, that have been discovered.' (Goodall, 1994: 6)

Definitions [See Appendix D for sources]

Plagiarism – the incorporation of the work of one person into the work of another without citing the source

Research report – a document that summarizes the main features of a study, including the research question … methods used to address it … findings … interpretation and implications

Annotations

2.97.1 Bailey, P.A. (2001) Academic misconduct: responses from deans and nurse educators. *Journal of Nursing Education* 40 (3) 124–31   16 References

Article describes what deans/chairs and faculty in baccalaureate nursing programmes perceive as academic misconduct among students. Results support the need for a clearer understanding among students of what constitutes plagiarism, and they need to be identified early so that appropriate action can be taken (CR 2.17).

2.97.2 Becker, H.S. (1986) *Writing for social scientists: how to start and finish your thesis, book or article.* Chicago, IL: University of Chicago Press ISBN 0226041085   References

This book aims to show students how to improve their writing skills. It focuses on the elusive work habits that contribute to good writing. Discussion on how to overcome others' criticisms, revise again and again, and develop the skills of writing clear prose are all discussed. A chapter is included on the personal and professional risks involved in scholarly writing.

2.97.3 Berry, R. (1994) *The research project: how to write it* (3rd edition). London: Routledge ISBN 0415110904   References

Designed for students at school, college or university, this book covers all aspects needed to develop, carry out and write up a research project. An example of a well-researched, well-written paper with full bibliography and notes is also included.

2.97.4 Browner, W.S. (1999) *Publishing and presenting clinical research.* Philadelphia, PA: Lippincott Williams and Wilkins ISBN 0683307452   References

Emphasizes concise writing, visually logical and simple graphical presentation, and focuses on the issues that trip up even experienced researchers.

2.97.5 Burnard, P. (2001) Writing skills: why nurses do not publish. *JCN Online* 15 (04) 337   7 References   www.jcn.co.uk/article.asp?ArticleID (Accessed 04/02/02)

Article considers some of the reasons why nurses do not publish and how they might be encouraged to do so (CR 2.99, 3.7).

2.97.6 Christensen, C. & Atweh, B. (1998) Collaborative writing in participatory action research. In Atweh, B., Kemmis, S. & Weeks, P. (eds) *Action research in practice: partnerships for social justice in education.* London: Routledge ISBN 0415171520   Chapter 16 329–41   2 References

Chapter discusses the process of collaborative writing in action research. The benefits of collaboration are outlined, as well as ways of writing and issues in learning and publishing action research stories (CR 2.15, 2.37.2).

2.97.7 Cormack, D.F.S. (1994) *Writing for health care professions.* Oxford: Blackwell Scientific   ISBN 0632034491   References

Gives advice to health care professionals on all aspects of writing papers. Publishing opportunities are also discussed (CR 2.99).

2.97.8 Crème, P. & Lea, M.R. (1997) *Writing at university: a guide for students.* Buckingham: Open University Press   ISBN 033519642X   References

Book provides university students and academic staff with strategies and approaches to academic writing. The whole process of writing assignments is considered, including attention to disciplinary diversity, the relationship between reading and writing, and the use of the personal and textual cohesion.

2.97.9 Cuba, L. (2002) *A short guide to writing about social science* (4th edition). New York: Longman   ISBN 032107842X   References

This writing guide is designed to help students prepare effective documents for their social sciences courses. Information is given on using the Internet as well as traditional information sources.

2.97.10 Daly, J. (2000) *Writer's guide to nursing periodicals.* London: Sage   ISBN 0761914927 References

This reference book is a single source of guidelines required by editors of 101 nursing journals. It also includes key journal facts and information of value when submitting articles for publication.

2.97.11 Davidhizar, R. & Dowd, S. (1998) Writing scholarly papers as a team. *Health Care Supervisor* 16 (4) 53–60   56 References

Identifies the advantages and disadvantages of writing in a team and how to go about selecting partners, topics and the importance of identifying roles and responsibilities.

2.97.12 Davis, M. (1997) *Scientific papers and presentations*. Oxford: Academic Press ISBN 0122063708 References

Provides a precise guide to writing proposals, literature reviews, theses, articles, slide presentations, posters and grants. Author also discusses methods for searching and citing scientific literature, composing reviews, preparing data presentations, communicating visually and public speaking (CR 2.12, 2.96, 2.99, 2.100, 3.19).

2.97.13 Ding, K. & Hu, P. (1999) Research studies in two health education journals, 1988–1997: targets and methodologies. *International Electronic Journal of Health Education* 2 (3) 101–10 22 References www.Kittle.siu.edu/iejhe/toc/2–3/vol 2–3 index. html (Accessed 14/11/03)

A content analysis was used to examine the general status of health education research and methodological applications of 336 articles, published by two major health education journals. Most studies reported information about research type and methods, sampling, target population, response rate, data collection instrumentation, data analysis and study purposes. Some articles failed to provide relevant information to enable readers to judge their quality (CR 2.88).

2.97.14 Dixon, N. (2001) Writing for publication – a guide for new authors. *International Journal for Quality in Health Care* 13 (5) 417–21 References

Author suggests that health care practitioners, who may be daunted by the publication process, can acquire experience in writing a paper by working through a systematic thought process that includes consideration of what journal readers and editors want. The most important part of writing is to think through key ideas and messages for readers and then to organize them into a logical structure. Writing clear answers to 10 key questions may be one way to start the process.

2.97.15 Ely, M., Vinz, R., Downing, M. & Anzol, M. (1997) *On writing qualitative research: living by words*. London: Falmer Press ISBN 0750706031 References

Written for beginners and experienced researchers, this book is about creating research writing that is useful, believable and interesting. Blending rigorous scholarship and a clear academic style, authors examine the process, rhetorical devices and other tools researchers use to evoke the complexity of their experience. Authors include accounts of their own research writing experiences to show how data can be presented in a meaningful way (CR 2.36).

2.97.16 Erlen, J.A., Siminoff, L.A., Sereika, S.M. & Sutton, L.B. (1997) Multiple authorship: issues and recommendations. *Journal of Professional Nursing* 13 (4) 262–70

Article discusses several issues relating to authorship, including the assignment of authorship credit, the increased pressure to publish, and the complexity of authorship issues associated with multi-site studies. Recommendations are made, and some guidelines developed by the authors early in their project are included.

2.97.17 Fairbairn, G. & Carson, A. (2002) Writing about nursing research: a storytelling approach. *Nurse Researcher: The International Journal of Research Methodology in Nursing and Health Care* 10 (1) 7–14 7 References

Authors argue that much of what is written by nurses is needlessly difficult, especially when it concerns research they have carried out. They suggest that consideration be given to writing as a form of story-telling. If they are to be successful in telling stories, nurse researchers must weave various elements together in coherent, interesting and easily understandable narratives, making clear their relationship to the intellectual landscape they inhabit.

2.97.18 Giltrow, J. (1995) *Academic writing: writing and reading across the disciplines* (2nd edition). Peterborough, Ontario: Broadview Press ISBN 1551110555 References

This text is designed to help students produce scholarly papers. Examples are included throughout which illustrate techniques for all stages of the process.

2.97.19 Glatthorn, A.A. (1998) *Writing the winning dissertation: a step-by step guide*. London: Corwin Press ISBN 0803966784 References

Book explains all the phases of writing a masters thesis or a doctoral dissertation and gives advice on laying foundations for the project, finding a research problem, developing the proposal, organizing and writing each chapter (CR 3.19).

2.97.20 Golden-Biddle, K. & Locke, K.D. (1997) *Writing matters: crafting theoretical points from qualitative research*. Thousand Oaks, CA: Sage ISBN 0803974310 References

Provides both theoretical and practical guidance for students and researchers who need to transform data organized around the metaphor of 'story'. Each chapter covers a different aspect of creating stories: disclosing, telling and revising for publication. Writing issues are addressed as the manuscript is taken from inception to publication (CR 2.89).

2.97.21 Goodman, N.W. & Edwards, M.B. (1997) *Medical writing: a prescription for clarity*

(2nd edition). Cambridge: Cambridge University Press   ISBN 0521498767   References

Provides practical help for authors when writing theses or material for publication. Each chapter has been updated and many examples of good and bad medical writing, drawn from published work, are used for illustration.

2.97.22   Holliday, A. (2002) *Doing and writing qualitative research*. London: Sage   ISBN 0761963928   References

Book offers students a primer in writing qualitative research. It provides clear guidance on how subjectivity is managed, and how scientific rigour is achieved by making the workings of written study apparent. Sensitive issues dealing with the proper use of identity in research settings are also discussed (CR 2.17, 2.36).

2.97.23   Huff, A.S. (1998) *Writing for scholarly publication*. Thousand Oaks, CA: Sage   ISBN 0761918051   References

In this guide to academic writing the author takes the reader step by step through the writing and publication process from choosing a subject, developing content and submitting the final manuscript for publication (CR 2.20).

2.97.24   Lea, M. & Stierer, B. (2000) *Student writing in higher education: new contexts*. Buckingham: Open University Press   ISBN 0335204074   References

Book brings together research carried out by practitioners in a number of international university contexts. Each chapter focuses on some aspect of new contexts, either by examining the writing and assessment practices of non-traditional university courses and settings, or by exploring attempts to introduce innovative practices in traditional academic subjects. The authors concentrate specifically on the implications for the work of university teachers.

2.97.25   Lester, J.D. & Lester, J.D. Jr (1999) *The essential guide to writing research papers*. New York: Longman   ISBN 0321024060   References

This text, intended for student researchers, includes discovery of a research topic, note taking, writing and formatting the finished manuscript to a specific style. Many examples are included (CR 2.18).

2.97.26   McGaghie, W.C., Bordage, G. & Shea, J.A. (2001) Manuscript introduction: problem statement, conceptual framework, and research question. *Academic Medicine* 76 (9) 923–4   8 References

Explains the importance of clearly conveying the problem statement, articulating an explicit conceptual framework and research hypothesis or question when writing a scholarly manuscript. Emphasizes the importance of presenting clearly identified variables.

2.97.27   McInerney, D.M. (2001) *Publishing your psychology research: a guide to writing for journals in psychology and related fields*. London: Sage   ISBN 0761973370   References

Book has bridged a gap in the literature, providing an expert view from both insider and outsider perspectives as to what it takes to be a credible author (CR 2.99).

2.97.28   McSherry, C. (2001) *Who owns academic work? Battling for control of intellectual property*. Cambridge, MA: Harvard University Press   ISBN 0674006291   References

Who owns academic work is provoking political and legal battles, fought on uncertain terrain for ever-higher stakes. The posting of faculty lecture notes on commercial websites is being hotly debated, even as faculty and university administrators square off in a battle for professional copyright. All but forgotten in ownership disputes is the more fundamental question – should academic work be owned at all? Once characterized as a kind of gift, academic work – and academic freedom – are now being framed as intellectual property. Drawing on legal, historical and qualitative research, the author explores the propertization of academic work and shows how this process is shaking the foundations of the university, the professoriate and intellectual property law.

2.97.29   Moriarty, M.F. (1997) *Writing science through critical thinking*. Sudbury, MA: Jones & Bartlett   ISBN 0867205105   References

This text addresses the need to assist students to write in the context of their field of study, in this case science. Although there are many 'how to' books, few address the central pedagogical issues underlying the process of learning to think and write scientifically.

2.97.30   Murrell, G., Huang, C. & Ellis, H. (1999) *Research in medicine: a guide to writing a thesis in the medical sciences* (2nd edition). Cambridge: Cambridge University Press   ISBN 0521626706   References

Provides advice for the beginner and covers all the steps involved from choosing a project to submitting a thesis. The practicalities of planning and financing a project are covered, and insights are given into the frustrations and satisfactions of doing research (CR 2.16, 3.13).

2.97.31   Muscari, M.E. (1998) Do the write thing: writing the clinically focused article. *Journal of Pediatric Health Care* 12 (5) 235–41   4 References

Encourages nurses (especially paediatric nurses) to write clinically-based articles, starting from the first ideas to the identification of the target audience and journal selection through to the publication process.

2.97.32 Oermann, M. (1999) Extensive writing projects: tips for completing them on time. *Nurse Author and Editor* 9 (1) 8–10   3 References

Outlines the planning involved in writing a book, grant application or thesis. Advises on developing the outline, setting targets, meeting deadlines and personal strategies that will assist in the successful completion of writing projects (CR 2.99).

2.97.33 Oermann, M.H. (2002) *Writing for publication in nursing.* Philadelphia, PA: Lippincott Williams and Wilkins   ISBN   0781725550   References

Book describes the process of writing for publication. Step-by-step guidance shows how to revise written work and submit the finished product for publication. Online writing tips are given at www.LWW.com/nursing/writing.

2.97.34 Oliver, P. (2003) *Writing your thesis.* London: Sage   ISBN 0761942998   References

Book is designed to help postgraduate and research students with the process, preparation, writing and examination of their theses.

2.97.35 Orna, E. & Stevens, G. (1995) *Managing information for research.* Buckingham: Open University Press   ISBN 0335193978   References

A book for first-time researchers that discusses transferring knowledge gained during research into written form. Also included is information on managing time, organizing and transferring data and coping with feelings of isolation and loss of confidence.

2.97.36 Peat, J., Elliott, E., Baur, L. & Keena, V. (2002) *Scientific writing: easy when you know how.* London: BMJ Books   ISBN   0727916254   References

Book covers the basics of grammar as well as how to write a grant application, abstracts, journal articles and reports. Guidance on referencing is also given.

2.97.37 Redman, P. (2001) *Good essay writing: a social sciences guide* (2nd edition). London: Sage/Open University Press   ISBN 0761972056   References

Book provides answers to key questions when writing essays. What do tutors look for when marking essays? What kinds of skill will be needed at different course levels? How can inadvertent plagiarism

be avoided? What are the protocols for referencing? Detailed guidelines on ways to support key arguments and address common worries are given, as well as examples of good practice.

2.97.38 Roberts, P. (2000) Practical issues in 'writing-up' a research thesis. *Nurse Researcher* 7 (4) 14–23   12 References

Paper describes three phases in managing the process of writing-up a research thesis: the input, process and output. Ideas and hints are given to make the process a more rewarding and developmental experience.

2.97.39 Rosser, B.R.S., Rugg, D.L. & Ross, M.W. (2001) Increasing research and evaluation productivity: tips for successful writing retreats. *Health Promotion Practice* 2 (1) 9–13   16 References

Relates the problems of disseminating research findings by publication and offers ten tips towards successful and productive writing opportunities (CR 2.98).

2.97.40 Sandelowski, M. (1998) Writing a good read: strategies for re-presenting qualitative data. *Research in Nursing and Health* 21 (4) 375–82   30 References

Author urges qualitative researchers to write with great clarity to enable the widest possible dissemination and utilization of their findings (CR 2.98, 2.102).

2.97.41 Sheridan, D.R. & Dowdney, D.L. (1997) *How to write and publish articles in nursing* (2nd edition). New York: Springer   ISBN 0826149812   References

Manual offers nurses a step-by-step approach to writing journal articles. Techniques, exercises, practical checklists and forms for each stage in the writing and marketing process are included. Guidance is given on using online databases, email and the Internet. Appendices include lists of nursing journals, publications for writers and writing and literary associations (CR 2.99).

2.97.42 Siebers, R. (2000) How accurate is data in abstracts of research articles? *New Zealand Journal of Medical Laboratory Science* 54 (1) April 22–3   10 References

Study aimed to determine the accuracy of abstracts of scientific articles in the *New Zealand Journal of Laboratory Science*, as a previous study had identified errors. All abstracts containing data from March 1995 to November 1999 were checked for accuracy. An error rate of 29.4 per cent was observed. Authors have a responsibility to ensure accuracy of their abstracts (CR 2.17, 2.99).

2.97.43   Skelton, J.R. & Edwards, S.J.L. (2000) The function of the discussion section in academic medical writings. *British Medical Journal* 320 (7244) 6 May 1269–70   15 References

Concerned about the tendency to speculate beyond reported results, the article advises caution when writing a discussion section. Guidelines are provided for potential authors as to how discussions should be written.

2.97.44   Taylor, D.McD. (2002) The appropriate use of references in a scientific research paper. *Emergency Medicine* 14 (2) 166–70   14 References

Discusses the value of accurate reference lists and provides guidelines for their preparation.

2.97.45   Thomas, R.M. (2003) *Blending qualitative and quantitative research methods in theses and dissertations.* London: Corwin Press ISBN 0761939326   References

Many students are opting for a mixed-method approach that combines qualitative and quantitative methods but no book exists that applies mixed methods to writing dissertations or theses. This book aims to fill the gap.

2.97.46   Tornquist, E.M. (1999) *From proposal to publication: an informal guide to writing about research.* Reading, MA: Addison-Wesley ISBN 0201080125   References

Covers writing a research proposal, theses and dissertations, research reports and articles. Suggested formats are given, together with advice on referencing, abstracts, presentations, organization of a grant proposal and aids to writing (CR 2.96, 2.99, 2.100).

2.97.47   Turabian, K.L. (1996) *A manual for writers of term papers, theses and dissertations* (6th edition). Chicago, IL: University of Chicago Press ISBN 0226816273   References

The British edition of an American *vade mecum,* intended to assist all those preparing academic work for advanced-level courses or presenting papers in scholarly journals. It gives comprehensive guidance on all aspects of style, presentation, reference styles, notes, bibliographical entries and provides annotated sample pages. Throughout, the needs of computer users are emphasized.

2.97.48   Williams, D. (2002) *Writing skills in practice: a practical guide for health professionals.* London: Jessica Kingsley ISBN 1853026492   References

Presents a guide to developing writing skills for students and practitioners. It covers the skills of record keeping, report writing and supplying clear,

written information for clients, as well as writing for teaching and learning and for publication.

2.97.49   Wolcott, H.F. (2001) *Writing up qualitative research* (2nd edition). Thousand Oaks, CA: Sage ISBN 0761924299   References

Book is full of 'how to do it' advice (CR 2.36).

2.97.50   Wolcott, H.F. (2002) Writing up qualitative research … better. *Qualitative Health Research* 12 (1) 91–103   13 References

Author presents his ideas for breaking free from the traditional order and segregation of topics – literature reviews, theory and method – in favour of integrating these components into a report only as needed. He urges researchers to consider alternative ways of satisfying the intent of a literature review and questions whether traditional requirements result in theories being forced or presented prematurely. Possible solutions are suggested to these dilemmas (CR 2.12, 2.36, 2.72).

2.97.51   Woods, P. (1999) *Successful writing for qualitative researchers.* London: Routledge ISBN 0415188474   References

Book discusses all aspects of the writing-up process, including getting started, keeping going, organizing one's work, coping with problems, editing, approaching publishers and getting published (CR 2.99).

2.97.52   Writer's Services.com *Michael Legat's factsheets* www.writerservices.com/wsres/r_legat_main.htm (Accessed 27/02/03)

These specially written fact sheets cover many aspects of writing that will be useful for authors.

2.97.53   Zeiger, M. (2000) *Essentials of writing biomedical papers.* New York: McGraw-Hill ISBN 0071345442   References

Specific principles of biomedical writing are presented and explained. A prototypical paper is systematically analysed and a full-length one is included for readers to evaluate.

2.98   DISSEMINATING RESEARCH FINDINGS

'… [T]he current way in which research findings are disseminated is the most important contributory factor to [the theory–practice] gap … dissemination [of research] is frequently neglected or fails to receive the time, planning and emphasis that it requires. Emphasis has been placed on carrying out the research, while strategic planning and funding for the dissemination of results has been neglected.' (Dickson, 1996: 5–6)

Definitions [See Appendix D for sources]

Diffusion – ... is haphazard, lacks a target and is generally unplanned and uncontrolled

Diffusion of innovations – the adoption, and the social processes involved in the adoption of technical innovations

Dissemination – ... it not only implies a more aggressive flow of information from the source ... but also targeting and tailoring the information for the intended audience

---

Example

Lewis, S.L., Prowant, B.F., Cooper, C.L. & Bonner, P.N. (1998) Nephrology nurses' perceptions of barriers and facilitators to using research to using research in practice ... including commentary by Lotas, M.J. *ANNA Journal* 25 (4) 397–406   25 References

Purpose of this study was to determine nephrology nurses' perceptions of barriers to research utilization and to identify effective ways to facilitate integration of research findings into practice. Authors concluded that additional nursing and non-nursing administrative support for research activities, designated time to read research and implement research-based clinical practices would contribute towards this goal.

Annotations

2.98.1   Anthony, D. (2000) Distance learning and research dissemination using online resources. *Nurse Researcher: The International Journal of Research Methodology in Nursing and Health Care* 8 (1) 53–64   27 References

Author analyses the opportunities for researchers and students offered by recent developments in information technology.

2.98.2   Beaumont, E. (1997) Dissemination of research-based knowledge among home care nurses: a Q methodology study. PhD Thesis (unpublished). Health Sciences Center, University of Illinois at Chicago   References

The purpose of this study was to describe, interpret and understand home care nurses' perceptions about key variables in research-based knowledge dissemination. Everett Rogers' Innovation Diffusion Model was the framework that guided interpretation of the study findings (CR 2.23, 2.74).

2.98.3   Brooten, D., Youngblut, J.M., Roberts, B.L., Montgomery, K., Standing, T., Hemstrom, M., Suresky, J. & Polis, N. (1999) Disseminating our breakthroughs: enacting a strategic framework. Papers from the 25th Anniversary of the American Academy of Nursing 'Breakthroughs in Nursing' 29 October–1 November, 1998. *Nursing Outlook* 47 (3) 133–7   8 References

A comprehensive framework to diffuse research findings is presented and its implementation by the Frances Payne Bolton School of Nursing is illustrated.

2.98.4   Cronenwett, L.R. (1995) Effective methods for disseminating research findings to nurses in practice. In Titler, M.G. & Goode, C.J. (eds) *The Nursing Clinics of North America: research utilization* 30 (3) Philadelphia, PA: W.B. Saunders ISSN 0029–6465 429–38   16 References

Discusses the challenges, goals and methods of disseminating research findings (CR 2.102.46).

2.98.5   Dooks, P. (2001) Diffusion of pain management research into nursing practice. *Cancer Nursing* 24 (2) 99–103   22 References

Pain management is a prime example of the practice research gap in the nursing of cancer patients. Rogers' Diffusion of Innovation Theory provides a framework for examining the issues and possible solutions to this complex problem. The theory examines how changes diffuse through a social system over time, and exposes some of the barriers and facilitators to this process. By examining adopters, the nature of innovation, the social system and patterns of communication, nurses may be helped to overcome some of the existing barriers (CR 2.102, 3.8).

2.98.6   Dunn, E.V., Norton, P.G., Stewart, M., Tudiver, F. & Bass, M.J. (eds) (1994) *Disseminating research/changing practice.* Thousand Oaks, CA: Sage ISBN 0803957068 References

Book covers general aspects of dissemination, issues of methodology and changing practitioner behaviour.

2.98.7   Forbes, D. & Phillipchuk, D. (2001) The dissemination and use of nursing research. *Canadian Nurse* 97 (7) 18–22 August   27 References

Reports a pilot project in which strategies for disseminating research findings were identified. The recommendations include involving those who would use the findings and targeting resources and funding specifically towards the dissemination of research (CR 2.23).

2.98.8 French, B. (2000) Networking for research dissemination: collaboration and mentorship. *Nurse Researcher* 7 (3) 13–23 50 References

Article examines the ways in which networks may function. The author believes networking can be a key agent in disseminating research and ensuring effective health care is incorporated into practice. The relationship between evidence-based practice and research is explored and the conflict of values is discussed (CR 2.15, 2.85).

2.98.9 Haines, A. & Donald, A. (eds) (1998) *Getting research findings into practice*. London: BMJ Books ISBN 0727912577 References

Guide aims to answer the question of why there is such a gap between research findings and what actually happens in practice. It suggests ways of deciding whether findings should be implemented and how this uptake may be promoted (CR 2.102, 3.8).

2.98.10 Hayward, S., Ciliska, D., DiCenso, A., Thomas, H. & Rafael, A. (1996) Evaluation research in public health: barriers to the production and dissemination of outcomes data. *Canadian Journal of Public Health* 87 (6) 413–17 87 References

Paper reviews methodological and socio-political barriers that impede the production and dissemination of outcome research in public health, with particular reference to nursing (CR 2.17, 2.29).

2.98.11 Kajermo, K.N., Nordstrom, G., Krusebrant, A. & Bjorvell, H. (2000) Perceptions of research utilization: comparisons between health care professionals, nursing students and a reference group of nurse clinicians. *Journal of Advanced Nursing* 31 (1) 99–109 31 References

Factors that determine the use of research findings in this study are highlighted. Education, support from managers and research presented in a user-friendly way were seen as facilitators. Isolation from knowledgeable colleagues with whom to discuss research was seen as a major barrier, and this indicates a need for positions in clinical practice for nurse researchers.

2.98.12 Meadows, A.J. (1997) *Communicating research*. London: Academic Press ISBN 0124874150 References

This book discusses the generation, transmission and use of scientific information.

2.98.13 Montgomery, K.S., Eddy, N.L., Jackson, E., Nelson, E., Reed, K., Stark, T.L. & Thomsen, C. (2001) Global research dissemination and utilization: recommendations for nurses and nurse educators. *Nursing and Health Care Perspectives* 22 (3) 124–9 24 References

Despite the Internet, a research–practice gap remains. This article offers seven strategies for increasing the dissemination and utilization of nursing research (CR 2.101, 2.102, 3.8).

2.98.14 Morse, J.M. (2000) The downside of dissemination. *Qualitative Health Research* 10 (3) May 291–2 Editorial

Editor considers the downside of disseminating research findings and the possible traps for researchers. Once published, research becomes beyond the original researcher's control. Material may be put on a website and distorted, copyright issues may occur and, even after publication, misrepresentations may spread over the Internet. There is also no control over how it is interpreted or used. Books and monographs, once traditional means for disseminating qualitative research, are no longer valued and publishers have introduced strict word limits, which reduce the rich descriptive aspects of qualitative research. Researchers are urged to consider ways to disseminate research to maintain its integrity (CR 2.17, 2.85, 2.99).

2.98.15 Mulhall, A. & Le May, A. (eds) (1999) *Bridging the gap: the dissemination and implementation of research in nursing*. Edinburgh: Churchill Livingstone ISBN 0443059845 References

Book includes and critically analyses the information currently available on dissemination and implementation of research in nursing, and debates the critical issues raised. The culture in which nursing, midwifery and health visiting operates are explained, and the key issues of dissemination, implementation and changing practice are discussed (CR 2.102).

2.98.16 Robinson, J. (2002) Research for whom? The politics of research dissemination and application. In Rafferty, A.M. & Traynor, M. (eds) *Exemplary research for nursing and midwifery*. London: Routledge ISBN 0415241634 Chapter 19 352–71 31 References

The editor's introduction to an important study highlights some of the problems experienced when undertaking sensitive research (3.21.5).

2.98.17 Scullion, P.A. (2002) Effective dissemination studies. *Nurse Researcher: The International Journal of Research Methodology in Nursing and Health Care* 10 (1) 65–77 26 References

Dissemination of research findings or other key messages is increasingly acknowledged as a vital yet complex process. The author explores and disentangles some of these complexities. The process of dissemination needs to be given greater emphasis by project-funding bodies, research supervisors, researchers and those responsible for implementing changes in clinical practice. Important initiatives are acknowledged and the concept of dissemination is explored – the source, message, medium and target groups are all examined. It is argued also that dissemination needs to be considered at the design stage of the research project. The author believes that the current commitment to research and evidence-based practice will have a limited impact on patient care until similar attention is paid to dissemination at corporate and individual levels (CR 2.14, 2.102, 3.13, 3.18).

2.98.18 Straus, S.E. & Sackett, D. (1998) Using research findings in clinical practice. *British Medical Journal* 317 (7154) 1 August 339–42   16 References

Provides an overview of the evidence-based practice process and discusses how clinicians can improve their skills in reading and applying evidence in practical situations (CR 2.95).

2.98.19 Tanner, J. & Hale, C. (2002) Research-active nurses' perception of the barriers to undertaking research in practice. *NT Research* 7 (5) 363–75   34 References

Most nursing literature focuses on barriers that prevent nurses from engaging in research. This article reports a study which identified how a small group of research-active clinical nurses perceived and overcame the reputed barriers to carrying out research in practice. It suggests that the main kind of support needed by nurses wanting to carry out research is that offered by facilitators who gave them confidence to carry it out and publish their findings.

2.98.20 Taylor-Piliae, R.E. (1998) Establishing evidence-based practice: issues and implications in critical care nursing. *Intensive and Critical Care Nursing* 14 (1) 30–7   43 References

The use of research findings to improve practice has been discussed and promoted for the last 20 years. The author argues that Rogers' theoretical model of the Diffusion of Innovations may prove useful in understanding the problem of the slow diffusion of the application of research evidence in clinical nursing practice. The diffusion of innovations in current critical care nursing practice at each stage of Rogers' theory is examined, with recommendations given to facilitate the establishment of evidence-based practice (CR 2.43).

2.98.21 Traynor, M. (1999) The problem of dissemination: evidence and ideology. *Nursing Inquiry* 6 (3) 187–97   71 References

Recent insights into the structure and function of the scientific paper have suggested that such texts are far from neutral channels of communication describing pre-existing objects, but are highly rhetorical texts originating from networks of scientists who are themselves socially situated and often different from the intended users of their research. Similarly, literary theory, and particularly feminist theory, has proposed that often when women read literature written by men they are positioned to 'identify against themselves' by an implicit or explicit male perspective masquerading as a general human experience. This has been said to account for a jarring, and possibly undermining, reading experience. This paper attempts to bring these two areas of theory to bear upon the 'problem' of dissemination among nurses (CR 2.10).

2.99   PUBLICATION PROCESSES

An increasing number of nurses are now writing for publication and it is the responsibility of all researchers to communicate their findings to colleagues. Many journals include instructions to authors regularly or periodically, and editors are available to give advice. Experts frequently referee papers submitted for publication to ensure the highest standards of scholarship. The general principles of copyright law do not vary greatly between countries. However, specific national legislation may differ. Please consult local librarians for guidance or the national copyright receipt office.

Definitions [See Appendix D for sources]

Abstract – a brief description of a completed or proposed investigation in research journals, usually located at the beginning of an article

Galley proofs – sheets of paper that show how an article or book will appear in typeset form

Peer review – a form of performance appraisal when, instead of the manager, a member of a team or of the profession appraises another's performance – giving both positive feedback and constructive criticism

Publication bias – a bias in published literature where the publication of research depends on the nature and direction of the study results. Studies in which an intervention is not found to be effective are sometimes not published [Because of this, systematic reviews that fail to include unpublished studies may overestimate the true effect of an intervention]

Query letter – a letter of inquiry sent to a journal to determine the editor's interest in publishing a manuscript [The letter usually contains an outline of the manuscript and important information about its content]

Refereed journal – a journal that makes decisions about the acceptance of manuscripts on the basis of recommendations from peer reviewers

Annotations

2.99.1   Alexander, A. & Potter, W.J. (eds) (2001) *How to publish your communication research.* Thousand Oaks, CA: Sage   ISBN 0761914544   References

Provides an 'insider's' guide to getting published in scholarly communication journals. The authors and journal editors explain what editors and reviewers look for when deciding which articles should be published and which should not.

2.99.2   American Psychological Association (2001) *Publication manual of the American Psychological Association* (5th edition). Washington, DC: APA Books   ISBN 1557987912   References

Gives detailed guidance to authors on the content and organization of a manuscript, expression of ideas, editorial style, typing instructions and a sample paper, submitting the paper, proof-reading and the journal programme of the association. The bibliography includes references to the history of the manual and suggested reading. Brief guidance is given on the preparation of materials other than journal articles. This new edition contains many revisions and has features on current technological tools, contemporary language issues and publishing standards. A full section on the ethics of scientific publishing is included, covering reporting results, the peer reviewer, plagiarism, author's and peer reviewer's responsibilities, duplicate publication of data and its verification and treatment of research participants (CR 2.17).

2.99.3   Banks, M. (1998) Get your book published. *British Medical Journal* 317 (7174) 19 December 1715–18   3 References

Provides some practical information about the book publishing industry and urges readers to ask themselves a series of questions before they start out. The article also gives advice on approaching a publisher and considering a contract.

2.99.4   Beyea, S.C. & Nicoll, L.H. (1998) Writing and submitting an abstract. *AORN Journal* 67 (1) 273–4

Addresses strategies for writing a competitive research abstract for congress or any other conference.

2.99.5   Bjørn, A. (2002) Peer review. *Scandinavian Journal of Caring Sciences* 16 (4) December 335–6 Editorial

Editor outlines the role of reviewers.

2.99.6   Bradigan, P.S., Powell, C.A & Van Brimmer, B. (eds) (1998) *Writer's guide to nursing and allied health journals.* Atlanta, GA: American Nurses Publishing   ISBN 1558101438

Guide provides essential information, including address, telephone and fax numbers, email and website addresses, audience, publication frequency, and manuscript acceptance rate for nearly 600 journals.

2.99.7   Bragadottir, H. (1998) Every nurse can be an author: on writing for publication. *Nursing Forum* 33 (4) 29–35   18 References

Identifies the barriers nurses might encounter when attempting to publish and provides guidelines and help for potential authors.

2.99.8   Butler, L. & Ginn, D. (1998) Canadian nurses' views on assignment of publication credit for scholarly and scientific work. *Canadian Journal of Nursing Research* 30 (1) 171–83   10 References

A total of 184 Canadian nurses were given 42 scenarios to determine their views on assignment of publication credit. Consensus greater than 80 per cent was achieved for seven of the 42 presented, but two recurrent themes were noted: that credit should be based entirely on contribution, rather than status; and that authorship and footnote acknowledgement should be discussed and resolved at an early stage. Disagreement concerning collaborative academic work was also highlighted. Results are discussed (CR 2.13, 2.15).

2.99.9   Chalmers, I. & Altman, D.G. (1999) How can medical journals prevent poor medical research? Some opportunities presented by electronic publishing. *The Lancet* 353 (9151) 6 February 490–3   59 References

Suggests that inadequate peer review of research reports has led to the publishing of poor medical research so it is recommended that journals publish research protocols as good scientific practice. Since the capacity for journals to do this is limited, electronic publishing is offered as an alternative.

2.99.10   Coeling, H. (2000) Electronic publishing: how, what and why? nursingworld.org/ojin/topic11/tpc11toc.htm (Accessed 16/11/03)

Provides links to articles, columns and web references on electronic publishing.

2.99.11   Committee on Publication Ethics *The COPE Report 1999: Guidelines on good publication practice*   www.publicationethics.org.uk/cope1999/gpp/gpp.phtml (Accessed 02/03/03)

COPE was founded in 1997 to address breaches of research and publication ethics. The guidelines created are intended to be advisory rather than prescriptive, and to evolve over time. They cover study design and ethical approval, data analysis, conflicts of interest, peer review, redundant publication, plagiarism, duties of editors, media relations and advertising (CR 2.17.62, 2.97).

2.99.12   Cummings, L.L. & Frost, P.J. (eds) (1995) *Publishing in the organizational sciences* (2nd edition). Thousand Oaks, CA: Sage   ISBN 0803971451   References

Book explains the entire context of scholarly publishing and how it should contribute towards advancing knowledge and successful management practice.

2.99.13   Curran, S. (1990) *How to write a book and get it published: a complete guide to the publishing maze.* London: Thorsons   ISBN 0722521464 References

A practical guide to the types of book that interest publishers. Advice is given on most aspects of book publishing (CR 2.97).

2.99.14   Davidoff, F., DeAngelis, C.D. Drazen, J.M., Hoey, J., Hojgaard, L., Horton, R., Koztin, S., Nicholls, M.G., Nylenna, M., Overbeke, A.J.P.M., Sox, H.C., Van Der Weyden, M.B. & Wilkes, M.S. (2001) Sponsorship, authorship and accountability. *Journal of the American Medical Association* 286 (20) 1232   6 References

Explains the requirement of authors to disclose conflicts of interest that may affect their research project, in particular, whether they had access to study data and to what extent they were involved in the decision to publish the data. Appended is a section from guidelines on publication ethics.

2.99.15   *Directory of European Nursing Journals* (1996) Edited by Anderson, Y. Copenhagen: Workgroup of European Nurse Researchers   ISBN 8772661879

Booklet provides information for nurse researchers who wish to extend their knowledge of nursing journals that publish research (CR Appendix B).

2.99.16   Dougherty, M.C. (2001) Nursing research reviewers. *Nursing Research* 50 (3) 135   Editorial

Outlines the processes undertaken by reviewers for the journal *Nursing Research*.

2.99.17   Duncan, A.M. (1999) Authorship, dissemination of research findings and related matters. *Applied Nursing. Research* 12 (2) 101–6   23 References

Sets out the criteria and obligations for first authorship and the role and responsibilities of co-authors and contributors. Discusses ethical and other problems that might arise from publications and recommends strategies to avoid them (CR 2.17, 2.98).

2.99.18   Earl-Slater, A. (2002) Peer reviewers' checklist. In Author *The handbook of clinical trials and other research.* Oxford: Radcliffe Medical Press   ISBN 1857754859 245–6

This *BMJ*-recommended checklist for reviewers aims to seek answers to the following questions for all papers submitted for publication. Is the paper important? Will it add enough to existing knowledge? And does the paper read well and make sense? (CR 2.2.13).

2.99.19   Elliott, R., Fischer, C.T. & Rennie, D.L. (1999) Evolving guidelines for publication of qualitative research studies in psychology and related fields. *British Journal of Clinical Psychology* 38 (3) 215–29   35 References

Proposes a set of continually evolving guidelines for reviewing qualitative research manuscripts which set out to legitimize qualitative research, ensure a more appropriate review, encourage better quality control and further the development of qualitative methodology.

2.99.20   Ernst, E. & Resch, K. (1999) Reviewer bias against the unconventional? A randomized double-blind study of peer review. *Complementary Therapies in Medicine* 7 (1) 19–23   22 References

Study tested the hypothesis that there is reviewer bias against publication of a test of an unconventional drug. A convenience sample of medical doctors was obtained from a list of conference participants. After analysing the evaluation sheets, the authors concluded that there was no evidence for a reviewer-bias against testing an unconventional drug. The low inter-rater reliability, however, suggested inadequate validity of the peer review (CR 2.24, 2.25, 2.27, 2.29).

2.99.21   Fitzpatrick, J.J. (2001) Scholarly publishing: current issues of cost and quality, fuelled by the rapid expansion of electronic publishing. *Applied Nursing Research Online* 14 (1) Editorial 7 pages   1 Reference   www2.appliednursingresearch.org/scripts/om.d11/serve?action=search DB& searchD… (Accessed 16/11/03)

Reports a set of principles generated to guide the transformation of the scholarly publishing system towards the goal of encouraging broad discussion and the endorsement of these principles.

2.99.22 Fonteyn, M. (1997) Successful publishing: debunking the myths. *Nurse Author and Editor* 7 (3) 4, 7–8   20 References

Identifies ten myths that might act as a barrier for those who would otherwise write for publication. It also explains the publication process.

2.99.23 Game, A. & West, M.A. (2002) Principles of publishing. *The Psychologist* 15 (3) 126–9   3 References

Combines recommendations on ethical publishing from various professional associations, including order of authorship, duplicate publication, plagiarism and accuracy of reporting. Includes five case studies as illustrations of the problems that can arise in writing for publication.

2.99.24 Godlee, F. & Jefferson, T. (eds) (1999) *Peer review in the health sciences.* London: BMJ Books   ISBN 0727911813   References

Book presents current knowledge about peer review, its influence on the publication or rejection of manuscripts, the quality of the literature and related issues.

2.99.25 Grant, J.S. (1998) Writing manuscripts for clinical journals. *Home Healthcare Nurse* 16 (12) 813–22   26 References

Advises on a range of aspects involved in the production of manuscripts, including selecting topics, developing content and writing tips and skills. Explains the review and publications process and includes a checklist of the points made for the potential author to measure her or success against.

2.99.26 Gunn, I.P. (2000) Commentary: issues and perspectives affecting CRNA practice. Death of a journal: lost opportunities, new challenges, or both? *CRNA – The Clinical Forum for Nurse Anaesthetists* 11 (4) 197–201   6 References

Reports the cessation of publication of a specialist journal and discusses some possible advantages and disadvantages of print versus electronic journals. There have been examples of poor research published in print, despite peer review, and it is too early to tell whether the process in online journals is any better. Authors and reviewers are urged to ensure that research published in print or online is valid and reliable so that findings may be appropriately applied in practice.

2.99.27 Hobbs, G. (2001) Academic journal publishing: past, present and future. *Journal of Education for Teaching* 27 (3) 215–19

Author looks at the past, present and future of the academic journal, but with a particular emphasis on the present. Ways in which the development of electronic journals have changed and revolutionized publishing in the last five years are examined.

2.99.28 Jackson, K. & Sheldon, L. (2000) Writing for publication. *Nurse Researcher* 7 (4) 68–74

Authors outline the key aspects of writing articles for publication in nursing journals (CR 2.97).

2.99.29 Legat, M. (1998) *Author's guide to publishing* (3rd edition). London: Robert Hale   ISBN 0709062273   References

This standard work has been extensively revised and updated and includes information on submitting work, contracts, author/publisher relationships, legal matters and the rewards of writing. The abandonment of the Net Book Agreement has caused changes in the publishing world as has the development in electronic publishing and these are discussed.

2.99.30 Legat, M. (2002) *Understanding publishers' contracts.* London: Robert Hale   ISBN 0709072899   References

The length and complexity of publishers' agreements can sometimes be confusing, especially for first-time authors. Typical contracts, from paperback houses, US and foreign publishers are analysed and each clause is explained and commented upon. There is also information on author/agent agreements, permissions letters, and where to go for further help in case of trouble.

2.99.31 Luey, B. (2002) *Handbook for academic authors* (4th edition). Cambridge: Cambridge University Press   ISBN 0521814774   References

This new edition gives answers to many questions that all authors ask, for example: What are you trying to do? Should you sign the publishing contract offered? Is it wise to publish in an electronic journal? How much can you expect to earn? What are your legal and ethical responsibilities as an author? What can you expect from your publisher? Practical advice is also given on negotiating a contract, preparing an electronic manuscript and seeking permission where appropriate. A new chapter evaluates various electronic media for different kinds of publication and suggests ways to use them to best advantage (CR 2.97).

2.99.32 Martin, P.A. (1998) Research peer review: a committee, when none is required. *Applied Nursing Research* 11 (2) May 90–2

Author suggests that researchers should choose colleagues who will give them constructive advice during the process of undertaking a research project.

2.99.33   McConnell, E.A. (2000) Nursing publications outside the United States. *Journal of Nursing Scholarship* 32 (1) 1st Quarter 87–92   8 References

Study replicated a 1992–93 examination of the characteristics of English-language nursing journals originating in countries other than the United States, and compared findings. Information about 82 journals from 13 countries was collected. In the earlier study the United Kingdom, Canada and Australia accounted for the largest number and the results of this new survey showed considerable similarity. Differences include a higher total circulation, changes in circulation among journal categories, and more publications offering services to authors. Reasons for manuscript rejection continue to be that a manuscript is poorly written or developed (CR 2.13, 2.97).

2.99.34   Meadows, A.J. (1998) *Communicating research.* San Diego, CA: Academic Press   ISBN 0124874150   References

Book examines ways in which chemists and sociologists write and publish their research and how these affect publication trends. It looks at publication strategies and their effectiveness in reaching the authors' targeted audiences. Two avenues are used to explore the communication of research findings – the medium used to convey the message and the needs of the research community (CR 2.97, 2.98).

2.99.35   Miracle, V.A. (2003) Writing for publication: you can do it! *Dimensions of Critical Care Nursing* 22 (1) 31–4   4 References

Discusses the barriers to writing articles for publication and how to overcome them.

2.99.36   Nemcek, M.A. (2000) Getting published online and in print: understanding the publication process. *AAOHN Journal* 48 (7) July 344–8   6 References

Author suggests that thoughtful selection of the target journal is time-consuming but can enhance the chances of publication. The article should be written in a clear, concise manner with as many ideas as possible expressed in the author's own words (CR 2.85).

2.99.37   Schulmeister, L. (1998) Quotation and reference accuracy of three nursing journals. *Image – The Journal of Nursing Scholarship* 30 (2) 143–6   16 References

Article reports on the accuracy of bibliographic citations in three widely circulated nursing journals: *RN, Nursing Management, and Image – The Journal of Nursing Scholarship.* Accurate citations facilitate retrieval of the cited documents and establish the judgement and credibility of authors. A random

sample of 60 references per journal published from July 1995 to June 1996 was reviewed for citation and quotation accuracy. Errors were classified as major or minor. Results are reported. The author concluded that the rates of errors were comparable to rates previously reported for medical and nursing journals. Errors of citation and quotation diminish the value of published papers (CR 2.17).

2.99.38   Sheldon, L. & Jackson, K. (1999) Demystifying the academic aura: preparing an abstract. *Nurse Researcher* 7 (1) 75–82   8 References

Authors present guidelines for preparing abstracts for submission as oral presentations during conference proceedings (CR 2.100).

2.99.39   Sibbald, B. (2000) COPE guidelines on good publication practice: an author's view. *Health and Social Care in the Community* 8 (6) 355–61   4 References   Guest Editorial

The Committee on Publication Ethics, a voluntary body of scientific editors and publishers, have issued 'Guidelines on Good Publication Practice'. While primarily targeted at journal editors, they will also be useful to authors. Topics covered include study design and ethical approval, data analysis, authorship, conflicts of interest, peer review, redundant publication, plagiarism, duties of editors, media relations, advertising and dealing with misconduct. The author comments on some of the guidelines, a copy of which is appended (CR 2.17, 2.99.11).

2.99.40   Smith, J.P. (1999) Plagiarists publish and perish. *Journal of Advanced Nursing* 30 (4) 777–8   Editorial

Editor examines the immoral, unethical and illegal activity of plagiarism, which can lead to professional suicide. Issues of copyright and the consequences of plagiarism are discussed (CR 2.17).

2.99.41   Song, F., Eastwood, A.J., Gilbody, S., Duley, L. & Sutton, A.J. (2000) Publication and related biases. *Health Technology Assessment* 4 (10) 115 pages

Reviews the evidence available on the causes and risk factors, existence and consequences of publication bias. Identifies the methods available for preventing and correcting biases.

2.99.42   Sparks, S.M. (1999) Electronic publishing and nursing research. *Nursing Research* 48 (1) 50–4   3 References

Article will assist nurses in taking advantage of the opportunities and minimizing the limitations of electronic publishing, especially on the World Wide Web.

Electronic publishing is described, together its advantages and disadvantages. Suggestions are made on how the Web may be woven into research (CR 2.85).

2.99.43 Taylor, E.W., Beck, J. & Ainsworth, E. (2001) Publishing qualitative adult educational research: a peer review perspective. *Studies in the Education of Adults* 33 (2) 163–79   44 References

Authors state that there are no standards for reporting qualitative data, which poses a confusing dilemma to those wanting to submit this type of research to scholarly journals. A rarely investigated resource offering insight into this challenge is peer review assessments of qualitative research. A study identified six major themes that are seen to be essential and these are discussed. Authors believe that these findings will assist scholars, together with encouraging future research into the peer review process.

2.99.44 Wager, E., Godlee, F. & Jefferson, T. (2002) *How to survive peer review*. London: BMJ Books   ISBN 0727916866

Book discusses peer review, what it is, how to be a reviewer and how to survive professional and informal reviews.

2.99.45 Wills, C.E. (2000) Strategies for managing barriers to the writing process. *Nursing Forum* 35 (4) 5–13   22 References

Identifies a range of barriers and constraints that prevent nurses from publishing and discusses strategies for managing them (CR 2.97).

2.100   TALKING ABOUT RESEARCH

In addition to writing about research, opportunities arise for students or experienced researchers to present their work to colleagues verbally. This may be in the classroom, to a small group of interested people or a formal presentation at a conference.

Annotations

2.100.1 Casey, A. *Preparing a conference poster* www.man.ac.uk/rcn/rs/poster.doc (Accessed 15/04/03)

Paper gives advice on preparing a conference poster. Hints are included for achieving an eye-catching return for the small amount of time and effort required.

2.100.2 Hall, G.M. (ed.) (2001) *How to present at meetings*. London: BMJ Books   ISBN 072791572X

Book handles all facets of preparing talks, from providing advice on how to use Powerpoint to step-by-step guidance on preparing for the lecture.

2.100.3 Jackson, K. & Sheldon, L. (2000) Demystifying the academic aura; preparing a poster. *Nurse Researcher* 7 (3) 70–3

Paper explores the art of producing and displaying a poster for a study day or conference (CR 2.99).

2.100.4 McCarthy, P. & Hatcher, C. (2002) *Presentation skills: the essential guide for students*. London: Sage   ISBN 0761940928   References

Book offers practical advice for students, giving presentations, a detailed explanation of how to conduct a successful presentation, and how to feel at ease with public speaking.

2.100.5 McConnell, E.A. (2002) Making outstandingly good presentations. *Dimensions of Critical Care Nursing* 21 (1) 28–30   References

Outlines the process of preparing and presenting in a variety of settings. It includes assessment, planning and the etiquette of delivering presentations.

2.100.6 Moore, L.W., Augspurger, P., King, M.O. & Proffitt, C. (2001) Insights on the poster preparation and presentation process. *Applied Nursing Research* 14 (2) May 100–4   References

Article presents insights derived from information shared by poster presenters regarding the preparation and presentation of their work.

2.100.7 Smith, R. (2000) How not to give a presentation. *British Medical Journal* 321 (7276) 23–30 December 1570–1

Light-hearted but cautionary advice on how avoid common mistakes when giving a presentation.

2.101   CREATING A RESEARCH UTILIZATION ENVIRONMENT

'Creation of a research utilization environment is a pre-condition to implementing appropriate research findings. Nurse managers, educators, researchers and clinicians all have responsibilities in relation to this. Creating support networks, providing opportunities for learning, communicating in a clear way and the willingness to participate in research are all required.' (Phillips, L.R.F., 1986: 462)

Definition [See Appendix D for source]

Research utilization – a process directed towards transferring specific research-based knowledge into actual clinical practice

Theory change – the study of methods used to incorporate new information into a knowledge base when the new information may conflict with existing information

Annotations

2.101.1 Camiletti, Y.A. & Huffman, M.C. (1998) Research utilization: evaluation of initiatives in a public health nursing division. *Canadian Journal of Nursing Administration* 11 (2) 59–77 25 References

Paper briefly describes the initiatives carried out to promote research in a public health nursing division and the results of an evaluation questionnaire. Results indicated that public health nurses valued research and felt comfortable with the concepts and phases of the research utilization model. They would engage in research activities if conducted at team meetings and when time was allotted. Administrative support and a supportive environment were positive facilitators to research utilization. Despite these findings, 67.5 per cent were not changing their practice. Difficulties identified were formulating the research question and critiquing articles, with lack of time being stated as the greatest deterrent.

2.101.2 Clarke, C. & Procter, S. (1999) Practice development: ambiguity in research and practice. *Journal of Advanced Nursing* 30 (4) 975–82 32 References

Practice development activity occupies an ambiguous position in relation to clinical practice and research. In practice it is seen at times as an added extra to normal work, while research fails to demonstrate the rigour of being generalizable because of its explicit location in a specific environment. This study explored the implications of this ambiguity with groups of practitioners. The authors argue for an appreciation of reflexive forms of research, such as action and practitioner research, so that these health care workers have a role in knowledge creation as well as its implementation.

2.101.3 Estabrooks, C.A. (1999) Mapping the research utilization field in nursing. *Canadian Journal of Nursing Research* 31 (1) 53–72 64 References

Article maps the field of research utilization and outcomes, proposing that we focus on major areas of inquiry: scientific, historical and philosophical foundations, synthesis, determinants, policy and interventions to increase research utilization. In so doing, alternative ways of viewing and conceptualizing this field are possible. In conducting the kinds of study and supporting the kinds of programme identified in this map, nursing, in collaboration with appropriate partners, can significantly advance the field of research dissemination and utilization studies and practice at many levels in the health system (CR 2.98).

2.101.4 Haines, A. & Donald, A. (eds) (2001) *Getting research findings into practice* (2nd edition). London: BMJ Books ISBN 0727915533 References

Written by international experts, this book covers all major areas in implementing research findings. These include: criteria for the implementation of research evidence in policy and practice; sources of information on clinical effectiveness and methods of dissemination; closing the gap between research and practice; implementing research findings in practice; evidence-based policy-making; barriers and bridges to evidence-based clinical practice; and implementing research findings in developing countries (CR 2.98, 2.102, 3.8, 3.11, 3.12, 3.22).

2.101.5 Janken, J.K., Blythe, G., Campbell, P.T. & Carter, R.H. (1999) Changing nursing practice through research utilization: consistent support for breastfeeding mothers. *Applied Nursing Research* 12 (1) 22–9 20 References

This research utilization project was designed to increase staff nurse support for four early postpartum breastfeeding practices. A before and after design was used to evaluate the extent to which the intended patient outcomes were achieved with the practice changes. Authors conclude that state-of-the-science nursing care was promoted and that the nurses involved became more adept in using research to guide practice (CR 2.30).

2.101.6 Kitson, A.L. (2001) Approaches used to implement research findings into nursing practice: report of a study tour to Australia and New Zealand. *International Journal of Nursing Practice* 7 (6) 392–405 29 References

Describes a study tour to investigate which models of research implementation were effective and what influences nurses in the implementation of research into practice. The views of staff responsible for its implementation were also elicited.

2.101.7 Lacko, L., Bryan, Y., Dellasega, C. & Salerno, F. (1999) Changing clinical practice through research: the case of delirium. *Clinical Nursing Research* 8 (3) 235–50 37 References

Reports a project which used change theory to include RNs in a research study on delirium and to use relevant findings. Results showed that staff nurses who used a standardized protocol were able to identify the presence and absence of delirium and asked to continue using this protocol after the study was terminated. Use of a theoretical model promoted the successful conduct of the research and the subsequent use of findings.

2.101.8   Morrison, E.F. (1998) Erroneous beliefs about research held by staff nurses. *Journal of Continuing Education in Nursing* 29 (5) 196–203 31 References

While working in clinical settings the researcher identified beliefs that may create unnecessary obstacles and limit nurses' research efforts. The article discusses these 11 beliefs, which have implications for nurses who are attempting to conduct clinical research. Examples are given.

2.101.9   Mulhall, A. & Le May, A. (2001) *Taking action: moving towards evidence-based practice.* Executive summary. London: Foundation of Nursing Studies   No ISBN

Over the last seven years the Foundation of Nursing Studies has assisted in the development, organization and evaluation of a number of activities to assist nurses to critically appraise and apply research/evidence in their everyday practice. This executive summary reports on the evaluation of this programme and comments on its implications for the current R&D agenda, education and professional development, Trust management, individual practitioners and the organization itself.

2.101.10   Omery, A. & Williams, R.P. (1999) The appraisal of research utilization across the United States. *Journal of Nursing Administration* 29 (12) December 50–6   35 References

Authors describe current and future nursing research utilization (RU) activities in various clinical agencies across the United States, and identify barriers and facilitators to those activities. The most frequent RU projects focused on pressure ulcers and pain management. Barriers included lack of resources, organizational culture, change and nurses' education. Facilitators were leadership commitment, available resources and a supportive organizational culture (CR 2.102).

2.101.11   Oranta, O., Routasalo, P. & Hupli, M. (2002) Barriers to and facilitators of research utilization among Finnish registered nurses. *Journal of Clinical Nursing* 11 (2) 205–13   33 References

Describes a survey of 316 Finnish nurses. Barriers to utilization included foreign language publications, non-co-operation by physicians and difficulty in interpreting statistics. Facilitators included nurses' positive attitudes, abilities and collaborative efforts.

2.101.12   Procter, S. & Renfrew, M. (2000) *Linking research and practice in midwifery: a guide*

to evidence-based practice. London: Ballière Tindall   ISBN 0702022977   References

Book explores how the links between midwifery research and practice can be strengthened in order to foster more effective care based on the best available evidence. Researchers, practitioners and consumers describe the key challenges and discuss how they can be met.

2.101.13   Radjenovic, D. & Chally, P.S. (1998) Research utilization by undergraduate students. *Nurse Educator* 23 (2) March–April 26–9   25 References

In order to assist baccalaureate students to critique research studies skilfully and determine their potential use in clinical practice, and encourage staff nurses to determine the appropriateness of implementing research findings into clinical practice, a research utilization component was incorporated into a senior-level clinical course. This is described, and the authors believe that this approach has implications for improving patient outcomes (CR 3.17).

2.101.14   Retsas, A. (2000) Barriers to using research evidence in nursing practice. *Journal of Advanced Nursing* 31 (3) 599–606   24 References

Barriers to the use of research evidence were identified by 400 registered nurses working in an Australian hospital. These were grouped under four main factors: accessibility of research findings, anticipated outcomes of using research, organizational support to use research and support from others. The most important factor was perceived to be organizational support, particularly in relation to providing time to use and conduct research (CR 2.102).

2.101.15   Sitzia, J. (2002) Barriers to research utilization: the clinical setting and nurses themselves. *Intensive Critical Care Nursing* 18 (4) August 230–43

This paper aims to encourage nurses to embrace the challenge of evidence-based practice. The known barriers to research utilization are outlined and some conceptual models in the implementation of research findings are introduced. A summary of key areas to be addressed is presented.

2.101.16   St Leger, A.S. & Walsworth-Bell, J. (1999) *Change-promoting research for health services: a guide for resource managers, research and development commissioners and researchers.* Buckingham: Open University Press   ISBN 0335202209   References

Book has been written for people who make decisions and bring about change at all levels and in a wide range of disciplines. These include clinicians, administrative staff and general managers of health care organizations. Research and development in a changing health service, commissioning research and putting it into practice, and doing and using research are all discussed.

2.101.17 Tranmer, J.E., Coulson, K., Holtom, D., Lively, T. & Maloney, R. (1998) The emergence of a culture that promotes evidence-based clinical decision-making within an acute care setting. *Canadian Journal of Nursing Administration* 11 (2) 36–58   17 References

Nursing research programmes within acute care hospitals are essential to the development and integration of nursing knowledge, are difficult to implement and are rarely evaluated. This paper describes the development, structures and processes of a nursing research programme within an acute care teaching hospital. Selected evaluation outcomes and future directions are discussed.

2.101.18 Tsai, S. (2000) Nurses' participation and utilization of research in the Republic of China. *International Journal of Nursing Studies* 37 (5) October 435–44   32 References

In order to improve understanding of nurses' participation in research activities a survey was undertaken in China, using a sample of 382 staff nurses and nurse managers. Although research participation was low overall, 64 per cent participated in some activities with data collection and conference presentations the most frequent activities. Nearly half had utilized research to change practice, but the main barriers to utilization were lack of time and staff. The findings provide directions for future training, education and managerial policy, especially for nurses in developing countries (CR 2.36, 2.52, 2.75, 2.98, 2.102, 3.1).

2.101.19 Van Mullem, C., Burke, L.J., Dohmeyer, K., Farrell, M., Harvey, S., John, L., Kraly, C., Rowley, F., Sebern, M., Twite, K. & Zapp, R. (1999) Strategic planning for research use in nursing practice. *Journal of Nursing Administration* 29 (12) 38–45   7 References

This study aimed to assess RN's knowledge, attitudes and practices of nursing research activities, assess factors that support a research environment and determine facilitating and challenging factors related to conducting regional nursing research. A 33-item instrument, the Iowa Model for Evidence-based Practice, was developed and utilized. Results are reported and their implications are discussed (CR 2.61).

2.101.20 Wright, S.G. (1997) *Changing nursing practice* (2nd edition). San Diego, CA: Singular Publishing Group Inc. ISBN 1565937589 References

Book explores the concept of change and discusses the complex skills that nurses need in order to become change agents. Many examples, which illustrate 'how to' change nursing practice, are included.

2.102   APPLYING RESEARCH TO PRACTICE

'The ultimate goal is not the use of research, it is to deliver high quality, cost-effective care to achieve desirable patient outcomes and to deliver care from a professional practice model.' (Crane, 1995: 575)

Definition [See Appendix D for source]

Implementing research findings – to use in practice

Example

Logan, J., Harrison, M.B., Graham, I.D., Dunn, K. & Bissonnette, J. (1999) Evidence-based pressure-ulcer practice: the Ottawa Model of Research Use. *Canadian Journal of Nursing Research* 31 (1) 37–52   39 References

Paper describes application of the Ottawa Model of Research Use (OMRU) to increase evidence-based practice relating to pressure ulcers across three health care settings. The barriers and supports encountered, and the strategies used, are described.

Annotations

2.102.1 Adamsen, L., Larsen, K., Bjerregaard, L. & Madsen, J.K. (2003) Danish research-active clinical nurses overcome barriers in research utilization. *Scandinavian Journal of Caring Sciences* 17 (1) March 57–65   46 References

Study investigated whether clinical nurses' own engagement in research had any impact on their perception of research utilization. Nurses who were research-active expressed more success in overcoming existing barriers. The research potential in others needed to be supported through training and guidance and taking up part-time research posts.

2.102.2 Bassett, C. (ed.) (2001) *Implementing research in the clinical setting*. London: Whurr Publications   ISBN 1861562845   References

Book addresses the issues of getting research findings into practice.

2.102.3 Bero, L.A., Grilli, R., Grimshaw, J.M., Harvey, E., Oxman, A.D.& Thomson, M.A. (1998) Closing the gap between research and practice: an overview of systematic reviews of interventions to promote the implementation of research findings. *British Medical Journal* 317 (7156) 15 August 465–8   31 References

Paper examines systematic reviews of different strategies for the dissemination and implementation of research findings. It aimed to identify evidence of the effectiveness of these strategies and also to assess the quality of the reviews. Recommendations are made for further work (CR 2.12, 2.98).

2.102.4 Blomfield, R. & Hardy, S. (2000) Evidence-based nursing practice. In Trinder, L. & Reynolds, S. (eds) *Evidence-based practice: a critical appraisal.* Oxford: Blackwell Science   ISBN 0632050586   Chapter 6 111–37   127 References

Chapter gives an overview of historical development of nursing as a profession. The notion of evidence-based practice in nursing is explored, together with its relevance to practice (CR 2.43.74, 3.8).

2.102.5 Brown, S.J. (1999) *Knowledge for health care practice: a guide to using research evidence.* Philadelphia, PA: W.B. Saunders ISBN 0721681085   References

This handbook guides readers, step by step, through the process of applying research evidence to clinical decision-making and patient care. It explores how to locate, understand and critically appraise research evidence and evaluate its clinical significance, applicability and scientific credibility.

2.102.6 Bryar, R.M. (1999) Using research in community nursing. In McIntosh, J. (ed.) *Research issues in community nursing.* Basingstoke: Macmillan   ISBN 0333735048   Chapter 1 6–28   68 References

Chapter explores factors that inhibit the utilization of research and identifies ways in which the use of research in community nursing practice, education and policy can be developed (CR 2.20.8).

2.102.7 Closs, S.J., Briggs, M. & Everitt, V.E. (1999) Implementation of research findings to reduce postoperative pain at night. *International Journal of Nursing Studies* 36 (1) February 21–31   44 References

Reports a study designed to introduce and evaluate a research-based intervention to improve night-time pain management. This involved the provision of patient information and the introduction of structured night-time pain assessment. Results are reported. These showed the intervention was associated with

statistically significant reductions in both average and worst overnight pain scores. The intervention required an investment in educational support but no additional resources for the successful reduction in pain scores (CR 2.29, 2.61).

2.102.8 Closs, S.J. & Bryar, R.M. (2001) The BARRIERS Scale: does it 'fit' the current NHS research culture? *NT Research* 6 (5) 853–65   12 References

Paper reports on part of a wider study aimed at producing a general picture of the underlying types of barrier to the implementation of research findings. Study used the BARRIERS Scale to identify the barriers, compare them with those identified in the USA, and identify under-reported and additional barriers not included in this scale. Authors concluded that it needed further development to maximize its use in the UK.

2.102.9 Craig, J. & Smyth, R. (2002) *Applying clinical evidence in nursing practice.* Edinburgh: Churchill Livingstone ISBN 1443070644   References

Book discusses evidence-based practice (EBP) and how nurses can apply these concepts to their work in any clinical setting. It also shows how clinical evidence can change nursing policies (CR 2.43, 3.11).

2.102.10 Crookes, P.A. & Davies, S. (eds) (1998) *Research into practice: essential skills for reading and applying research in nursing and health care.* Edinburgh: Ballière Tindall ISBN 0702020680   References

Book does not focus on how to do research but rather it concentrates on the retrieval, analysis and application of existing research in order to identify and develop good practice.

2.102.11 Curzio, J. & McCowan, M. (2000) Evidence-based practice. Getting research into practice: developing oral hygiene standards. *British Journal of Nursing* 9 (7) 13–26 April 434–8   18 References

Reports the work done in one trust in the UK following the establishment of a nursing research and practice development committee. This included a survey to identify existing or ongoing projects, the establishment of a link-nurse system and educational seminars. Oral hygiene was the first trust-wide topic tackled and a standard of practice was developed. Results are reported and pointers for the future are identified.

2.102.12 Earl-Slater, A. (2001) Barriers to applying clinical trial evidence in practice. *British Journal of Clinical Governance* 6 (4) 279–82   22 References

Suggests some learning exercises and techniques to enable the removal of some of the main barriers to clinical practice (CR 2.2.13, 2.29).

2.102.13   Eisnberg, J.M. (2001) Putting research to work: reporting and enhancing the impact of health services research. *Health Services Research* 36 (2) 10–17   6 References

Discusses the importance of translating research findings into practice and highlights the difficulty in assessing the impact of research. Identifies levels of impact, either for further research or policy practice and outcomes, and reminds health services researchers that the purpose of research is to improve health (CR 3.10).

2.102.14   Farquhar, C.M., Stryer, D. & Slutsky, J. (2002) Translating research into practice: the future ahead. *International Journal for Quality in Health Care* 14 (3) 233–49   24 References

Article summarized and analysed the focus and methodologies of the Translating into Practice (TRIP) projects, funded in 1999–2000 by the US Agency for Healthcare Research Quality (AHRQ). AHRQ funded 27 grants and a wide variety of providers, settings and patients were targeted. The most common studies used randomized controlled trials and the major interventions were educational frameworks using adult learning or organizational theory.

2.102.15   Fealy, G.M. (1999) Research utilization. In Treacy, M.P. & Hyde, A. (eds) *Nursing research: design and practice.* Dublin: University College Dublin Press   ISBN 1900621290   Part 1 Research Design   Chapter 6 75–92   62 References

Chapter explores research utilization both as a concept and a practical endeavour. It discusses the nature of utilization and explores the factors influencing it. The roles and responsibilities of key personnel in the process of implementing findings of research in clinical practice are discussed (CR 2.14.30).

2.102.16   Fitzpatrick, J., Stevenson, J.S. & Polis, N.S. (eds) (1994) *Nursing research and its utilization.* New York: Springer   ISBN 0826180906   References

Book includes sections on how research has been used in various specialist areas; perspectives on the delivery of care; and research training and guidance for those wishing to have a career in research. International perspectives include nursing research in the Western Pacific region and in Holland, and challenges that exist in conducting cross-national nursing research (CR 3.3, 3.16, 3.17, 3.22).

2.102.17   Garner, P., Kale, R., Dickson, R., Dans, T. & Salinas, R. (1998) Implementing research findings in developing countries. *British Medical Journal* 317 (7157) 22 September 531–5   27 References

Acknowledges that health care systems in other countries may not be efficient and outlines political, financial and other constraints in the implementation of research findings. Discusses the use of evidence-based initiatives in order to make the best use of health care resources.

2.102.18   Granger, B. (1999) *Research strategies for clinicians.* Norwalk, CT: Appleton-Lange   ISBN 0838515398   References

Book is intended for nurses who want to learn or refine research skills in the clinical setting. It provides information on how to apply basic research concepts in practice. It is designed in a textbook/workbook format, allowing 'hands on' use.

2.102.19   Haines, A. & Donald, A. (eds) (2002) *Getting research findings into practice* (2nd edition). London: BMJ Books   ISBN 0727915533   References

Book addresses ways in which evidence from research is applied in health care research and clinical settings. This new edition addresses changes in thinking and policy, paying particular attention to the demand for clinical governance and new ideas on implementing economic evaluations.

2.102.20   Hamer, S. & Collinson, G. (eds) (1999) *Achieving evidence-based practice: a handbook for practitioners.* London: Ballière Tindall   ISBN 0702023493   References

Achieving evidence-based practice is complex and challenging for health care professionals. From understanding and interpreting research findings, through to implementing and managing change, this book addresses all the key dimensions necessary for success – looking for, reflecting upon and applying the evidence where appropriate (CR 2.95).

2.102.21   Haynes, B. & Haines, A. (1998) Barriers and bridges to evidence-based clinical practice. *British Medical Journal* 317 (7153) 25 July 272–6   29 References

Iterates the aim of evidence-based practice and the problems that practitioners may encounter when searching and evaluating evidence. Provides a strategy to harness evidence and integrate it into health care policy.

2.102.22   Hjalte, L. (2000) It is not my world. Nurses' (working clinically) ideas of scientific research on nursing and application of the results in practical work. *Vard I Norden. Nursing Science and Research in the Nordic Countries* 20 (4) 32–7   27 References

Study describes some nurses' ideas of scientific research on nursing, and the application of the results in practical work. Ten nurses were interviewed and results showed that the traditions influencing the notions of the nurse are a practical approach to knowledge, demand for conformity and women's rights. Scientific research was utilized during study periods, but was not considered useful in clinical work. It was believed that scientists work in another world and use language that it is impossible to understand. This attitude is a deliberate choice and four areas were identified to make the nurses' work related to science: their education, occupational group, the organization and the research institution (CR 2.36, 2.68, 3.7, 3.17).

2.102.23 Hockey, L. (2000) Research. In Lawton, S., Cantrell, J. & Harris, J. (eds) *District nursing: providing care in a supportive context.* Edinburgh: Churchill   Livingstone   ISBN 0443062501   Chapter 6 101–12   43 References

Chapter aims to bring research as a concept and an activity right into the heart of district nursing as the author believes that it must be at the centre of practice. The need for research is defended and some basic principles and approaches are discussed.

2.102.24 Horsley, J.A. (1983) U*sing research to improve nursing practice: a guide. CURN project.** Orlando, PL: Grune & Stratton   ISBN 080891510X References

*Conduct and Utilization of Research in Nursing project, Michigan Nurses' Association

Book attempts to move research and practice closer together by describing the processes involved in incorporating research-based knowledge into practice. Emphasis is put on the activities undertaken by the organization involved in change, rather than by individuals. These are creating a climate for practice change, planning, implementing and then evaluating the processes.

2.102.25 Kajermo, K.N., Nordstrom, G., Krusebrant, A. & Bjorvell, H. (1998) Barriers to and facilitators of research utilization, as perceived by a group of registered nurses in Sweden. *Journal of Advanced Nursing* 27 (4) 798–807   35 References

Authors describe six major barriers to research utilization and state that nurses who had studied research methods in their basic education seemed to perceive fewer barriers than those who had not. Facilitating factors suggested were: diverse models of education; the allocation of resources for education and implementation of findings in clinical practice;

and special positions in clinical practice for nurses with scientific qualifications (CR 2.101).

2.102.26 Kendall, S. (1999) Evidence-based health visiting: the utilization of research for effective practice. In McIntosh, J. (ed.) *Research issues in community nursing.* Basingstoke: Macmillan   ISBN 0333735048   Chapter 2 29–52   51 References

Chapter explores conceptual and practical issues surrounding the need for evidence-based health visiting (CR 2.20.8, 3.11).

2.102.27   Kitson, A. (1998) Research utilization: knowledge for practice. In: *Knowledge development: clinicians and researchers in partnership.* Helsinki: The Finnish Federation of Nurses   ISSN 0251–4753   Proceedings of the Workgroup of European Nurse Researchers (9th Biennial Conference 5–8 July 1998 Helsinki, Finland) Volume 1 52–64   52 References

Paper assesses the way existing information is used, what works and what does not, when attempts are made to get research findings into practice. It describes research evidence which identifies factors known to inhibit and promote research utilization. Some of the theoretical and conceptual frameworks used to explain how findings are or are not used in practice are explored, and a multidimensional conceptual framework is suggested which may help to move research utilization forward.

2.102.28   Le May, A., Alexander, C. & Mulhall, A. (1998) Research-based practice: practitioners' and managers' view. *Managing Clinical Nursing* 2 (3) 87–92   15 References

Paper reports findings of a study that focused on senior managers' views compared to those of practitioners and clinical managers of research-based nursing practice. Findings showed similarities and differences between the two groups' experiences, perceptions and views on the impact and potential of research for individuals, professional groups and organizations. These have implications for the development of evidence-based practice and clinical governance (CR 3.7).

2.102.29   Le May, A., Alexander, C. & Mulhall, A. (1998). Research utilization in nursing: barriers and opportunities. *Journal of Clinical Effectiveness* 3 (2) 59–63   15 References

Paper reports on the research culture of a small group of nurses and managers in three Trusts in England. The opportunities for, and barriers to, research-based practice are discussed, and the findings emphasize the complexity of creating and sustaining this culture.

2.102.30   Lilford, R.J., Pauker, S.G., Braunholtz, D.A. & Chard, J. (1998) Decision analysis and the implementation of research findings. *British Medical Journal* 317 (7155) 8 August 405–9 22 References

Explains how decision analysis reconciles evidence-based medicine with patient preferences. Articulates the difficulty in separate analysis for individual patients, which may be overcome by computer programming, but stresses that decision analysis can provide guidelines for managing groups of patients with similar clinical features.

2.102.31 MacVicar, M. (1999) Integrating research into nursing practice. In Perkins, E.R., Simnett, I. & Wright, L. (eds) *Evidence-based health promotion.* Chichester: John Wiley & Sons ISBN 0471978515 Section 13.2 298–308 20 References

Discusses the application of research to practice, ways of knowing, the place of scientific knowledge in nursing and building knowledge about student learning (CR 2.6, 2.8).

2.102.32 Mateo, M.A. & Kirchhoff, K.T. (1999) *Using and conducting nursing research in the clinical setting* (2nd edition). Philadelphia, PA: W.B. Saunders ISBN 0721671659 References

This resource explores how to conduct and use research in a variety of clinical settings. It shows how research is used in practice and how it affects quality assurance and clinical problem-solving. It discusses practice outcomes, examines the forces influencing today's focus on outcomes, and provides guidelines for evaluating programmes and avoiding pitfalls in data collection. Strategies for facilitating research, gaining access to a clinical setting, acquiring funding, collaborating with other researchers and conducting a study are provided. Chapters are also included on writing the report and disseminating research through presentation and publication (CR 2.15, 2.43, 2.95, 2.97, 3.13).

2.102.33 McSherry, R., Simmons, M., Abbott, P. (eds) (2001) *Evidence-informed nursing: a guide for clinical nurses.* London: Routledge ISBN 0415204976 References

This introduction provides students with an understanding of why they should use research information as a basis for high-quality patient care, and how this should be used in the clinical setting.

2.102.34 Middlewood, D., Coleman, M. & Lumby, J. (eds) (1999) *Practitioner research in education: making a difference.* London: Paul Chapman Publishing ISBN 1853963925 References

Authors explore the effects of teachers' and lecturers' research and its impact on organizational

improvement. Whether affecting whole school/college cultures, or influencing practice through an individual's research, the accounts in this book show how research can make a difference. Although material in this book is chiefly applied to schools, it also has relevance for nurses.

2.102.35 Morin, K.H., Bucher, L., Plowfield, L., Hayes, E., Mahoney, P. & Armiger, L. (1999) Using research to establish protocols for practice: a state-wide study of acute care agencies. *Clinical Nurse Specialist* 13 (2) 77–84 33 References

This study examined research utilization practices relative to developing practice protocols in acute care agencies in Delaware. Examples of research-based protocols, defined as those supported by research citations, were obtained and examined. Although most were referenced, they were not research-based. Most institutions used textbooks and standards to support nursing practice protocols. The authors concluded that those responsible for developing protocols were not familiar with the use of research findings to guide their development or revision, and were unsure what constituted the 'use of research' (CR 2.17, 3.7, 3.8).

2.102.36 Mulhall, A. (2001) Nursing research and nursing practice: an exploration of two different cultures. *European Journal of Oncology Nursing* 5 (2) 121–7 21 References

Explores the research/practice gap and examines the differences in culture between research and practitioners in the UK. Advocates that differences should be made explicit and strategies should be employed by researchers to facilitate research in practice (CR 3.8).

2.102.37 Parahoo, K. (1998) Research utilization and research-related activities of nurses in Northern Ireland. *International Journal of Nursing Studies* 35 (5) 283–91 25 References

Discusses data from a large-scale survey that included nurses' own reports of research utilization, their attitudes to research, projects carried out and their frequency of accessing research information. The implications are discussed (CR 2.52).

2.102.38 Parent, N. & Fortin, F. (1999) Use of research in the clinical practice support programme for the benefit of heart patients (French). *Rechérche en Soins Infirmiers* 57 June 50–6 16 References

Using an example of nursing care for heart patients, this article presents the application of a model of use of research results. This consists of six phases in support of a critical judgement on the value of scientific work: preparation, validation, comparative evaluation, decision-making, adoption/application and evaluation. Each phase applies the model criteria, not only to the research results but also to the whole research process followed by the author. This model of research use can provide nurses with the means of proposing changes in practice.

2.102.39   Radjenovic, D. & Chally, P.S. (1998) Research utilization by undergraduate students. *Nurse Educator* 23 (2) 26–9   25 References

Authors describe the introduction of a research utilization component into a senior-level clinical course. This was because students and staff nurses, who had completed an introductory course, were not able to critique research studies skilfully and determine their use in practice. Authors believe this approach has implications for improving patient outcomes (CR 3.17).

2.102.40   Retsas, A. & Nolan, M. (1999) Barriers to nurses' use of research: an Australian hospital study. *International Journal of Nursing Studies* 36 (4) August 335–43   27 References

149 nurses working in an Australian hospital identified barriers to the use of research in clinical practice. These were the perceived usefulness of research to clinical practice, the perceived ability of the practitioner to generate change and their accessibility to research. Authors believe that fundamental changes need to take place in the education system to improve the teaching of research (CR 3.17).

2.102.41   Sheldon, T.A., Guyatt, G.H. & Haines, A. (1998) When to act on the evidence. *British Medical Journal* 317 (7151) 11 July 139–142   40 References

Emphasizes that not all research findings could or should be implemented, but suggests that practitioners judge the quality and findings of available research, their relevance to the clinical setting, the potential benefit versus harm, and consideration of costs and resources. It concludes that researchers should design studies that take into account potential users and the need to convince decision-makers to use the intervention studied.

2.102.42   Sing-Ling, T. (1998) An exploratory study for nurses' participation and utilization of nursing research. In: *Knowledge development: clinicians and researchers in partnership.* Helsinki: The Finnish Federation of Nurses   ISSN 0251–4753 Proceedings of the Workgroup of European Nurse Researchers (9th Biennial Conference 5–8 July 1998 Helsinki, Finland)   Volume 2   899–913   22 References

Reports a study that explored factors affecting nurses' participation in research activities and those influencing whether research results are used in practice. Findings are discussed.

2.102.43   Sterling, Y.M. & McNally, J.A. (1999) Clinical practice of doctorally prepared nurses. *Clinical Nurse Specialist* 13 (6) November 296–302 31 References

The major themes identified in this study showed the value of doctoral education to advanced practice. The nurses were actively involved in patient care, patient outcomes were affected, cost-effective care was promoted and clinical research was utilized (CR 3.17).

2.102.44   Thompson, C., McCaughan, D., Cullum, N., Sheldon, T. & Raynor, P. (2002) The value of research in decision making. *Nursing Times* 98 (42) 15–21 October 30–4   22 References

Examines the application of research-based information in clinical decision-making. It draws on findings (and work in progress) of two projects that seek to contribute to establishing the potential for evidence-based approaches to nursing. Authors believe that understanding the types of clinical decision made, their clinical uncertainties and unanswered questions are of value to researchers, policy-makers and practitioners.

2.102.45   Tiffany, C.R. & Lutjens, L.R.J. (1998) *Planned change theories for nursing: review, analysis and implications.* Thousand Oaks, CA: Sage ISBN 076190235X   References

Book is designed to enable nurses to understand the process of planned change. It presents overviews of three widely accepted change theories as well as new systems-oriented change theory, and shows the implications of these for research-based nursing practice (CR 2.7, 2.98).

2.102.46   Titler, M.G. & Goode, C.J. (eds) (1995) *The Nursing Clinics of North America: research utilization.* 30 (3) Philadelphia, PA: W.B. Saunders   ISSN 0029–6465

Gives an overview of the theoretical aspects of research utilization, describing what is known about the barriers and facilitators. The differences between evaluating the impact of using research findings in practice and conducting the research itself are also described. Different research utilization models are reviewed, compared and critiqued, and methods for effective dissemination are outlined. A selection of examples which represent the complexities of research utilization activities is given.

2.102.47   Vaughan, B. & Edwards, M. (1996) *Interface between research and practice.* London: King's Fund Centre   ISBN 1857170849   References

Paper gives examples of how research can be utilized in practice and how projects may be developed from practice. Material is based on work carried out in Nursing Development Units.

2.102.48 Walsh, D. (2001) Evidence-based care: and finally … how do we put all the evidence into practice? *British Journal of Midwifery* 9 (2) 74–80 27 References

Author makes suggestions as to how the evidence-based practice agenda may become a reality.

PART 3: THE BACKGROUND TO RESEARCH IN NURSING

Development of Nursing Research

3.1   AFRICA, AMERICA (SOUTH & CENTRAL) AND ASIA

The history of nursing research development in some parts of the world shows varying levels of progress and sophistication. Positive and rapid growth is reported in some countries, whereas in others the process is in its early stages.

Annotations

3.1.1   Ehrenfeld, M. (1998) Nursing research in Israel. In: *Knowledge development: clinicians and researchers in partnership*. Helsinki: The Finnish Federation of Nurses   ISSN 0251–4753   Proceedings of the Workgroup of European Nurse Researchers (9th Biennial Conference 5–8 July 1998 Helsinki, Finland) Volume 1 236–40   No References

Report outlines education for and in nursing, dissemination of research, funding, the role of the Israeli Nurses' Association, completed and ongoing research during 1997–98 and future developments.

3.1.2   Glazer, G. & DeKeyser, F. (1998) Prerequisites and priorities for nursing research in Israel. *Online Journal of Issues in Nursing* 5 (2) 10 pages   12 References   www.nursingworld.org/ojin/topic12/tpc12_4.htm (Accessed 17/11/03)

Article describes prerequisites and priorities for nursing research in Israel. The historical development of nursing research details shifts in types of research by decade from the 1960s through to the 1990s. Prerequisites for the development of research include individual, professional, institutional and federal commitments. Priorities for Israeli nursing research include development of a master plan that reflects its unique culture and geography (CR 3.20).

3.1.3   Kim, M. (1998) Nursing research in Asia. *International Nursing Review* 45 (1) January–February 21–2

The status of nursing research in eight Asian countries was presented at a meeting convened by the World Health Organization (WHO) West Pacific Regional Office and organized by Yonsei University's WHO Collaborating Centre for Nursing/Midwifery. The aim was to discuss the establishment of an Asian Research and Training Network.

3.1.4   Lange, I. & Campos, C. (1998) Nursing research in Chile … Presented at ICN's 21st Quadrennial Congress, Vancouver, Canada 15–20 June 1997. *International Nursing Review* 45 (1) January–February 23–5   10 References

A 1989 Pan-American Health Organization (PAHO) study on nursing research trends in seven Latin American countries (Brazil, Colombia, Chile, Ecuador, Honduras, Mexico and Peru) showed that most nursing research is conducted in Brazil, followed by Colombia and Chile.

3.1.5   Neves, E.P. & Mauro, M.Y.C. (2000) Nursing in Brazil: trajectory, conquests and challenges. *Online Journal of Issues in Nursing* 5 (2) 15 pages   27 References   www.nursingworld.org/ojin/topic12/tpc12_6htm (Accessed 16/11/03)

Describes the development of modern nursing for each decade from the 1920 s to date in Brazil. Those in education and research are highlighted. The current status of nursing, the workforce, professional organizations and research priorities are all reported (CR 3.15, 3.20).

3.1.6   Opare, M. & O'Brien, B. (2002) Strengthening qualitative nursing research in Ghana. *Clinical Nursing Research* 11 (4) November 359–62   Editorial

Discusses ways in which qualitative research can be further developed in Ghana.

3.1.7   Primomo, J. (2000) Nursing around the world: Japan – preparing for the century of the elderly. *Online Journal of Issues in Nursing* 5 (2) 21 pages 53 References www.nursingworld.org/ ojin/admin/tocvsn2/htm (Accessed 14/11/03)

Nursing education, practice, research and demographic trends are described.

3.1.8 Sajiwandani, J. (1998) Capacity building in the new South Africa: contribution of nursing research. *Nursing Standard* 12 (40) 34–7   16 References

Describes the reconstruction of South Africa following the collapse of the apartheid regime, including developments in health care that have led to a growth in nursing research. Outlines the initiatives that are being used to meet the countries needs.

3.1.9 Tlou, S.D. (1998) Nursing research in Africa. *International Nursing Review* 45 (1) January–February 20

The research priorities outlined are based on input from colleges of nursing and national nurses' associations throughout the African region and from nurses attending a consultative meeting at ICN's 21st Quadrennial Congress in Vancouver, Canada (CR 3.20).

3.1.10 Webb, C. (1998) Nursing research in a developing country: a different edge. *Journal of Clinical Nursing* 7 (6) November 485–7   Editorial

Highlights the difficulties of developing nursing research and publishing as reported by Professor Leana Uys of the University of Natal, South Africa.

3.2   AUSTRALIA AND NEW ZEALAND

Development of nursing research in Australia and New Zealand has gained momentum and literature here reports some of the achievements and hopes for the future.

Annotations

3.2.1 Anonymous (1999) Nursing bits and bytes. CYBERNURSE–Government sites. *Australian Journal of Advanced Nursing* 16 (3) 31

Websites

www.aph.gov.au/ Parliament of Australia
www.statistics.gov.au/ Australian Department of Health and Aged Care
www.aihw.gov.au/ Australian National Agency for Health and Welfare Statistics and Information
www.dva.gov/main2.htm Department of Veteran's Affairs
www.health.gov.au/nhmrc/ National Health and Medical Research Council

3.2.2 Lyneham, J. (1998) CYBERNURSE– Nursing research. *Australian Journal of Advanced Nursing* 16 (2) 25

Websites

www.joannabriggs.edu.au/activities.html The Joanna Briggs Institute
www.health.gov.au/hfs/nhmrc/index.htm NH & MRC
www.leeds.ac.uk/rdinfo
www.atlasti.de ATLAS/ti
www.redgum.bendigo.labrobe.edu.au/~obrien/ NursResearch/
www.langara.bc.ca/vnc/nursres.htm

3.2.3 New Zealand Nurses' Organization *NZ nurse researchers database* www.nursingresearch. co.nz/researches/researches.php3 (Accessed 23/02/03)

This database provides a resource for researchers to identify and contact NZ nurse researchers. It also provides a resource for those seeking to fund research. Nurse researchers are invited to submit their details for inclusion.

3.2.4 New Zealand Nursing Research *Index of NZ nursing research* www.nursingresearch.co.nz/ research/research.php3 (Accessed 23/02/03)

Website describes the Index of NZ Nursing Research that at present contains 284 entries. Authors are asked to submit information about their research so that a more complete picture may be obtained.

3.2.5 Stein-Parbury, J. (2000) Nursing around the world: Australia. *Online Journal of Issues in Nursing* 5 (2) 11 pages   7 References www. nursingworld.org/ojin/topic12/tpc12_3htm (Accessed 16/11/03)

Traces the influence of the British model in the development of early nursing in Australia. Discusses the current Australian health care system, workforce, professional organizations and research issues.

3.2.6 Wilkes, L., Borbasi, S., Hawes, C., Stewart, M. & May, D. (2002) Measuring the outputs of nursing research and development in Australia: the researchers. *Australian Journal of Advanced Nursing* 19 (4) June–September 15–20 References

This paper reports on an investigation of the nursing research published by Australian authors from 1995 to 2000 in 11 nursing journals based in Australia, the UK and the USA. The focus of the article is on the researchers drawn from a total of 509 articles that were content analysed and categorized according to topic of the research, paradigm, methods used and funding acknowledgement. The researchers were analysed on the basis of gender, discipline, employment and location. Results of the investigation are reported.

3.2.7   Yates, P., Baker, D., Barrett, L., Christie, L., Dewar, A.-M., Middlemore, D., Stallan, G. & Bennetto, G. (2002) Cancer nursing research in Queensland, Australia: barriers, priorities and strategies for progress. *Cancer Nursing* 25 (3) 167–80

This study describes the research experience, attitudes and opinions of nurses in Queensland, Australia, about their research knowledge, skills, experience and priorities in cancer nursing. A mixed picture is reported and strategies are identified for developing research, including providing information, support, mentorship and resources (CR 2.52, 2.96, 3.17, 3.20).

3.3   EUROPE

The progress of nursing research in Europe continues to show exciting developments. Van Maanen (1998) reports in a survey that 'nursing research appears to have become an integral part of clinical nursing as well as of nursing education'. Also reported was that nurses had access to professional nursing literature in 24 countries, 23 indicating that English literature was used and in 16 countries languages other than English and the mother tongue were accessed in terms of the professional literature (van Maanen, 1998: 69/70) (CR 3.3.14).

Annotations

3.3.1   Carlos III Health Institute *Intranet unifies medical research community* www.microsoft.com/resources/casestudies/CaseStudy.asp?CaseStudyID=13108 (Accessed 15/11/03)

Reports the development of an intranet infrastructure from previously unconnected organizations that came together in 1988 to form Spain's primary medical institute. The institute conducts research into all aspects of health care (CR 3.14).

3.3.2   Council of Europe (1996) *Nursing research*. Strasbourg: Council of Europe Publishing ISBN 9287131120   References

Following a conference of European Health Ministers in Nicosia, Cyprus, in 1990, a decision was made to conduct a study on nursing research. An international group of experts met and reported on the difficulties that had been encountered during its

development. The report covers nursing and nursing research, priorities and methodological issues, building up a national strategy and international co-operation. A series of recommendations are made.

3.3.3   Crow, R. (2001) Building knowledge in nursing and midwifery – European Academy of Nursing Science. *International Journal of Nursing Studies* 38 (4) August 373–4

Discusses formation of the European Academy of Nursing Science whose aim is to sustain a forum of European nurse scientists, to develop and promote knowledge in nursing science, and to recognize research and scholarly achievement in the pursuit of excellence. Its objectives are outlined and brief information is given about its membership (CR 2.6).

3.3.4   Hackmann, M. (2000) Development of nursing research in Germany in the European context. *International Journal of Nursing Practice* 6 (5) 222–8   38 References

Describes the evolution of nursing research in Europe, noting the differences found between research development in Europe and Germany, together with an analysis of why this might be so.

3.3.5   Hale, C. (1999) *Building a European nursing research strategy*. Salamanca, Spain 13–17 March 1999 www.man.ac.uk/rcn/europe/salrntchale.htm (Accessed 27/12/01)

This Euro-conference in Spain aimed to ascertain what progress had been made in the European Union countries since publication of a committee report in 1993–94, and further develop some of the ideas and create a strategy for their implementation. The participants, structure, process, outcome and impressions are outlined. Particular points that emerged are that there is a wide diversity of nursing research capacity in the European Community, the UK has the most sophisticated infrastructure and it was difficult for the workgroups not to be dominated by the opinions of the UK representatives. An important point to note is that the development of nursing research within the UK and USA has brought problems in terms of the split between theory and practice, and countries now developing their programmes may wish to organize their activities to keep research and practice moving forward in tandem.

3.3.6   Kearney, N., Campbell, S. & Sermeus, W. (1998) Practising for the future: utilizing information technology in cancer nursing practice ... workflow information systems for European nursing care. *European Journal of Oncology Nursing* 2 (3) 169–75   29 References

The development of pan-European nursing research is in its infancy as nurses across the continent struggle to deal with numerous barriers that prevent collaborative projects. Through a European Community-funded study a group of researchers are examining the Workflow Information Systems for European Nursing Care to see how this may add to the body of knowledge (CR 2.15, 2.85).

3.3.7   McCarthy, M. (2003) Public health in the new European Union Research Programme. *Journal of Epidemiology and Community Health* 57 (4) 236–7 5 References Editorial europa. eu.int/comm/research/fp6/index_en.html (Accessed 14/11/03)

Reports on the EU Council and Parliament's 6th Framework Programme for Research from 2003 to 2008.

3.3.8   Moreno-Casba, T. & de Frutos-Sánchez, D. (2002) Developing a national strategy to promote and extend nursing research in Spain. *NT Research* 7 (4) 263–71

The main objective of the Centre for Co-ordinating and Developing Nursing Research, as part of the Institute of Health Carlos III, is to develop a national strategy to organize and facilitate the integration of nursing research into clinical practice. Plans include the dissemination of research; fostering the development and training of future nurse researchers; providing opportunities for international exchange of research knowledge and experience; and promoting pan-European nursing research collaboration.

3.3.9   Pardo, C., Reolid, M., Delicado, M., Mallebrera, E. & Garcia-Meseguer, M. (2001) Nursing research in Spain: bibliometrics of references of research papers in the decade 1985–1994. *Journal of Advanced Nursing* 35 (6) 933–43 44 References

Paper describes bibliographic references in Spanish nursing research papers and their evolution over a decade. The authors believe that now the study of nursing is totally incorporated into the university sector, bibliometric studies may help to consolidate nursing research. When compared to *Nursing Research* and publications in other national and international science areas, references in Spanish nursing research papers are scarce and not very specific. But now there has been a slight increase in references in English (CR 2.99).

3.3.10   Smith, L.N. (1999) Workgroup of European Nurse Researchers (WENR) *Annual report for the United Kingdom*. University of Glasgow: WENR   12 References   www.man.ac. uk/rcn/europe/wenr99rpt.htm (Accessed 27/12/01)

Report covers the context, historical summary, education for/in research, completed and ongoing

research, dissemination and utilization, involvement of the Royal College of Nursing, funding and future developments in the UK (CR 2.98, 2.102, 3.17).

3.3.11   Tallberg, M. (1998) Finnish nurses strive for knowledge. In: *Knowledge development: clinicians and researchers in partnership*. Helsinki: The Finnish Federation of Nurses   ISSN 0251–4753 Proceedings of the Workshop of European Nurse Researchers (9th Biennial Conference 5–8 July 1998 Helsinki, Finland) Volume 1 81–7   42 References

Paper gives a condensed picture of how knowledge development has evolved in Finland during more than 100 years (CR 2.6).

3.3.12   Tierney, A.J. (1998) Nursing research in Europe. *International Nursing Review* 45 (1) January–February 15–19   12 References

Nursing research has been developing in Europe for over 30 years. Yet it is still a relatively new activity in some countries and extremely variable in a region where countries vary greatly in size, language, culture, politics and socio-economic status, and in the role and status of nursing and health care systems. While such diversity limits a comprehensive account of nursing research throughout Europe in a short article, an overall view is given, based on experience in the UK and participation in the Workgroup of European Nurse Researchers (WENR) (CR 3.20).

3.3.13   United Kingdom Research Office (UKRO) (2003) *News on EU Research policy and programmes*. British Council On-line Bulletin Issue: E1 03: 01–1 January 2003 Brussels   www. ukro.ac.uk/public/pub/aboutukr.htm   (Accessed 15/11/03)

Discusses various EU policies, research news, education, training and culture, external collaboration, events and awards, new publications, online resources and a glossary (CR 2.2).

3.3.14   van Maanen, H. (1998) Two decades WENR: did history write nursing research – or did nursing research write history? In: *Knowledge development: clinicians and researchers in partnership*. Helsinki: The Finnish Federation of Nurses ISSN 0251–4753   Proceedings of the Workgroup of European Nurse Researchers (9th Biennial Conference Helsinki, Finland) Volume 1 65–80

Paper discusses the outcomes of a survey in which many National Nursing Associations in membership with the International Council of Nurses participated. It presents a preliminary analysis of 20 years of WENR conference proceedings, a historical record of what research nurses have accomplished over the years and an overview of the vision of the scientific nursing community within the countries in Europe.

3.3.15 Vehvilainen-Julkunen, K. (2000) International column. Finnish nursing research: issues and challenges … including commentary by Kesselring, A., Shin, K.R. & Grypdonck, M. *Applied Nursing Research Online* 13 (4) 218–21 6 References www2.appliednursingresearch.org/scripts/om.d11/serve?action=searchDB&searchD… (Accessed 19/11/03)

Article provides an overview of Finnish nursing using the results of recently published evaluation reports of nursing research, education and nursing organizations.

3.3.16 Willman, A. & Stoltz, P. (2002) Yes, no, or perhaps: reflections on Swedish human science nursing research development. *Nursing Science Quarterly* 15 (1) 66–70 46 References

Traces the development of Swedish nursing from its roots in medical science and compares theoretical developments with international views. Determines whether Swedish nursing now belongs in a human science perspective.

3.3.17 Workgroup of European Nurse Researchers www.wenr.org (Accessed 27/10/2002)

Website provides information about the organization, its meetings, conferences, publications and country reports.

3.3.18 Zanotti, R. (1999) Nursing research in Italy. *Annual Review of Nursing Research* 17 295–322 127 References

Reports the development of research in Italy through an examination of literature covering 14 years from 1983 to 1995. It is the first attempt to identify the main characteristics of Italian nursing research published in Italian journals.

3.4 UNITED KINGDOM

Most nurses in the United Kingdom now have the opportunity to learn about research during their university studies and this is gradually leading to an increase in publications and increased awareness that it is the foundation for good practice.

Annotations

3.4.1 Biley, F.C. & Freshwater, D. (1999) Trends in nursing and midwifery research and the need for change in complementary therapy

research. *Complementary Therapies in Nursing and Midwifery* 5 (4) 99–102 47 References

Reviews trends in nursing and midwifery research and the growth of naturalistic inquiry. Provides a summary of the seminal contribution to nursing theory and qualitative methodology, which, it is suggested, might form a basis for furthering complementary therapies research (CR 2.36).

3.4.2 Crow, S. & Le Var, R. (1998) Developing a national research strategy: evaluating education and the development of professional knowledge. In: *Knowledge development: clinicians and researchers in partnership.* Helsinki: The Finnish Federation of Nurses ISSN 0251–4753 Proceedings of the Workgroup of European Nurse Researchers (9th Biennial Conference 5–8 July 1998 Helsinki Finland) Volume 1 198–204 21 References

Paper explores key aspects of the process and outcomes of the development of a national R&D strategy to evaluate pre- and post-registration education. It argues for a national perspective of education and practice in the continuing development and critical evaluation of professional knowledge.

3.4.3 Fyffe, T. & Hanley, J. (2002) Scoping nursing and midwifery research and development capa-city in Scotland to inform the development of a future strategy. *NT Research* 7 (4) 255–62 11 References

Presents the findings of a scoping exercise into nursing and midwifery research capacity which, together with further consultation, has been used to develop a research strategy for Scotland.

3.4.4 Rafferty, A.M., Traynor, M. & Lewison, G. (2000) *Measuring the outputs of nursing R&D.* London: Centre for Policy in Nursing Research No ISBN 42 References

Paper reports the mapping of published nursing research from 1988 to 1995 using the Wellcome Trust's Research Outputs Database, and makes recommendations to enhance the profile and performance of nursing research. Authors recommend a publication strategy, including topics and approaches, and collaboration likely to result in high-impact research or funding success (CR 3.13).

3.4.5 Rafferty, A., Newell, R. & Traynor, M. (2002) Nursing and midwifery research in England: working towards establishing a dedicated fund. *NT Research* 7 (4) 243–54 26 References

Examines the current condition of nursing and midwifery research in respect of capacity and strategy. Proposes a strategic fund for both which focuses on impact of patient care rather than the professional community (CR 3.13).

3.5   UNITED STATES OF AMERICA AND CANADA

The development of nursing research is at its most advanced in the United States of America and nurses from all over the world can continue to learn from their prolific literature. Although nursing practice and research operate within varying 'political' systems, we all have much to learn and share for the benefit of patients and clients.

Annotations

3.5.1   Canadian   International   Nurse Researcher Database (CNRD) *About the CNRD: background and frequently asked questions for potential supporters and members* www.causn. org/Databases/international_nurse_researcher_data base.htm (Accessed 17/11/03)

This free-to-the-user, web-based system was designed to promote excellence in nursing practice through research and evaluation, strengthen linkages between those responsible for health care delivery, promote and support research networks, and educate others about nursing research. Paper provides information about the database and its users.

3.5.2   Gortner, S.R. (2000) Knowledge development in nursing: our historical roots and future opportunities. *Nursing Outlook* 48 (2) 60–7   66 References

Traces the historical development of nursing research in North America and offers six themes for future nursing investigation (CR 3.20).

3.5.3   Stolley, J.M., Buckwalter, K.C. & Garand, L. (2000) The evolution of nursing research. *Journal of the Neuromusculoskeletal System* 8 (1) 10–15   38 References

Summarizes 150 years of nursing research, educational advancement, research funding and support, and the development of the National Institute of Nursing Research (CR 3.14).

3.6   STATE OF THE ART

The development of nursing research has and is taking place over varying periods of time in different countries, but reported progress is ongoing and exciting in some parts of the world, and frustrating in others. To take stock of 'where we are' from time to time can help to consolidate the efforts being made to improve practice.

Annotations

3.6.1   Cotter, A. & Smith, P. (1998) Epilogue: setting new research agendas. In Smith, P. (ed.) *Nursing research: setting new agendas*. London: Arnold   ISBN 0340661941   Chapter 10 212–28   30 References

Chapter examines nursing and nursing research, new paradigms, the concept of paradox, new research roles, whether nursing should develop its own methodology, the quantitative/qualitative distinction and the future of nursing research (CR 2.9, 2.16, 3.7.7, 3.16, 3.20).

3.6.2   Donaldson, S.K. (2000) Breakthroughs in scientific research: the discipline of nursing, 1960–1999. *Annual Review of Nursing Research* 18 247–311   266 References

This review presents the milestones or scientific breakthroughs in the context of the prevailing thinking within and beyond the discipline of nursing. The nature of each scientific breakthrough in nursing is characterized as to the trans-disciplinary change in thinking that has been brought about. Opportunities for future scientific breakthroughs in nursing are presented.

3.6.3   Fawcett, J. (1999) Scholarly dialogue. The state of nursing science: hallmarks of the 20th and 21st centuries … including commentary by Rawnsley, M.M. *Nursing Science Quarterly* 12 (4) 311–18   15 References

Discusses the hallmarks of twentieth-century nursing, current trends in nursing science and makes predictions for the twenty-first century, including the need to save our discipline by detaching ourselves from non-nursing disciplines.

3.6.4   Hinshaw, A.S., Feetham, S.L. & Shaver, J.L.F. (eds) (1999) *Handbook of clinical nursing research*. Thousand Oaks, CA: Sage   ISBN 080395784X   References

Book assesses the current range of scientific progress in the discipline of nursing, explores the depth of knowledge to date and provides specific direction to advance science for nursing in the future. The content is divided into two sections. Part 1 examines theoretical and methodological issues and Part 2 presents syntheses of defined areas of clinical nursing research. Future directions are also outlined (CR 2.6, 2.7, 2.102).

3.6.5   Morse, J.M. (1999) Qualitative methods: the state of the art. *Qualitative Health Research* 9 (3) 393–406   17 References

The example of the experience of traumatic injury is used to explore research possibilities in qualitative research and to convey an appreciation for methodological diversity (CR 2.36).

3.6.6 Munhall, P.L. (2001) Preface. In Author *Nursing research: a qualitative perspective* (3rd edition). Sudbury, MA: Jones & Bartlett and National League for Nursing   ISBN 0763711357 ix–xvii

Author discusses the current state of the art of qualitative research (CR 2.36.98).

3.6.7 Raisler, J. (2000) Midwifery care research: what questions are being asked? What lessons have been learned? *Journal of Midwifery and Women's Health* 45 (1) 20–36   173 References

Purpose of this study was to create and critically evaluate a research database about midwifery care that identifies topics studied, research methods, results, funding, publication data, and implications for a future midwifery research agenda. The review covered American literature between 1984 and 1998. Results are reported and key areas for future research are suggested (CR 2.12, 3.20).

3.6.8 Watson, J. & Platt, S. (eds) (2000) *Researching health promotion*. London: Routledge ISBN 0415215919   References

Reviews the current state of health promotion research and maps out the key debates and major themes. It contributes to ongoing epistemological, theoretical and methodological debates in health promotion research. Some examples of practice are included (CR 3.11, 3.12).

A Profession's Responsibility

3.7 RESEARCH, PRACTICE AND PROFESSIONAL RESPONSIBILITY

In many countries today there is an increasing emphasis on cost-effectiveness when there seems to be an unlimited demand for health care. All nurses want to give their patients and clients the best possible research-based care, but 'political' pressures from within and outside care settings can sometimes make this very difficult. Literature in this section highlights some of the problems, including the poor quality of some research.

Definition [see Appendix D for source]

Journal club – a group that meets regularly (usually in clinical settings) to discuss and critique research reports appearing in research journals, often with the goal of assessing the utilization potential of the findings

---

Annotations

3.7.1 Björkström, M.E., Johansson, I.S., Hamrin, E.K.F. & Athlin, E.E. (2003) Swedish nursing students' attitudes to and awareness of research and development within nursing. *Journal of Advanced Nursing* 41 (4) 393–402   32 References

Identified factors that may have an impact on nurses' attitudes and awareness of research and development.

3.7.2 Chen, H. (2000) Factors holding up the development of nursing scientific research in traditional Chinese medicine and its countermeasures (Chinese). *Chinese Nursing Research* 14 (5) 192–3   6 References

Paper examines the status of nursing research in a Chinese hospital from the point of view of both nurses and administrative personnel. Problems that emerged were nurses with a lower record of formal schooling, poor elementary knowledge of Chinese medicine, lack of awareness of scientific research,

difficulties in reading specialty literature and lack of leadership. Most nursing administrators paid no attention to scientific research and were unable to act as leaders in this area.

3.7.3 Hancock, H., Emden, C., Schubert, S. & Haller, A. (2000) They were different and few: an Australian study of midwives' attitudes to research and computerised research findings. *Australian College of Midwives Journal* 13 (1) 7–13   18 References

Study sought to determine factors influencing the utilization of research findings before and after exposure to an online research database. The small group that was sampled rated research as highly important to providing quality midwifery care, and saw themselves as key players. These findings are not in keeping with previous research, and were largely accounted for by the small number of volunteers who took part.

3.7.4 MacVicar, M.H.M. (1998) Intellectual development and research: student nurses' and student midwives' accounts. *Journal of Advanced Nursing* 27 (6) 1305–16   19 References

Describes the way in which student nurses and midwives experience research in practice, based on a series of in-depth interviews. The author reports an impressionistic model of their intellectual development that is believed to offer a new line of inquiry on the research to practice problem (CR 2.68).

3.7.5 Mazuryk, M., Daeninck, P., Neumann, C.M. & Bruera, E. (2002) Daily journal club: an educational tool in palliative care. *Palliative Medicine* 16 (1) 57–61   10 References

Describes a daily journal club for medical education and presents the results of a trainee satisfaction survey. The survey demonstrates an increased emphasis on evidence-based practice and suggests that journal clubs are a useful educational tool.

3.7.6 Smith, P. (ed.) (1997) *Research-mindedness for practice: an interactive approach for nursing and health care.* New York: Churchill Livingstone ISBN 044305293X   References

Book aims to help nurses become research-minded, decode research jargon, explore and explode myths, and to increase confidence by asking questions and thinking analytically and critically. It also encourages them to apply research-mindedness to practice.

3.7.7 Smith, P. (ed.) (1998) *Nursing research: setting new agendas*. London: Arnold ISBN 0340661941 References

Book explores the relationship between nursing research and practice. It is written from the combined perspective of educators, researchers and practitioners, and discusses ways in which research can be taken forward.

3.8 RESEARCH/PRACTICE GAP

'Professional accountability demands that nurses utilize the findings of research to perform their roles' (Polit & Hungler, 1999: 3). Ways are suggested in this section as to how the gap may be narrowed.

Definition [See Appendix D for source]

Research/practice gap – the lag between the rate at which research results are produced and utilized

Example

Mulhall, A., Le May, A. & Alexander, C. (1999) Bridging the research–practice gap: a reflective account of research work ... including commentary by Hunt, J. *NT Research* 4 (2) 119–31 30 References

Describes the process by which the culture of three NHS Trusts was reflected on. The authors attempted to expose hitherto hidden factors that affected the work. Because the context and researchers may affect the types of question posed, the methodologies used and the interpretation of results, the authors suggest that more structured reflection on the studies conducted would be beneficial and may assist in bridging the gap between academics and practitioners.

Annotations

3.8.1 Fox, N.J. (2003) Practice-based evidence: towards collaborative and transgressive research. *Sociology* 37 (1) 81–102 74 References

Rehearses the arguments pertaining to post-structuralism and post-modernism and cites their contribution to the research–practice gap. Applies the principles of practice-based research to elements of the research process to provide a more integrated and usable model (CR 2.4, 2.7, 2.8, 2.15, 2.102).

3.8.2 Fox, R.D. (2000) Using theory and research to shape the practice of continuing professional development. *Journal of Continuing Education in the Health Professions* 20 (4) 238–46 13 References

Paper describes some of the factors that have led to the gap between theory and practice and makes suggestions on how to reduce it. Among the factors are the different perspectives of practitioners and scholars as to the purposes of research, the appropriate foci of studies and the attributes of quality of studies related to continuing professional development. A system of research and development that can ensure a tighter link between research and practice is proposed (CR 2.7, 2.101, 2.102).

3.8.3 Hicks, C. (1999) Incompatible skills and ideologies: the impediment of gender attributions on nursing research. *Journal of Advanced Nursing* 30 (1) 129–39 25 References

Despite initiatives to increase research output in nursing there is evidence for a continuing research/practice rift. One explanation for this is the perceived conflict between the skills and ideologies associated with clinical nursing and research. Characteristics necessary for high-quality nursing is diametrically opposed to those required by research. The question of gender roles is discussed as this may also contribute to stereotypes of nursing associated largely with being a female occupation and research requiring attributes associated with masculinity (CR 2.13, 2.43, 3.16).

3.8.4 Hill, S., Beattie, R.S. & McDougall, M. (1999) Conducting qualitative health research in the health sector: researcher issues and dilemmas. *Health Services Management Research* 12 (3) 183–9 15 References

Article contributes to bridging the gap between research activity and the practical implementation of management decision-making. The methodological and ethical issues that emerge are discussed (CR 2.14, 2.17, 2.36).

3.8.5 King, K.M. & Teo, K.K. (2000) Integrating clinical quality improvement strategies with nursing research. *Western Journal of Nursing Research* 22 (5) 596–608 27 References

The challenge in linking research and practice is for practitioners to use consistently the best available evidence in their clinical practice, and for researchers to engage in clinically relevant research that provides practitioners with the evidence to do so. The authors advocate that blending Clinical Quality Improvement (CQI) strategies with research methodology is a means of bridging the research/ practice gap. The process of doing this is described.

3.8.6 McCarthy, H. & Leierer, S. (1999) Grey matter. Seven habits of highly effective qualitative researchers and rehabilitation counselors. *Rehabilitation Education* 13 (2) 153–62   30 References

Many students and practitioners in the fields of counselling and rehabilitation perceive clinical skills and activities with clients as quite different from, and much more appealing than, the experience of doing research. As a learning tool designed to reduce the perceived gap between clinical and research endeavours, the authors highlight seven dimensions that the qualitative or interpretative approach has in common with counselling practice. The message of the article is to uncover the fundamental connectedness among the variety of ways of knowing (e.g. research) and doing (e.g. practice) in the discipline of rehabilitation counselling (2.36, 3.17).

3.8.7 Mulhall, A. (2001) Bridging the research–practice gap: breaking new ground in health care. *International Journal of Palliative Nursing* 7 (8) 389–94   28 References

This article explores what the research/practice gap is and discusses five important reasons for it. The issue is then raised as to whether or not there is a gap between evidence and practice, despite the existence of the gap between research and practice. The potential conflict between the 'know how' knowledge, important in practice, and the 'know that' knowledge, important in academia, is discussed. The concept of practitioner-centred research is suggested as a strategy, which would solve the present problem.

3.8.8 Rafferty, A.M. & Traynor, M. (1999) The research–practice gap in nursing: lessons from the research policy debate … including commentary by Lathlean, J. *NT Research* 4 (6) 458–66   50 References

The combined effect of the evidence-based movement, the introduction of the NHS research and development programme, and policies intended to modernize the management of knowledge have heightened the force of the 'implementation impulse' in research. New and experimental ways are being sought to close the conjunction between research and practice. Nurses are the key 'interface' workers in health care, therefore the NHS needs to create a research-rich nursing culture if it is to influence the quality and outcomes of patient care. Much depends on the policies crafted to build capacity in areas of need and the conditions under which the conduct and commissioning operate. Rarely have

discussions on the research/practice gap been informed by insights from research policy literature. This paper aims to bring the two together; to use insights from one to interrogate the other (CR 3.11).

3.8.9 Rolfe, G. (1996) *Closing the theory–practice gap: a new paradigm for nursing.* Oxford: Butterworth-Heinemann   ISBN 075062616X References

Book approaches the problems of integrating nursing theory, research and education with the realities of nursing practice. Examples of initiatives make the book relevant for qualified nurses across a wide spectrum of the profession.

3.8.10 Rolfe, G. (1998) The theory–practice gap in nursing: from research-based practice to practitioner-based research. *Journal of Advanced Nursing* 28 (3) 672–9   50 References

Argues that the application of generalizable research findings to individual, unique, person-centred practice is one of the main causes of the theory/practice gap. It is suggested that a paradigm of clinical research is required in order to complement the existing sociological paradigm and if it is to make a difference to practice, research must be practitioner-based (CR 2.6, 2.28).

3.8.11 Schmitt, M.H. (1999) Closing the gap between research and practice: strategies to enhance research utilization. *Research in Nursing and Health* 22 (6) 433–44   12 References Editorial

Discusses some of the literature on strategies to enhance research utilization.

3.8.12 Shriver, M., De Burger, R., Brown, C., Simpson, H.L. & Meyerson, B. (1998) Bridging the gap between science and practice: insight to researchers from practitioners. *Public Health Reports* 113 (Supplement 1) 189–93   4 References

Five policy advocates and practitioners provide recommendations to researchers to make research data more usable, accessible and applicable for the field of human immunodeficiency virus (HIV) prevention for injecting and other drug users. Translating research into usable information will facilitate its use within political and policy discussions (CR 3.11).

3.8.13 Stark, S., Cooke, P. & Stronach, I. (2000) Minding the gap: some theory–practice disjunctions in nursing education research. *Nurse Education Today* 20 (2) 155–63   42 References

This paper deconstructs three influential ENB-sponsored research projects. It is argued that these reports introduce forms of 'Utopianism', re-inserting theory/practice gaps they sought to close down.

As a result of the idealism revealed by the deconstruction, five key issues for the future development in nursing research are discussed.

3.8.14   Thomson, M.A. (1998) Closing the gap between nursing research and practice. *Evidence-Based Nursing* 1 (1) 7–8   33 References Editorial

Editorial summarizes what is known about the effectiveness of continuing professional education and behaviour change strategies. Suggestions are made for choosing appropriate activities to help nurses close the research/practice gap (CR 3.17).

3.8.15   Tretini, M. & Paim, L. (2001) Caring and research in nursing: a convergent approach (Portuguese). *Texto & Contexto Enfermagem* 10 (1) 11–31   18 References

Authors describe a research method, called 'The Research and Caring Convergent Method', that can be used at the same time as nursing activities in the clinical area, and would help to overcome the research/practice gap.

3.8.16   Upton, D.J. (1999) How can we achieve evidence-based practice if we have a theory–practice gap in nursing today? *Journal of Advanced Nursing* 29 (3) 549–55   46 References

Paper discusses how nursing can achieve evidence-based practice when a theory/practice gap exists today. The concept of evidence-based practice is discussed, together with the relationships between theory, practice and the theory/practice gap. An analysis is made of these concepts within the four pillars of nursing – management, practice, research and education. The author discusses whether evidence-based practice can be achieved (CR 3.7, 3.17).

3.8.17   Youngblut, J.M. & Brooten, D. (2000) Commentary: moving research into practice: a new partner. *Nursing Outlook* 48 (2) 55–6   1 References

Reports the establishment of the Sarah Hirsh Institute for Best Nursing Practices Based on Evidence in 1998 at the Frances Payne Bolton School of Nursing, Case Western Reserve University. Its aim is to address the gap between research and practice through the production of State of the Evidence reviews, and provision of consultation services to help health care facilities to implement practice recommendations (CR 3.14).

The Role of Government

3.9   UNITED KINGDOM

Papers in this section document some aspects of the part the UK government has played in the development of nursing research, and the wider context within which it operates.

Definition [See Appendix D for source]

Research governance – ... a system of control in an area [for example, the NHS in general, local hospitals, primary care trusts, community clinics, or private, voluntary or charitable sectors]

Annotations

3.9.1   Alderman, G. (2000) Teaching and research in higher education. *Reflections on Higher Education* 11 January 26–34

Discusses some of the problems of the Research Assessment Exercise and its effects on teaching and research in universities. These are the distinction between research and non-research active staff, the narrowness of which research 'counts', ways in which it must be published and a premium on short-termism. The impact of Teacher Quality Assessment is also discussed and the author believes that both systems should be made into one.

3.9.2   Baker, M.R. & Kirk, S. (eds) (2001) *Research and development for the NHS: evidence, evaluation and effectiveness* (3rd edition). Oxford: Radcliffe Medical Press   ISBN 1857754026   References

Book gives an overview of the continuing progress of the NHS Research and Development Programme. Three changes are of particular significance: the establishment of the Service Delivery and Organization Programme; the linking of some of the outputs of the Health Technology Assessment Programme to the work of the National Institute of Clinical Excellence to develop the links between theory and practice; and changes in funding ensuring greater transparency

and a greater sensitivity to the priorities and needs of the NHS.

3.9.3   Brocklehurst, N. (1999) Capitulation or consultation? A way forward for nursing research. *NT Research* 4 (3) 167–9   8 References Guest Editorial

Author outlines the development of nursing research in the UK and discusses some of its current problems.

3.9.4   Department of Health *Research governance index* www.doh.gov.uk/research/rd1/researchgovernance/researchgovindex.htm (Accessed 15/11/03)

Provides links to information on research governance, research ethics and intellectual property (CR 2.17).

3.9.5   Department of Health (2000) *Towards a strategy for nursing research and development: proposals for action.* London: Department of Health   No ISBN   9 References

Reports on the outcomes of a workshop held in York designed to explore how best to give effect to the *Making a Difference* commitment. Paper provides a brief discussion of the background and context and goes on to identify a number of areas where strategic action is needed. It makes firm recommendations for a coherent strategy to strengthen the nursing contribution to research and development.

3.9.6   Earl-Slater, A. (2002) National Research Register. In Author *The handbook of clinical trials and other research.* Oxford: Radcliffe Medical Press   ISBN 1857754859   213–15

Briefly describes the government-funded database of research projects (see www.doh.gov.uk/research/nrr.htm) (CR 2.2.13).

3.9.7   Earl-Slater, A. (2002) Research governance and the fate of research. *Journal of Clinical Governance* 7 (1) 57–62   12 References

Addresses the key skills needed to improve research skills and capabilities and provides a template for gauging the value of money spent. Provides learning points for those sponsoring, managing or hosting research (CR 2.2.13).

3.9.8   Earl-Slater, A. (2002) Research governance: baseline assessment/implementation plan in the NHS. In Author *The handbook of clinical trials and other research*. Oxford: Radcliffe Medical Press   ISBN 1857754859   297–302

Briefly explains the British government's proposals for developing the research base in health and social care (CR 2.2.13).

3.9.9   Fyffe, T. & Hanley, J. (2002) Scoping the nursing and midwifery research and development capacity in Scotland to inform the development of a future strategy. *NT Research* 7 (4) 255–62   11 References

Scotland is developing a nursing and midwifery research strategy and the paper briefly describes the process and the groundwork carried out so far. The strategy was launched in autumn 2002.

3.9.10   Rolfe, G. (ed.) (2000) Project 2000: nursing in the third millennium. In Author *Research, truth, authority: postmodern perspectives on nursing*. Basingstoke: Macmillan   ISBN 0333776372 Epilogue 192–204   33 Notes and References

Epilogue discusses the relationship between power and knowledge in the context of research commissioned/funded by the UK Department of Health. It highlights problems nurses face in trying to obtain funding, much of which is not seen as 'real' research. The promotion of evidence-based practice by government is similarly discussed (CR 2.5.19, 2.43, 3.13).

3.9.11   Shuldham, C.M. (2001) Towards a strategy for nursing research: where to next …? *Nurse Researcher: The International Journal of Research Methodology in Nursing and Health Care* 8 (4) 49–52   7 References

Reports the discussions at a workshop where nurse executive directors of trusts and academic staff examined the way forward for research in nursing. The implications of government and European papers on research and development for trusts are highlighted and ways forward are suggested.

3.9.12   Stevens, A. (2001) *Issues in methodological research: perspectives from researchers and commissioners* 5 (8) www.nechta.org/project. asp?pjtld=1102 (Accessed 1711/03)

Outlines the principal research question, factors of interest, methods, sample groups, findings, conclusions and implications for further research in a project set up to obtain researchers' and others' views on the innovative projects on research methodology under the NHS Health Technology Assessment Programme and the usefulness of the research.

3.9.13   Taylor, M. (2002) Research governance. *Health and Social Care in the Community* 10 (1) 6–9   Editorial

Editorial presents the Department of Health's summary of good practice in research and development, which sums up in one place how people and organizations in health and social care research need to work together (CR 2.14, 2.16, 2.17).

3.9.14   Thompson, D.R. (1999) Making nursing research visible. *NT Research* 4 (5) 325–6   6 References   Guest Editorial

Author explains his role in the development of nursing research in the UK. The three main tasks are: influencing the NHS R&D agenda, strengthening the R&D workforce capacity and implementing research findings.

3.9.15   Traynor, M. & Rafferty, A.M. (1999) Nursing and the research assessment exercise: past, present and future. *Journal of Advanced Nursing* 30 (1) 186–92   17 References

Paper examines approaches to undertaking nursing research and building its capacity in Higher Education institutions in the UK. Responses to the last two Research Assessment Exercises (RAE) are reviewed, findings of a small study of nursing departments which entered the last RAE are reported, and the authors speculate on the likely future of nursing research in light of recent education and health policy (CR 3.11).

3.9.16   United Kingdom, Department of Health, NHS Management Executive (1998) *Achieving effective practice: a clinical effectiveness and research information pack for nurses, midwives and health visitors*. London: NHS Executive   No ISBN References

Booklet explains key activities in clinical effectiveness and how they work together to lead to improved patient care. It also includes sections on searching the literature, critically appraising research findings, designing a research study and preparing a proposal (CR 2.12, 2.14, 2.95, 2.96).

3.10   UNITED STATES OF AMERICA AND CANADA

Institutes in the US and Canada fund many research projects and they work to promote research activity in advancing nursing practice to establish priorities and make grants available.

Annotations

3.10.1   Abdellah, F.G. (1998) Interview with Faye, G. Abdellah on nursing research and health policy. *Journal of Nursing Scholarship* 30 (3) 215–19

This major interview by Maura McAuliffe with Faye Abdellah examines nursing theory, nursing models, educating nurses, cost containment, international nursing, health policy in the US and the lessons learned, and provides a glimpse into the future (CR 2.7, 3.11, 3.17, 3.22).

3.10.2   Grady, P.A. (2001) Research partnership program to address health disparities. *Nursing Outlook Online* 49 (5) September/October www.nih.gov/ninr/new_info/pubs/outlook.septol.html (Accessed 15/11/03)

Outlines a pilot initiative to enhance current partnerships between minority-serving nursing schools and more research-intensive university nursing research programmes. Its goals are to increase the number of minority researchers, to increase the minority health research conducted at the partnering schools and to help establish the research area of health disparities as an important and desirable field of study. Websites of suggested resources are given (CR 2.15, 3.20).

3.10.3   Hinshaw, A.S. (1999) Evolving nursing research traditions: influencing factors. In Hinshaw, A.S., Feetham, S.L. & Shaver, J.L.F. (eds) *Handbook of clinical nursing research*. Thousand Oaks, CA: Sage   ISBN 080395784X   Part 1   Chapter 2 19–30   46 References

Chapter examines the 'accepted' traditions that have evolved in the recent history of the discipline of nursing and considers future developing traditions. These trends are examined within the context of the factors that have facilitated their growth (CR 3.6.4).

3.10.4   Institute of Health Services and Policy Research (IHSPR) www.cihr-irsc.gc.ca/e/institutes/ihspr/ihspr_strategic_plan_e.pdf (Accessed 17/11/03)

This Canadian institute supports innovative research, capacity-building and knowledge translation initiatives designed to improve the way health services are managed and delivered.

3.10.5   National Institutes of Health www.nih.gov/ (Accessed 17/11/03)

The home page of the National Institute of Health includes news, events, health information, grants and contracts, scientific resources, institutes and offices, and information for employees (CR 3.13).

3.10.6   National Institute of Nursing Research www.nih.gov/ninr/ (Accessed 17/11/03)

The home page of the NINR includes details about the Institute, its staff, mission, history, news and information, legislative activities, research programmes,

grants and funding, training, scientific advances and other resources (CR 3.13).

3.10.7   Wood, M.J. (2001) Canadian nursing research in the millennium. *Clinical Nursing Research* 10 (3) 227–32   1 Reference

Outlines the history of nursing research in Canada and documents the development of two major research agendas. These are a capacity-building programme in the health service and nursing at $6.5 million (Canadian dollars), and a programme with the following features: 12 Chairs in Health Service and Nursing Research, regional training centres, career research awards for 100 researchers, postdoctoral awards for 120 scholars and regional partnerships for those with underdeveloped applied research capacity.

3.11   RESEARCH AND POLICY-MAKING

Research is essential to policy-makers for planning appropriate facilities to improve the health care of all patients and clients. The nature of research into nursing with all its complexities and potential cost implications has meant that both personnel and funds have not always been available. Decisions have sometimes been made without sufficient background information, resulting in wasted resources and less than satisfactory care.

Definition [See Appendix D for source]

Operational research – a process of offering aid to organizational decision-making through the construction of a model representing the interactions of relevant factors that can be used to clarify implications of choice

Example

Ciliska, D., Hayward, S., Dobbins, M., Brunton, G. & Underwood, J. (1999) Transferring public health nursing research to health-system planning: assessing the relevance and accessibility of systematic reviews. *Canadian Journal of Nursing Research* 31 (1) 23–6   15 References

This study was designed to gain an understanding of research needs, perceptions of barriers to research utilization, and attitudes towards systematic reviews of decision-makers in public health at the level of systems planning. A total of 242 people in positions of public health policy and decision-making participated. Respondents reported a great, largely unmet, need for research evidence. They viewed systematic reviews as likely to overcome the barriers to research use related to critical appraisal, time, timeliness, availability, cost and credibility, but not the barriers related to policy climate, authority or implementation resources (CR 2.12, 2.98, 2.101, 2.102).

Annotations

3.11.1 Black, N. (2001) Evidence-based policy: proceed with care. *British Medical Journal* 323 (7307) 4 August 275–9   28 References (Commentary by Donald, A.)

Paper discusses the relationships between policy-making and research and asks: what is the implied model of policy-making?; is health care policy evidence based?; what other models of policy-making exist? Reasons are given why research evidence has little influence on service policies and ways in which it could become more influential (CR 2.43).

3.11.2 Bond, M. (1999) Policy analysis. *Nurse Researcher* 7 (1) 66–74   14 References

Paper explores various writers' definitions of the term 'policy analysis' and looks at its aspects. This is a form of research in its own right as well as one element in the mixed bag of research approaches (CR 2.86, 2.91).

3.11.3 Centre for Policy in Nursing Research/ Royal College of Nursing/Research Forum for Allied Health Professionals/Association of Commonwealth Universities (2001) *Promoting research in nursing and the allied health professions: a report to Task Group 3 by the CPNR, CHEMS Consulting, The Higher Education Consultancy Group and the Research Forum for Allied Health Professions* 01/64 November London: Higher Education Funding Council for England   2 Volumes

Paper maps the present position of university research in nursing, midwifery, health visiting and the allied health professions, examined the demand for such research, and explored the case for further investment by HEFCE and the Department of Health. Findings are presented in two volumes: the main report focuses on the demand and on the business case, while the Technical Annex discusses research activity in the disciplines concerned.

3.11.4 Davies, H. (2001) *Health services research: avoiding common pitfalls, hospital medicine monograph.* Dinton, Nr. Salisbury: Quay Books   ISBN 1856421953   References

Contains articles previously published in *Hospital Medicine*.

3.11.5 Hall, V.K. (2001) Playing in the 'mud' of government. In Byrne-Armstrong, H., Higgs, J. & Horsfall, D. (eds) *Critical moments in qualitative research.* Oxford: Butterworth-Heinemann   ISBN 0750651598   Chapter 9 115–27   16 References

Chapter gives an account of the author's experiences while working as a research consultant for the Australian government. It is about the 'messy parts' and critical moments of playing in the mud. The nitty-gritty realities of hard politics compete against many vested interests and lobby groups, so that social justice does not always win (CR 2.36.17).

3.11.6 Hammersley, M. (2002) *Educational research: policy making and practice.* London: Paul Chapman Publishing   ISBN 0761974202   References

Book deals with some basic and controversial issues about educational research and its relationship with policy-making and practice. It explores whether there can be harmony in the relationship between researchers and educational policymakers; do increases in knowledge always lead to practical improvement and never undesirable consequences? Would educational research flourish if it were subjected to more central and external control? And what is the role of research reviews in making the results of research publicly available?

3.11.7 Hamric, A.B. (1998) Using research to influence the regulatory process. *Advanced Nursing Practice Quarterly* 4 (3) 44–50   14 References

Article presents two case examples of the effective use of research findings to influence regulatory policy in two different states. Factors involved in using research to shape policy are discussed, including recommendations for nursing policy-makers and researchers (CR 2.102).

3.11.8 Lavis, J.N., Ross, S.E., Hurley, J.E., Hohenadel, J.M., Stoddart, G.L., Woodward, C.A. & Abelson, J. (2002) Examining the role of health services research in public policy making. *The Millbank Quarterly* 80 (1) 125–54   48 References

Article used organizing frameworks and analytic insights from three research fields to study the role of health services research in public policy-making. It discusses which types of policy are amenable to being researched and suggests the need to look at research and competing influences on policy-making in order to make better use of health services research (CR 3.5).

3.11.9 Lee, M.B., Tinevez, L. & Saeed, I. (2002) Linking research and practice: participation of nurses in research to influence policy. *International Nursing Review* 49 (1) 20–6   3 References

Authors describe research conducted by the Pakistan Nursing Council in Islamabad. To raise awareness of the importance of research in policy-making a special experience was planned for eight nurses completing a one-year postgraduate diploma in teaching administration (CR 2.15, 3.17).

3.11.10 Lohr, K.N. & Steinwachs, D.M. (2002) Health services research: an evolving definition of the field. *Health Services Research* 37 (1) 7–9   3 References

Discusses the new definition for health services research, which encompasses the need for health services, receipt of care, quality and cost, and health outcomes.

3.11.11 Lomas, J. (2000) Connecting research and policy. *Canadian Journal of Policy Research* 1 (1) 140–4   12 References

Examines the ways in which researchers and policymakers would benefit from a greater understanding of each other's perspectives.

3.11.12 Marsh, D. (ed.) (1998) *Comparing policy networks*. Buckingham: Open University Press ISBN 0335196462

Although not directly related to research, this book addresses the current theoretical and methodological agenda in the policy networks debate. The funding, undertaking, publishing and implementation of research findings are all linked to government and institutional policies, and how well these local and international networks function is important for research.

3.11.13 Mason, D., Leavitt, J. & Chaffee, M. (2002) *Policy and politics in nursing and health care* (4th edition). Philadelphia, PA: W.B. Saunders   ISBN 0721695345   References

Book is designed to raise nurses' awareness and understanding of health policy and political issues, enabling them to analyse policy issues, enhance their political knowledge and skills, and prepare them for leadership roles in policy-making and public health. Over 100 well-known nurses explore strategies for policy development and political action, and their application in the workplace, government, organizations and community.

3.11.14 Ozga, J. (2000) *Policy research in educational settings: contested settings*. Buckingham: Open University Press   ISBN 0335202950   References

Book argues for independent, critical research on education policy in the context of attacks on the quality and usefulness of educational research in general. The author takes issue with the argument, promoted by government departments and agencies, that education policy research should be limited to work that assists policy-makers. It offers guidance on the theoretical and methodological resources available to practitioners and others, and discusses some of the main issues and problems in doing policy research in education.

3.11.15 Roos, N.P. & Shapiro, E. (1999) From research to policy: what have we learned? *Medical Care* 37 (6) 291–305   37 References

Summarizes eight years of experience at the academic/policy-making interface. Analyses this experience in the light of validity; simplicity versus complexity and time frameworks and assesses the impact of research on health care policy.

3.11.16 Rosenhead, J. (2001) Operational research. In Fulop, N., Allen, P., Clarke, A. & Black, N. (eds) *Studying the organization and delivery of health services: research methods*. London: Routledge   ISBN 0415257638   Chapter 10 154–71   29 References

Discusses one of the key elements that will enable health service managers to respond to some of the pressing current issues of organization and delivery. Its theoretical basis is discussed and examples are given (CR 3.12.3).

3.11.17 Scott, C. & West, E. (2000) Nursing in the public sphere: health policy research in a changing world. *Journal of Advanced Nursing* 33 (3) 387–95   87 References

Reviews a selection of the literature to identify trends in health policy and the implications for nursing research. Article concludes that there is a move away from university-based models of the production of knowledge towards employers, practitioners and users.

3.11.18 Thomas, A., Chataway, J. & Wuyts, M. (eds) (1998) *Finding out fast: investigative skills for policy and development*. London: Sage/Open University   ISBN 0761958371   References.

This definitive guide to research informs policy and public action, particularly on issues of development. The editors recognize that policy decisions are often required quickly, while researchers usually struggle with incomplete data or limited resources. The book provides ideas and guidance on how to research, evaluate and use information fast, while also discussing the dangers of misusing methods which interpret the need for speed as an excuse for not allocating proper resources to analysis and investigation (CR 2.102).

3.11.19 Vaughan, R.J. & Buss, T.F. (1998) *Communicating social science research to policy makers*. London: Sage   ISBN 0803972164   References

This practical guide to doing policy analysis is for academics who want to bring their research to the attention of the decision-makers in the public sector, or who want to train their students in the skills necessary to undertake policy-relevant research.

3.11.20   Wood, M.J. (2000) Influencing health policy through research. *Clinical Nursing Research* 9 (3) August 213–16   2 References Editorial

Discusses the role of evaluation research in policy-making and identifies several important criteria for increasing its value, including developing partnerships between nurses and policy-makers (CR 2.43).

3.12   RESEARCH IN HEALTH CARE

Health services research is an area where many governments spend a considerable amount of money, albeit far less than that spent on defence. All health professionals have the responsibility to read, assess the value of and implement research findings to ensure the highest standards of care.

Annotations

3.12.1   Agency for Healthcare Research and Quality (1999) *Research methodology* www.ahcpr.gov/research/dec99/1299ra18.htm (Accessed 17/11/03)

Reports on a journal supplement that explores the use of qualitative methods in health services research (CR 2.36).

3.12.2   Charlton, B.G. (1999) Clinical research methods for the new millennium. *Journal of Evaluation in Clinical Practice* 5 (2) 251–63   28 References

Laments the decline in discovery of new treatments over the last 35 years, citing ethics committees that exceed their terms of reference and the emergence of health economics as key to this decline. Suggests ways in which clinical research can overcome inhibitors by promoting partnerships between professionals and clients (CR 2.17, 3.4)

3.12.3   Fulop, N., Allen, P., Clarke, A. & Black, N. (eds) (2001) *Studying the organization and delivery of health care services: research methods.* London: Routledge   ISBN 0415257638   References

Reader introduces research methods from a wide range of disciplines and applies them to research on the organization and delivery of health services.

3.12.4   McCarthy, T. & White, K.L. (2000) Origins of health services research. *Health Services Research* 35 (2) 375–87   18 References

Traces the development of research concerning populations, outcomes and other issues that has evolved into the term 'health services research'. Argues that this type of research should be held as equally important as biomedical research (CR 3.5).

3.12.5   Mechanic, D. (2001) Lessons from the unexpected: the importance of data infrastructure, conceptual models, and serendipity in health services research. *The Millbank Quarterly* 79 (3) 459–77   34 References

Debates the growth, changes and developments in the US health service, together with the advances in methodology and research techniques. Identifies a need to build a strong data structure and a conceptual model of the health service that reflects its complexity. Uses three examples, including research undertaken in the UK, to illustrate arguments, and outlines the challenges facing health service research (CR 3.5, 3.11).

3.12.6   Oliver, S. & Peersman, G. (2001) *Using research for effective health promotion.* Buckingham: Open University Press   ISBN 0335208703   References

This book bridges the gap between research and practice in health promotion. It advances evidence-based care by illustrating how service providers and researchers can change their practices to benefit the public. It advances the debate about the relative values of qualitative and experimental research, and encourages an increased participation of service users in their development and evaluation. It provides health promotion specialists with timesaving tools to draw upon research quickly and critically (CR 2.9, 3.8, 3.11).

3.12.7   Perrin J.M. (2002) Health services research for children with disabilities. *The Millbank Quarterly* 80 (2) 303–24   70 References

Identifies the epidemiology and characteristics of children and adolescents with disabilities and highlights the difficulties in researching them. Discusses a range of issues affecting their care and proposes ways in which gaps in research can be addressed.

3.12.8   Rafferty, A.M. & Traynor, M. (1999) Building and benchmarking research capacity for nursing. *NT Research* 4 (1) 5–7   Guest Editorial

Considers some of the issues around building and benchmarking research, using nursing as a focus or case study. The performance of nursing research from existing sources is described as well as the implications this may have for further work.

3.12.9   Wilson-Barnett, J. (2001) Research capacity in nursing. *International Journal of Nursing Studies* 38 (3) 241–2   2 References Editorial

Guest authors are invited to expand on research development strategies that have been successful in different contexts and national settings.

Funding for Research

3.13 FUNDING FOR RESEARCH

Probably the most crucial issue relating to research is the amount of funding available. Governments, private institutions, industry and individual donors all have many calls on the funds that they may be willing to allocate to research. Nursing has frequently been fairly low on the list of priorities.

Annotations

3.13.1 American Nurses Foundation (annual) *Nursing research grants program*. Washington, DC: American Nurses Foundation www.nursingworld.org/anf/nrggrant.htm (Accessed 17/11/03)

Outlines information on these annual awards, provides dates for application and guidance on obtaining an application package.

3.13.2 *Annual register of grant support 2003: a directory of funding sources.* Edited by Bowker staff (2002) 36th edition. New Providence, NJ: Bowker & Ingram ISBN 1573871265

Book is the standard reference source on non-repayable financial support in the United States that will be of value to hospitals, community service groups, medical research facilities and other institutional applicants. Information given includes name, address, telephone, fax, name of programmes, type of programmes, purpose, legal basis, eligibility, financial data, awards and application information.

3.13.3 AORN research grant program www.aorn.org/research/grantguidelines.htm (Accessed 17/11/03)

Website gives an overview of this grant programme for members of the AORN. Funding opportunities, levels, guidelines for grants, funding sources and application deadlines are included.

3.13.4 Canadian Institutes of Health Research *Grants and awards guides* www.cihr-irsc.gc.ca/e/services/17209.shtml (Accessed 17/11/03)

Website gives advice on grant writing and general guidelines for all research funding programmes.

3.13.5 Center for Systems Science *CIHR funding opportunities* css.sfu.ca/grants/cihr.html (Accessed 14/06/03)

Lists regular, special, strategic initiatives and partnership programmes and CIHR institutes' websites.

3.13.6 Corti, L. (1999) Economic and Social Science Research Council funding and oral history: a short guide for applicants. *Oral History* 27 (2) Autumn 93–6

Provides information on the strategies operated by the ESRC when providing funding for social science research. Practical information is given to prospective applicants (see www.esrc.ac.uk) (Accessed 14/06/03).

3.13.7 Crofts, L. & McMahon, A. (2002) Raising the profile of nursing research among medical research charities. *NT Research* 7 (5) 378–89 12 References

Paper investigates the involvement of nurses with medical research charities, and identifies ways in which they could improve their chances of obtaining funds from such sources.

3.13.8 Crombie, I.K. & du V Florey, C. (1998) The pocket guide to grant applications. London: BMJ Books ISBN 0727912194

Book gives advice on how to approach organizations and includes a floppy disk with guidelines on drawing up grant applications.

3.13.9 Department of Health *NHS R&D funding* www.doh.gov.uk/research/rd3/nhsrandd/funding-mainpage.htm (Accessed 14/06/03)

Gives the latest information on funding allocations, background and links to government papers and reports on research and development.

3.13.10 Department of Health *R&D in the NHS: Implementing the Culyer Report.* London: Department of Health www.open.gov.uk/doh/culyer2.htm (Accessed 14/06/03)

Outlines the new strategy for funding R&D in the National Health Service and lists documents that are available on the Internet.

3.13.11   Directory of biomedical and health care grants 2003 (2002) 17th edition. Phoenix, AZ: Oryx Press   ISBN 1573565695

Covers over 3,000 funding sources, including 500 new additions from all levels of government, corporations and foundations.

3.13.12 Economic and Social Research Council (ESRC) *Research funding* www.esrc.ac.uk/esrccontent/researchfunding/index.asp (Accessed 17/11/03)

Outlines current and forthcoming opportunities for research funding and lists commissioning updates.

3.13.13 European Commission *Grants and loans* europa.eu.int/comm/secretariat_general/sgc/aides/index_en.htm (Accessed 14/06/03)

Provides information on how Commission funding operates and gives links to relevant websites.

3.13.14 Foundation Center (1997) *The Foundation directory 1997*. New York: Foundation Centre   ISBN 0614300401

This is a standard reference work for information about 8,729 private and community grant-making foundations in the United States. Sources for nursing are included. Information is given on donors, type of grant, financial data, fields of interest, limitations, publications and application information.

3.13.15   Goldblatt, D. (1998) How to get a grant funded. *British Medical Journal* 317 (7173) 12 December 1647–8

Gives advice on how to write a grant application.

3.13.16   Grants Register 2003 (2002) 21st edition. Edited by Austin, R. London: Macmillan   ISBN 0333964748   www.macmillanonline.net (Accessed 14/06/03)

A comprehensive guide to postgraduate grants and professional funding worldwide.

3.13.17   Kenner, C. & Walden, M. (2001) *Grant writing tips for nurses and other health professionals*. Atlanta, GA: American Nurses Publishing ISBN 155810173X

Describes the major kinds of grant, with an emphasis on federal sources. Each step of the grant-writing process is discussed. Advice is given on adhering to one's institution's internal requirements, managing the paper trail and dealing with rejection (CR 2.96).

3.13.18   Kerr, J.C. (1996) *Canadian nursing: issues and perspectives* (3rd edition). St Louis, MO: Mosby ISBN 0815152256 Chapter 11 135–45 20 References

Discusses Federal support for nursing research, research supported by university schools of nursing and in health care agencies.

3.13.19   Kovner, C.T. (2002) A new US president: an opportunity for nurses to have a voice in research funding priorities. *Applied Nursing Research Online* 13 (4) November 2 pages Editorial   www2.appliednursingresearch.org/scripts/om.d11/serve?action=searchDB&searchD…

Discusses the problems and opportunities for nurses to serve at the highest levels of government and gain positions where the decisions about funding are made.

3.13.20   Lauffer, A. (1997) *Grants, etc.* (2nd edition). Beverly Hills, CA: Sage ISBN 0803954689 References

Book includes a step-by-step checklist of project design essentials, a section on Internet access filled with key website links and information on creating web pages. A wide range of examples will assist fund seekers of all kinds (CR 2.96).

3.13.21   Miner, L.E. (ed.) (1997) *Directory of research grants 1997 with a guide to proposal planning and writing* (22nd edition). Phoenix, AZ: Oryx Press   ISBN 0897749480

This directory offers factual and concise descriptions of nearly 6,000 research funding programmes. Listings are non-repayable research funding for projects in medicine, the physical and social sciences, the arts, humanities and education. Information included is programme focus and goals, restrictions, eligibility, funding amounts, deadlines and sponsor name and address. Also included is a list of website addresses for those organizations that have established a presence on the Internet (CR 1.7, 2.96).

3.13.22 National Center for Research Resources *Research funding opportunities*. Bethesda, MD: National Institutes of Health www.ncrr.nih.gov/ (Accessed 14/06/03)

Website provides information about NIH and NCRR grants programmes. Other relevant information relating to research may also be accessed.

3.13.23 National Institute of Nursing Research *Research and funding programs* www.nih.gov/ninr/research.html (Accessed 14/06/03)

This website enables nurses to search for grants awarded by the National Institute of Nursing Research.

3.13.24   Perrin, L. (2001) The Wellcome Trust and oral history. *Oral History* 29 (1) Spring 106–9

Article describes the main grant schemes offered by the Wellcome Trust History of Medicine Grants Programme. Details are given to applicants and the Trust's policies relating to oral history projects are outlined (see www.wellcome.ac.uk) (CR 2.47).

3.13.25   Picard, C. (2002) Gold standards and hierarchies: should we shift to circles of knowledge? *NT Research* 7 (4) 241–2   4 References Editorial

Author makes a plea for the award of a greater proportion of research money from the National Institutes of Health for qualitative studies. Seventy-five per cent of funding goes to 'gold standard' (i.e. quantitative) studies, which are of course important, but there is a risk that the patient and his/her views may be lost (CR 3.10).

3.13.26   Rafferty, A.M., Bond, S. & Traynor, M. (2000) Does nursing, midwifery and health visiting need a research council? *NT Research* 5 (5) 325–35   32 References

Authors believe that a more secure funding base for nursing research could strengthen the position of nursing in higher education, address the issues of research capacity and problems over research careers, as well as improve the focus of nursing research as a whole. Different options for funding are considered and it is argued that a current policy convergence exists that makes arguments for a dedicated fund more compelling than hitherto (CR 3.9, 3.11, 3.16).

3.13.27   RDINFO *A digest of health-related research funding and training opportunities* www.rdinfo.org.uk/ (Accessed 14/06/03)

Provides researchers with up-to-date information on health research funding and training opportunities.

3.13.28   Ries, J.B. & Leukefeld, C.G. (1995) *Applying for research funding: getting started and getting funded*. Thousand Oaks, CA: Sage   ISBN 0803953658   References

Book covers the components needed when applying for research funding: key connections, research in the real world, what and when to write, checking for infractions and dealing with the reviewer's decision (CR 2.96).

3.13.29   Ries, J.B. & Leukefeld, C.G. (1997) *The research funding guidebook: getting it, managing it, and renewing it*. Thousand Oaks, CA: Sage   ISBN 0761902317   References

Book begins with rejection and makes suggestions on how to re-submit applications to make them more competitive. The practical issues after funding is obtained are discussed. There is a progress checklist to keep you or track and guidance on time management is also given.

3.13.30   Smith, M. (2000) Making the most of research funding opportunities. *Nurse Researcher: The International Journal of Research Methodology in Nursing and Health Care* 8 (1) 4–18   14 References/websites

Author offers guidance to new researchers on obtaining funds for health-related projects and outlines the support available.

3.13.31   UCSD Biomedical and Medical Center Libraries *Grants* scilib.ucsd.edu/bml/static/grants. htm (Accessed 14/06/03)

Lists resources about grants and foundations. Additional sources are: grants and how to get them; grants as sources of funding; information on awarded grants; online databases; and electronic resources.

3.13.32   United Kingdom, Department of Health Research *NHS R&D funding* www.doh. gov.uk/research/rd3/nhsrandd/fundingmainpage.htm (Accessed 14/06/03)

Reports the latest developments in funding allocations.

3.13.33   University of Newcastle-Australia *Searching for funding* www.newcastle.edu.au/ research/grants/search.html (Accessed 14/06/03)

The Sponsored Programs Information Network (SPIN) Australia is a database containing information about thousands of funding opportunities. It provides details of the sponsor, funding limits, eligibility, closing dates, locations tenable, programme synopses, objectives, restrictions and keywords.

3.13.34   Worldwide Nurse *Nursing research – funding information* www.wwnurse.com/nursing/ research-funding.shtml (Accessed 14/06/03)

Website lists sources of funding.

3.13.35   Youngblut, J.M. & Brooten, D. (2002) Institutional research responsibilities and needed infrastructure. *Journal of Nursing Scholarship* 34 (2) 159–64   9 References

Article describes research granting institutions' responsibilities to the funding agencies, research participants and investigators. It also identifies the infrastructure and resources necessary for the successful completion of funded projects.

Useful websites for funding (Accessed 17/11/03)

www.amrc.org.uk   Association of Medical Research Charities

britac.ac.uk/   British Academy

www.esrc.ac.uk/   Economic and Social Research Council

www.europaneu.int/comm/index-en.htm European Commission

www.leverhulme.org.uk   Leverhulme Trust

www.mrc.ac.uk/   Medical Research Council

www.nuffieldfoundation.org   Nuffield Foundation

www.wellcome.ac.uk   Wellcome Trust

Research Centres/Institutes

3.14 RESEARCH CENTRES/INSTITUTES

Probably one of the major ways in which a consistent research programme can be carried out is for units, centres or departments in colleges or universities to establish their priorities and obtain private funding or be financed by government sources. Staff members will usually be engaged in research as well as having teaching commitments, although this can cause conflicts in terms of time.

Annotations

3.14.1   Centre for Policy in Nursing Research www.lshtm.ac.uk/php/hsru/cpnr.htm   (Accessed 14/06/03)

Website presents the aims of this new centre, established jointly by the Department of Public Health and Policy at the London School of Hygiene and Tropical Medicine and the Royal College of Nursing. These are: to help develop a co-ordinated strategy for nursing research in the UK; disseminate models of good research practice; identify current needs for research and training; and to help set a national agenda for nursing research (CR 3.17, 3.20).

3.14.2   Centre for Research in Nursing and Midwifery Education www.eihms.surrey.ac.uk/Centre%20for%20Research%20N&M%20Ed.htm (Accessed 14/06/03)

This interdisciplinary centre is situated in the European Institute of Health and Medical Sciences at the University of Surrey, Guildford. Its aims are to provide a focus for research in nursing and midwifery education, and will include the investigation of the development of nursing and midwifery knowledge skills and the effectiveness of educational strategies. Activities will involve networking with local, national and international organizations in order to develop a research programme that encompasses multicultural and global contexts.

3.14.3   Christ, G.H. & Weinstein, L. (1995) Developing a research unit within a hospital social work department. *Health and Social Work* 20 (1) 60–9   23 References

Article describes the establishment of a research unit as an integral part of a hospital social work department. Methods are discussed for building support within the institution, the process of initiation, deciding on study topics and bridging the gap between clinical and research staff. The evolution of the relationship between clinical and research staff was characterized by four different phases: curiosity, competitiveness, co-operation and collaboration. The benefits and costs of the unit are also discussed.

3.14.4   CORDIS: Community Research and Development Information Service www.cordis.lu/en/home.html (Accessed 14/06/03)

Provides links to European Union-funded research, a research and development gateway, together with national and regional research and development and innovation services.

3.14.5   Flinders Institute for Health Research *Nursing research units* www.nursing.sturt.flinders.edu.au/research/pages/nru.htm (Accessed 14/06/03)

Institute has consolidated its research efforts by establishing five units that will develop interdisciplinary, professional and community research links. These are: nursing and midwifery practice; alcohol, tobacco and other drugs; mental health; nursing education; and gerontological nursing research units.

3.14.6   Foundation of Nursing Studies *Dissemination series* www.fons.org/projects/dissemination/index.htm (Accessed 07/02/03)

The Foundation is committed to making practice development information available to all nurses and the first set of reports have been distributed to all nursing/medical libraries and to all nurse executive directors in the UK. All the initiatives reported on in the series aim to improve the care of patients by using research findings and evidence to develop and change practice (CR 2.98, 2.102).

3.14.7   Gillebrand, W.P., Burton, C. & Watkins, G.G. (2002) Clinical networks for nursing research. *International Nursing Review* 49 (3) September 188–93   20 References

Details a new initiative from the Clinical Practice Research Unit that aims to support programmatic research in clinical practice.

3.14.8 Institute of Education, University of London *Social Science Research Unit (SSRU)* ioewebserver.ioe.ac.uk/ioe/cms/get.asp?cid=807&807_0=810 (Accessed 15/04/03)

The context for the Unit's work is the range of challenges facing education, health and welfare services today. These include financial and social costs, questions about the effectiveness and appropriateness of these services in improving people's well-being, and the way such services operate and are perceived by providers, users and policy-makers. The work is also concerned with the related issues of values, attitudes, beliefs and behaviour, and the complex relationship between research findings and policy initiatives.

3.14.9 Institute of Education, University of London *SSRU research areas: evidence-based policy practice (EPPI-Centre)* ioewebserver/ioe.ac.uk/ioe/cms/get.asp?cid=1514 (Accessed 01/05/03)

Outlines its programme of work that includes health promotion research and dissemination of information relating to the evaluation of health promotion interventions; education – a centre for evidence-informed policy and practice in education; and user involvement investigating the generation and use of evidence of effectiveness as seen by people using health and education services.

3.14.10 International Council of Nurses (1990) *Directory of nursing research units* (2nd edition). Geneva: International Council of Nurses No ISBN ICN/89/202

Directory cites 115 nursing research units worldwide which were identified by national nurses' associations in membership with the International Council of Nurses. Information included is unit name and address, contact person, type of setting, number of professional staff, disciplines included, research activities and support, and conducted research. The latter are reported under the following categories: recipients of care, nursing practice, theory, education, research on nurses, organizations, management and administration and research methodology. Also included are methodological approaches used, additional research activities, and whether consultancy is provided to outside professionals with or without fees.

3.14.11 International Council of Nurses (2003) *Nursing research: a tool for action*. Geneva: International Council of Nurses

This 'Nursing Matters' fact sheet provides quick reference information on international perspectives relating to the nursing profession. Priorities and strategies are briefly discussed (see www.icn.ch/matters_research.htm) (Accessed 14/06/03)

3.14.12 International Nursing Review (1994) Germany's first and only research unit. *International Nursing Review* 41 (1) Issue 313 6 News

Reports the setting-up of the Agnes Karll Institute for nursing research in 1991. Its focal points of research are based on World Health Organization 'Health for all' objectives (CR 3.3).

3.14.13 McKeown, M. (2001) Directions: research into practice. *Mental Health Care & Learning Disabilities* 4 (8) 276–7

Reports on the new nursing research unit at the University of Central Lancashire that seeks to bridge the gap between academia and clinical practice (CR 3.8).

3.14.14 McMillan, I. (1992) Research development. *Nursing Times* 88 (50) 9 December 19

Reports the creation of a new mental health nursing research unit in London. Links have been made with two universities and a medical school, and two topics have been identified as priorities (CR 3.21).

3.14.15 National Centre for Social Research (NatCen) www.natcen.ac.uk (Accessed 15/04/03)

NatCen is the largest independent social research institute in Britain. It conducts social research among members of the public to provide information on a range of social policy issues.

3.14.16 Netherlands Institute for Health Services Research *Health services for Europe: What NIVEL Has to Offer* www.nivel.nl (Accessed 07/03/03)

Describes the work of NIVEL, The Netherlands Institute for Health Services Research. It is aimed principally at policy-makers, planners, decision-makers and advisors concerned with health services in Europe. It will also be of interest to potential research partners, for example, other research institutes, professional organizations and consumer groups. It can offer expertise, experience and extensive collaborative research networks (CR 2.15, 3.3).

3.14.17 *Network for Psychiatric Nursing Research* www.man.ac.uk/rcn/ukwide/npnr.html (Accessed 15/04/03)

This network is a UK-based service offering a comprehensive search and information service for health professionals working in mental health nursing research. Its aim is to disseminate and develop research and practice initially within the United Kingdom.

3.14.18   Oguisso, T. (1990) How ICN is promoting research. *International Nursing Review* 37 (4) Issue 292   9 References

Examines the role of the International Council of Nurses in promoting research. Its historical background is discussed, together with study seminars held and the statement and guidelines published on research. Health research was the theme for discussion at the World Health Assembly and the ICN statement is included in the article. The Task Force was given a mandate to provide for each country a history of nursing research, up-to-date figures of nursing researchers and where they were prepared, types of education programme, research being undertaken, funded posts available, numbers of nurses employed to undertake research, the greatest needs, and trends and priorities for nursing research (CR 3.22).

3.14.19   Queensland University of Technology *The Centre for Nursing Research* www.hlth.qut. edu.au/nrs/research/index.jsp (Accessed 15/04/03)

Website outlines the major objectives of this centre and the range of services that it provides.

3.14.20   Royal College of Nursing *Research and Development Co-ordinating Centre* www.man.ac. uk/rcn/ (Accessed 14/06/03)

Centre is a showcase for resources available for nursing research and development. It provides a framework for sharing information about research networks, policy issues, governance, funding, training and support units, dissemination and practice development. The site will be permanently 'under construction' so that it develops in line with the needs of professional nurses endeavouring to conduct relevant research and keep abreast of current activities (CR 2.98, 3.13).

3.14.21   *Royal College of Nursing Research Society* www.man.uk/rcn/rs/index.htm (Accessed 15/04/03)

This website provides information on all activities of the society. It aims to support nurses who identify and practise research, disseminate research findings, supervise research, conduct research, critically appraise research reports and utilize research.

3.14.22   *Russell Sage Foundation* www.russell-sage.org/ (Accessed 15/04/03)

This American Foundation is devoted exclusively to research in the social sciences. It is a funding source for studies by scholars at other academic and research institutions, and an active member of the nation's social science community. It also publishes books that derive from the work of its grantees and Visiting Scholars (CR 3.13).

3.14.23   University of Birmingham *The National Co-ordinating Centre for Research Methodology* www.publichealth.bham.ac.uk/nccrm/ (Accessed 28/02/03)

The core mission of the methodology programme is to promote identification, development and use of appropriate methods so that health and social care can be built on the best possible evidence base. Its core tasks are promoting active debate on methodology, identifying key questions for methodological research, prioritizing research questions, commissioning and managing research, disseminating findings and ensuring all procedures are carried out to the highest standards.

3.14.24   University of Central Lancashire, Faculty of Health, Department of Nursing www. uclan.ac.uk/ (Accessed 14/06/03)

Reports the activities of the Clinical Practice Research Unit that will bring together practitioners and academics in specific clinical areas with the aim of advancing clinical nursing knowledge and science.

3.14.25   University of Newcastle – Australia *Centre for Health Services Research* www.newcastle. edu.au/research/centres/chsr.html (Accessed 14/06/03)

The activities of the Centre are described.

3.14.26   University of Newcastle – Australia *Centre for Mental Health Studies* www.newcastle.edu.au/ research/centres/mhs.html (Accessed 15/04/03)

This multidisciplinary Centre seeks to promote excellence in mental health research, education and service evaluation. It provides a focus for many professionals, including nurses.

3.14.27   University of Newcastle – Australia *Centre for Nursing Research and Practice Development* www.newcastle.edu.au/faculty/health/research/ nurse-research.html (Accessed 14/06/03)

Reports the activities of the Centre and includes information on human research ethics, grants and fellowships, research centres and support units.

3.14.28   University of Newcastle upon Tyne, Faculty of Medical Sciences *Health services research* medical.faculty.ncl.ac.uk/research/groupinfo? GroupCode=HSR (Accessed 19/06/03)

Gives the history, mission and key objectives of the Centre, together with its position in the university, and an outline of its collaboration with other institutions. Current research themes are presented.

3.14.29 *University of Sheffield, School of Health and Related Research (ScHARR)* www.shef.ac.uk/uni/academic/R-Z/scharr/about.htm (Accessed 14/06/03)

Brings together a wide range of health-related skills, including health economics, operational research, management sciences, epidemiology, medical statistics and information science. It acts as a partner to the NHS and has links with other institutions in the UK, Europe and the Far East.

3.14.30 **University of York** *Centre for Evidence-based Nursing.* York: Department of Health Studies www.york.ac.uk/depts/hstd/centres/evidence/ev-intro.htm (Accessed 14/06/03)

This website gives the background and objectives of the Centre for Evidence-based Nursing, current projects, recent publications, the Cochrane Wounds Group and links to external information sources.

3.14.31 **University of York** *Social Policy Research Unit* york.ac.uk/inst/spru/welcome.htm (Accessed 14/06/03)

This unit carries out policy-related research using methodological skills, academic knowledge and understanding of policy-making. It focuses on two major areas – health and social care and social security. Basic details of objectives, approach, research programmes and staffs are given (CR 3.11).

3.14.32 **Ward, M.F.** (2000) Developing a mental health nursing network to support research. *Nurse Researcher* 7 (3) 24–31   8 References

Paper describes the development and management of the Network for Psychiatric Nursing Research, which was specifically set up to counter the professional isolation of those wishing to undertake or implement research for practice. It is affiliated with other mental health research organizations in the USA, Canada, Australia and Scandinavia (see www.man.ac.uk/rcn/ukwide/npnr.html).

Professional Groups/Organizations

Professional groups have played, and continue to play, major roles in the development of nursing research.

Annotations

3.15.1 American Academy of Family Physicians *Federation of Practice Based Research Networks* www.aafp.org/research/fpbrn (Accessed 14/06/03)

Website outlines the mission of the Federation and its role in the development of research networks.

3.15.2 Anonymous *American Association of Colleges of Nursing (AACN).* Washington, DC: American Association of Colleges of Nursing www.aacn.nche.edu/ (Accessed 14/06/03)

The AACN website offers information about the organization and its services, including conferences and publications. Programme areas include education, research, governmental advocacy and data collection. Resources include curriculum standards, key statistics, links for prospective students and newsletter issues. It also includes information about the *Journal of Professional Nursing*, and a list of member institutions with web links.

3.15.3 European Honour Society of Nursing and Midwifery *Scholarship in Nursing Practice, Education and Midwifery* www.shef.ac.uk/~stti/society.htm (Accessed 14/06/03)

Reports that this new society is being established across Europe for the purpose of advancing knowledge through scholarly activity in nursing and midwifery practice, education and research. Information is given on joining, activities, the board, enursing (newsletter), members and publications.

3.15.4 Felton, G., McCorkle, M.R. & Redman, B. (1998) The coming of age of military nursing research. *Journal of Professional Nursing* 14 (2) 85–91 11 References

Provides a historical perspective of military nursing research and addresses the challenge facing military nursing researchers, which includes the development of programmes of research (CR 3.5).

3.15.5 Freda, M.C. & Lewis, J.A. (2001) The Society for Women's Health research. *Nursing Outlook Online* 49 (5) September/October www. women's-health.org (Accessed 16/12/01)

Outlines the functions of the Society for Women's Health Research, which comprises health care professionals, health advocates and physicians. Its main purpose is to bring to national attention the full spectrum of women's health issues and to call for funding for research. It is especially concerned with how medical conditions and pharmaceuticals affect women differently from men. Pressure is exerted nationally via the National Institutes of Health and Congress. Journal editors are urged to strengthen their criteria by requiring gender analysis in papers accepted for publication, and conferences are also organized. An Annual Congress is held. The Society also publishes the *Journal of Women's Health* and *Gender-based Medicine*, and a website gives further information.

3.15.6 Rhodes, P., Nocon, A., Booth, M., Chowdrey, M.Y., Fabian, A., Lambert, N., Mohammed, F. & Walgrove, T. (2002) A service users' research advisory group from the perspectives of both service users and researchers. *Health and Social Care in the Community* 10 (5) 402–9 26 References

Provides an account of the experiences of service users' involvement in the research process and describes the positive outcomes derived from participating in such research.

3.15.7 Royal College of Nursing *Research and Development Co-ordinating Centre – International* www.man.ac.uk/rcn/international/intindex.html (Accessed 14/06/01)

Lists websites on networks, policy/strategy, ethics, funding, training and support units. Gives details of research in progress, the dissemination of this research and practice development (CR 2.17, 2.98, 3.11, 3.13).

3.15.8 Shaw, T. (1999) The work of the Foundation of Nursing Studies. *Nursing Standard* 13 (50) 31–2   1 Reference

The Foundation of Nursing Studies is an independent, registered charity that seeks to bridge the gap between research and health care delivery. The work of the Foundation is described and the author outlines how nurses can get involved with its work (CR 3.8).

Research Roles and Careers

3.16 RESEARCH ROLES AND CAREERS

There are a variety of roles that nurses may have in relation to research and all are important to ensure that professional practice is based on firm foundations. Some nurses will conduct research, others will facilitate this process and most will be informed consumers. Each role will require different levels of knowledge and skill that nurses may acquire at varying periods in their professional careers.

Definition [See Appendix D for source]

Research assistant – the individual who assists the principal investigator with such activities as subject recruitment, data collection and data analysis

---

Annotations

3.16.1 Andre, R. & Frost, P.J. (eds) (1996) *Researchers hooked on teaching: noted scholars discuss the synergy's of teaching and research.* London: Sage   ISBN 0761906223   References

International contributors describe their experiences of balancing the tension between teaching and research. The themes which emerge are teachers as models for each other and their students, individualism versus collectivism in the institution and classroom, integrating individual research interests into the classroom and finding one's voice.

3.16.2 Beresford, P. & Evans, C. (1999) Research note: research and empowerment. *British Journal of Social Work* 29 (5) 671–7   5 References

Discusses the emergence of the evidence-based movement against the development of the 'role and relations' of research. Seeks to involve the users of research in all parts of the process and illustrates with two examples.

3.16.3 Chesney, M. (2000) Interaction and understanding: 'me' in the research. *Nurse Researcher* 7 (3) 58–69   25 References

Author focuses on herself as the researcher, in the context of research with women who have given birth in Pakistan. Insights are shared which open up a theoretical window on the relationships between researcher and the women in the study (CR 2.42).

3.16.4 Chesney, M. (2001) Dilemmas of self in the method. *Qualitative Health Research* 11 (1) January 127–35   24 References

Author focuses on the researcher in research. Some personal dilemmas encountered during years of doing research are explored. These concern the position of the researcher and honesty, the criticism of Western dominance and how the research process has changed the author (CR 2.16).

3.16.5 Clare, J. & Hawes, C. (2001) Engendering change: empowering nurse academics to take part in a university research culture. *Australian Journal of Advanced Nursing* 18 (4) June–August 32–6   References

This paper outlines a strategic approach to creating a research culture in one university school of nursing and midwifery in Australia. A climate to facilitate change was put in place, together with a research support structure. The success of this strategy can be seen by the increased participation in research activities, enhanced productivity and the increasing confidence of the staff (CR 2.10, 2.101, 3.2).

3.16.6 Coulson, S. & Phelan, L. (2000) Clinical research in paediatric oncology and the role of the research nurse in the UK. *European Journal of Oncology Nursing* 4 (3) 154–61   40 References

Discusses the role of the research nurse when undertaking clinical trials in conjunction with scientific and medical staff (CR 2.17, 2.29, 3.23).

3.16.7 Cusick, A. (2001) The experience of clinician-researchers in occupational therapy. *American Journal of Occupational Therapy* 55 (1) January–February 9–18   72 References

Study examined the experience of 15 occupational therapy clinicians who analysed their own roles in relation to research, the processes involved, and the outcomes. The qualitative approach of grounded theory was used in acute care hospitals in one

Australian city. Results from in-depth interviews were analysed, and one core category emerged. This encompassed a process of role change from clinician to clinician-researcher. Conditions for this change were identified and three key concepts were derived to elaborate the core category. The person was active in identifying research as significant, constructing actions in relation to research, and evaluating the experience. These findings further the understanding of the role of clinician-researchers (CR 2.22, 2.45, 2.68, 3.16).

3.16.8 Daley, L.L. & Wright, L.K. (2000) The role of a clinical outcome research evaluator: a graduate nursing student's experience. *Clinical Nurse Specialist* 14 (3) 127–32   13 References

Article describes a graduate nursing student's supervised research experience. The study evaluated an intervention that consisted of telephone counselling of caregivers responsible for elders with dementia. The student's preparation for the role of evaluator is reported and the processes involved are discussed (CR 2.43).

3.16.9 Edwards, A. (2002) Responsible research: ways of being a researcher. *British Educational Research Journal* 28 (2) 157–68   51 References

Being an educational researcher is not an easy option. We are practitioners in an engaged social science, which makes particular demands, including responsibility to the field of study. It is argued that close-to-the-field research is an important part of this responsibility. Because examinations of individual agency and responsibility must take into account contexts, their values and opportunities, this presidential address also examines how the British Educational Research Association, as a learned society, can sustain the identities of engaged researchers and how their revelations from the field can inform educational policy and the methodologies which shape educational inquiry.

3.16.10 Emden, C. (1998) Establishing a 'track record': research productivity and nursing academe. *Australian Journal of Advanced Nursing* 16 (1) 29–33   26 References

Many nursing academics in Australia are finding to their dismay that an outstanding teaching career and exemplary contribution to their field – and a PhD – are not enough to achieve promotion within their university, or secure a new academic post. One must also possess a proven or established 'track record' in research and publication. The operational funding arrangements for Australian universities rely in part on the research productivity of academic staff members. This puts special expectation on the way academics conduct their scholarly work. This paper reviews relevant research, draws on personal

experience and highlights how nursing academics may most strategically establish a research and publication record with a view to career advancement.

3.16.11 Ghersi, D. (2002) Making it happen: approaches to involving consumers in Cochrane Reviews. *Evaluation and the Health Professions* 25 (3) 270–82   12 References

Article discusses consumer involvement in the Cochrane review process in relation to the ten key principles that guide the work of the Cochrane Collaboration (CR 2.12).

3.16.12 Glesne, C. (1999) *Becoming qualitative researchers: an introduction* (2nd edition). New York: Longman   ISBN 0801316332

3.16.13 Jarvis, P. (2000) The practitioner-researcher in nursing ... including commentary by Yerrell, P., Thompson, D.R., Burnard, P. & Draper, P. *Nurse Education Today* 20 (1) 30–44   34 References

Knowledge is changing rapidly in late modern society, which has led to the recognition that no two practice situations are the same. This has been implicit in the perceived gap between theory and practice. Research is best undertaken by practitioners. This is especially important in the developing world where practice situations are so different from those in the West (CR 3.8).

3.16.14 Kenkre, J.E. & Foxcroft, D.R. (2001) Career pathways in research: pharmaceuticals. *Nursing Standard* 16 (8) 7 November 36–9   5 References

Article describes the pharmaceutical pathway as a way for nurses to develop clinical research roles.

3.16.15 Luker, K. (1999) The dilemma concerning the nurse's role in a multi-disciplinary research agenda. *NT Research* 4 (2) 85–6   Guest Editorial

Explores the opportunities and problems in trying to raise the research skills base of nursing. Powerful tensions exist relating to the quality of research in practice disciplines, and what is considered to be the role of nurses in a multidisciplinary research agenda.

3.16.16 Middlewood, D., Coleman, M. & Lumby, J. (1999) *Practitioner research in education: making a difference*. London: Paul Chapman Publishing   ISBN 1853963925   References

Authors explore the effects of teachers' and lecturers' research and its impact on organizational improvement. Whether affecting whole school cultures or influencing practice through individual research, the accounts in this book show how research *can* make a difference (CR 2.102).

3.16.17   Moch, S.D. & Gates, M.F. (eds) (1999) *The researcher experience in qualitative research.* Thousand Oaks, CA: Sage   ISBN 0761913424 References

This book, which is aimed across disciplines, shows how researchers must consider their own place when undertaking research. Various populations and settings in which research takes place are examined, as well as ways in which researcher experience can be processed and reported (CR 2.16, 2.36).

3.16.18   Mueller, M. (2001) From delegation to specialization: nurses and clinical trial co-ordination. *Nursing Inquiry* 8 (3) September 182–90   51 References

Paper considers an area of clinical research that has been delegated by physician-researchers to nurses and others in the United States, that of clinical trials co-ordination. Interviews were used to explore the processes by which the boundaries and definitions of work have been established. The processes that have been established to formalize a role for nurses in clinical work are discussed, and the question is raised as to whether specialization alone will distinguish nursing from other occupational groups engaged in clinical research work (CR 2.29, 2.68).

3.16.19   Newell, R. (2002) Research and its relationship to nurse education: focus and capacity. *Nurse Education Today* 22 (4) May 278–84   14 References

Paper argues that nursing is currently in a weak position with regard to creating a future workforce that will have the capacity to understand, undertake, disseminate and utilize research findings. A key government document setting out the future of nursing contains little reference to the role of R&D either in clinical practice or in the preparation of the workforce. However, a recent publication that sets out a potential strategy for research in nursing gives hope for the future, but the profession will need to be on its guard to ensure it is translated into action (CR 3.9).

3.16.20   Owen, S. & Maslin-Prothero, S.E. (2001) Developing your research profile. *Nurse Education in Practice.* 1 (1) 5–11   16 References

Paper addresses nurse teachers and lecturers who are interested in developing their research profile but are unsure of how to go about it. Issues addressed include valuing your own experience, writing for publication, time management, learning from others, considering a sideways move, finding an academic mentor, becoming a reviewer, attending conferences and seeking research funding. Developing a research profile is a long process and there is growing interest in having a more clearly defined career pathway to support aspiring researchers (CR 2.99, 3.7, 3.13, 3.18).

3.16.21   Robinson, J. (1999) Taking the initiative: supporting nursing research in an acute trust. *Nurse Researcher* 6 (4) 41–50   14 References

Paper outlines three initiatives that have brought a group from the Royal Hospital for Sick Children in Edinburgh from their first hesitant steps in nursing research to a thriving research-active body of nurses with over 20 projects in progress. The initiatives are shared governance, joint hospital/university lectureship appointments and pump-priming funding.

3.16.22 Royal College of Nursing *The clinical research nurse in NHS trusts and GP practices: guidance for nurses and their employers.* Employment Brief 22/98 www.man.ac.uk/rcn/clinresgrades.htm (Accessed 01/05/03)

Brief gives advice on defining terms, codes of conduct and regulations, job descriptions, suggested grading criteria, education and careers for nurses in clinical research, further reading and compares NHS pay scales with those of researchers in other settings.

3.16.23   Royal College of Nursing – RCN Research Society *Career pathways for research nurses* www.man.ac.uk/rcn/rs/career.htm (Accessed 07/02/03)

Reports work done by the Research Society of the Royal College of Nursing to develop five potential career pathways for nurses to develop their skills and expertise. These are: academic, clinical, clinical research nurse, pharmaceutical and management. Each pathway is presented as a matrix, to demonstrate the facility to develop a career along a single pathway or by developing a greater knowledge by moving between them. The information described includes the typical role, experience, knowledge, training, skills and qualifications expected at each stage along each pathway.

3.16.24   Ryan, S. (2001) Consultant nurses: pioneers of a new world. *NT Research* 6 (3) 645–7   8 References

Discusses the roles and skills required in the consultant nurse. Included among these is the ability to bridge the research/practice divide and take the lead in demystifying the process of research.

3.16.25   Secrist, J. & Fitzpatrick, J. (2000) *What else you can do with a PhD.* Thousand Oaks, CA: Sage   ISBN 0761919708   References

Book provides practical advice and support for readers moving out of academia.

3.16.26   Serrant-Green, L. (2002) Black on black: methodological issues for black researchers working in minority ethnic communities. *Nurse Researcher: The International Journal of Research Methodology in Nursing and Health Care* 9 (4) 30–44   20 References

Author explores some of the issues relating to conducting qualitative research in black and ethnic minority communities. Some of the personal tensions encountered as a black researcher are discussed (CR 2.16, 2.36).

3.16.27   Sterling, Y.M. (2001) The clinical imperative in clinical nursing research. *Applied Nursing Research* 14 (1) February 44–7   23 References

Author believes that clinical nurse investigators cannot generate relevant questions to study phenomena with which they are not experienced. The nurse researchers' early involvement in the clinical world is therefore a prerequisite of proposal development and subsequent design of the study if it is to have rigour and significance.

3.16.28   Tolve, C.J. (1999) Nursing scholarship: role of faculty practice. *Clinical Excellence for Nurse Practitioners* 3 (1) 28–33   6 References

As nursing education has moved into the academic setting, nursing faculty has focused on the traditional components of scholarship in the faculty role: research and publication, teaching and service. Many changes in higher education and health care

have necessitated a re-examination of this position. Principal findings of a study showed that nursing deans and faculty view scholarship as the generation, dissemination, application and advancement of nursing knowledge. The strongest theme to emerge was the role conflict and fragmentation as they tried to balance all the components of scholarship. Faculty practice was considered to be an important issue in nursing but many nurses were working in environments where it is not accommodated, mandated or formally expected. Other findings suggested that faculty practice roles could be considered a component as long as scholarly outcomes are demonstrated.

3.16.29   Vesilind, P.A. (1999) *So you want to be a professor? A handbook for graduate students.* Thousand Oaks, CA: Sage   ISBN 0761918973 References

Book begins with a discussion of jobs in academia and how to find them. Chapters cover a wide range of political skills for future academic success, including lecturing, organizing a course, meeting your first class, testing, maintaining a research programme, and writing for publication.

3.16.30   Wilson-Barnett, J. (2001) Research capacity in nursing. *International Journal of Nursing Studies* 38 (3) June 241–2   Editorial

Editorial examines the research capacity in nursing from a British perspective.

Research Education

3.17 RESEARCH EDUCATION

Most nurses now have a research component/module as part of their studies that will enable them to appreciate the importance of the subject in underpinning all practice. The level of study will differ but all nurses need to have the skills of reading research papers and the ability to make judgements about its application to their own practice.

Annotations

3.17.1 Alves, D.B. & Santos, L.A. (1998) The truth about research on DEN/UFS (Portuguese). *Revista Brasileira de Enfermagem* 51 (4) 561–70 9 References

Examines professors' conceptions about groups, areas and research projects, scientific production, difficulties and possibilities related to research activity, strategies being used for the development of research and how students are being initiated into the 'scientific' world.

3.17.2 Attia, J. & Page, J. (2001) A graphic framework for teaching critical appraisal of randomized controlled trials. *ACP Journal Club* 134 (3) A11–12 3 References

Describes a five-step framework that can be used to teach critical appraisal of randomized controlled trials using flow diagrams to aid understanding (CR 2.29).

3.17.3 Ax, S. & Kincade, E. (2001) Nursing students' perceptions of research: usefulness, implementation and training. *Journal of Advanced Nursing* 35 (2) 161–70 40 References

Study explored students' perceptions of the usefulness of research for nursing practice, beliefs about difficulties in implementing research on the wards and their satisfaction with the research training received. Several students in one institution disagreed with their training, and authors suggest that educational and organizational improvements need to be introduced to transform nursing into a research-active profession (CR 2.3, 2.102).

3.17.4 Barrett, E. & Lally, V. (2000) Meeting new challenges in educational research training: the signposts for educational research CDROM. *British Educational Research Journal* 26 (2) 271–90 25 References

Article describes the development and evaluation of an interactive multimedia resource. It is designed to be used by postgraduate students on a wide range of courses, especially those on part-time and distance learning programmes. The impact of this type of resource is discussed. Also included are whether research students can become 'critical' in a multimedia environment, and some methodological difficulties in evaluating its use in supporting learning.

3.17.5 Benson, A. & Blackman, D. (2003) Can research methods ever be interesting? *Active Learning in Higher Education* 4 (1) 29–55 41 References

Describes the creation of an activity-based research methods module that was developed in response to poor student evaluations, which led to an improvement in engagement and understanding from students.

3.17.6 Boswell, C. & Sevcik, L. (2002) Start a clinical research project (invest in yourself). *Nursing Forum* 37 (1) 30–3 2 References

Suggests that associating with a seasoned researcher is a useful way of developing research skills. Points out the potential pitfalls of doing research, but argues that it is a challenge that nurses should undertake (CR 3.19).

3.17.7 Brock, A. & Butts, J.B. (1998) On target: a model to teach baccalaureate nursing students to apply critical thinking. *Nursing Forum* 33 (3) July–September 5–10 10 References

Article presents an education model that faculty members can use to teach nursing students to think critically and incorporate research findings into clinical practice. The model offers a four-semester plan that can be integrated into programmes of study (CR 2.102).

3.17.8 Centre for Policy in Nursing Research (1998) *Nursing research and the higher education context: a second working paper.* London: Centre for Policy in Nursing Research No ISBN References.

Paper provides various contexts for understanding the dilemmas faced by nurses involved in higher education. The political context of higher education policy and issues facing medical education in the UK are discussed, together with a brief history of nurse education, UK events in an international context and the performance of nursing in the last two Research Assessment Exercises. The findings of a study examining the foundations of nursing knowledge, the level of supervision in a study of PhDs and current academic activity of the UK's university nursing departments, together with their views and experiences, are all reported. Points for consideration by heads of university departments, National Health Service (NHS) research commissioners, managers, education commissioners and the NHS Executive of the Department of Health are given (CR 2.6, 3.9, 3.11, 3.18).

3.17.9 Cheek, J. (2002) Advancing what? Qualitative research, scholarship, and the research imperative. *Qualitative Health Research* 12 (8) 1130–40   20 References

Analyses the notion of scholarship and explores the role it plays in shaping and advancing scholarship (CR 2.36).

3.17.10 Cobb, A.K. & Hoffart, N. (1999) Teaching qualitative research through participatory coursework and mentorship. *Journal of Professional Nursing* 15 (6) 331–9   38 References

Authors discuss the challenge of adequately preparing new qualitative researchers while there is a lack of faculty expertise and mentorship, student unfamiliarity with qualitative research when entering the doctoral programme, and uncertainty of appropriate teaching methods. The methods used to address these issues are discussed, including a two-course qualitative research sequence. This provided evidence of the suitability of this approach and the ideas could serve as the basis for others teaching qualitative research (CR 2.36, 3.18).

3.17.11 Connolly, B.H., Lupinnaci, N.S. & Bush, A.J. (2001) Changes in attitudes and perceptions in physical therapy among professional physical therapy students and new graduates. *Physical Therapy* 81 (5) 1127–34   31 References

A longitudinal study was conducted with physical therapy students prior to a research methods course, immediately after completion of the course and after a year of practice. The aim was to ascertain their perception of knowledge with respect to research, which sources should be used (evidence-based practice or traditional protocols) for clinical decision-making, and what should be used in a clinical setting for patient management (CR 2.52, 3.7).

3.17.12 Cooke, A. & Green, B. (2000) Developing the research capacity of departments of nursing and midwifery based in higher education: a review of the literature. *Journal of Advanced Nursing* 32 (1) 57–65   47 References

Reviews the literature to identify factors that might affect the research capacity of nursing and midwifery departments. Concludes that there is no formula for success because of the complexity of the situation but there is much advice that can be drawn upon in developing research capacity (CR 2.12).

3.17.13 Crookes, P.A. & Bradshaw, P.L. (2002) Developing scholarship in nursing – steps within a strategy. *Journal of Nursing Management* 10 (3) 177–81   9 References

Explores the differences between the institutional policies in the UK and Australia concerning the generation of scholarship and makes suggestions about research capacity and capacity-building in nursing. Discusses how educational managers can promote nursing scholarship and identifies roles and responsibilities that might be taken by individuals to develop their activity (CR 3.16).

3.17.14 Daley, B.J., Shaw, C.R., Balistrieri, T., Glasenapp, K. & Piacentine, L. (1999) Concept maps: a strategy to teach and evaluate critical thinking. *Journal of Nursing Education* 38 (1) 42–7   11 References

Authors describe a study that implemented concept maps as a methodology to teach and evaluate critical thinking.

3.17.15 Desaulles, C. (1998) Learning by doing research: nurse teachers and practising nurses study the communication about patient's pain in the wards. In: *Knowledge development: clinicians and researchers in partnership*. Helsinki: The Finnish Federation of Nurses ISSN 0251–4753 Proceedings of the workgroup of European Nurse Researchers (9th Biennial Conference 5–8 July 1998 Helsinki, Finland) Volume 1 205–16

Reports a study that describes how nurses from a school of nursing and clinical areas co-operated to develop research skills. The implications for researchers, teachers and care in the clinical area are all discussed.

3.17.16 Dobratz, M.C. (2003) Putting the pieces together: teaching undergraduates research from a theoretical perspective. *Journal of Advanced Nursing* 41 (4) 383–92   61 References

Paper evaluates teaching and learning outcomes of an undergraduate research course designed around a conceptual or theoretical approach (CR 2.7).

3.17.17 Duggelby, W. (1998) Improving undergraduate nursing research education: the effectiveness of collecting and analyzing oral histories. *Journal of Nursing Education* 37 (6) 247–52   19 References

Trained senior nursing students in their nursing research class collected nine oral histories from retired RNs. Both subjects and the control group completed a pre-test and post-test Attitudes Towards Nursing Research Questionnaire. The former had significantly positive changes in their attitudes towards nursing research after collecting and analysing oral history data. The author concluded that this was an effective experiential learning strategy (CR 2.30, 2.47, 2.61, 2.75).

3.17.18 Fazzone, P.A. (2001) An experiential method for teaching research to graduate nursing students. *Journal of Nursing Education* 40 (4) 174–9   16 References

Article describes a creative and interactive method that embraces both naturalistic and positivistic approaches to research. It consists of five elements: creating a non-threatening environment, using guided imagery, teaching research along the 'Continuum of Inquiry', take-home and mid-term exams based on hypothetical clinical situations and developing a research proposal (CR 2.96).

3.17.19 Fonseca, T. & King, M. (2000) Incorporating the Internet into traditional library instruction. *Computers in Libraries* 20 (2) 38–42   5 References

Authors describe a blueprint for effectively teaching Internet research methods to librarians and users (CR 2.85).

3.17.20 Gassner, L., Wotton, K., Clare, J., Hofmeyer, A. & Buckman, J. (1999) Theory meets practice. *Collegian: Journal of the Royal College of Nursing, Australia* 6 (3) 14–21, 28   29 References

The difficulty nursing students experience in making the transition from the university to the clinical context is attributed to the gap between theory and practice, and education and service. Collaboration between academics and clinicians in the provision of undergraduate education is considered to be a strategy for overcoming these problems. A collaborative model was developed and evaluated by illuminative research methods. Findings showed that the model was effective in facilitating relationships necessary for the successful development and implementation of reality-based learning for students (CR 2.11, 2.15, 3.8).

3.17.21 Heinrich, K.T. (2001) Doctoral women as passionate scholars: an exploratory inquiry of passionate dissertation scholarship. *Advances in Nursing Science* 23 (3) 88–103   23 References

Although doctoral students who are passionate about their dissertation research, and are more likely to make innovative contributions to nursing knowledge, little is written about such scholarship in the literature. This article describes an exploratory inquiry involving two focus groups of self-described passionate dissertation scholars. Underlining the passion, participants called passionate scholarship exciting and risky, personally meaningful and socially relevant life's work (CR 2.6, 2.69).

3.17.22 Heylings, D.J.A. & Tariq, V.N. (2001) Reflection and feedback on learning: a strategy for undergraduate research project work. *Assessment and Evaluation in Higher Education* 26 (2) 153–64   13 References

Paper describes how students and staff worked collaboratively to develop a structured scheme for use with undergraduate research project work.

3.17.23 Hitchcock, B.W. & Murphy, E. (1999) A triad of research roles: experiential learning in an undergraduate research course. *Journal of Nursing Education* 38 (3) 120–7   34 References

This article describes an innovative approach to teaching undergraduate research content involving students in a faculty research study, and a student project undertaken in a nursing research course. Junior-level students participated as subjects, data collectors and consumers of the research by analysing the findings and their clinical relevance. Positive results of the experience are reported (CR 3.16).

3.17.24 Holloway, I. & Walker, J. (1999) *Getting a PhD in health and social care*. Oxford: Blackwell Science.   ISBN 0632050578   References

Written by two academics in the field of health care, this book offers practical advice on preparation, progress and procedures when undertaking advanced studies. It takes students through the necessary stages of a research degree, assists in forward planning and pre-empting potential pitfalls along the way.

3.17.25 Julliard, K.N., Gujral, J.K., Hamil, S.W., Oswald, E., Smyk, A. & Testa, N. (2000) Art-based evaluation in research education. *Art Therapy: Journal of the American Art Therapy Association* 17 (2) 118–24   8 References

Reports on a study that used art to evaluate an all-day seminar for graduate students on research methods. The authors explored students' feelings about research concepts, and hoped to foster understanding of these concepts in a holistic and relevant way.

3.17.26   Kenty, J.R. (2001) Weaving undergraduate research into practice-based experiences. *Nurse Educator* 26 (4) 182–6   10 References

Because most nursing education programmes fail to link research to practice-based courses, thus contributing to the research/practice gap, the Collaborative Learning project was designed and implemented. The learning activities that linked research to practice-based experiences in an adult health course, and the outcomes of the strategy, are discussed (CR 3.8).

3.17.27   Lau, F. & Hayward, R. (2000) Building a virtual network in a community health research training program. *Journal of the American Medical Informatics Association* 7 (4) 361–77   60 References

Describe the processes, experiences, lessons and implications of building a virtual network as part of a two-year community heath research training programme in a Canadian province. Ten key lessons from this work are discussed and the authors believe that virtual networks can be used as the basis for future research and as a practical guide for managers (CR 2.85).

3.17.28   Leasure, A.R., Davis, L. & Thievon, S.L. (2000) Comparison of student outcomes and preferences in a traditional vs. world wide web-based baccalaureate nursing research course. *Journal of Nursing Education* 39 (4) 149–54   8 References

Reports on the student outcomes when comparing traditional vs web-based learning about nursing research. There was no significant difference in examination scores or course grades. The web-based course provided opportunities for methods of communication that are not traditionally nurtured in classroom settings, students gained confidence in using computers, and their writing skills improved (CR 2.85).

3.17.29   Lehna, C. & Pfoutz, S. (1999) Teaching nursing research: integrating quantitative and qualitative methods. *Nurse Educator* 24 (6) 24–7   9 References

The authors, each an expert in either quantitative or qualitative methods, describe how they designed and co-taught a course in research methods for graduate nursing students (CR 2.9).

3.17.30   Leonard, D. (2001) *A woman's guide to doctoral studies*. Buckingham: Open University Press   ISBN 0335202527   References

Book aims to help women undertake and enjoy serious scholarly work while recognizing the wider 'rules' of the academic game. The situation in the UK is compared with that of North America and Australia, and the pros and cons of PhDs and the new professional doctorates are discussed. Practical questions are addressed, for example: where to study; finding the right supervisor; finding time, money and space; getting off to a good start; how to access work on gender; keeping going; completion, the viva and life after the doctorate.

3.17.31   Lucas, B. & Lidstone, G. (2000) Ethical issues in teaching about research ethics. *Evaluation and Research in Education* 14 (1) 53–64   References

Authors relate their experience of teaching this subject using a simulation programme. Students' reactions to the use of simulation at emotional and intellectual levels are described and discussed (CR 2.17, 2.51).

3.17.32   Morrison-Beedy, D. & Cote-Arsenault, D. (2000) The Cookie Experiment revisited: broadened dimensions for teaching nursing research. *Nurse Educator* 25 (6) 294–6   5 References

The Cookie Experiment, a unique teaching strategy developed more than a decade ago by Thiel, has been refined and expanded to include hands-on quantitative and qualitative components while also serving as a way to lessen students' phobias about research. The authors present this strategy and discuss its applicability to undergraduate and graduate courses.

3.17.33   Mulhall, A., Le May, A. & Alexander, C. (2000) Research-based nursing practice – an evaluation of an educational programme. *Nurse Education Today* 20 (6) 435–43   20 References

Paper describes a series of nine workshops on research utilization undertaken in England. Their purpose was to help nurses, midwives and health visitors to critically appraise research and implement research in their workplace. Results are reported and the implications are discussed (CR 2.101, 2.102).

3.17.34   Northway, R., Davies, P., Lado, A. & Williams, R. (2001) Involving pre-registration nursing students in a research project. *Nurse Researcher: The International Journal of Research Methodology in Nursing and Health Care* 8 (4) 53–64   12 References

Authors describe how they invited students to be involved as data collectors in a research project planned and managed by lecturers. The various processes involved are discussed, as this approach has not been widely written about (CR 2.17, 3.16, 3.18).

3.17.35   Papadopoulos, I. & Lees, S. (2002) Developing culturally competent researchers. *Journal of Advanced Nursing* 37 (3) 258–64   18 References

Paper discusses the need for the development of culturally competent health researchers in all areas of research and proposes a model to achieve this aspiration.

3.17.36 Pelayo-Alvarez, M., Albert-Ros, X., Gil-latorre, G. & Gutierrez-Sigler, D. (2000) Feasibility analysis of a personalized training plan for learning research methodology. *Medical Education* 34 (2) 139–45   15 References

Reports a study that determined performance in learning research methodology by means of the Keller Plan, to assess its impact on attitudes towards research and to estimate its acceptability. Third-year family residents took part and results showed that those using the Keller Plan obtained better knowledge, were motivated in studying and it was positively accepted as a method of learning (CR 3.7).

3.17.37 Petracchi, H.E. & Patchner, M.E. (2001) A comparison of live instruction and interactive televised teaching: a 2-year assessment of teaching an MSW research methods course. *Research on Social Work Practice* 11 (1) 108–17   22 References

Reports a study that evaluated the performance and experiences of distance learning students enrolled in a graduate-level foundation social work research methods course. Results showed that interactive television appeared to be a viable option when compared with face-to-face teaching.

3.17.38 Porter, E.J. (2001) Teaching undergraduate nursing research: a narrative view of evaluation studies and a typology for further research. *Journal of Nursing Education* 40 (2) 53–62   45 References

A narrative review using Cook and Campbell's validity framework for experimental and quasi-experimental studies was done to appraise the validity of eight studies in which teaching strategies for undergraduate research had been evaluated. The research reports emphasized the teaching strategy's 'contextual validity' rather than their internal of external validity. A typology consisting of four categories of evaluation studies that vary according to purpose, methodological assumptions, types of validity emphasized and student sample size was proposed. These categories, minimally represented in current literature, are complementary approaches for further evaluation studies (CR 2.25, 2.35).

3.17.39 Royse, D. (2000) Teaching research online: a process evaluation. *Journal of Teaching in Social Work* 20 (1/2) 145–58   21 References

Article reports on a research methods course taught over the Internet to an off-campus social work programme in 1997. The pilot test of the computer-based instruction is evaluated with both quantitative and qualitative data. Results showed that students learned as much research content as those in traditional classes, although there was no decrease in their anxieties over statistics (CR 2.23, 2.85).

3.17.40 Sigmon, H.D. & Grady, P.A. (2001) Increasing nursing post-doctoral opportunities: National Institute of Nursing Research spring science work group. *Nursing Outlook* 49 (4) July–August 179–81

Reports a meeting that considered ways to increase post-doctoral opportunities for nurse researchers. The present gaps and strengths were identified and strategies and collaborative approaches for the future were suggested. The group believed that nurse scientists have critical roles to play in basic laboratory studies, translational research, clinical investigations, care delivery and outcome evaluations (CR 2.15, 3.10).

3.17.41 Steele, L.L. (2001) Incorporating research application into nurse practitioner education. *The Online Journal of Knowledge Synthesis for Nursing* Document Number 3E September 10   5 References www.stti.iupui.edu/Virginia Hendersonlibrary/PDFs/ ec_doc3e.pdf (Accessed 16/11/03).

Outlines the problem of teaching research utilization and presents a strategy designed to enhance nurse practitioners' application of research findings (CR 2.95, 2.102).

3.17.42 Tooley, J. & Darby, D. (1998) *Educational research, a critique: a survey of published educational research*. London: Office for Standards in Education   No ISBN

Research set out to examine a small sample of educational research studies. This was to ascertain whether criticisms made by Professor David Hargreaves that educational research is poor value for money, remote from educational practice and often of indifferent quality were justified. Its conclusions are disturbing, in particular in terms of the general health of the academic educational research community and its potential influence in the training and education of future teachers.

3.17.43 Traynor, M. (1998) Survey looks at problems in university nursing research. *Nursing Times* 94 (29) 22–28 July   66–7   2 References

Author reports the findings of a survey that examined the contradictory pressures experienced by nurse teachers, and the effects this has on research (CR 2.52).

3.17.44 Tsai, S.-I. (2003) The effects of a research utilization in-service program on nurses.

International Journal of Nursing Studies 40 (2) February 105–13   26 References

This quasi-experimental study evaluated an eight-week course of research utilization training for nurses. Research instruments used included a scale of attitudes towards research, a scale of perceived support for research, a research participation and research utilization questionnaires (CR 2.35).

3.17.45   University of Rochester, School of Nursing *Medical Center cybercourse: nursing research NUR 301* www.urmc.rochester.edu/son/academics/nur301 (Accessed 07/03/03)

This undergraduate research course is now offered in traditional and distance learning formats. Students will acquire a familiarity with the process of scientific inquiry and the application of qualitative and quantitative research to the development of nursing knowledge. In addition, skills developed will be information retrieval, a knowledge of statistics (this is a pre- or co-requisite of the course), and the ability to undertake critical reviews of evidence-based literature.

3.17.46   Wilkes, L., Cooper, K., Lewin, J. & Batts, J. (1999) Concept mapping: promoting science learning in BN learners in Australia. *Journal of Continuing Education in Nursing* 30 (1) 37–44 17 References

The authors used concept mapping as a methodology to teach science to two classes of students. Positive outcomes are reported, and issues arising out of the process related to how to balance science content and the techniques of concept mapping, and how to assess the students' learning outcomes. The technique can link science and nursing practice, be used in the clinical area to teach patients, and in staff development programmes (CR 2.86).

3.17.47   Wood, M.J. (2002) The post-doctoral fellowship. *Clinical Nursing Research* 11 (2) 123–5 Editorial

Discusses aspects of post-doctoral fellowships and the reasons why some fail to make research part of their life's work.

3.18   RESEARCH SUPERVISION AND MENTORSHIP

Providing students with appropriate and constructive supervision demands different skills from those of doing research. Teachers themselves may therefore need guidance and, in addition to studying for research degrees and doctorates, institutions may offer short courses or the opportunity to learn from each other.

Definition [See Appendix D for source]

Research supervisor – ... an experienced researcher or academic trainer who advises students or employees in independent research

Annotations

3.18.1   Crofts, L. (1999) Research in the raw: research supervision in a busy trust. *Nurse Researcher* 6 (4) 29–39   6 References

Author describes her role as Director of Nursing Research and Development in a London NHS Trust. The realities and problems of conducting and overseeing research projects in clinical areas are discussed. The practice of allowing undergraduates to do research in clinical areas is questioned because of the demands made on patients and staff. Most projects are small-scale and are not likely to generate new knowledge, so many universities are moving towards replacing the traditional dissertation with an extended literature critique (CR 2.16, 3.16, 3.17).

3.18.2   Delamont, S., Atkinson, P. & Parry, O. (1997) *Supervising the PhD: a guide to success.* Buckingham: Open   University   Press   ISBN 0335195164   References

Provides 'everything you wanted to know about PhD supervision but were afraid to ask'. Book is written to assist both novice and experienced supervisors.

3.18.3   Fletcher, C. (2002) Supervising activists for research degrees: responsibilities, rights and freedoms. *Active Learning in Higher Education* 3 (1) 88–103   30 References

Discusses the role of supervisors of students undertaking research degrees who are attempting to achieve change in work or social roles. Presents some ideas developed from experience of supervising doctoral candidates.

3.18.4   Gillibrand, W.P., Burton, C. & Watkins, G.G. (2002) Clinical networks for nursing research. *International Nursing Review* 49 (3) 188–93   20 References

Details an initiative to support programmatic research in nursing practice through clinical networks for nursing research. Gives examples of how this has resulted in a number of evaluative studies.

3.18.5   Hawkins, P. & Shohet, R. (2000) *Supervision in the helping professions* (2nd edition).

Buckingham: Open University Press ISBN 0335201172   References

Book offers a comprehensive and practical guide to the complex issues inherent in the supervision of health and social services personnel. It explores the purposes, models and different forms of supervision in many disciplines, including nursing.

3.18.6   Jack, B. (1999) Staying the course: the supervisee's personal experience of the supervision relationship. *Nurse Researcher* 6 (4) 19–27   5 References

Paper focuses on the author's experiences when undertaking a part-time PhD. The responsibilities of supervisor and student are outlined, together with how to get started and keeping going through the inevitable 'ups and downs' of the process.

3.18.7   Jones, A. (1999) Significant relationships: planning for effective research supervision. *Nurse Researcher* 6 (4) 5–17   1 References

Paper explores the relationship between supervisor and supervisee and guidelines are offered to encourage professional, ethical and academically suitable exchanges. Both parties will gain if personal compatibility and carefully structured supervision relationships are established.

3.18.8   Katz, E. & Coleman, M. (2001) Induction and mentoring of beginning researchers at academic colleges of education in Israel. *Mentoring and Tutoring* 9 (3) 223–9   36 References

Describes an initiative to introduce a mentoring system for teachers, including the rationale and benefits to professional development (CR 3.16).

3.18.9   Marrow, C. (1998/99) Keeping above the surface in an action research study. *Nurse Researcher* 6 (2) 57–70   28 References

Author describes some experiences of leading and participating in an action research project. The main issues considered include the importance of facilitating the preparation and development of those involved, and collaborating with them on all aspects of the research process. Critical reflections on the part of the supervisor about the whole process are also included (CR 2.16, 2.67, 2.69, 2.77).

3.18.10   Medoff-Cooper, B. & Dekeyser, F. (1998) Developing a research mentoring partnership in Israel. *Journal of Obstetric, Gynaecological and Neonatal Nursing* 27 (2) 197–202   5 References

Describes a relationship developed between two universities that began with a student exchange and mentoring programme. Explains that the goal of the

partnership is to develop research expertise and capacity.

3.18.11   Smith, D. (2001) Learning through supervising. In Byrne-Armstrong, H., Higgs, J. & Horsfall, D. (eds) *Critical moments in qualitative research*. Oxford: Butterworth-Heinemann   ISBN 0750651598   Chapter 10 128–35

Giving a personal view, the author discusses the nature of supervision, the importance of research candidature experiences and their learning in the spiral of supervision (CR 2.36.17).

3.18.12   Styles, I. & Radloff, A. (2001) The synergistic thesis: student and supervisor perspectives. *Journal of Further and Higher Education* 25 (1) 97–106   20 References

Provides a model incorporating motivation, beliefs, management strategies and preferences which the author conceptualizes as a framework for supervisors and students in the production of a successful thesis.

3.19   STUDENT GUIDES TO RESEARCH

Books in this section will guide students through the various stages of doing and writing about research.

Annotations

3.19.1   Allan, G. & Skinner, C. (eds) (1991) *Handbook for research students in the social sciences*. London: Falmer Press   ISBN 1850009368   References

Discusses the nature of research degrees, study skills, management of research and research strategies in the social sciences (CR 3.17).

3.19.2   Allison, B. (1997) *The students' guide to preparing dissertations and theses*. London: Kogan Page   ISBN 0749421932   References

Book is a detailed guide to all aspects of preparing dissertations and theses and covers contents, presentation and style.

3.19.3   Barnes, R. (1996) *Successful study for degrees* (2nd edition). London: Routledge   ISBN 0415127416   References

Book gives advice on many elements required for undergraduate and postgraduate study. Sections cover study skills, developing higher order questioning, reading academic texts, essays, seminars, dissertations, reliability, validity and meaning (CR 2.24, 2.25).

3.19.4 Bell, J. (1999) *Doing your research project: a guide for first-time researchers in education and social science* (3rd edition). Buckingham: Open University Press ISBN 0335203884 References

Book is a source of reference and a guide to good practice for all novice researchers. This edition reflects advances in technology and methodology and includes new material on narrative inquiry, supervision, intellectual property, ethics, finding and searching information sources and the production of literature reviews (CR 2.12, 2.17, 2.78, 3.18).

3.19.5 Berry, R. (1994) *The research project: how to write it* (3rd edition). London: Routledge ISBN 0415110904 References

This guide is for novices and those who are more experienced. Topics include choosing a subject, using the library, taking notes, shaping and developing the project (CR 1.1).

3.19.6 Clough, P. & Nutbrown, C. (2002) *A student's guide to methodology: justifying enquiry.* London: Sage ISBN 0761974229 References

Authors present a perspective on methodology as a process which begins from the moment curiosity about a topic is aroused. Although in dissertations and theses methodology is usually reported within a single chapter, the authors show how every element of the account – from the framing of research questions to the drawing of conclusions – is a function of methodology.

3.19.7 Cryer, P. (2000) The *research student's guide to success* (2nd edition). Buckingham: Open University Press ISBN 0335206867 References

Author provides a practical guide to all elements surrounding research at postgraduate level, particularly the needs of the growing number of part-time students taking research for higher studies. New chapters are included on options for postgraduate study, research, skills development and employment issues.

3.19.8 Fairbairn, G.J. & Fairbairn, S. (2001) *Reading at university: a guide for students.* Buckingham: Open University Press ISBN 033520385X References

Book urges students to think about reading and about themselves as readers. Advice is given about all aspects of the subject to enable students become more efficient in this important aspect of university work.

3.19.9 Fitzpatrick, J., Secrist, J. & Wright, D.J. (1998) *Secrets for a successful dissertation.* Thousand Oaks, CA: Sage ISBN 0761912517 References

Authors take students through the process from the doctoral proposal to formal defence of their dissertation. Advice is also given on the emotional and mental stress caused by the process itself (CR 2.97).

3.19.10 Higgins, R. (1996) *Approaches to research: a handbook for those writing dissertations.* London: Jessica Kingsley ISBN 1853023078 References

Takes a step-by-step approach to what is involved in choosing, organizing and presenting a research project.

3.19.11 Howard, K. & Sharp, J.A. (1996) *The management of a student research project* (2nd edition). Aldershot: Gower ISBN 056607706X References

This practical guide is for students intending to write up and present for examination the results of research projects.

3.19.12 Johnson, M. & Burnard, P. (2002) The 'pear-shaped' doctoral thesis and how to avoid it! *Nurse Education Today* 22 (5) July 355–7 5 References Guest Editorial

Authors identify some of the problems associated with undertaking a PhD in the UK and discuss ways in which they can be minimized.

3.19.13 Madsen, D. (1992) *Successful dissertations and theses: a guide to graduate student research from proposal to completion* (2nd edition, reprint). San Francisco, CA: Jossey-Bass ISBN 0783725507 References

Book gives practical advice on all aspects of writing dissertations and theses. This includes starting and completing the work, working with one's advisors, selecting the topic, preparing the proposal, following research procedures, organizing and writing the work, defending it, adapting it for publication and using the library. Two sample proposals are included, one using a historical approach and the other an experimental approach (CR 2.96, 3.18).

3.19.14 Murray, L. & Lawrence, B. (2000) *Practitioner-based enquiry: principles for postgraduate research.* London: Falmer Press ISBN 0750707712 References

Book provides conceptual and methodological insights into small-scale, applied, educational research activity. It is more than an A-Z of how to do research, and gives useful background material to help advanced students.

3.19.15 Phillips, E.M. & Pugh, D.S. (2000) *How to get a PhD: a handbook for students and their supervisors* (3rd edition). Buckingham: Open University Press ISBN 033520550X References

This practical text provides a realistic understanding of the process of doing research for a doctoral degree. Its main aim is to help students understand and achieve the necessary skills, and assist supervisors in planning and executing appropriate research programmes. New material includes information technology, publishing and working towards a PhD in a practice discipline (CR 2.99, 3.18).

3.19.16　Piantanida, M. & Garman, N. (1999) *The qualitative dissertation: a guide for students and faculty*. Thousand Oaks, CA: Corwin Press ISBN 080396689X　References

Authors describe the entire processes involved in a qualitative dissertation. Helpful advice is given on the rough patches that may be encountered (CR 2.97).

3.19.17　Quaratiello, A.R. (2000) *The college student's research companion* (2nd edition). New York: Neal-Schuman　ISBN 0335202209　References

Book explains the fundamental principles of academic library research. Students are guided through the maze of resources available, and taken through all stages of the research process. The use of electronic sources comprises about half of the text.

3.19.18　Redman, P. (2001) *Good essay writing: a social sciences guide* (2nd edition). London: Sage/Open University ISBN 0761972056 References

Book provides answers to the key questions that need to be considered when preparing an essay. Examples of student essays are included.

3.19.19　RCN Research Society *PhD student network* www.man.ac.uk/rcn/rs.phd.htm (Accessed 01/05/03)

Aim of this student network is to provide a forum for nurses (and other health professionals) undertaking doctorates to network, discuss issues and support each other (CR 3.17, 3.18).

3.19.20　Rudestam, K.E. & Newton, R.R. (2000) *Surviving your dissertation: a comprehensive guide*

to content and process (2nd edition). Thousand Oaks, CA: Sage　ISBN 0761919627　References

Book is intended as a 'how to' guide for graduate students at all stages of their research. Described as a handbook, most elements relating to planning, completing and writing up projects are included.

3.19.21　Shwarz McCotter, S. (2001) The journey of a beginning researcher. *The Qualitative Report* (On-line serial) 6 (2) 103 paragraphs 42 References www.nova.edu/ssss/QR/QR6-2/mccotter.html (Accessed 16/11/03)

Outlines the obstacles in undertaking qualitative research and offers some personal solutions to novice researchers. Includes how to integrate theory with the data, how to deal with being a participant and researcher simultaneously and how to represent participants faithfully (CR 2.16).

3.19.22　Smith, R.V. (1990) *Graduate research: a guide for students in the sciences* (2nd edition). New York: Plenum Press　ISBN 0306434652 References

Students in a wide variety of disciplines can use this workbook for self-instruction. Chapters cover the whole process of undertaking research and include getting started, commitment, making choices, time management, ethics, developing library and writing skills, presenting papers, obtaining funds and getting a job.

3.19.23　Walliman, N.S.R. (2000) *Your research project: a step-by-step guide for the first-time researcher*. London: Sage　ISBN 0761965394 References

Book systematically explains the theory of and approaches to research while also helping the student/practitioner develop their topic and acquire the necessary research skills to complete a research project. It encourages the formation of critical analysis, rigour and independence of thought, and develops the crucial writing skills required in writing research proposals, reports and theses (CR 2.96).

Research Priorities

3.20 RESEARCH PRIORITIES

There have been many studies that aimed to establish priorities for nursing research in clinical practice. Governments, institutions, funding bodies and local personnel all contribute to this debate, and may control what is actually achieved, particularly through the allocation of funding.

Annotations

3.20.1 Aylott, M. (2000/2001) Research priorities: a Delphi survey. *Paediatrc Nursing* 12 (10) 16–20 51 References

Reports a three-round Delphi survey that aimed to establish nursing research priorities on children's intensive care units where extra-corporeal membrane oxygenation was used. Resulting themes identified were: labour intensity, consumerism, ethical issues and clinical issues. All of these have implications for planning and organizing a nursing research strategy within paediatric intensive care (CR 2.66).

3.20.2 Bakker, D.A. & Fitch, M.I. (1998) Oncology nursing research priorities: a Canadian perspective. *Cancer Nursing* 21 (6) 394–401 14 References

Reports a survey among oncology nurse researchers and nurses working in oncology clinical settings to establish their care priorities. The findings provided the basis for developing a Canadian national oncology nursing research agenda. In addition, the findings provide direction for practice and education strategic plans as well as information to guide decision-making around research funding.

3.20.3 Barrett, S., Kristjanson, L.J., Sinclair, T. & Hyde, S. (2001) Priorities for adult cancer nursing research: a west Australian replication. *Cancer Nursing* 24 (2) 88–98 22 References

Based on two previous surveys, undertaken in the USA and Canada to identify cancer nursing research priorities, this replication study aimed to see whether it was possible to establish possible changes in priorities and account for cultural difference in health care systems. Results are reported that the authors anticipate will stimulate discussion and a re-assessment of priorities in other settings (CR 2.13, 2.66).

3.20.4 Canada Research Chairs *Research priorities in Canadian universities* www.chairs.gc.ca/english/research/strategic/ (Accessed 07/02/03)

This website lists the Strategic Research Plan (SRP) summaries prepared by Canadian universities participating in the Canada Research Chairs programme. These provide an overview of the main research directions of each university.

3.20.5 Commonwealth of Australia, Department of Education, Science and Training *Promoting and maintaining good health* www.dest.gov.au/priorities/good_health.htm (Accessed 07/02/03)

Outlines the goals of this national research priority that aims to promote and maintain good health, and prevent disease particularly among younger and older Australians (CR 3.2).

3.20.6 Daniels, L. & Ascough, A. (1999) Developing a strategy for cancer nursing research: identifying priorities. *European Journal of Oncology Nursing* 3 (3) 161–9 31 References

Reports a collaborative study between a university and regional cancer centre that aimed to facilitate a strategic approach to cancer nursing research. The Delphi technique was used to identify the views of health care professionals regarding research priorities. Results provided a framework for the formulation of a strategy and enabled comparison of current priorities with those previously identified (CR 2.15, 2.66).

3.20.7 Fochtman, D. & Hinds, P.S. (2000) Identifying nursing research priorities in a pediatric clinical trials co-operative group: the pediatric oncology nursing experience. *Journal of Pediatric Oncology Nursing* 17 (2) April 83–7 15 References

Using a Delphi technique, 87 research ideas were generated by nurses from the Pediatric Oncology Group that were then reviewed by a panel of experts. The top ten nursing research priorities are listed (CR 2.66).

3.20.8   Hamrin, E., Eriksson, K., Akademi, A., Ehrenfeld, M., Mucha, K., Lorensen, M., Tierney, A. & Hinshaw, A.S. (1998) Priorities in nursing science beyond the year 2000 – which way Europe? In: *Knowledge development: clinicians and researchers in partnership.* Helsinki: The Finnish Federation of Nurses   ISSN 0251–4753 Proceedings of the Workgroup of European Nurse Researchers (9th Biennial Conference 5–8 July 1998 Helsinki, Finland) Volume 1   313–17   4 References

Paper discusses which areas in European health care should be considered as priorities for the future, whether research education for nurses today is adequate for those areas, and how European collaboration to develop more effective nursing research priorities can be achieved (CR 2.15).

3.20.9   Heartfield, M. (2000) Research directions for specialist practice. *Accident and Emergency Nursing* 8 (4) 214–22   38 References

Paper identifies the research priorities necessary to advance emergency nursing as a specialist area of nursing practice. Nurses working in nine Australian hospital emergency departments identified 44 core topics relevant to their knowledge base. Four highest-ranked priorities were education needs and opportunities, specialist roles of triage, trauma and practitioners' and nurses' coping mechanisms.

3.20.10   Hirschfield, M.J. (1998) WHO priorities for a common nursing research agenda. *International Nursing Review* 45 (1) January–February 13–14   2 References

In September 1997 a high-powered research team was brought to Geneva by the International Council of Nurses (ICN) to set priorities and recommend strategies for ICN leadership roles. Extracts from country and regional reviews of nursing research have been published, beginning with the WHO Nursing Unit analysis of research at nursing/midwifery collaborating centres, together with future foci for nursing research.

3.20.11   Im, E., Meleis, A.I. & Park, Y.S. (1999) A feminist critique of research on menopausal experience of Korean women. *Research in Nursing and Health* 22 (5) 410–20   74 References

Taking a feminist stance that the menopausal experience of Asian women does not come from pure biology but from their continuous interactions with their environment, the authors propose directions for future research on the menopause. A search of 158 studies showed that there were many methodological problems suggesting that interpretation, understanding and generalization of findings should be undertaken with caution (CR 2.10, 2.12, 2.28).

3.20.12   Ironside, P.M. (2001) Creating a research base for nursing education: an interpretive review of conventional, critical, feminist, postmodern and phenomenologic pedagogies. *Advances in Nursing Science* 23 (3) 72–87   50 References

The National League for Nursing Priorities for Nursing Education Research calls on educators to increase their pedagogic literacy to meet the challenges of the changing social, health care and educational worlds, and to develop research-based pedagogies for nursing. The elements that are necessary are described, and an example – narrative pedagogy – is discussed (CR 2.10, 2.49, 3.17).

3.20.13   Lewis, S.L., Cooper, C.L., Cooper, K.G., Bonner, P.N., Parker, K. & Frauman, A. (1999) Research priorities for nephrology nursing: American Nephrology Nurses' Association's Delphi study. *ANNA Journal* 26 (2) 215–25   24 References

Study identified and prioritized research topics of importance for nephrology. A three-round Delphi study was used and five main areas emerged as priorities (CR 2.66).

3.20.14   Maman, S., Campbell, J., Sweat, M.D. & Gielen, A.C. (2000) The intersections of HIV and violence: directions for future research and interventions. *Social Science & Medicine* 50 (4) 459–78 52 References

Paper reviews the available literature on the intersections between HIV and violence and presents an agenda for future research to guide policy and programmes (CR 3.11).

3.20.15   McGuire, D.B. & Ropka, M.E. (2000) Research and oncology nursing practice. *Seminars in Oncology Nursing* 16 (1) 35–46   64 References

Article traces the evolution of oncology nursing research and discusses its contribution to oncology nursing practice. Placing research in perspective will help to show where the speciality should go and suggest directions for research priorities and for conceptual, methodologic and health policy activities (CR 3.6).

3.20.16   National Institutes of Health *Setting research priorities at the National Institutes of Health* www.nih.gov/about/researchpriorities.htm (Accessed 22/01/03)

This website gives an overview of the National Institutes of Health (NIH); how science works; the NIH's history; how the NIH funds medical research; assessing health needs and scientific opportunities; the Institutes and the role of the NIH Director. An appendix lists the Institutes and Centres of the National Institutes of Health.

3.20.17 Nieswiadomy, R.M. (2002) Research priorities for the future. In Author *Foundations of nursing research* (4th edition). Upper Saddle River, NJ: Prentice-Hall ISBN 0130339911 Chapter 1 17–18 53 References

Author documents the organizations, societies and authors who have identified research priorities in their respective fields since 1980 (CR 2.1.55).

3.20.18 Oliver, S. (1999) Users of health services: following their agenda. In Hood, S., Mayall, B. & Oliver, S. (eds) *Critical issues in social research: power and prejudice*. Buckingham: Open University Press ISBN 0335201407 Chapter 10 139–53 42 References

Author explores how health services could be reshaped if they were to draw on the insights of service users, and could thereby respond to their circumstances and priorities. Involving service users as equals to plan and conduct research is revolutionary, but it will only reach its potential when lay people take leading roles in such partnerships and in their evaluation.

3.20.19 Pullen, L., Tuck, I. & Wallace, D.C. (1999) Research priorities in mental health nursing. *Issues in Mental Health Nursing* 20 (3) 217–27 27 References

Study determined research priorities that focused on mental health nursing in the published literature from 1990 to 1996. Experts, organizations and individual research projects were also consulted and examined. Six categories emerged from a content analysis: support, holism, mental health nursing practice, quality care outcomes, mental health aetiology and mental health delivery systems. Identifying these elements will assist in knowledge development (CR 2.12, 2.88, 3.13).

3.20.20 Rosenfeld, P., Duthie, E., Bier, J., Bowar-Ferres, S., Fulmer, T., Iervolino, L., McClure, M.L., McGivern, D.O. & Roncoli. M. (2000) Engaging staff nurses in evidence-based research to identify nursing practice problems and solutions. *Applied Nursing Research* 13 (4) November 197–203 15 References

Article describes how one academic health science centre engaged its nursing staff in devising an action plan for change. A second objective was to design a survey instrument that would be easy to complete and distribute, collect and analyse. This enabled specific action plans to be developed around the identified problems. The process promoted interest in advancing nursing research and evidence-based practice among the clinicians and administrators (CR 2.52, 2.69, 3.17).

3.20.21 Royal College of Nursing *Priorities for R&D in nursing* www.man.ac.uk/rcn/policy/ index. htm (Accessed 28/02/03)

Website brings together work from the UK that focuses on the identification of priorities in nursing. The background, priorities and the R&D infrastructure and capacity, and capacity-building are outlined and links are given.

3.20.22 Rudy, S.F., Wilkinson, M.A., Dropkin, M.J. & Stevens, G. (1998) Otorhinolaryngology nursing research priorities: results of the 1996/1997 SOHN Delphi survey. *ORL–Head & Neck Nursing* 16 (1) Winter 14–20 14 References

This study aimed to establish research priorities for the specialty of otorhinolaryngology (ORL). The Delphi technique was utilized and nurses experienced in ORL care took part. The top five research priorities were: care of neck stomas and related equipment; quality of life in head and neck cancer patients; impact of managed care on ORL nursing delivery; value of ORL specialty/nursing units; and effective techniques to promote cessation of substance abuse in adolescents (CR 2.36, 2.66).

3.20.23 Rustoen, T. & Schjolberg, T. (2000) Cancer nursing research priorities: a Norwegian perspective. *Cancer Nursing* 23 (5) 375–81 23 References

Study aimed to determine research priorities among Norwegian nurses and to investigate implications these may have for future planning. Differences between cancer nurse specialists and other nurses working in this field were also evaluated. Results are reported and possible topics for future research were identified.

3.20.24 Scott, E., McMahon, A., Kitson, A. & Rafferty, A.M. (1999) A national initiative to set priorities for research and development in nursing, midwifery and health visiting: investigating the method. *NT Research* 4 (4) 283–90 8 References

Paper provides a progress report of the first phase of the national initiative established to identify priorities for R&D for the nursing professions. The methods used and the primary and secondary results achieved are described, and an outline is given of how it is proposed to more the initiative forward.

3.20.25 Soanes, L., Gibson, F., Bayliss, J. & Hannan, J. (2000) Establishing nursing research priorities on a paediatric haematology, oncology, immunology and infectious diseases unit: a Delphi survey. *European Journal of Oncology Nursing* 4 (2) 108–17 42 References

Authors reports a Delphi survey, conducted by the Nurses' Research Group, devised as a first step towards developing a strategy for evidence-based nursing. A detailed account is given of the method, procedures and outcomes of a Delphi survey.

Priorities, identified and owned by staff working on this unit, would be more likely to be implemented in practice if staff had been involved in the research (CR 2.66).

3.20.26 Sowell, R.L. (2000) Identifying HIV/AIDS research priorities for the next millennium: a Delphi study with nurses in AIDS care. *Journal of the Association of Nurses in AIDS Care* 11 (3) 42–52   42 References

Using the Delphi technique, nurses from the Association of Nurses in AIDS Care, initially identified more than 2,000 potential research topics. The overall priorities were: HIV community-led education and prevention; development of more tolerable drugs; prevention, focusing on individual or specific group behaviour; vaccine development and research related to an adherence to drug therapy (CR 2.66).

Research Reviews

3.21 RESEARCH REVIEWS

Books in this section give examples of research in practice, which aim to help nurses understand its value when caring for patients and clients.

Annotations

3.21.1 Alexander, J., Levy, V. & Roch, S. (eds) (1993) *Midwifery practice: a research-based approach*. Basingstoke: Macmillan ISBN 0333576179 References

Provides a broad-ranging survey and analysis of key research literature placed in the context of clinical practice.

3.21.2 Ford, P. & Walsh, M. (1994) *New rituals for old: nursing through the looking glass*. Oxford: Butterworth-Heinemann ISBN 0750615818 References

Some accepted concepts in nursing are subjected to rigorous scrutiny, and selected research findings are analysed to open them up to debate. Authors believe that critical questioning will enable a sound knowledge base to be developed. Areas covered are concepts of empowerment and delivery of care.

3.21.3 Macleod Clark, J. & Hockey, L. (1979) *Research for nursing: a guide for the enquiring nurse*. Aylesbury, Buckinghamshire: HM+M Publishers ISBN 085602077X References

Book is divided into four major sections: understanding research; studies relating to patient care; studies of nurses, nursing management and education; and research and the future.

3.21.4 Macleod Clark, J. & Hockey, L. (eds) (1989) *Further research for nursing*. London: Scutari ISBN 1871364140 References

A companion volume to *Research for Nursing: A Guide for the Enquiring Nurse*, this book aims to help nurses understand the value of research in their practice. A general introduction to research is given, together with its relevance to nursing and an overview of research processes. The remainder of the book contains overviews of research in 12 topic areas. Each is illustrated by a précis of one or two specific studies. Several chapters are devoted to studies about specific patient groups and others to more general nursing issues.

3.21.5 Rafferty, A.M. & Traynor, M. (eds) (2002) *Exemplary research for nursing and midwifery*. London: Routledge ISBN 0415241634 References

This book, which is organized under three headings–research classics, conceptualizing practice and clinical effectiveness – includes 19 classic and influential accounts of nursing research selected by a panel of senior nurse researchers and teachers. Each paper is accompanied by editorial commentary explaining the significance of the research in question, how it relates to the research tradition, its influences and impact.

3.21.6 Walsh, M. & Ford, P. (1990) *Nursing rituals, research and rational actions*. Oxford: Butterworth-Heinemann ISBN 0750600977 References

Book highlights key areas of nursing practice where research evidence is available but in many instances is not being used. Rituals of clinical practice and organization are explored and recommendations for good practice are given.

3.21.7 Wilson-Barnett, J. & Batehup, L. (1988) *Patient problems: a research base for nursing care*. London: Scutari Press ISBN 1871364108 References

Book reviews research relating to some of the major challenges in patient care: problems with adjustment to illness and recovery, depression, communication problems, pain and sleep disturbance. Authors' aim has been to describe research which assists in providing assessment tools to explore patients' responses to health problems and evaluate interventions aimed to solve them. The authors hope that similar books will be developed as the body of research knowledge increases (CR 2.12, 2.20, 2.55, 3.20).

3.21.8 Wilson-Barnett, J. & Clark, J.M. (eds) (1993) *Research in health promotion and nursing*. Basingstoke: Macmillan ISBN 0333601343 References

Book provides a research-based perspective on the vital relationship between health promotion and nursing practice. It focuses on ethical and theoretical issues, health promotion in practice, developing the nurses' health promotion role in healthy lifestyles, and future directions. The vital importance of empirical research and evaluation of practice is highlighted.

International Nursing Research

3.22 INTERNATIONAL NURSING RESEARCH

'Individual research projects that are disconnected and scattered around the world may not have the necessary impact. The collaboration of a community of researchers, organized to explore and answer a set of related questions and considered from different socio-political and cultural perspectives, could empower nurses to make a difference in the health and health care of those who need it most.' (Meleis, 1989: 139) [adapted]

Annotations

3.22.1 Costello, A. & Zumla, A. (2000) Moving to research partnerships in developing countries. *British Medical Journal* 321 (7264) 30 September 827–9   9 References

Article rejects the semi-colonial nature of research in developing countries, asserting that nationals should lead research projects partnered by technical support from outsiders. It is argued that such research needs monitoring by funding authorities, but is more likely to result in changes to national policy and practice (CR 3.1).

3.22.2 Fitzpatrick, J.J. (2002) International partnerships for research. *Applied Nursing Research Online* 15 (4) Editorial www2.appliednursingresearch.org/scripts/om.d11/serve?action=searchDB&searchD … (Accessed 07/02/03)

Author shares a set of guiding principles for international projects to facilitate their success.

3.22.3 Freda, M.C. (1998) International nursing and world health. *MCN: The American Journal of Maternal/Child Nursing* 23 (6) 329–32   References

Article describes some of the reasons why all nurses should become more knowledgeable about international health issues, the practice of nursing in other countries, international nursing research and nursing education in other countries.

3.22.4 Fry, M. & McAlpine, A. (1998) Bridging the gap: international nursing consultancy – the lived experience. *Australian Emergency Nursing Journal* 1 (5) 22–3

Describes the experience of being involved in two international nursing projects, highlighting the exciting nature of the work and the benefits it can generate. When undertaking this type of research particular factors need to be considered, including an understanding of the tendering process, clinical setting, cultural diversity and the resources available (CR 3.8).

3.22.5 Hakim, C. (2000) National comparative studies. In Author *Research designs: successful designs for social and economic research* (2nd edition). London: Routledge   ISBN 041522313X   Chapter 13 200–10

Chapter includes the logic of comparative analysis, organization of research work, funding and practical problems which may be encountered in cross-national studies (CR 2.21.4).

3.22.6 Hantrais, L. (1999) Contextualization in cross-national comparative research. *International Journal of Social Research Methodology: Theory and Practice* 2 (2) 93–108   References

Paper tracks the shift in cross-national comparisons in the social sciences away from universalistic culture-free approaches to culture-boundedness, which has placed the theory and practice of contextualization at the nexus of cross-national comparative studies. A number of recurring questions are addressed: the selection of appropriate contextual frames of reference, the impact of the researcher's own cultural traditions and issues of equivalence of concepts and interpretation.

3.22.7 Kitua, A.Y., Mashalla,Y.J.S. & Shija, J.K. (2000) Co-ordinating health research to promote action: the Tanzanian experience. *British Medical Journal* 321 (7264) 30 September 821–3   11 References

The failure of developing countries to co-ordinate their health research activities is discussed and Tanzanian efforts to overcome this by identifying research priorities and an ethical framework are explained (CR 3.20).

3.22.8 McConnell, E.A. (1998) International nursing. In Deloughery, G. (ed.) *Issues and trends in nursing* (3rd edition). St Louis: Mosby ISBN 0815126085   Chapter 14 368–89   48 References

Chapter discusses factors that affect international nursing and the impact of international trends in nursing education on primary health care. It compares the mission of some organizations and describes ways in which they can affect and influence nursing and health care worldwide. A plan for involvement and some activities are suggested.

3.22.9 Ogilivie, M. (2002) Ethical decision making in international nursing research. *Qualitative Nursing Research* 12 (6) 807–15   References

Author urges researchers in international settings to continually examine cross-cultural ethical issues to ensure that their work is sound. The process of ethical decision-making is discussed (CR 2.17, 2.53).

3.22.10 Sochalski, J., Aiken, L.H., Rafferty, A.M., Shamian, J., Müller-Mundt, G., Hunt, J., Giovannelli, P. & Clarke, H. (1998) Building multinational research. *Reflections* 24 (3) 20–3   13 References

Reports on the background to a multinational research project involving teams from the USA, Canada, England, Scotland and Germany. Its aim is to investigate how nurse staffing influences patient outcomes. Three sub-scales, derived from an instrument entitled 'The Nursing Work Index', measure nurse autonomy, control over practical resources and relations with physicians, all of which have been found to be significant predictors of both patient satisfaction, hospital mortality rates, and nurse outcomes such as stress and needle-stick injury rates. The researchers believe that the research will create a body of knowledge, encourage a new way of thinking about patient care and health services, and establish a cadre of international investigators.

3.22.11 Tan-Torres Edejer, T. (1999) North–south research partnerships: the ethics of carrying out research in developing countries. *British Medical Journal* 319 (7207) 14 August 438–41   35 References

Discusses the inequity in research funding and differing ethical standards of research in developing countries. Argues that the burdens and benefits of health research should be shared among north and south partners. Identifies the principles of research partnerships (CR 2.17).

References

References recorded here relate to books and articles consulted during the development of this book. Page numbers of quotations are included in the main text.

Agger, B. (1991) Critical theory, post-structuralism, post-modernism: their sociological relevance. *Annual Review of Sociology* 17

Apps, J. & Yeomans, M. (1995) Ethical issues in nursing research. In Henry, K. & Pashley, G. (eds) *Community ethics and health care research*. Dinton, Nr. Salisbury: Mark Allen

Bernard, J. (1973) My four revolutions: an autobiographical history of the American Sociological Association. *American Journal of Sociology* 78: 782

Breakwell, G.M., Hammond, S. & Fife-Schaw, C. (eds) (2000) *Research methods in psychology* (2nd edition). London: Sage

Brown, S.R. (1996) Q methodology and qualitative research. *Qualitative Health Research* 6 (4)

Burns, N. & Grove, S.K. (1997) *The practice of nursing research: conduct, critique and utilization*. Philadelphia, PA: W.B. Saunders

Centre for Advanced Research in Phenomenology www.phenomenologycenter.org

Crane, J. (1995) The future of research utilization. In Titler, M.G. & Goode, C.J. (eds) *The nursing clinics of North America: research utilization*. 30 (3) Philadelphia, PA: W.B. Saunders

Cresswell, J.W. (1998) *Qualitative inquiry and research design: choosing among five traditions*. Thousand Oaks, CA: Sage

Denzin, N.K. & Lincoln, Y.S. (eds) (1994) *Handbook of qualitative research*. Thousand Oaks, CA: Sage

Dickson, R. (1996) Dissemination and implementation: the wider picture. *Nurse Researcher* 4 (1)

Dictionary of Social Science Methods (1983) Edited by Miller, P.McC. and Wilson, M.J. Chichester: John Wiley

Evans, D. (2003) Hierarchy of evidence: a framework for ranking evidence evaluating healthcare interventions. *Journal of Clinical Nursing* 12 (1)

Fife-Schaw, C. (2000) Introduction. In Breakwell, G.M., Hammond, S. & Fife-Schaw, C. (eds) *Research methods in psychology* (2nd edition). London: Sage

Fox, D. (1982) *Fundamentals of research in nursing* (4th edition). Norwalk, CT: Appleton-Century-Crofts

Goodall, C.J. (1994) Writing and research: an introduction. *Nurse Researcher* 2 (1)

Hek, G., Judd, M. & Moule, P. (1996) *Making sense of research: an Introduction for nurses*. London: Cassell

Howarth, K. (1998) *Oral history*. Stroud, Glos: Sutton Publishing Co.

Krippendorf, K. (1980) *Content analysis: an introduction to its methodology*. Beverly Hills, CA: Sage

Leininger, M.M. (1985) *Qualitative research methods in nursing*. Orlando, FL: Grune & Stratton

Leininger, M.M. (1987) Importance and uses of ethno-methods: ethnography and ethnonursing research. *Recent Advances in Nursing*

Lindlof, T.R. (1995) *Qualitative communication research methods*. Thousand Oaks, CA: Sage

Linstone H.A. & Turoff, M. (eds) (1975) *The Delphi method: techniques and applications*. Reading, MA: Addison-Wesley

Mackenzie, J., Husband, C. & Gerrish, K. (1995) Researching in collaboration: a guide to successful partnerships. *Nurse Researcher* 3 (1)

Meleis, A.I. (1989) International research: a need or luxury? *Nursing Outlook* 37 (3)

Millward, L.J. (2000) Focus groups. In Breakwell, G.M., Hammond, S. & Fife-Schaw, C. (eds) *Research methods in Psychology* (2nd edition). London: Sage

Nieswiadomy, R.M. (2002) *Foundations of nursing research* (4th edition). Upper Saddle River, NJ: Prentice-Hall

Omery, A., Kasper, C.E. & Page, G.G. (eds) (1995) *In search of nursing science*. Thousand Oaks, CA: Sage

Phillips, D.C. (1987) *Philosophy, science and social inquiry: contemporary methodological controversies in social science and related applied fields of research*. Oxford: Pergamon

Phillips, L.R.F. (1986) *A clinician's guide to the critique and utilization of nursing research*. Norwalk, CT: Appleton-Century-Crofts

Polit, D.F. & Hungler, B.P. (1991) *Nursing research: principles and methods* (4th edition). Hagerstown, MD: Lippincott

Polit, D.F. & Hungler, B.P. (1995) *Nursing research: principles and methods* (5th edition). Philadelphia, PA: Lippincott

Polit, D.F. & Hungler B.P. (1999) *Nursing research: principles and methods* (6th edition). Philadelphia, PA: Lippincott

Rafferty, A.M. (1997/98) Writing, researching and reflexivity in nursing history. *Nurse Researcher* 5 (2)

Reason, P. & Rowan, J. (eds) (1981) *Human inquiry: a sourcebook of new paradigm research*. Chichester: John Wiley

Treece, E.W. & Treece, J.W. Jr (1986) *Elements of research in nursing* (4th edition). St Louis, MO: Mosby van Maanen, H. (1998) Two decades WENR: did history write nursing research – or did nursing research write history? In: *Knowledge development: clinicians and researchers in partnership*. Helsinki: The Finnish Federation of Nurses ISSN 0251–4753 Proceedings of the Workgroup of European Nurse Researchers (9th Biennial Conference Helsinki, Finland) Volume 1

van Teijlingen, E.R. & Hundley, V. *The importance of pilot studies*. Social Research Update Issue 35 Guildford: Department of Sociology, University of Surrey www. soc.surrey.ac.uk/sru/SRU35.html (Accessed 13/11/03)

Wakefield, J.C. (1995) When an irresistible epistemology meets an immovable ontology. *Social Work Research* 19 (1)

Waltz, C.F., Strickland, O.L. & Lenz, E.R. (1984) *Measurement in nursing research*. Philadelphia, PA: F.C. Davis

Wilson, S.L. (2000) Single-case experimental designs. In Breakwell, G.M., Hammond, S. & Fife-Schaw, C. (eds) *Research methods in psychology* (2nd edition). London: Sage

Woods, N.F. & Catanzaro, M. (1988) *Nursing research: theory and practice*. St Louis, MO: Mosby

Yin, R.K. (1984) *Case study research: design and methods*. Beverly Hills, CA: Sage

Appendix A: Computer Programs for Design and Analysis

AnSWR 6.4
Purpose: A software system for co-ordinating and conducting large-scale, team-based analysis projects that integrate qualitative and quantitative techniques. It allows the collection of data from different sources, including observational notes, interview transcriptions, historical documents and standardized questionnaires. Includes tools for controlling access to the database and assigning different levels of user rights to the research team.
Publisher: Division of HIV/AIDS Prevention. Centers for Disease Control (CDC) Atlanta GA 30333 USA
www.cdc.gov/hiv/software/answr.htm

ANTHROPAC 4.98
Purpose: Menu-driven DOS program for collecting and analysing data on cultural domains. Collects and analyses structured qualitative and quantitative data, performs consensus analysis and multiple regression. Includes techniques that are unique to anthropology.
Publisher: Analytic Technologies. 11 Ohlin Lane Harvard MA 01451 USA
www.analytictech.com/

AQUAD v5.8
Purpose: Interprets text using one- or two-step coding and analyses words using single word counts and lists. Differentiates between speakers and will copy text segments, retrieve text by number line, code or key words.
Publisher: Verlag Ingeborg Huber. Postfach 46 Schwangau, Germany
www.aquad.de

ATLAS ti
Purpose: Visual qualitative analysis of large bodies of textual, graphical, audio or video data. Includes a variety of tools for accomplishing the tasks associated with a systematic approach to qualitative data.
Publisher: Scolari. Sage Publications 1 Oliver's Yard 55 City Road London EC1Y 1SP
www.sagepublications.com

BEST (Behavioural Evaluation Strategy and Taxonomy Software)
Purpose: Two separate but integrated modules that facilitate the real-time collection and analysis of observational category system data. Records multiple, mutually exclusive and overlapping events, creates categories, can be used to formulate different observation systems and records information live or on synchronized videotape.
Publisher: Scolari. Sage Publications 1 Oliver's Yard 55 City Road London EC1Y 1SP
www.sagepublications.com

CDC EX Text
Purpose: Creates, manages and analyses semi-structured qualitative databases from templates tailored to researchers questionnaires. Online codebooks can be created which allow the application of codes to specific responses and data may be exported in a variety of formats for further analysis with other software programs. Software may be downloaded from CDC website.
Publisher: Division of HIV/AIDS Prevention. Centers for Disease Control (CDC) Atlanta GA 30333 USA
www.cdc.gov/hiv/software/ez-text.htm

C-I-SAID
Purpose: Facilitates the study and analysis of documents usually based on interviews or dialogues. Supports quantitative and qualitative analysis of sound, video or text, and provides different methods for coding source data.
Publisher: Scolari. Sage Publications 1 Oliver's Yard 55 City Road London EC1Y 1SP
www.sagepublications.com

CODE-A-TEXT
Purpose: A multimedia system for the analysis of recorded dialogues, interview transcripts and protocols with individuals or groups.
Publisher: Scolari. Sage Publications 1 Oliver's Yard 55 City Road London EC1Y 1SP
www.sagepublications.com

DECISION EXPLORER 3.1
Purpose: Generates a map of issues involved in complex situations which can then be explored and analysed.
Publisher: Scolari. Sage Publications 1 Oliver's Yard 55 City Road London EC1Y 1SP
www.sagepublications.com

DICTION 5.0
Purpose: A Windows-based program that searches a passage for five general features and can determine the tone of a verbal message.
Publisher: Scolari. Sage Publications 1 Oliver's Yard 55 City Road London EC1Y 1SP
www.sagepublications.com

ENDNOTE 5.0
Purpose: 'Cite while you write' bibliographic software. Can be used to search online databases, organize references and create instant bibliographies. Integrates with Microsoft Word so that citations can be located and inserted without leaving a Word document.
Publisher: ISI ResearchSoft 3501 Market Street Philadelphia, PA 19104 USA
www.endnote.com/

EPI INFO
Purpose: Epidemiological program for word processing, data management and analysis designed for health care professionals. Has questionnaire design function and can generate geographical maps with data.
Publisher: Division of Surveillance, Epidemiology and Prevention. Center for Disease Control (CDC) Atlanta GA 30333 USA
www.cdc.gov/epo/epi/epiinfo.htm

ETHNOGRAPH 5.0
Purpose: Codes and analyses textual qualitative data.
Publisher: Scolari. Sage Publications 1 Oliver's Yard 55 City Road London EC1Y 1SP
www.sagepublications.com

GBSTAT 6.5
Purpose: Statistics and graphics package, which can manipulate and analyse data from virtually any source and export them to familiar graphics packages. [Available in both Macintosh and Windows versions.]
Publisher: Scolari. Sage Publications 1 Oliver's Yard 55 City Road London EC1Y 1SP
www.sagepublications.com

GENSTAT
Purpose: A sophisticated package for the manipulation and analysis of experimental data.
Publisher: VSN International Ltd. 5 The Waterhouse Waterhouse Street Hemel Hempstead Herts P1 1ES UK
www.vsn-intl.com/genstat/

HyperRESEARCH
Purpose: A qualitative data analysis tool for Mackintosh and PC which works with text or multimedia data. The hypothesis tester presents data for examination similar to statistical analysis.

Publisher: Scolari. Sage Publications 1 Oliver's Yard 55 City Road London EC1Y 1SP
www.sagepublications.com

MAXqda
Purpose: Analyses qualitative textual data and interfaces with Internet Explorer and MS Office applications to edit existing documents.
Publisher: Scolari. Sage Publications 1 Oliver's Yard 55 City Road London EC1Y 1SP
www.sagepublications.com

METHODOLOGIST'S TOOLCHEST 3.0
Purpose: Consists of nine modules which each address a specific aspect of the research process – developing a sound research design, funding proposal, thesis or dissertation. It is fully integrated and accessed through a single application.
Publisher: Scolari. Sage Publications 1 Oliver's Yard 55 City Road London EC1Y 1SP
www.sagepublications.com

MINITAB 13
Purpose: Statistical analysis and graphics software, which will perform a wide range of analyses from the simple to the complex.
Publisher: Minitab Inc. Quality Plaza 1829 Pine Hall Road State College PA 16801–3008 USA
www.minitab.com/products/13/INDEX.HTM

PROCITE
Purpose: For the management and access of references, including search and web-based facilities.
Publisher: Adept Scientific plc. Amor Way Letchworth Herts SG6 1ZA
www.adeptscience.co.uk

QSR N6
Purpose: Designed for researchers making sense of complex data, N6 offers a complete toolkit for rapid coding, thorough exploration and rigorous management and analysis. With a full command language for automating, coding and searching, and a Command Assistant that formats the command for you. Coded material is displayed for reflection, revision of coding and coding-on to new categories. With searches of coding or text accessed by visual displays, the researcher can test hypotheses, locate patterns or pursue a line of inquiry to a confident conclusion.
Publisher: Scolari. Sage Publications 1 Oliver's Yard 55 City Road London EC1Y 1SP
www.sagepublications.com

QSR Nvivo 2.0
Purpose: For qualitative research, combines rich, editable text with code-based theorizing, searches and the ability to embed sound, image and other files into documents.

Publisher: Scolari. Sage Publications 1 Oliver's Yard 55 City Road London EC1Y 1SP
www.sagepublications.com

REFERENCE MANAGER
Purpose: Database software for the creation of references and bibliographies.
Publisher: Adept Scientific plc. Amor Way Letchworth Hertfordshire SG6 1ZA
www.adeptscience.co.uk

RESULTS FOR RESEARCH
Purpose: Interviewing software.
Publisher: Scolari. Sage Publications 1 Oliver's Yard 55 City Road London EC1Y 1SP
www.sagepublications.com

SPHINX SURVEY 4.0
Purpose: A package for the design and production of questionnaires and the conduct of surveys on the Internet. Also assists with the collection of responses, analysis of data and report generation.
Publisher: Scolari. Sage Publications 1 Oliver's Yard 55 City Road London EC1Y 1SP
www.sagepublications.com

SPSS 12.0
Purpose: SPSS is a modular product for the analytical process, including planning, data collecting, data access, data management and preparation, analysis, reporting and deployment. Generates decision-making information quickly using statistics, effectively presents results with tabular and graphical output. Uses a variety of reporting methods, including secure Web publishing.
Publisher: SPSS Inc. 233 S. Wacker Drive 11th floor Chicago, IL 60606-6307
www.SPSS.com

winMax
Purpose: A tool for text analysis that can be used for Grounded Theory oriented 'code and retrieve' analysis as well as for more sophisticated text analysis, enabling both qualitative and quantitative procedures to be combined. Codes can be weighted to give a measure of the significance of a piece of coding, making it possible to retrieve only the most important segments given a particular coding. Codes can easily be copied, merged, split or deleted as your requirements become clearer while you explore the text.
Publisher: Scolari. Sage Publications 1 Oliver's Yard 55 City Road London EC1Y 1SP
www.sagepublications.com

Appendix B: Journals

A number of journals regularly report on or present research findings or discuss methodology. This list is not comprehensive, rather it should be seen as an indicator of the breadth of specialist journals and reflects the sources used in this bibliography.

AACN Clinical Issues: Advanced Practice in Acute & Critical Care (USA)
AAOHN Journal (American Association of Occupational Health Nurses)
Academic Medicine (USA)
Accident and Emergency Nursing (USA)
ACP Journal Club (USA)
Active Learning in Higher Education (UK)
Adapted Physical Activity Quarterly (USA)
Addiction (UK)
Advanced Nursing Practice Quarterly (USA)
Advances in Nursing Science (USA)
Affilia – Journal of Women & Social Work (USA)
Aging Today (USA)
Aihaj (USA)
AJIC: American Journal of Infection Control
Alternative Therapy in Health & Medicine (USA)
American Journal of Clinical Nutrition
American Journal of Epidemiology
American Journal of Evaluation
American Journal of Health Behavior
American Journal of Hospice and Palliative Care
American Journal of Occupational Therapy
American Journal of Physical Medicine and Rehabilitation
American Journal of Psychiatry
American Journal of Public Health
American Journal of Sports Medicine
ANNA Journal (American Nephrology Nurses' Association)
Annals of Epidemiology (USA)
Annual Review of Nursing Research (USA)
Annual Review of Psychology (USA)
Anthropology and Medicine (UK)
AORN Journal – Association of Operating Room Nurses (USA)
Applied Nursing Research (USA)
Applied Nursing Research Online (USA)
Applied Statistics (UK)
Archives of Psychiatric Nursing (USA)
Art Therapy – Journal of the American Art Therapy Association
ASHA Leader (USA)

Assessment and Evaluation in Higher Education (UK)
Australian & New Zealand Journal of Mental Health Nursing
Australian College of Midwives Journal
Australian Critical Care
Australian Emergency Nursing Journal
Australian Health Review
Australian Journal of Advanced Nursing
Australian Occupational Therapy Journal
Avante (Canada)

Behavioral Medicine (USA)
Bibliotheca Medica Canadiana
Bioethics (UK)
British Educational Research Journal
British Journal of Clinical Governance
British Journal of Family Planning
British Journal of Guidance and Counselling
British Journal of Learning Disabilities
British Journal of Midwifery
British Journal of Nursing
British Journal of Occupational Therapy
British Journal of Perioperative Nursing
British Journal of Social Work
British Medical Journal
Bulletin de Méthodologie Sociologique (France)
Bulletin of Medical Ethics (UK)
Bulletin of the Medical Library Association (USA)

Cambridge Quarterly of Health Care Ethics (UK)
Canadian Journal of Community Mental Health
Canadian Journal of Nursing Administration
Canadian Journal of Nursing Leadership
Canadian Journal of Nursing Research
Canadian Journal of Occupational Therapy
Canadian Journal of Policy Research
Canadian Journal of Public Health
Canadian Journal of Rehabilitation (ceased publication)
Canadian Nurse
Canadian Oncology Nursing Journal
Cancer Nursing (USA)
Cannt Journal (Canada)
Chart (USA)
Child: Care, Health and Development (UK)
Children and Society (UK)
Children and Youth Services Review (UK)
Chinese Nursing Research (China)
Chronolog (USA)

CINAHLnews (USA)
Clinical Effectiveness in Nursing (UK)
Clinical Excellence for Nurse Practitioners (USA)
Clinical Nurse Specialist (USA)
Clinical Nursing Research (USA)
Clinical Rehabilitation (UK)
CMAJ: Canadian Medical Association Journal
Cochrane Library (UK)
Collegian: Journal of the Royal College of
   Nursing, Australia
Community Mental Health Journal (USA)
Community Practitioner (UK)
Complementary Therapies in Medicine (UK)
Complexity and Chaos in Nursing (USA)
Computers in Libraries (USA)
Computers in Nursing (USA)
Contemporary Nurse: a Journal for the Australian
   Nursing Profession
Crime and Delinquency (USA)
Critical Care Nurse (USA)
CRNA – the Clinical Forum for Nurse
   Anesthetists (USA)
Cross-cultural Research – The Journal of
   Comparative Social Science (USA)
Cultura de Los Cuidados (Spain)
Curationis: South African Journal of Nursing
Current Paediatrics (UK)
Current Sociology (UK)
Cyberskeptic's Guide to Internet Research (USA)

Death Studies (USA)
Developmental Review (USA)
Diabetes Educator (USA)
Disability and Society (UK)

Educational Action Research: an International
   Journal (UK)
Educational Management
Educational Research (UK)
Educational Researcher (USA)
Educational Review (UK)
Emergency Medicine (USA)
Enfermería Clínica (Spain)
Ethnography (UK)
EUNurse
European Journal of Oncology Nursing (UK)
Evaluation (UK)
Evaluation and Research in Education (UK)
Evaluation and the Health Professions (USA)
Evaluation: the International Journal of Theory,
   Research and Practice (UK)
Evidence-based Nursing (UK)

Family Journal: Counseling & Therapy for
   Couples and Families (USA)
Family Practitioner
Feminism and Psychology (UK)
Feminist Review (UK)

Gastroenterology Nursing (USA)
General Hospital Psychiatry (USA)
Graduate Research in Nursing Online (USA)

Hastings Center Report (USA)
Health (USA)
Health and Social Care in the Community (UK)
Health and Social Work (UK)
Health Care on the Internet (USA)
Health Care Supervisor
Health Education (USA)
Health Education Journal (UK)
Health Education Research (UK)
Health Expectations (UK)
Health Informatics (UK)
Health Information for Libraries (UK) (formerly
   Health Libraries Review)
Health Libraries Review (UK)
Health Promotion Practice (USA)
Health Services Management Research (UK)
Health Services Research (USA)
Health Technology Assessment (UK)
Health Visitor (UK)
Health: Interdisciplinary Journal for the Social
   Study of Health, Illness and Medicine (UK)
Hoitotiede (Finland)
Home Healthcare Nurse (USA)
Hospice Journal (USA)
Hospital and Health Service Administration

Icus and Nursing Web Journal (Greece)
Image: Journal of Nursing Scholarship (USA)
   (now Journal of Nursing Scholarship)
Information World Review (UK)
Inquiry (USA)
Inside Case Management (USA)
Intensive and Critical Care Nursing (USA)
Interdisciplinary Science Reviews (UK)
International Electronic Journal of Health
   Education (USA)
International History of Nursing Journal (UK)
International Journal for Quality in Health
   Care (UK)
International Journal of Qualitative Studies in
   Education (USA)
International Journal of Clinical Practice (UK)
International Journal of Eating Disorders (USA)
International Journal of Health Promotion and
   Education (UK)
International Journal of Nursing Studies (UK)
International Journal of Palliative Nursing (UK)
International Journal of Qualitative Studies in
   Education (UK)
International Journal of Quality Science (UK)
International Journal of Social Research
   Methodology: Theory and Practice (UK)
International Journal of Sociology and Social
   Policy (UK)

International Nursing (Switzerland) (formerly International Nursing Review)
Internet Medicine (USA)
Internet Reference Services Quarterly (USA)
Issues in Mental Health Nursing (USA)

JAMA: Journal of the American Medical Association
JCN Online (UK)
Journal of Accident and Emergency Medicine (UK)
Journal of Advanced Nursing (UK)
Journal of Allied Health (USA)
Journal of Alternative and Complementary Medicine (USA)
Journal of Applied Research in Clinical & Experimental Therapeutics (USA)
Journal of Audiological Medicine (UK)
Journal of Cardiovascular Pharmacology and Therapeutics (USA)
Journal of Clinical Effectiveness (UK)
Journal of Clinical Epidemiology (USA)
Journal of Clinical Governance (UK)
Journal of Clinical Nursing (UK)
Journal of Community Nursing (UK)
Journal of Community Practice (USA)
Journal of Consulting and Clinical Psychology (USA)
Journal of Contemporary Ethnography (UK)
Journal of Continuing Education in Nursing (USA)
Journal of Continuing Education in the Health Professions (USA)
Journal of Education for Teaching (UK)
Journal of Epidemiology and Community Health (UK)
Journal of Ethnic and Migration Studies (UK)
Journal of Evaluation in Clinical Practice (UK)
Journal of Family Nursing (USA)
Journal of Health Service Research and Policy (UK)
Journal of Law and Health (USA)
Journal of Management in Medicine (UK)
Journal of Management Studies (UK)
Journal of Manipulative and Physiological Therapeutics (USA)
Journal of Medical Ethics (UK)
Journal of Mental Health and Aging (USA)
Journal of Mental Health Counseling (USA)
Journal of Midwifery and Women's Health (USA)
Journal of Neonatal Nursing (UK)
Journal of Nursing Administration (USA)
Journal of Nursing Care Quality (USA)
Journal of Nursing Education (USA)
Journal of Nursing Management (UK)
Journal of Nursing Scholarship (USA) (formerly Image: Journal of Nursing Scholarship)
Journal of Paediatrics & Child Health (UK)
Journal of Pediatric Health Care (USA)
Journal of Pediatric Nursing (USA)

Journal of Phenomenological Psychology (USA)
Journal of Professional Nursing (USA)
Journal of Prosthetic Dentistry (USA)
Journal of Quality in Clinical Practice (Australia)
Journal of Rheumatology (Canada)
Journal of Social Issues (USA)
Journal of Teaching in Social Work (USA)
Journal of the American Academy of Nurse Practitioners
Journal of the American Dietetic Association
Journal of the American Informatics Association
Journal of the American Medical Association
Journal of the American Medical Informatics Association
Journal of the American Society for Information Science & Technology
Journal of the Association of Nurses in AIDS Care (JANAC) (USA)
Journal of the Medical Library Association (USA)
Journal of the Neuromusculoskeletal System (USA)
Journal of the Society of Pediatric Nurses (USA)
Journal of the WOCN (Wound, Ostomy and Continence Nurses Society) (USA)
Journal of Transcultural Nursing (USA)
Journal of Women's Health (USA)

Lancet (UK)

Managing Clinical Nursing (UK)
MCN: The American Journal of Maternal/Child Nursing
Medical Education (UK)
Medical Reference Services Quarterly (USA)
Mental Health Care and Learning Disabilities (UK)
Mentoring and Tutoring (UK)
Metas de Enfermeria (Spain)
Midirs Midwifery Digest (UK)
Millbank Quarterly (USA)
Modern Midwife (UK)

National Academies of Practice Forum: Issues in Interdisciplinary Care (USA)
National Network (USA)
New England Journal of Medicine (USA)
New Zealand Journal of Medical Laboratory Sciences
New Zealand Journal of Physiotherapy
NLM Technical Bulletin (USA)
NT Research (UK)
Nurse Author & Editor (USA)
Nurse Education in Practice (UK)
Nurse Education Today (UK)
Nurse Educator (USA)
Nurse Researcher: the International Journal of Research Methodology in Nursing and Health Care (UK) (formerly Nurse Researcher)
Nursing (USA)
Nursing & Residential Care (UK)

Nursing and Health Care Perspectives (USA)
Nursing and Health Sciences (Australia)
Nursing Diagnosis (USA)
Nursing Ethics: an International Journal for Health
   Care Professionals (UK)
Nursing Forum (USA)
Nursing Inquiry (Australia)
Nursing Outlook (USA)
Nursing Philosophy (UK)
Nursing Research (China)
Nursing Research (USA)
Nursing Review (Ireland)
Nursing Science Quarterly (USA)
Nursing Spectrum (New England edition) (USA)
Nursing Standard (UK)
Nursing Standard Online (UK)
Nursing Times (UK)
Nursing Times Learning Curve (UK)

Occupational Therapy: Journal of Research (USA)
Oncology Nursing Forum (USA)
Online (USA)
Online and CDROM Review (UK)
Online Journal of Issues in Nursing (USA)
Online Journal of Knowledge Synthesis for
   Nursing (USA)
Oral History (UK)
Organizational Research Methods (USA)
ORL – Head and Neck Nursing (USA)
Orthopedic Nursing Journal (USA)
Ostomy Wound Management (USA)
Outcomes Management in Nursing Practice (USA)

Paediatric Nursing (UK)
Pan American Journal of Public Health (USA)
Pflege (Germany)
Philosophy of the Social Sciences (USA)
Physical Therapy (USA)
Physiotherapy Research International (UK)
Physiotherapy Theory and Practice (USA)
Practising Midwife (UK)
Primary Health Care – Research and
   Development (UK)
Professional Nurse (UK)
Professioni Infermieristiche (Italy)
Psychoanalytic Psychology (USA)
Psychological Bulletin (USA)
Psychologist (UK)
Public Health Nursing (USA)
Public Health Reports (USA)

Qualitative Health Research (USA)
Qualitative Research (UK)

Radiologic Technology (USA)
Recherche en Soins Infirmiers (France)
Reflections (USA)
Reflections on Higher Education (UK)
Rehabilitation Education (USA)
Rehabilitation Psychology (USA)
Research in Education (UK)
Research in Nursing and Health (USA)
Research on Social Work Practice (USA)
Research Practitioner (USA)
Revista Brasileira de Enfermagem (Brazil)
RN (USA)

Scandinavian Journal of Caring Sciences (Norway)
Scholarly Inquiry for Nursing Practice (USA)
Scientometrics (USA)
Searcher: the Magazine for Database
   Professionals (USA)
Seminars in Oncology Nursing (USA)
Social Research Update (UK)
Social Science and Medicine (UK)
Social Science Computer Review (USA)
Social Sciences in Health – International Journal
   of Research and Practice (UK)
Social Work (USA)
Social Work Research (USA)
Sociological Methodology (USA)
Sociological Research Online (UK)
Studies in the Education of Adults (UK)
Systematic Practice and Action Research

Texto & Contexto Enfermagem (Portuguese)
The Laryngoscope (USA)
The Qualitative Report (online)
Third World Quarterly (UK)
Topics in Geriatric Rehabilitation (USA)
Topics in Health Information Management (USA)

Value in Health (USA)
Vard I Norden Nursing Science and Research in
   the Nordic Countries (Denmark)
Visions: the Journal of Rogerian Nursing
   Science (USA)

Western Journal of Nursing Research (USA)
Women and Health (USA)
Work: American Journal of Prevention,
   Assessment & Rehabilitations

Appendix C: Sage Publications

This appendix gives details of five series of books relating to research methodology, some of which have been included in the text.

The information has been provided by Sage Publications and indicates books in print and forthcoming as at 2004.

For up-to-date information please visit:

www.sagepublications.com

APPLIED SOCIAL RESEARCH METHODS SERIES

Methods for Policy Research. Ann Majchrzak, 1984
Paper (0–8039–2060–1)

Linking Auditing and Meta-Evaluation: Enhancing Quality in Applied Research. Thomas A. Schwandt and Edward S. Halpern, 1988
Paper (0–8039–2968–4)

Ethics and Values in Applied Social Research. Allan Kimmel, 1988
Paper (0–8039–2632–4)

On Time and Method. Janice R. Kelly and Joseph E. McGrath, 1988
Paper (0–8039–3047-X)

Synthesizing Research: a Guide for Literature Reviews (3rd edition). Harris M. Cooper, 1998
Paper (0–7619–1348–3)

Research in Health Care Settings. Kathleen E. Grady and Barbara Strudler Wallstro, 1988
Paper (0–8039–2875–0)

Ethnography: Step by Step (2nd edition). David M. Fetterman, 1998
Paper (0–7619–1385–8)

Participant Observation: a Methodology for Human Studies. Danny L. Jorgensen, 1989
Paper (0–8039–2877–7)

Ethnography: Step by Step. David M. Fetterman, 1989
Paper (0–8039–2891–2)

Integrating Research: a Guide for Literature Reviews (2nd edition). Harris M. Cooper, 1989
Paper (0–8039–3431–9)

Standardized Survey Interviewing Minimizing Interviewer-related Error. Floyd J. Fowler Jr. and Thomas W. Mangione, 1990
Paper (0–8039–3093–3)

Productivity Measurement: a Guide for Managers and Evaluators. Robert O. Brinkerhoff and Dennis E. Dressler, 1990
Paper (0–8039–3152–2)

Focus Groups: Theory and Practice. David W. Stewart and Prem N. Shamdasani, 1990
Paper (0–8039–3390–8)

Practical Sampling. Gary T. Henry, 1990
Paper (0–8039–2959–5)

Decision Research: a Field Guide. John S. Carroll and Eric J. Johnson, 1990
Paper (0–8039–3269–3)

Research with Hispanic Populations. Gerardo Marin and Barbara Vanoss, 1991
Paper (0–8039–3721–0)

Internal Evaluation: Building Organizations from Within. Arnold J. Love, 1991
Paper (0–8039–3201–4)

Computer Simulation Applications: an Introduction. Marcia Lynn Whicker and Lee Sigelman, 1991
Paper (0–8039–3246–4)

Studying Families. Anne P. Copeland and Kathleen M. White, 1991
Paper (0–8039–3248–0)

Event History Analysis. Kazuo Yamaguchi, 1991
Paper (0–8039–3324-X)

Meta-analytic Procedures for Social Research. Robert Rosenthal, 1991
Paper (0–8039–4246-X)

Research in Educational Settings. Geoffrey M. Maruyama and Stanley Deno, 1992
Paper (0–8039–4208–7)

Researching Persons with Mental Illness. Rosalind J. Dworkin, 1992
Paper (0–8039–3604–4)

Planning Ethically Responsible Research: a Guide for Students and Internal Review Boards. Joan E. Sieber, 1992
Paper (0–8039–3964–7)

Applied Research Design: a Practical Guide. Terry E. Hedrick, Leonard Bickman and Debra J. Rog, 1993
Paper (0–8039–3234–0)

Doing Urban Research. Gregory D. Andranovich and Gerry Riposa, 1993
Paper (0–8039–3989–2)

Secondary Research: Information Sources and Methods (2nd edition). David W. Stewart and Michael A. Kamins, 1993
Paper (0–8039–5037–3)

Telephone Survey Methods: Sampling Selection, and Supervision (2nd edition). Paul J. Lavrakas, 1993
Paper (0–8039–5307–0)

Diagnosing Organizations: Methods, Models, and Processes (2nd edition). Michael I. Harrison, 1994
Paper (0–8039–5645–2)

Group Techniques for Idea Building (2nd edition). Carl M. Moore, 1994
Paper (0–8039–5643–6)

Introduction to Facet Theory: Content Design and Intrinsic Data Analysis in Behavioral Research. Samuel Shye and Dov Elizur with Michael Hoffman, 1994
Paper (0–8039–5671–1)

Graphing Data: Techniques for Display and Analysis. Gary T. Henry 1994
Paper (0–8039–5675–4)

Research Methods in Special Education. Donna M. Mertens and John McLaughlin, 1994
Paper (0–8039–4809–3)

Improving Survey Questions: Design and Evaluation. Floyd J. Fowler Jr., 1995
Paper (0–8039–4583–3)

Data Collection and Management: a Practical Guide. Magda Stouthamer-Loeber and Welmoet Bok van Kammen, 1995
Paper (0–8039–5657–6)

Mail Surveys: Improving the Quality. Thomas W. Mangione, 1995
Paper (0–8039–4663–5)

Qualitative Research Design: an Interactive Approach. Joseph A. Maxwell, 1996
Paper (0–8039–7329–2)

Analyzing Costs, Procedures, Processes, and Outcomes in Human Services: an Introduction. Brian T. Yates, 1996
Paper (0–8039–4786–0)

Doing Legal Research: a Guide for Social Scientists and Mental Health Professionals. Roberta Morris, Bruce D. Sales and Daniel W. Shuman, 1997
Paper (0–8039–3429–7)

Randomized Experiments for Planning and Evaluation: a Practical Guide. Robert F. Boruch, 1997
Paper (0–8039–3510–2)

Measuring Community Indicators: a Systems Approach to Drug and Alcohol Problems. Paul J. Gruenewald, Andrew J. Treno, Gail Taff and Michael Klitzner, 1997
Paper (0–7619–0685–1)

Mixed Methodology: Combining Qualitative and Quantitative Approaches. Abbas Tashakkori and Charles Teddlie, 1998
Paper (0–7619–0071–3)

Narrative Research: Reading, Analysis and Interpretation. Amia Lieblich, Rivka Tuval-Mashiach and Tamar Zilber, 1998
Paper (0–7619–1043–3)

Communicating Social Science Research to Policymakers. Roger J. Vaughan and Terry F. Buss, 1998
Paper (0–8039–7216–4)

Practical Meta-Analysis. Mark W. Lipsey and David B. Wilson, 2000
Paper (0–7619–2168–0)

Survey Research Methods (3rd edition). Floyd J. Fowler Jr., 2001
Paper (0–7619–2191–5)

Interpretive Interactionism (2nd edition). Norman K. Denzin, 2001
Paper (0–7619–1514–1)

Applications of Case Study Research (2nd edition). Robert K. Yin, 2003
Paper (0–7619–2551–1)

Case Study Research: Design and Methods (3rd edition). Robert K. Yin, 2003
Paper (0–7619–2553–8)

Scale Development: Theory and Applications (2nd edition). Robert F. DeVellis, 2003
Paper (0–7619–2605–4)

Need Analysis: Tools for the Human Services and Education (2nd edition). Jack McKillip, 2004
Paper (0–7619–2618–6)

INTRODUCING QUALITATIVE METHODS SERIES

Doing Conversation Analysis: A Practical Guide. Paul ten Have, 1998
Paper (0–7619–5586–0)

Using Foucault's Methods. Gavin Kendall and Gary Wickham, 1998
Paper (0–7619–5717–0)

Qualitative Evaluation. Ian Shaw, 1999
Paper (0–7619–5690–5)

Researching Life Stories and Family Histories. Robert L. Miller, 1999
Paper (0–7619–6092–9)

The Quality of Qualitative Research. Clive Seale, 1999
Paper (0–7619–5598–4)

Categories in Text and Talk. Georgia Lepper, 2000
Cloth (0–7619–5666–2) (hardback only)

Focus Groups in Social Research. Michael Bloor, Jane Frankland and Michelle Thomas, 2000
Paper (0–7619–5743-X)

Researching the Visual. Michael Emmison and Philip Smith, 2000
Paper (0–7619–5846–0)

Methods of Critical Discourse Analysis. Ruth Wodak and Michael Meyer, 2001
Paper (0–7619–6154–2)

Qualitative Research in Social Work. Ian Shaw and Nick Gould, 2001
Paper (0–7619–6182–8)

Qualitative Research Through Case Studies. Max Travers, 2001
Paper (0–7619–6806–7)

Qualitative Research in Information Systems: A Reader. Michael D. Myers and David Avison, 2002
Cloth (0–7619–6632–3) (hardback only)

Gender and Qualitative Methods. Helmi Järviluoma, Pirkko Moisala and Anni Vilkko, 2003
Paper (0–7619–6585–8)

Qualitative Research in Education. Peter R. Freebody, 2003
Paper (0–7619–6141–0)

Using Documents in Social Research. Lindsay Prior, 2003
Paper (0–7619–5747–2)

Doing Research in Cultural Studies. Paula Saukko, 2003
Paper (0–7619–6505–X)

Qualitative Research in Sociology. Amir Marvasti, 2003
Paper (0–7619–4861–9)

Narratives in Social Science Research. Barbara Czarniawska, 2004
Paper (0–7619–4195–9)

Criminological Research. Lesley Noaks and Emma Wincup, 2004
Paper (0–7619–7407–5)

Qualitative Methods for Health Research. Judith Green and Nicki Thorogood, 2004
Paper (0–7619–4771–X)

METHODS IN NURSING RESEARCH SERIES

Ethnography in Nursing Research. Janice M. Roper and Jill Shapira, 1999
Paper (0–7619–0874–9)

Hermeneutic Phenomenological Research. Marlene Zichi Cohen, David L. Kahn and Richard H. Steeves, 2000
Paper (0–7619–1720–9)

Meta-Study of Qualitative Health Research. Barbara L. Paterson, Sally E. Thorne and Connie Canam, 2001
Paper (0–7619–2415–9)

QUALITATIVE RESEARCH METHODS SERIES

Reliability and Validity in Qualitative Research. Jerome Kirk and Marc L. Miller, 1986
Paper (0–8039–2470–4)

Speaking of Ethnography. Michael H. Agar, 1986
Paper (0–8039–2492–5)

The Politics and Ethics of Fieldwork: Muddy Boots and Grubby Hands. Maurice Punch, 1986
Paper (0–8039–2517–4)

Linking Data. Nigel G. Fielding and Jane Fielding, 1986
Paper (0–8039–2518–2)

The Clinical Perspective in Fieldwork. Edgar H. Schein, 1987
Paper (0–8039–2976–5)

Membership Roles in Field Research. Peter Adler, 1987
Paper (0–8039–2578–6)

Semiotics and Fieldwork. Peter K. Manning, 1987
Paper (0–8039–2640–5)

Analyzing Field Reality. Jaber F. Gubrium, 1988
Paper (0–8039–3096–8)

Systematic Data Collection. Susan C. Weller and A. Kimball Romney, 1988
Paper (0–8039–3074–7)

Meta-Ethnography: Synthesizing Qualitative Studies. George W. Noblit and R. Dwight Hare, 1988
Paper (0–8039–3023–2)

Ethnostatistics: Qualitative Foundations for Quantitative Research. Robert P. Gephart Jr., 1988
Paper (0–8039–3026–7)

The Long Interview. Grant McCracken, 1988
Paper (0–8039–3353–3)

Microcomputer Applications in Qualitative Research. Bryan Pfaffenberger, 1988
Paper (0–8039–3120–4)

Knowing Children: Participant Observation with Minors. Gary Alan Fine and Kent L. Sandstrom, 1988
Paper (0–8039–3365–7)

Interpretive Biography. Norman K. Denzin, 1989
Paper (0–8039–3359–2)

Psychoanalytic Aspects of Fieldwork. Jennifer C. Hunt, 1989
Paper (0–8039–3474–4)

Ethnographic Decision Tree Modeling. C.H. Gladwin, 1989
Paper (0–8039–3487–4)

Writing up Qualitative Research. Harry F. Wolcott, 1990
Paper (0–8039–3793–8)

Writing Strategies: Reaching Diverse Audiences. Laurel Richardson, 1990
Paper (0–8039–3522–6)

Living the Ethnographic Life. Dan Rose, 1990
Paper (0–8039–3999-X)

Selecting Ethnographic Informants. Edited by Jeffrey C. Johnson, 1991
Paper (0–8039–3587–0)

Analyzing Visual Data. Michael S. Ball and Gregory W.H. Smith, 1992
Paper (0–8039–3435–1)

Understanding Ethnographic Texts. Paul Atkinson, 1992
Paper (0–8039–3937-X)

Archival Strategies and Techniques. Michael R. Hill, 1993
Paper (0–8039–4825–5)

Case Study Methods. Jacques Hamel, Stephane Dufour and Dominic Fortin, 1993
Paper (0–8039–5416–6)

Doing Critical Ethnography, Jim Thomas, 1993
Paper (0–8039–3923-X)

Ethnography in Organizations. Helen B. Schwartzman, 1993
Paper (0–8039–4379–2)

Secrecy and Fieldwork. Richard G. Mitchell Jr., 1993
Paper (0–8039–4385–7)

Narrative Analysis. Catherine Kohler Riessman, 1993
Paper (0–8039–4754–2)

Emotions and Fieldwork. Sherryl Kleinman and Martha A. Copp, 1993
Cloth (0–8039–4721–6)
Paper (0–8039–4722–4)

Strategies for Interpreting Qualitative Data. Martha S. Feldman, 1994
Paper (0–8039–5916–8)

Dangerous Fieldwork. Raymond M. Lee, 1994
Paper (0–8039–5661–4)

Conversation Analysis: the Study of Talk-in-Interaction. George Psathas, 1994
Paper (0–8039–5747–5)

Ethnomethodology. Alain Coulon, 1995
Paper (0–8039–4777–1)

The Active Interview. James A. Holstein and Jaber F. Gubrium, 1995
Paper (0–8039–5895–1)

Qualitative Media Analysis. David L. Altheide, 1996
Paper (0–7619–0199-X)

Studying Organizational Symbolism: What, How, Why? Michael Owen Jones, 1996
Paper (0–7619–0220–1)

Insider/Outsider Team Research. Jean M. Bartunek and Meryl Reis Louis, 1996
Paper (0–8039–7159–1)

Working with Sensitizing Concepts: Analytical Field Research. Will C. van den Hoonaard, 1997
Paper (0–7619–0207–4)

Doing Team Ethnography: Warnings and Advice. Ken Erickson and Donald Stull, 1997
Paper (0–7619–0667–3)

Focus Groups as Qualitative Research (2nd edition). David L. Morgan, 1997
Paper (0–7619–0343–7)

A Narrative Approach to Organization Studies. Barbara Czarniawska, 1998
Paper (0–7619–0663–0)

The Life Story Interview. Robert Atkinson, 1998
Paper (0–7619–0428-X)

Employing Qualitative Methods in the Private Sector. Marilyn L. Mitchell, 1998
Paper (0–8039–5981–8)

The Ethnographer's Method. Alex Stewart, 1998
Paper (0–7619–0394–1)]

Conducting Interpretive Policy Analysis. Dvora Yanow, 1999
Paper (0–7619–0827–7)

Gender Issues in Ethnography (2nd edition). Carol A.B. Warren and Jennifer Kay Hackney, 2000
Paper (0–7619–1717–9)

Exploratory Research in the Social Sciences. Robert A. Stebbins, 2001
Paper (0–7619–2399–3)

Systematic Self-Observation. Noelie Rodriguez and Alan Ryave, 2002
Paper (0–7619–2308–X)

Discourse Analysis. Nelson Phillips and Cynthia Hardy, 2002
Paper (0–7619–2362–4)

QUANTITATIVE APPLICATIONS IN THE SOCIAL SCIENCES SERIES

Analysis of Ordinal Data. David K. Hildebrand, James D. Laing and Howard Rosenthal, 1970
Paper (0–8039–0795–8)

Analysis of Nominal Data (2nd edition). H.T. Reynolds, 1977
Paper (0–8039–0653–6)

Canonical Analysis and Factor Comparison. Mark S. Levine, 1977
Paper (0–8039–0655–2)

Causal Modeling (2nd edition). Herbert B. Asher, 1977
Paper (0–8039–0654–4)

Cohort Analysis. Norval D. Glenn, 1977
Paper (0–8039–0794-X)

Operations Research Methods: as Applied to Political Science and the Legal Process. Stuart S. Nagel with Marian Neef, 1977
Paper (0–8039–0651-X)

Tests of Significance 4. Ramon E. Henkel, 1977
Paper (0–8039–0652–8)

Ecological Inference. Laura Irwin Langbein and Allan J. Lichtman, 1978
Paper (0–8039–0941–1)

Multidimensional Scaling 11. Joseph B. Kruskal and Myron Wish, 1978
Paper (0–8039–0940–3)

Analysis of Covariance. Albert R. Wildt and Olli T. Ahtola, 1979
Paper (0–8039–1164–5)

Factor Analysis: Statistical Methods and Practical Issues. Jae-On Kim and Charles W. Mueller, 1979
Paper (0–8039–1166–1)

Introduction to Factor Analysis: What it is and How to do it. Jae-On Kim and Charles W. Mueller, 1979
Paper (0–8039–1165–3)

Multiple Indicators: an Introduction. John L. Sullivan and Stanley Feldman, 1980
Paper (0–8039–1369–9)

Exploratory Data Analysis. Frederick Hartwig and Brian E. Dearing, 1980
Paper (0–8039–1370–2)

Reliability & Validity. Edward G. Carmines and Richard A. Zeller, 1980
Paper (0–8039–1371–0)

Analyzing Panel Data. Gregory B. Markus, 1980
Paper (0–8039–1372–9)

Discriminant Analysis. William R. Klecka, 1980
Paper (0–8039–1491–1)

Log-Linear Models. David Knoke, 1980
Paper (0–8039–1492-X)

Interrupted Time Series Analysis. David McDowall, Richard McCleary, Errol E. Meidinger and Richard A. Hay Jr., 1980
Paper (0–8039–1493–8)

Applied Regression: an Introduction. Michael S. Lewis-Beck, 1980
Paper (0–8039–1494–6)

Research Designs. Paul E. Spector, 1981
Paper (0–8039–1709–0)

Unidimensional Scaling. John P. McIver and Edward G. Carmines, 1981
Paper (0–8039–1736–8)

Magnitude Scaling: Quantitative Measurement of Opinions. Milton Lodge, 1981
Paper (0–8039–1747–3)

Multiattribute Evaluation. Ward Edwards and J. Robert Newman, 1982
Paper (0–8039–0095–3)

Dynamic Modeling: an Introduction. R. Robert Huckfeldt, C.W. Kohfeld and Thomas W. Likens, 1982
Paper (0–8039–0946–2)

Network Analysis. David Knoke and James H. Kuklinski, 1982
Paper (0–8039–1914-X)

Interpreting and Using Regression. Christopher H. Achen, 1982
Paper (0–8039–1915–8)

Test Item Bias. Steven J. Osterlind, 1983
Paper (0–8039–1989–1)

Mobility Tables. Michael Hout, 1983
Paper (0–8039–2056–3)

Measures of Association. Albert M. Liebetrau, 1983
Paper (0–8039–1974–3)

Confirmatory Factor Analysis: a Preface to LISREL. J. Scott Long, 1983
Paper (0–8039–2044-X)

Covariance Structure Models: an Introduction to LISREL. J. Scott Long, 1983
Paper (0–8039–2045–8)

Introduction to Survey Sampling. Graham Kalton, 1983
Paper (0–8039–2046–6)

Achievement Testing: Recent Advances. Isaac I. Bejar, 1983
Paper (0–8039–2047–4)

Nonrecursive Causal Models. William D. Berry, 1984
Paper (0–8039–2053–9)

Matrix Algebra: an Introduction. Krishnan Namboodiri, 1984
Paper (0–8039–2052–0)

Introduction to Applied Demography: Data Sources and Estimation Techniques. Norfleet W. Rives Jr. and William J. Serow, 1984
Paper (0–8039–2134–9)

Game Theory: Concepts and Applications. Frank C. Zagare, 1984
Paper (0–8039–2050–4)

Using Published Data: Errors and Remedies. Herbert Jacob, 1985
Paper (0–8039–2299-X)

Bayesian Statistical Inference. Gudmund R. Iversen, 1985
Paper (0–8039–2328–7)

Cluster Analysis. Mark S. Aldenderfer and Roger K. Blashfield, 1985
Paper (0–8039–2376–7)

Linear Probability, Logit, and Probit Models. John H. Aldrich and Forrest D. Nelson, 1985
Paper (0–8039–2133–0)

Event History Analysis: Regression for Longitudinal Event Data. Paul D. Allison, 1985
Paper (0–8039–2055–5)

Canonical Correlation Analysis: Uses and Interpretation. Bruce Thompson, 1985
Paper (0–8039–2392–9)

Models for Innovation Diffusion. Vijay Mahajan and Robert A. Peterson, 1985
Paper (0–8039–2136–5)

Multiple Regression in Practice. William D. Berry and Stanley Feldman, 1985
Paper (0–8039–2054–7)

Stochastic Parameter Regression Models. Paul Newbold and Theodore Bos, 1985
Paper (0–8039–2425–9)

Using Microcomputers in Research. Thomas W. Madron, C. Neal Tate and Robert G. Brookshire, 1985
Paper (0–8039–2457–7)

Secondary Analysis of Survey Data. K. Jill Kiecolt and Laura E. Nathan, 1986
Paper (0–8039–2302–3)

Multivariate Analysis of Variance. James H. Bray and Scott E. Maxwell, 1986
Paper (0–8039–2310–4)

The Logic of Causal Order. James A. Davis, 1986
Paper (0–8039–2553–0)

Introduction to Linear Goal Programming. James P. Ignizio, 1986
Paper (0–8039–2564–6)

Understanding Regression Analysis: an Introductory Guide. Larry D. Schroeder, David L. Sjoquist and Paula E. Stephan, 1986
Paper (0–8039–2758–4)

Randomized Response 58: a Method for Sensitive Surveys. James Alan Fox and Paul E. Tracy, 1986
Paper (0–8039–2309–0)

Meta-Analysis: Quantitative Methods for Research Synthesis. Fredric M. Wolf, 1986
Paper (0–8039–2756–8)

Linear Programming 60: an Introduction. Bruce R. Feiring, 1986
Paper (0–8039–2850–5)

Multiple Comparisons. Alan J. Klockars and Gilbert Sax, 1986
Paper (0–8039–2051–2)

Information Theory: Structural Models for Qualitative Data. Klaus Krippendorff, 1986
Paper (0–8039–2132–2)

Survey Questions: Handcrafting the Standardized Questionnaire. Jean M. Converse and Stanley Presser, 1986
Paper (0–8039–2743–6)

Latent Class Analysis. Allan L. McCutcheon, 1987
Paper (0–8039–2752–5)

Analysis of Variance (2nd edition). Gudmund R. Iversen and Helmut Norpoth, 1987
Paper (0–8039–3001–1)

Microcomputer Methods for Social Scientists (2nd edition). Edited by Philip A. Schrodt, 1987
Paper (0–8039–3043–7)

Three Way Scaling: a Guide to Multidimensional Scaling and Clustering. Phipps Arabie, Douglas Carroll and Wayne S. Desarbo, 1987
Paper (0–8039–3068–2)

Q Methodology. Bruce McKeown, 1988
Paper (0–8039–2753–3)

Analyzing Decision Making: Metric Conjoint Analysis. Jordan J. Louviere, 1988
Paper (0–8039–2757–6)

Rasch Models for Measurement. David Andrich, 1988
Paper (0–8039–2741–X)

Principal Components Analysis. George H. Dunteman, 1989
Paper (0–8039–3104–2)

Pooled Time Series Analysis. Lois W. Sayrs, 1989
Paper (0–8039–3160–3)

Analyzing Complex Survey Data. Eun Sul Lee, Ronald N. Forthofer and Ronald J. Lorimor, 1989
Paper (0–8039–3014–3)

Time Series Analysis: Regression Techniques (2nd edition). Charles W. Ostrom Jr., 1990
Paper (0–8039–3135–2)

Understanding Significance Testing. Lawrence B. Mohr, 1990
Paper (0–8039–3568–4)

Experimental Design and Analysis. Steven R. Brown and Lawrence E. Melamed, 1990
Paper (0–8039–3854–3)

Metric Scaling: Correspondence Analysis. Susan C. Weller and A. Kimball Romney, 1990
Paper (0–8039–3750–4)

Basic Content Analysis (2nd edition). Robert Philip Weber, 1990
Paper (0–8039–3863–2)

Expert Systems. Robert A. Benfer, Edward E. Brent Jr. and Louanna Furbee, 1991
Paper (0–8039–4036–X)

Data Theory and Dimensional Analysis. William G. Jacoby, 1991
Paper (0–8039–4178–1)

Regression Diagnostics: an Introduction. John Fox, 1991
Paper (0–8039–3971–X)

Computer-assisted Interviewing. Willem E. Saris, 1991
Paper (0–8039–4066–1)

Contextual Analysis. Gudmund R. Iversen, 1991
Paper (0–8039–4272–9)

Summated Rating Scale Construction: an Introduction. Paul E. Spector, 1992
Paper (0–8039–4341–5)

Central Tendency and Variability. Herbert F. Weisberg, 1992
Paper (0–8039–4007–6)

ANOVA: Repeated Measures. Ellen R. Girden, 1992
Paper (0–8039–4257–5)

Processing Data: the Survey Example. Linda B. Bourque and Virginia A. Clark, 1992
Paper (0–8039–4741–0)

Logit Modeling: Practical Applications. Alfred DeMaris, 1992
Paper (0–8039–4377–6)

Analytic Mapping and Geographic Databases. G. David Garson and Robert S. Biggs, 1992
Paper (0–8039–4752–6)

Working with Archival Data: Studying Lives. Glen H. Elder Jr., Eliza K. Pavalko and Elizabeth C. Clipp, 1992
Paper (0–8039–4262–1)

Multiple Comparison Procedures. Larry E. Toothaker, 1992
Paper (0–8039–4177–3)

Nonparametric Statistics: an Introduction. Jean Dickinson Gibbons, 1992
Paper (0–8039–3951–5)

Nonparametric Measures of Association. Jean Dickinson Gibbons, 1993
Paper (0–8039–4664–3)

Understanding Regression Assumptions. William D. Berry, 1993
Paper (0–8039–4263-X)

Regression with Dummy Variables. Melissa A. Hardy, 1993
Paper (0–8039–5128–0)

Loglinear Models with Latent Variables. Jacques A. Hagenaars, 1993
Paper (0–8039–4310–5)

Bootstrapping: a Nonparametric Approach to Statistical Inference. Christopher Z. Mooney and Robert D. Duval, 1993
Paper (0–8039–5381-X)

Maximum Likelihood Estimation: Logic and Practice. Scott R. Eliason, 1993
Paper (0–8039–4107–2)

Ordinal Log-Linear Models. Masako Ishii-Kuntz, 1994
Paper (0–8039–4376–8)

Random Factors in ANOVA. Sally E. Jackson and Dale E. Brashers, 1994
Paper (0–8039–5090-X)

Univariate Tests for Time Series Models. Jeff B. Cromwell, Walter C. Labys and Michel Terraza, 1994
Paper (0–8039–4991-X)

Multivariate Tests for Time Series Models. Jeff B. Cromwell, Walter C. Labys, Michael J. Hannan and Michel Terraza, 1994
Paper (0–8039–5440–9)

Interpreting Probability Models: Logit, Probit, and Other Generalized Linear Models. Tim Futing Liao, 1994
Paper (0–8039–4999–5)

Typologies and Taxonomies: an Introduction to Classification Techniques. Kenneth D. Bailey, 1994
Paper (0–8039–5259–7)

Data Analysis: an Introduction. Michael S. Lewis-Beck, 1995
Paper (0–8039–5772–6)

Multiple Attribute Decision Making: an Introduction. K. Paul Yoon and Ching-Lai Hwang, 1995
Paper (0–8039–5486–7)

Causal Analysis with Panel Data. Steven E. Finkel, 1995
Paper (0–8039–3896–9)

Chaos and Catastrophe Theories. Courtney Brown, 1995
Paper (0–8039–5847–1)

Basic Math for Social Scientists: Concepts. Timothy M. Hagle, 1995
Paper (0–8039–5875–7)

Basic Math for Social Scientists: Problems and Solutions. Timothy M. Hagle, 1996
Paper (0–8039–7285–7)

Calculus. Gudmund R. Iversen, 1996
Paper (0–8039–7110–9)

Regression Models: Censored, Sample Selected, or Truncated Data. Richard Breen, 1996
Paper (0–8039–5710–6)

Tree Models of Similarity and Association. James E. Corter, 1996
Paper (0–8039–5707–6)

Computational Modeling. Charles S. Taber and Richard John Timpone, 1996
Paper (0–8039–7270–9)

LISREL Approaches to Interaction Effects in Multiple Regression. James Jaccard and Choi K. Wan, 1996
Paper (0–8039–7179–6)

Analyzing Repeated Surveys. Glenn Firebaugh, 1997
Paper (0–8039–7398–5)

Monte Carlo Simulation. Christopher Z. Mooney, 1997
Paper (0–8039–5943–5)

Statistical Graphics for Univariate and Bivariate Data. William G. Jacoby, 1997
Paper (0–7619–0083–7)

Interaction Effects in Factorial Analysis of Variance. James Jaccard, 1998
Paper (0–7619–1221–5)

Odds Ratios in the Analysis of Contingency Tables. Tam[ac]as Rudas, 1998
Paper (0–7619–0362–3)

Statistical Graphics for Visualizing Multivariate Data. William G. Jacoby, 1998
Paper (0–7619–0899–4)

Applied Correspondence Analysis: an Introduction, Sten Erik Clausen, 1998
Paper (0–7619–1115–4)

Game Theory Topics: Incomplete Information, Repeated Games and N-Player Games. Evelyn C. Fink, Scott Gates and Brian D. Humes, 1998
Paper (0–7619–1016–6)

Social Choice: Theory and Research. Paul E. Johnson, 1998
Paper (0–7619–1406–4)

Neural Networks. Hervé Abdi, Dominique Valentin and Betty Edelman, 1999
Paper only (0–7619–1440–4)

Relating Statistics and Experimental Design. Irwin P. Levin, 1999
Paper only (0–7619–1472–2)

Latent Class Scaling Analysis. C. Mitchell Dayton, 1999
Paper (0–7619–1323–8)

Sorting Data. A.P.M. Coxon, 1999
Paper only (0–8039–7237–7)

Analyzing Documentary Accounts. Randy Hodson, 1999
Paper only (0–7619–1743–8)

Effect Size for ANOVA Designs. Jose M. Cortina and Hossein Nouri, 1999
Paper only (0–7619–1550–8)

Nonparametric Simple Regression. John Fox, 2000
Paper only (0–7619–1585–0)

Logistic Regression. Fred C. Pampel, 2000
Paper only (0–7619–2010–2)

Translating Questionnaires and Other Research Instruments. Orlando Behling and Kenneth S. Law, 2000
Paper only (0–7619–1824–8)

Multiple and Generalized Nonparametric Regression. John Fox, 2000
Paper only (0–7619–2189–3)

Generalized Linear Models. Jeff Gill, 2000
Paper only (0–7619–2055–2)

Interaction Effects in Logistic Regression. James Jaccard, 2001
Paper only (0–7619–2207–5)

Missing Data. Paul D. Allison, 2001
Paper only (0–7619–1672–5)

Applied Logistic Regression Analysis (2nd edition). Scott Menard, 2001
Paper only (0–7619–2208–3)

Spline Regression Models. Lawrence C. Marsh and David R. Cormier, 2001
Paper only (0–7619–2420–5)

Logit and Probit. Vani Kant Borooah, 2002
Paper only (0–7619–2242–3)

Correlation. Peter Y. Chen and Paula M. Popovich, 2002
Paper only (0–7619–2228–8)

Longitudinal Research (2nd edition). Scott Menard, 2002
Paper only (0–7619–2209–1)

Confidence Intervals. Michael J. Smithson, 2003
Paper (0–7619–2499–X)

Interaction Effects in Multiple Regression (2nd edition). James Jaccard, 2003
Paper only (0–7619–2742–5)

Internet Data Collection. Samuel J. Best and Brian S. Krueger, 2004
Paper only (0–7619–2710–7)

Appendix D: Sources of Definitions

'Selection of terms and definitions is difficult because of indistinct lines between methodological issues and philosophical terms and debates.' (*Dictionary of Social Science Methods*, 1983: vii)

Each definition included in this book has been obtained from published papers, glossaries or dictionaries and readers will note the variety of sources. Many different ones could have been included, but the authors have chosen those that appeared to be the most clear and concise.

Section no.	Definition	Author(s)	Page in source text
2.3	Applied research	Polit, D.F. & Hungler, B.P. (1995) *Nursing research: principles and methods* (5th edition). Philadelphia, PA: Lippincott	636
	Basic research	*Dictionary of nursing theory & research* (1995) 2nd edition. Edited by Powers, B.A. & Knapp, T.R. Thousand Oaks, CA: Sage	12
	Clinical research	Denzin, N.K. & Lincoln, Y.S. (eds) (1994) *Handbook of qualitative research*. Thousand Oaks, CA: Sage	342 (adapted)
	Community health nursing research	Hockey, L. (1995) Implications for research: progress, problems and possibilities. *Asian Journal of Nursing Studies* 2 (4) 17–25	17
	Comparative research	Ovretveit, J. (1998) *Cross-cultural nursing: anthropological approaches to nursing research: a practical guide*. Oxford: Radcliffe Medical	6
	Empirical research	Williamson, Y.M. (ed.) (1981) *Research methodology and its application to nursing research*. New York: John Wiley	418
	Fixed-design research	Robson, C. (2000) *Real world research: a resource for social scientists and practitioner-researchers* (2nd edition). Oxford: Blackwell	547
	Flexible-design research	Robson, C. (2000) *Real world research: a resource for social scientists and practitioner-researchers* (2nd edition). Oxford: Blackwell	547
	Methodological research	Baker, M.R. & Kirk, S. (eds) *Research and development for the NHS: evidence, evaluation and effectiveness* (3rd edition). Oxford: Radcliffe Medical Press	187
	Nursing research	Hockey, L. (1995) Implications for research: progress, problems and possibilities. *Asian Journal of Nursing Studies* 2 (4) 17–25	17
	Research	Hockey, L. (1995) Implications for research: progress, problems and possibilities. *Asian Journal of Nursing Studies* 2 (4) 17–25	17
	Research methodology	Abdellah, F.G. & Levine, E. (1994) *Preparing nursing research for the 21st century: evolution, methodologies, challenges*. New York: Springer	157

Sec-tion no.	Definition	Author(s)	Page in source text
	Research-mindedness	Royal College of Nursing of the United Kingdom (1982) *Research mindedness and nurse education*. London: RCN	not known
2.4	Research approaches	Abdellah, F.G. & Levine, E. (1994) *Preparing nursing research for the 21st century: evolution, methodologies, challenges*. New York: Springer	25
	Research processess	Treece, E.W. & Treece, J.W. Jr (1986) *Elements of research in nursing* (4th edition). St Louis, MO: Mosby	510
2.5	Cartesianism	*The Oxford English dictionary* (2002) 2nd edition on CDROM Version 3.0. Oxford University Press Electronic Publishing Department ISBN 0198613423	
	Concept	Nieswiadomy, R.M. (2002) *Foundations of nursing research* (4th edition). Upper Saddle River, NJ: Prentice-Hall	357
	Conceptual framework	Nieswiadomy, R.M. (2002) *Foundations of nursing research* (4th edition). Upper Saddle River, NJ: Prentice-Hall	357
	Conceptual model	Nieswiadomy, R.M. (2002) *Foundations of nursing research* (4th edition). Upper Saddle River, NJ: Prentice-Hall	357
	Constructivism	Schwandt, T.A. (1997) *Qualitative inquiry: a dictionary of terms*. Thousand Oaks, CA: Sage	19–20
	Critical realism	Collier, A. (1994) *Critical realism: an introduction to Roy Bhaskar's philosophy*. London: Verso	24
	Hermeneutics	*New international Webster's comprehensive dictionary of the English language* (1996) Naples, FL: Trident Press International	591
	Modernism	*Blackwell dictionary of sociology: a user's guide to sociological language* (1995). Edited by Johnson, A.G. Oxford: Blackwell	182
	Ontology	*Blackwell dictionary of sociology: a user's guide to sociological language* (1995). Edited by Johnson, A.G. Oxford: Blackwell	195
	Operationalization	Baker, T.L. (1994) *Doing social research* (2nd edition). New York: McGraw-Hill	479
	Paradigm	*Blackwell dictionary of sociology: a user's guide to sociological language* (1995). Edited by Johnson, A.G. Oxford: Blackwell	296
	Philosophy	*Reader's Digest universal dictionary* (1987) London: Reader's Digest Association	1161
	Positivism	Blackwell dictionary of sociology: *a user's guide to sociological language* (1995). Edited by Johnson, A.G. Oxford: Blackwell	207
	Positivist	*The Oxford English Dictionary* (2002) 2nd edition on CDROM Version 3.0. Oxford University Press Electronic Publishing Department ISBN 0198613423	
	Post-modern thought	*The Oxford English Dictionary* (2002) 2nd edition on CDROM Version 3.0. Oxford University Press Electronic Publishing Department ISBN 0198613423	

Sec-tion no.	Definition	Author(s)	Page in source text
	Post-modernism	Ward, G. (1997) *Postmodernism*. London: Hodder Headline	1
	Post-positivism	Schwandt, T.A. (1997) *Qualitative Inquiry: dictionary of terms*. Thousand Oaks, CA: Sage	121
	Post-structuralism	*Encylopedia of feminist theories* (2000). Edited by Code, L. London: Routledge	397
	Realism	*Blackwell dictionary of sociology: a user's guide to sociological language* (1995). Edited by Johnson, A.G. Oxford: Blackwell	226
	Relativism	*New international Webster's comprehensive dictionary of the English language* (1996) Naples, FL: Trident Press International	1063
	Spatial ability	McVey, M.D. (2001) Understanding concepts in research methodology: the role of spatial ability. *Research in Education* 65 May 100–2	101
	Structuralism	Schwandt, T.A. (1997) *Qualitative inquiry: a dictionary of terms*. Thousand Oaks, CA: Sage	146–7
2.6	Empiricism	Thompson, I.E., Melia, K.M. & Boyd, K.M. (2000) *Nursing ethics* (4th edition). Edinburgh: Churchill Livingstone	364
	Epistemology	*Dictionary of nursing theory and research* (1995) 2nd edition. Edited by Powers, B.A. & Knapp, T.R. Thousand Oaks, CA: Sage	51
	Human Becoming Theory	Parse, R.R. (1997) Transforming research and practice with the human becoming theory. *Nursing Science Quarterly* 10 (4) 171–4	171
	Praxis	*Reader's Digest universal dictionary* (1987) London: Reader's Digest Association	1212
	Science of unitary human beings	Gunther, M.E. Marriner-Tomey, A. & Alligood, M.R. (2001) *Nursing theorists and their work* (5th edition). St Louis, MO: Mosby	228
2.7	Chaos theory	Lett, M. (2001) A case for chaos theory in nursing. *Australian Journal of Advanced Nursing* 18 (3) 14–19	15
	Critical theory	*Blackwell dictionary of sociology: a user's guide to sociological language* (1995). Edited by Johnson, A.G. Oxford: Blackwell	61
	Facet theory	Breakwell, G.M., Hammond, S. & Fife-Schaw, C. (eds) (2000) *Research methods in psychology* (2nd edition). London: Sage	116
	Functionalism	Schwandt, T.A. (1997) *Qualitative inquiry: a dictionary of terms*. Thousand Oaks, CA: Sage	56
	Grand theories	Nieswiadomy, R.M. (2002) *Foundations of nursing research*. (4th edition). Upper Saddle River, NJ: Prentice-Hall	360
	Middle-range theory	Nieswiadomy, R.M. (2002) *Foundations of nursing research* (4th edition). Upper Saddle River, NJ: Prentice-Hall	363
	Reductionism	Thompson, I.E., Melia, K.M. & Boyd, K.M. (2000) *Nursing ethics* (4th edition). Edinburgh: Churchill Livingstone	368

Sec- tion no.	Definition	Author(s)	Page in source text
	Taxonomy	*Reader's Digest universal dictionary* (1987) London: Reader's Digest Association	1551
	Theoretical frameworks	*Dictionary of social science methods* (1990) Edited by Miller, P.McC. & Wilson, M.J. Chichester: John Wiley	112
	Theoretical substruction	McQuiston, C.M. & Campbell, J.C. (1997) Theoretical substruction: a guide for theory testing research. *Nursing Science Quarterly* 10 117–23	117
	Theory	*Dictionary of nursing theory and research* (1995) 2nd edition. Edited by Powers, B.A. & Knapp, T.R. Thousand Oaks, CA: Sage	170
2.8	Applied science	*Dictionary of nursing theory and research* (1995) 2nd edition. Edited by Powers, B.A. & Knapp, T.R. Thousand Oaks, CA: Sage	157
	Basic science	*Dictionary of nursing theory and research* (1995) 2nd edition. Edited by Powers, B.A. & Knapp, T.R. Thousand Oaks, CA: Sage	157
	Deductive reasoning	*Dictionary of nursing theory and research* (1995) 2nd edition. Edited by Powers, B.A. & Knapp, T.R. Thousand Oaks, CA: Sage	64
	Inductive reasoning	Polit, D.F. & Hungler, B.P. (1995) *Nursing Research: principles and methods* (5th edition). Philadelphia, PA: Lippincott	643
	Objectivity	Thompson, I.E., Melia, K.M. & Boyd, K.M. (2000) *Nursing ethics* (4th edition). Edinburgh: Churchill Livingstone	369
	Science	*Dictionary of nursing theory and research* (1995) 2nd edition. Edited by Powers, B.A. & Knapp, T.R. Thousand Oaks, CA: Sage	157
	Scientific method	Williamson, Y.M. (ed.) (1981) *Research methodology and its application to nursing*. New York: John Wiley	424
	Scientism	*New international Webster's comprehensive dictionary of the English language* (1996) Naples, FL: Trident Press International	1127
	Subjectivity	Thompson, I.E., Melia, K.M. & Boyd, K.M. (2000) *Nursing ethics* (4th edition). Edinburgh: Churchill Livingstone	369
2.9	Qualitative research	Bryman, A. (1992) *Quantity and quality in social research*. London: Routledge	94
	Quantitative research	Bryman, A. (1992) *Quantity and quality in social research*. London: Routledge	94

Section no.	Definition	Author(s)	Page in source text
2.10	Feminism	*Encyclopedia of feminist theories* (2000). Edited by Code, L. London: Routledge	195
	Feminist research	*Dictionary of nursing theory and research* (1995) 2nd edition. Edited by Powers, B.A. & Knapp, T.R. Thousand Oaks, CA: Sage	65
2.11	New paradigm research	Reason, P. & Rowan, J. (eds) (1981) *Human inquiry: sourcebook of new paradigm research*. Chichester: Wiley	Back cover
2.12	Cochrane review	Clarke, M. & Oxman, A. (eds) (2002) *The Cochrane reviewers' handbook glossary*. Version 4.1.4 [Updated March 2001] In The Cochrane Library Issue 2. Oxford: Update Software. Updated Quarterly	5
	ejournals	Nieswiadomy, R.M. (2002) *Foundations of nursing research*. (4th edition). Upper Saddle River, NJ: Prentice-Hall	81
	ezines	Nieswiadomy, R.M. (2002) *Foundations of nursing research* (4th edition). Upper Saddle River, NJ: Prentice-Hall	81
	Grey literature	Earl-Slater, A. (2002) *The handbook of clinical trials and other research*. Oxford: Radcliffe Medical Press	147
	Integrative literature review	Stevens, K.R. & Cassidy, V. (eds) (1999) *Evidence-based teaching: current research in nursing education*. Sudbury, MA: Jones & Bartlett	11
	Literature review	Stevens, K.R. & Cassidy, V. (eds) *Evidence-based teaching: current research in nursing education*. Sudbury, MA: Jones & Bartlett	11
	Primary source	Nieswiadomy, R.M. (2002) *Foundations of nursing research* (4th edition). Upper Saddle River, NJ: Prentice-Hall	366
	Secondary source	Nieswiadomy, R.M. (2002) *Foundations of nursing research* (4th edition). Upper Saddle River, NJ: Prentice-Hall	368
	Systematic review	Stevens, K.R. & Cassidy, V. (eds) *Evidence-based teaching: current research in nursing education*. Sudbury, MA: Jones & Bartlett	11
2.13	Replication study	Nieswiadomy, R.M. (2002) *Foundations of nursing research* (4th edition). Upper Saddle River, NJ: Prentice-Hall	367
2.14	Gatekeeper	Oliver, P. (1997) *Research for business, marketing and education*. London: Hodder & Stoughton	186
	Research protocol	*Dictionary of nursing theory and research* (1995) 2nd edition. Edited by Powers, B.A. & Knapp, T.R. Thousand Oaks, CA: Sage	131
2.15	Collaborative research	*New international Webster's comprehensive dictionary of the English language* (1996) Naples, FL: Trident Press International	257
	Cross-disciplinary research	Epton, S.R., Payne, R.L. & Pearson, A.W. (eds) (1983) *Managing inter-disciplinary research*. Chichester: Wiley	9

Sec-tion no.	Definition	Author(s)	Page in source text
	Multi- and interdisciplinary research	Epton, S.R., Payne, R.L. & Pearson, A.W. (eds) (1983) *Managing inter-disciplinary research*. Chichester: Wiley	9
	Networking	*Reader's Digest universal dictionary* (1987) London: Reader's Digest Association	1036
2.17	Anonymity	Baker, T.L. (1994) *Doing social research* (2nd edition). New York: McGraw-Hill	473
	Autonomy	*Reader's Digest universal dictionary* (1987) London: Reader's Digest Association	116
	Beneficence	Thompson, I.E., Melia, K.M. & Boyd, K.M. (2000) *Nursing ethics* (4th edition). Edinburgh: Churchill Livingstone	363
	Confidentiality	Williamson, Y.M. (ed.) (1981) *Research methodology and its application to nursing*. New York: John Wiley	416
	Covert research	Baker, T.L. (1994) *Doing social research* (2nd edition). New York: McGraw-Hill	474
	Deception	Medical Research Council of Canada (1987) *Guidelines on research involving human subjects*. Ottawa: Supplies and Services, Canada	26
	Equipoise	Earl-Slater, A. (2002) *The handbook of clinical trials and other research.* Oxford: Radcliffe Medical Press	124
	Ethics	Williamson, Y.M. (ed.) (1981) *Research methodology and its application to nursing*. New York: John Wiley	416
	Informed consent	*Dictionary of nursing theory and research* (1995) 2nd edition. Edited by Powers, B.A. & Knapp, T.R. Thousand Oaks, CA: Sage	86
	Institutional Review Boards	Polit, D.F. & Hungler, B.P. (1995) *Nursing research: principles and methods* (5th edition). Philadelphia, PA: Lippincott	643
	Interference	Commission on Research Integrity (1995) *Integrity and misconduct in research. Report of the Commission on Research Integrity*. Washington, DC: US Department of Health and Human Services	15
	Justice	*New international Webster's comprehensive dictionary of the English language* (1996) Naples, FL: Trident Press International	693
	Maleficence	*The Oxford English Dictionary* (2002) 2nd edition on CDROM Version 3.0. Oxford University Press Electronic Publishing Department ISBN 0198613423	
	Misappropriation	Commission on Research Integrity (1995) *Integrity and misconduct in research. Report of the Commission on Research Integrity*. Washington, DC: US Department of Health and Human Services	15

Sec-tion no.	Definition	Author(s)	Page in source text
	Misrepresentation	Commission on Research Integrity (1995) *Integrity and misconduct in research. Report of the Commission on Research Integrity*. Washington, DC: US Department of Health and Human Services	15–16
	Research misconduct	Commission on Research Integrity (1995) *Integrity and misconduct in research. Report of the Commission on Research Integrity*. Washington, DC: US Department of Health and Human Services	15
2.18	Problem statement	Polit, D.F. & Hungler, B.P. (1995) *Nursing research: principles and methods* (5th edition). Philadelphia, PA: Lippincott	650
2.19	Construct	Williamson, Y.M. (ed.) (1981) *Research methodology and its application to nursing*. New York: John Wiley	416–17
	Dependent variable	Phillips, L.R.F. (1986) *A clinician's guide to the critique and utilization of nursing research*. Norwalk, CT: Appleton-Century-Crofts	456
	Extraneous variable	Williamson, Y.M. (ed.) (1981) *Research methodology and its application to nursing*. New York: John Wiley	419
	Independent variable	Phillips, L.R.F. (1986) *A clinician's guide to the critique and utilization of nursing research*. Norwalk, CT: Appleton-Century-Crofts	458
	Intervening variable	Baker, T.L. (1994) *Doing social research* (2nd edition). New York: McGraw-Hill	477
	Mediating variable	Ovretveit, J. (1998) *Cross-cultural nursing: anthropological approaches to nursing research: a practical guide*. Oxford: Radcliffe Medical Press	114
	Variable	Holm, K. & Llewellyn, J.G. (1986) *Nursing research for nursing practice*. Philadelphia, PA: W.B. Saunders	274
2.20	Alternative hypothesis	*Dictionary of nursing theory and research* (1995) 2nd edition. Edited by Powers, B.A. & Knapp, T.R. Thousand Oaks, CA: Sage	4
	Conceptual definition	Leary, M.R. (2001) *Introduction to behavioral research methods* (3rd edition). Boston, MA: Allyn & Bacon	400
	Critical multiplism	Leary, M.R. (2001) *Introduction to behavioral research methods* (3rd edition). Boston, MA: Allyn & Bacon	400
	Hypothesis	*Dictionary of social science methods* (1990). Edited by Miller, P.McC. & Wilson, M.J. New York: John Wiley	91
	Hypothetico-deductive method	*Blackwell dictionary of sociology: a user's guide to sociological language* (1995). Edited by Johnson, A.G. Oxford: Blackwell	135
	Null hypothesis	Clarke, M. & Oxman, A. (eds) (2002) *The Cochrane reviewers' handbook glossary*. Version 4.1.4 [Updated March 2001] In The Cochrane Library Issue 2. Oxford: Update Software. Updated Quarterly	17

Sec-tion no.	Definition	Author(s)	Page in source text
	Operational definition	Leary, M.R. (2001) *Introduction to behavioral research methods* (3rd edition). Boston, MA: Allyn & Bacon	406
	Research hypothesis	Nieswiadomy, R.M. (2002) *Foundations of nursing research* (4th edition). Upper Saddle River, NJ: Prentice-Hall	368
	Research objective	Bouma, G.D. & Atkinson, G.B.J. (1995) *A handbook of social science research* (2nd edition). Oxford: Oxford University Press	48
2.21	Research design	*Dictionary of social science methods* (1990). Edited by Miller, P.McC. & Wilson, M.J. New York: John Wiley	72
2.22	Cluster sample	Williamson, Y.M. (ed.) (1981) *Research methodology and its application to nursing.* New York: John Wiley	171
	Convenience (accidental) sample	Williamson, Y.M. (ed.) (1981) *Research methodology and its application to nursing.* New York: John Wiley	171
	Population	Williamson, Y.M. (ed.) (1981) *Research methodology and its application to nursing.* New York: John Wiley	171
	Population element	Williamson, Y.M. (ed.) (1981) *Research methodology and its application to nursing.* New York: John Wiley	171
	Population stratum	Williamson, Y.M. (ed.) (1981) *Research methodology and its application to nursing.* New York: John Wiley	171
	Purposive sample	Williamson, Y.M. (ed.) (1981) *Research methodology and its application to nursing.* New York: John Wiley	172
	Quota sample	Williamson, Y.M. (ed.) (1981) *Research methodology and its application to nursing.* New York: John Wiley	172
	Sampling	*Dictionary of nursing theory and research* (1995) 2nd edition. Edited by Powers, B.A. & Knapp, T.R. Thousand Oaks, CA: Sage	164
	Sampling error	Earl-Slater, A. (2002) The *Handbook of clinical trials and other research.* Oxford: Radcliffe Medical Press	307
	Simple random sample	Williamson, Y.M. (ed.) (1981) *Research methodology and its application to nursing.* New York: John Wiley	172
	Snowball sample	Williamson, Y.M. (ed.) (1981) *Research methodology and its application to nursing.* New York: John Wiley	172
	Stratified random sample	Williamson, Y.M. (ed.) (1981) *Research methododology and its application to nursing* New York: John Wiley	172
	Subject	*Dictionary of nursing theory and research* (1995) 2nd edition. Edited by Powers, B.A. & Knapp, T.R. Thousand Oaks, CA: Sage	164
	Systematic random sample	Williamson, Y.M. (ed.) (1981) *Research methodology and its application to nursing.* New York: John Wiley	172
	Target population	Williamson, Y.M. (ed.) (1981) *Research methodology and its application to nursing.* New York: John Wiley	171

Sec-tion no.	Definition	Author(s)	Page in source text
	Universe	Williamson, Y.M. (ed.) (1981) *Research methodology and its application to nursing*. New York: John Wiley	172
2.23	Feasibility study/tests	Smith, C.E., Cha, J.J., Kleinbeck, S.V.M., Clements, F.A., Cook, D. & Koehler, J. (2002) Feasibility of in-home telehealth for conducting nursing research. *Clinical Nursing Research* 11 (2) 220–33	223
	Pilot study	*Dictionary of social science methods* (1990). Edited by Miller, P.McC. & Wilson, M.J. New York: John Wiley	97
2.24	Inter-rater (inter-observer) reliability	Polit, D.F. & Hungler, B.P. (1995) *Nursing research: principles and methods* (5th edition). Philadelphia, PA: Lippincott	705
	Intra-observer (rater) reliability	Litwin, M.S. (1995) *How to measure reliability and validity. Volume 7: The Survey Kit*. Thousand Oaks, CA: Sage	83
	Reliability	*Dictionary of social science methods* (1990). Edited by Miller, P.McC. & Wilson, M.J .New York: John Wiley	96
	Split-half reliability	Leininger, M.M. (1985) *Qualitative research methods in nursing*. Orlando, FL: Grune & Stratton	68
	Test–retest reliability	Holm, K. & Llewellyn, J.G. (1986) *Nursing research for nursing practice*. Philadelphia, PA: W.B. Saunders	270
2.25	Concurrent validity	Polit, D.F. & Hungler, B.P. (1995) *Nursing research: principles and methods* (5th edition). Philadelphia, PA: Lippincott	638
	Construct validity	Leininger, M.M. (1985) *Qualitative research methods in nursing*. Orlando, FL: Grune & Stratton	69
	Content validity	*Dictionary of social science methods* (1990). Edited by Miller, P.McC. & Wilson, M.J. New York: John Wiley	21
	Convergent validity	*Dictionary of social science methods* (1990). Edited by Miller, P.McC. & Wilson, M.J. New York: John Wiley	23
	Criterion-related validity	Phillips, L.R.F. (1986) *A clinician's guide to the critique and utilization of nursing research*. Norwalk, CT: Appleton-Century-Crofts	454
	External validity	Phillips, L.R.F. (1986) *A clinician's guide to the critique and utilization of nursing research*. Norwalk, CT: Appleton-Century-Crofts	455
	Face validity	Black, T.R. (1999) *Doing quantitative research in the social sciences: an integrated approach to research design, measurement and statistics*. London: Sage	195
	Internal validity	Phillips, L.R.F. (1986) *A clinician's guide to the critique and utilization of nursing research*. Norwalk, CT: Appleton-Century-Crofts	457
	Member validation	Miller, G. & Dingwall, R. (eds) (1997) *Context and method in qualitative research*. London: Sage	41

Section no.	Definition	Author(s)	Page in source text
	Predictive validity	Polit, D.F. & Hungler, B.P. (1995) *Nursing research: principles and methods* (5th edition). Philadelphia, PA: Lippincott	649
	Qualitative validity	Leininger, M.M. (1985) *Qualitative research methods in nursing*. Orlando, FL: Grune & Stratton	68
	Validity	Polit, D.F. & Hungler, B.P. (1995) *Nursing research: principles and methods* (5th edition). Philadelphia, PA: Lippincott	656
2.26	Analysis triangulation	Kimchi, J., Polivka, B. & Stevenson, J.S. (1991) Triangulation: operational definitions. *Nursing Research* 40 (6) 364–6	365
	Between-methods triangulation	Rees, C.E. & Bath, P.A. (2001) The use of between-methods triangulation in cancer nursing research: a case study examining information sources for partners of women with breast cancer. *Cancer Nursing* 24 (2) 104–11	104
	Data triangulation	Denzin, N.K. & Lincoln, Y.S. (eds) (1994) *Handbook of qualitative research*. Thousand Oaks, CA: Sage	214 (adapted)
	Interdisciplinary triangulation	Denzin, N.K. & Lincoln, Y.S. (eds) (1994) *Handbook of qualitative research*. Thousand Oaks, CA: Sage	215 (adapted)
	Investigator triangulation	Denzin, N.K. & Lincoln, Y.S. (eds) (1994) *Handbook of qualitative research*. Thousand Oaks, CA: Sage	215 (adapted)
	Methodological triangulation	Denzin, N.K. & Lincoln, Y.S. (eds) (1994) *Handbook of qualitative research*. Thousand Oaks, CA: Sage	215 (adapted)
	Multiple triangulation	Mitchell, E.S. (1986) Multiple triangulation: a methodology for nursing science. *Advances in Nursing Science* 8 (3) 18–26	23
	Theory triangulation	Denzin, N.K. & Lincoln, Y.S. (eds) (1994) *Handbook of qualitative research*. Thousand Oaks, CA: Sage	215 (adapted)
	Triangulation	*Dictionary of social science methods* (1990). Edited by Miller, P.McC. & Wilson, M.J. New York: John Wiley	102
2.27	Attrition bias	Clarke, M. & Oxman, A.D. (eds) (2003) *Cochrane reviewers' handbook*. Version 4.1.6 [Updated January 2003] In The Cochrane Library Issue 3. Oxford: Update Software. Updated Quarterly	42
	Bias	Gillis, A. & Jackson, W. (2002) *Research for nurses: methods and interpretation*. Philadelphia, PA: F.A. Davis	298
	Detection bias	Clarke, M. & Oxman, A.D. (eds) (2003) *Cochrane reviewers' handbook*. Version 4.1.6 [Updated January 2003] In The Cochrane Library Issue 3. Oxford: Update Software. Updated Quarterly	42–3
	Methodological quality	Clarke, M. & Oxman, A. (eds) (2002) *The Cochrane reviewers' handbook glossary*. Version 4.1.4 [Updated March 2001] In The Cochrane Library Issue 2. Oxford: Update Software. Updated Quarterly	16

Section no.	Definition	Author(s)	Page in source text
	Observational bias	*Encyclopedia of feminist theories* (2000). Edited by Code, L. London: Routledge	41
	Performance bias	Clarke, M. & Oxman, A.D. (eds) (2003) *Cochrane reviewers' handbook*. Version 4.1.6 [Updated January 2003] In The Cochrane Library Issue 3. Oxford: Update Software. Updated Quarterly	42
	Research bias	Gillis, A. & Jackson, W. (2002) *Research for nurses: methods and interpretation*. Philadelphia, PA: F.A. Davis	298
	Selection bias	Clarke, M. & Oxman, A.D. (eds) (2003) *Cochrane reviewers' handbook*. Version 4.1.6 [Updated January 2003] In The Cochrane Library Issue 3. Oxford: Update Software. Updated Quarterly	40
2.28	Empirical generalization	Ritchie, J. & Lewis, J. (2003) *Qualitative research practice: a guide for social science students*. London: Sage	264
	Fuzzy generalization	Bassey, M. (1999) *Case study research in educational settings*. Buckingham: Open University Press	12
	Generalizability	Clarke, M. & Oxman, A. (eds) (2002) *The Cochrane reviewers' handbook glossary*. Version 4.1.4 [Updated March 2001] In The Cochrane Library Issue 2. Oxford: Update Software. Updated Quarterly	12
	Inferential generalization	Ritchie, J. & Lewis, J. (2003) *Qualitative research practice: a guide for social science students*. London: Sage	267
	Representational generalization	Ritchie, J. & Lewis, J. (2003) *Qualitative research practice: a guide for social science students*. London: Sage	268
	Scientific generalization	Bassey, M. (1999) *Case study research in educational settings*. Buckingham: Open University Press	12
	Statistical generalization	Bassey, M. (1999) *Case study research in educational settings*. Buckingham: Open University Press	45
	Theoretical generalization	Ritchie, J. & Lewis, J. (2003) *Qualitative research practice: a guide for social science students*. London: Sage	264
	Theory building	Ritchie, J. & Lewis, J. (2003) *Qualitative research practice: a guide for social science students*. London: Sage	264
2.29	CONSORT	Earl-Slater, A. (2002) *The handbook of clinical trials and other research*. Oxford: Radcliffe Medical Press	84
	Control group	Phillips, L.R.F. (1986) *A clinician's guide to the critique and utilization of nursing research*. Norwalk, CT: Appleton-Century-Crofts	462
	Controlled clinical trial	Clarke, M. & Oxman, A. (eds) (2002) *The Cochrane reviewers' handbook glossary*. Version 4.1.4 [Updated March 2001] In The Cochrane Library Issue 2. Oxford: Update Software. Updated Quarterly	8

Sec-tion no.	Definition	Author(s)	Page in source text
	Cross-over trial	Clarke, M. & Oxman, A. (eds) (2002) *The Cochrane reviewers' handbook glossary*. Version 4.1.4 [Updated March 2001] In The Cochrane Library Issue 2. Oxford: Update Software. Updated Quarterly	8
	Double-blind trial	*Dictionary of social science methods* (1990). Edited by Miller, P.McC. & Wilson, M.J. New York: John Wiley	34
	Dual-blind trial	Caspi, O., Millen, C. & Sechrest, L. (2000) Integrity and research: introducing the concept of dual blindness. How blind are double-blind clinical trials in alternative medicine? *Journal of Alternative and Complementary Medicine 6 (6) 493–8*	493
	Experiment	Holm, K. & Llewellyn, J.G. (1986) *Nursing research for nursing practice*. Philadelphia, PA: W.B. Saunders	262
	Multi-centre trials	Abdellah, F.G. & Levine, E. (1994) *Preparing nursing research for the 21st century: evolution, methodologies, challenges*. New York: Springer	67
	Placebo	Clarke, M. & Oxman, A. (eds) (2002) *The Cochrane reviewers' handbook glossary*. Version 4.1.4 [Updated March 2001] In The Cochrane Library Issue 2. Oxford: Update Software. Updated Quarterly	19
	Placebo effect	Clarke, M. & Oxman, A. (eds) (2002) *The Cochrane reviewers' handbook glossary*. Version 4.1.4 [Updated March 2001] In The Cochrane Library Issue 2. Oxford: Update Software. Updated Quarterly	19
	Randomized clinical trial	Abdellah, F.G. & Levine, E. (1994) *Preparing nursing research for the 21st century: evolution, methodologies, challenges*. New York: Springer	76
	Run-in period	Clarke, M. & Oxman, A. (eds) (2002) *The Cochrane reviewers' handbook glossary*. Version 4.1.4 [Updated March 2001] In The Cochrane Library Issue 2. Oxford: Update Software. Updated Quarterly	24
	Sequential trial	Clarke, M. & Oxman, A. (eds) (2002) *The Cochrane reviewers' handbook glossary*. Version 4.1.4 [Updated March 2001] In The Cochrane Library Issue 2. Oxford: Update Software. Updated Quarterly	25
	Single-blind trial	Clarke, M. & Oxman, A. (eds) (2002) *The Cochrane reviewers' handbook glossary*. Version 4.1.4 [Updated March 2001] In The Cochrane Library Issue 2. Oxford: Update Software. Updated Quarterly	25
	Tracker trials	Lilford, R.J., Braunholtz, D.A., Gennhalgh, R. & Edwards, S.J.L. (2000) Trials and fast-changing technologies: the case for tracker studies. *British Medical Journal 320 (7226)* 1 January 43–6	1–2

Sect ion no.	Definition	Author(s)	Page in source text
	Trials register	Clarke, M. & Oxman, A. (eds) (2002) *The Cochrane reviewers' handbook glossary*. Version 4.1.4 [Updated March 2001] In The Cochrane Library Issue 2. Oxford: Update Software. Updated Quarterly	27
	Zelen consent design	Homer, C.S.E. (2002) Using the Zelen design in randomized controlled trials: debate and controversies. *Journal of Advanced Nursing* 38 (2) 200–7	200
2.33	Factorial designs	*Dictionary of statistics and methodology: a non-technical guide for the social sciences* (1993). Edited by Vogt, W.P. Newbury Park, CA: Sage	90
2.34	Single-case design	Polgar, S. & Thomas, S.A. (1991) *Introduction to research in the health sciences* (2nd edition). Melbourne: Churchill Livingstone	84
2.35	Interrupted time-series designs	Woods, N.F. & Catanzaro, M. (1988) *Nursing research theory and practice*. St Louis, MO: Mosby	564
	Non-equivalent control group	Woods, N.F. & Catanzaro, M. (1988) *Nursing research theory and practice*. St Louis, MO: Mosby	564
	Quasi-experiment	Woods, N.F. & Catanzaro, M. (1988) *Nursing research theory and practice*. St Louis, MO: Mosby	564
2.36	Bricolage	Schwandt, T.A. (1997) *Qualitative inquiry: a dictionary of terms*. Thousand Oaks, CA: Sage	10–11
	Bricoleur	Schwandt, T.A. (1997) *Qualitative inquiry: a dictionary of terms*. Thousand Oaks, CA: Sage	10–11
	Field experiment	Baker, T.L. (1994) *Doing social research* (2nd edition). New York: McGraw-Hill	476
	Field notes	Polit, D.F. & Hungler, B.P. (1995) *Nursing research: principles and methods* (5th edition). Philadelphia, PA: Lippincott	642
	Field study	Polit, D.F. & Hungler, B.P. (1995) *Nursing research: principles and methods* (5th edition). Philadelphia, PA: Lippincott	642
	Fieldwork	*Dictionary of nursing theory and research* (1995) 2nd edition. Edited by Powers, B.A. & Knapp, T.R. Thousand Oaks, CA: Sage	69
	Imagework method	Edgar, I.R. (1999) The imagework method in health and social sciences research. *Qualitative Health Research* 9 (2) 198–211	199
	Interactionism	*New international Webster's comprehensive dictionary of the English language* (1996) Naples, FL: Trident Press International	661
	Naturalistic inquiry	Schwandt, T.A. (1997) *Qualitative inquiry: a dictionary of terms*. Thousand Oaks, CA: Sage	101
	Qualitative research	Denzin, N.K. & Lincoln, Y.S. (eds) (1994) *Handbook of qualitative research*. Thousand Oaks, CA: Sage	2

Section no.	Definition	Author(s)	Page in source text
	Queer theory	Jary, D. & Jary, J. (2000) *Collins dictionary of sociology* (3rd edition). Glasgow: Harper Collins	501
	Theme	De Santis, L. & Ugarriza, D.N. (2000) The concept of theme as used in qualitative nursing research. *Western Journal of Nursing Research* 22 (3) 351–72	362
	Trajectory model	Weiner, C., Strauss, A.L., Fagerhaug, S. & Suczek, B. (1997). Trajectories biographies and the evolving medical technical scene – labor and delivery and the intensive care nursery. In strauss, A.L. & Corbin, J. (eds) *Grounded theory in practice*. Thousand Oaks, CA: Sage. Chapter 9	229–50
2.37	Action research	*Dictionary of social science methods* (1990). Edited by Miller, P.McC. & Wilson, M.J. New York: John Wiley	119
	Participatory action research	Atweh, B., Kemmis, S. & Weeks, P. (eds) *Action research in practice: partnerships for social justice in education*. London: Routledge	23
2.38	Atheoretical research	Phillips, L.R.F. (1986) A *clinician's guide to the critique and utilization of nursing research*. Norwalk, CT: Appleton-Century-Crofts	453
2.39	Case study	Polit, D.F. & Hungler, B.P. (1995) *Nursing research: principles and methods* (5th edition). Philadelphia, PA: Lippincott	636
2.40	Causal comparative	*Dictionary of nursing theory and research* (1995) 2nd edition. Edited by Powers, B.A. & Knapp, T.R. Thousand Oaks, CA: Sage	20
	Correlational research	Polit, D.F. & Hungler, B.P. (1995) *Nursing research: principles and methods* (5th edition). Philadelphia, PA: Lippincott	638–9
2.41	Case control study	*Dictionary of nursing theory and research* (1995) 2nd edition. Edited by Powers, B.A. & Knapp, T.R. Thousand Oaks, CA: Sage	17
	Cross-sectional study	Clarke, M. & Oxman, A. (eds) (2002) *The Cochrane reviewers' handbook glossary*. Version 4.1.4 [Updated March 2001] In The Cochrane Library Issue 2. Oxford: Update Software. Updated Quarterly	8
	Epidemiological research	*Dictionary of nursing theory and research* (1995) 2nd edition. Edited by Powers, B.A. & Knapp, T.R. Thousand Oaks, CA: Sage	50
	Epidemiology	Clarke, M. & Oxman, A. (eds) (2002) *The Cochrane reviewers' handbook glossary*. Version 4.1.4 [Updated March 2001] In The Cochrane Library Issue 2. Oxford: Update Software. Updated Quarterly	11
	Retrospective study	Clarke, M. & Oxman, A. (eds) (2002) *The Cochrane reviewers' handbook glossary*. Version 4.1.4 [Updated March 2001] In The Cochrane Library Issue 2. Oxford: Update Software. Updated Quarterly	23
2.42	Culture	Hodgson, I. (2001) Engaging with cultures: reflections on entering the ethnographic field. *Nurse Researcher* 9 (1) 41–51	42

Section no.	Definition	Author(s)	Page in source text
	Emic	*Dictionary of nursing theory and research* (1995) 2nd edition. Edited by Powers, B.A. & Knapp, T.R. Thousand Oaks, CA: Sage	49
	Ethnography	Leininger, M.M. (1985) *Qualitative research methods in nursing*. Orlando, FL: Grune & Stratton	35
	Ethnology	Schwandt, T.A. (1997) *Qualitative inquiry: a dictionary of terms*. Thousand Oaks, CA: Sage	44
	Ethnomethodology	Schwandt, T.A. (1997) *Qualitative inquiry: a dictionary of terms*. Thousand Oaks, CA: Sage	44
	Ethnonursing	Leininger, M.M. (1985) *Qualitative research methods in nursing*. Orlando, FL: Grune & Stratton	38
	Ethnoscience	Leininger, M.M. (1985) *Qualitative research methods in nursing*. Orlando, FL: Grune & Stratton	237
	Ethology	Morse, J.M. & Field, P.A. (1996) *Nursing research: the application of qualitative approaches* (2nd edition). London: Chapman & Hall	23
	Etic	Polit, D.F. & Hungler, B.P. (1995) *Nursing research: principles and methods* (5th edition). Philadelphia, PA: Lippincott	641
	Ideographic research	Jary, D. & Jary, J. (2000) *Collins dictionary of sociology* (3rd edition). Glasgow: Harper Collins	287
	Nomothetic research	Brewer, J.D. (2000) *Ethnography*. Buckingham: Open University Press	190
	Reflexivity	Schwandt, T.A. (1997) *Qualitative inquiry: a dictionary of terms*. Thousand Oaks, CA: Sage	135–6
2.43	Benchmark	*New international Webster's comprehensive dictionary of the English language* (1996) Naples, FL: Trident Press International	129
	Evaluation research	Polit, D.F. & Hungler, B.P. (1995) *Nursing research: principles and methods* (5th edition). Philadelphia, PA: Lippincott	641
	Evidence-based medicine/nursing	Sackett, D.L., Straus, S.E., Richardson, W.S., Rosenberg, W. & Haynes, R.B. (2000) *Evidence-based medicine: how to practice and teach* (2nd edition). Edinburgh: Churchill Livingstone	2
	Gold standard	Clarke, M. & Oxman, A. (eds) (2002) *The Cochrane reviewers' handbook glossary*. Version 4.1.4 [Updated March 2001] In The Cochrane Library Issue 2. Oxford: Update Software. Updated Quarterly	12–13
	Hierarchy of evidence	Earl-Slater, A. (2002) *The handbook of clinical trials and other research*. Oxford: Radcliffe Medical Press	154
	Intervention research	Burns, N. & Grove, S.K. (1999) *Understanding nursing research* (2nd edition). Philadelphia, PA: W.B. Saunders	801
	Outcomes research	Slater, C.H. (1997) What is outcomes research and what can it tell us? *Evaluation and the Health Professions* 20 (3) 243–64	245

Sec-tion no.	Definition	Author(s)	Page in source text
2.44	Ex-post facto research	Baker, T.L. (1994) *Doing social research* (2nd edition). New York: McGraw-Hill	475
2.45	Dimensional analysis	Kools, S., McCarthy, M., Durtham, R. & Robrect, L. (1996) Dimensional analysis: broadening the conception of grounded theory. *Qualitative Health Research* 6 (3) 312–30	314
	Grounded theory	Polit, D.F. & Hungler, B.P. (1995) *Nursing research: principles and methods* (5th edition). Philadelphia, PA: Lippincott	643
	Heuristic research	*Dictionary of nursing theory and research* (1995) 2nd edition. Edited by Powers, B.A. & Knapp, T.R. Thousand Oaks, CA: Sage	79–80
	Symbolic interaction	Lindlof, T.R. (1995) *Qualitative communication research methods*. Thousand Oaks, CA: Sage	40
2.46	External criticism (appraisal, examination)	Nieswiadomy, R.M. (2002) *Foundations of nursing research* (4th edition). Upper Saddle River, NJ: Prentice-Hall	360
	Historical research	Woods, N.F. & Catanzaro, M. (1988) *Nursing research theory and practice*. St Louis, MO: Mosby	558
	Historicism	*Blackwell dictionary of sociology: a user's guide to sociological language* (1995). Edited by Johnson, A.G. Oxford: Blackwell	131
	Historiography	*New international Webster's comprehensive dictionary of the English language* (1996) Naples, FL: Trident Press International	599
	History	*New international Webster's comprehensive dictionary of the English language* (1996) Naples, FL: Trident Press International	599
	Internal criticism	Nieswiadomy, R.M. (2002) *Foundations of nursing research* (4th edition). Upper Saddle River, NJ: Prentice-Hall	361
2.47	Oral history	Grele, R.J. (1998) Movement without aim: methodological and theoretical problems in oral history. In Perks, R. & Thomson, A. (eds) *The oral history reader*. London: Routledge	63
2.48	Cohort	Whitney, J.D. (2000) Comparative, observational designs: case-control and cohort studies. *Journal of the wound, ostomy and continence nurses society* 27 (3) May 191–3	192
	Cohort study	Clarke, M. & Oxman, A. (eds) (2002) *The Cochrane reviewers' handbook glossary*. Version 4.1.4 [Updated March 2001] In The Cochrane Library Issue 2. Oxford: Update Software. Updated Quarterly	6
	Developmental research	Williamson, Y.M. (ed.) (1981) *Research methodology and its application to nursing*. New York: John Wiley	418
	Longitudinal designs	Baker, T.L. (1994) *Doing social research* (2nd edition). New York: McGraw-Hill	477

Sec-tion no.	Definition	Author(s)	Page in source text
2.49	Bracketing	Nieswiadomy, R.M. (2002) *Foundations of nursing research* (4th edition). Upper Saddle River, NJ: Prentice-Hall	356
	Phenomenography	Barnard, A., McCosker, H. & Gerber, R. (1999) Phenomenography: a qualitative research approach for exploring understanding in health care. *Qualitative Health Research* 9 (2) 212–26	212
	Phenomenology	Woods, N.F. & Catanzaro, M. (1988) *Nursing research theory and practice.* St Louis, MO: Mosby	563
2.50	Prescriptive theory	Thomas, C. (2002) TiChi introduction www.cs.umd/edu/class/fall2002/cmsc838s/ tichi/	
2.51	Monte Carlo simulation	*Dictionary of statistics and methodology: a non-technical guide for the social sciences* (1993). Edited by Vogt, W.P. Thousand Oaks, CA: Sage	180
	Role play	*New international Webster's comprehensive dictionary of the English language* (1996) Naples, FL: Trident Press International	1968
	Simulation	*New international Webster's comprehensive dictionary of the English language* (1996) Naples, FL: Trident Press International	2122
2.52	Comparative survey	Treece, E.W. & Treece, J.W. Jr (1986) *Elements of research in nursing* (4th edition). St Louis, MO: Mosby	178–81
	Cross-cultural survey	Treece, E.W. & Treece, J.W. Jr (1986) *Elements of research in nursing* (4th edition). St Louis, MO: Mosby	178–81
	Cross-sectional survey	Treece, E.W. & Treece, J.W. Jr (1986) *Elements of research in nursing* (4th edition). St. Louis, MO: Mosby	178–81
	Evaluation survey	Treece, E.W. & Treece, J.W. Jr (1986) *Elements of research in nursing* (4th edition). St Louis,MO: Mosby	178–81
	Field survey	Treece, E.W. & Treece, J.W. Jr (1986) *Elements of research in nursing* (4th edition). St Louis, MO: Mosby	178–81
	Long-term/longitudinal survey	Treece, E.W. & Treece, J.W. Jr (1986) *Elements of research in nursing* (4th edition). St Louis, MO: Mosby	178–81
	Short-term survey	Treece, E.W. & Treece, J.W. Jr (1986) *Elements of research in nursing* (4th edition). St Louis, MO: Mosby	178–81
	Survey	Phillips, L.R.F. (1986) *A clinician's guide to the critique and utilization of nursing research.* Norwalk, CT: Appleton-Century-Crofts	464
2.53	Cross-cultural analysis	*Encyclopedia of feminist theories* (2000). Edited by Code, L. London: Routledge	111
	Cross-cultural method	Reber, A.S. & Reber, E. (2001) *The Penguin dictionary of psychology* (3rd edition). London: Penguin	167
2.54	Criterion-referenced measures	Woods, N.F. & Catanzaro, M. (1988) *Nursing research theory and practice.* St Louis, MO: Mosby	555
	Measurement	Woods, N.F. & Catanzaro, M. (1988) *Nursing research theory and practice.* St Louis, MO: Mosby	560

Sec-tion no.	Definition	Author(s)	Page in source text
	Norm-referenced measures	Woods, N.F. & Catanzaro, M. (1988) *Nursing research theory and practice.*St Louis, MO: Mosby	562
	Outcome measures	Abdellah, F.G. & Levine, E. (1994) *Preparing nursing research for the 21st century:evolution, methodologies, challenges.* New York: Springer	25
2.55	Instrument	Polit, D.F. & Hungler, B.P. (1995) *Nursing research: principles and methods* (5th edition). Philadelphia, PA: Lippincott	643
	Methodological studies	Nieswiadomy, R.M. (2002) *Foundations of nursing research* (4th edition). Upper Saddle River, NJ: Prentice-Hall	363
2.64	Data	Polit, D.F. & Hungler, B.P. (1995) *Nursing research: principles and methods* (5th edition). Philadelphia, PA: Lippincott	639
	Data cleaning	Earl-Slater, A. (2002) *The handbook of clinical trials and other research.* Oxford: Radcliffe Medical Press	100
	Data collection	Polit, D.F. & Hungler, B.P. (1995) *Nursing research: principles and methods* (5th edition). Philadelphia, PA: Lippincott	639
	Data set	*Dictionary of statistics and methodology: a non-technical guide for the social sciences* (1993). Edited by Vogt, W.P. Newbury Park, CA: Sage	61
	Database	*Dictionary of statistics and methodology: a non-technical guide for the social sciences* (1993). Edited by Vogt, W.P. Newbury Park, CA: Sage	59
	Multiple imputation	Patrician, P.A. (2002) Multiple imputation for missing data. *Research in Nursing and Health* 25 (1) 76–84	79
2.65	Critical incident	Flanagan, J.C. (1954) The critical incident technique. *Psychological Bulletin* 51 (4)	327–58
	Critical incident technique	Flanagan, J.C. (1947) *The Aviation Psychology Program in the Army Air Forces.* AAF Psychology Program Research Report No. 1. Washington, DC: Government Printing Office	No known
2.66	Consensus methods	Jones, J. & Hunter, D. (1995) Nominal group technique (expert panel): consensus methods for medical and health services research. *British Medical Journal* 311 (7001) 376–80	376
	Delphi technique	*Dictionary of nursing theory and research* (1995) 2nd edition. Edited by Powers, B.A. & Knapp, T.R. Thousand Oaks, CA: Sage	41
2.67	Diaries	Field, P.A. & Morse, J.M. (1985) *Nursing research: the application of qualitative approaches.* Rockville, MD: Aspen	85
2.68	Depth interview	*Dictionary of social science methods* (1990). Edited by Miller, P.McC. & Wilson, M.J. New York: John Wiley	62

Sec-tion no.	Definition	Author(s)	Page in source text
	Exploratory interview	*Dictionary of social science methods* (1990). Edited by Miller, P.McC. & Wilson, M.J. New York: John Wiley	62
	Interview	*Dictionary of social science methods* (1990). Edited by Miller, P.McC. & Wilson, M.J. New York: John Wiley	62
	Interview schedule	Baker, T.L. (1994) *Doing social research* (2nd edition). New York: McGraw-Hill	477
	Pilot interview	*Dictionary of social science methods* (1990). Edited by Miller, P.McC. & Wilson, M.J. New York: John Wiley	62
	Semi-structured interview	*Dictionary of social science methods* (1990). Edited by Miller, P.McC. & Wilson, M.J. New York: John Wiley	62
	Shadowed data	Morse, J.M. (2001) Editorial *Qualitative Health Research* 11 (3) 291–2	291
	Standardized/ structured interview	*Dictionary of social science methods* (1990). Edited by Miller, P.McC. & Wilson, M.J. New York: John Wiley	62
	Transcript	Oliver, P. (1997) *Research for business, marketing and education*. London: Hodder & Stoughton	190
2.69	Focus group	Baker, T.L. (1994) *Doing social research* (2nd edition). New York: McGraw-Hill	476
2.70	Telephone interview	Seaman, C.H. (1987) *Research methods: principles, practice and theory for nursing* (3rd edition). Norwalk, CT: Appleton & Lange	433
2.71	Biographical method	Denzin, N.K. (1989) *The research act: a theoretical introduction to sociological methods*. Thousand Oaks, CA: Sage	269
	Biography	*New international Webster's comprehensive dictionary of the English language* (1996) Naples, FL: Trident Press International	139
	Interpretative biography	Cresswell, J.W. (1998) *Qualitative inquiry and research design: choosing among five traditions*. Thousand Oaks, CA: Sage	232
	Life history	Polit, D.F. & Hungler, B.P. (1995) *Nursing research: principles and methods* (5th edition). Philadelphia, PA: Lippincott	645
	Self-report	Grady, K.E. & Wallston, B.S. (1988) *Research in health care settings*. Newbury Park, CA: Sage	112
2.72	Non-participant observation	Seaman, C.H. (1987) *Research methods: principles, practice and theory for nursing* (3rd edition). Norwalk, CT: Appleton & Lange	434
	Observation	Seaman, C.H. (1987) *Research methods: principles, practice and theory for nursing* (3rd edition). Norwalk, CT: Appleton & Lange	434

Section no.	Definition	Author(s)	Page in source text
	Participant observation	Seaman, C.H. (1987) *Research methods: principles, practice and theory for nursing* (3rd edition). Norwalk, CT: Appleton & Lange	434
	Structured observation	www.insightexpress.com/ix/smartTag.asp? chapter = 8	
	Unobtrusive measures	*Blackwell dictionary of sociology: a user's guide to sociological language* (1995). Edited by Johnson, A.G. Oxford: Blackwell	304
	Unstructured observation	Polit, D.F. & Hungler, B.P. (1999) *Nursing research: principles and methods* (6th edition). Philadelphia, PA: Lippincott	717
	Vignettes	Hughes, R. & Huby, M. (2002) The application of vignettes in social and nursing research. *Journal of Advanced Nursing* 37 (4) 382–6	382
2.73	Projective techniques	*Dictionary of social science methods* (1990). Edited by Miller, P.McC. & Wilson, M.J. New York: John Wiley	88
2.74	Q sort	Phillips, L.R.F. (1986) *A clinician's guide to the critique and utilization of nursing research*. Norwalk, CT: Appleton-Century-Crofts	462
2.75	Questionnaire	Holm, K. & Llewellyn, J.G. (1986) *Nursing research for nursing practice*. Philadelphia, PA: W.B. Saunders	270
2.76	Archival research	Baker, T.L. (1994) *Doing social research* (2nd edition). New York: McGraw-Hill	473
	Archives	*New international Webster's comprehensive dictionary of the English language* (1996) Naples, FL: Trident Press International	76
	Records	Treece, E.W. & Treece, J.W. Jr (1986) *Elements of research in nursing* (4th edition). St Louis, MO: Mosby	318
2.77	Personal construct	*Penguin dictionary of psychology* (1985). Edited by Reber, A.S. Harmondsworth: Penguin	532
	Repertory grid	*Lexicon of psychology, psychiatry and psychoanalysis* (1988). Edited by Kuper, L. London: Routledge	298
2.78	Conversation	*Reader's Digest universal dictionary* (1987) London: Reader's Digest Association	347
	Discourse	*Blackwell dictionary of sociology: a user's guide to sociological language* (1995). Edited by Johnson, A.G. Oxford: Blackwell	82
	Narrative	*New international Webster's comprehensive dictionary of the English language* (1996) Naples, FL: Trident Press International	844
	Storyline graph	Sandelowski, M. (1999) Time and qualitative research. *Research in Nursing and Health* 22 (1) 79–87	83
	Talk	*Reader's Digest universal dictionary* (1987) London: Reader's Digest Association	1543

Sec-tion no.	Definition	Author(s)	Page in source text
2.79	Analytic induction	Johnson, P. (1998) Analytic induction. In Symon, G., Cassell, C. (eds) *Qualitative methods and analysis in organizational research: a practical guide*. London: Sage Chapter 3 28–50	28
	Clinical significance	Earl-Slater, A. (2002) *The handbook of clinical trials and other research*. Oxford: Radcliffe Medical Press	57
	Coding	*Blackwell dictionary of sociology: a user's guide to sociological language* (1995). Edited by Johnson, A.G. Oxford: Blackwell	41
	Data analysis	Phillips, L.R.F. (1986) *A clinician's guide to the critique and utilization of nursing research*. Norwalk, CT: Appleton-Century-Crofts	455
	Non-parametric statistics	Portney, L.G. & Watkins, M.P. (1993) *Foundations of clinical research: applications to practice*. Norwalk, CT: Appleton & Lange	687
	Parametric statistics	Portney, L.G. & Watkins, M.P. (1993) *Foundations of clinical research: applications to practice*. Norwalk, CT: Appleton & Lange	688
	Raw data	*Dictionary of social science methods* (1990). Edited by Miller, P.McC. & Wilson, M.J. New York: John Wiley	30
	Statistical significance	Earl-Slater, A. (2002) *The handbook of clinical trials and other research*. Oxford: Radcliffe Medical Press	315
2.81	Descriptive statistics	*Dictionary of social science methods* (1990). Edited by Miller, P.McC. & Wilson, M.J. New York: John Wiley	30
2.82	Inferential statistics	Phillips, L.R.F. (1986) *A clinician's guide to the critique and utilization of nursing research*. Norwalk, CT: Appleton-Century-Crofts	459
2.86	Concept map	www.graphic.org/concept.html	
	Concept mapping	www.graphic.org/concept.html	
	Constant comparison	*Evidence-based Nursing* (1998) 1 (1) Glossary	Inside back cover
	Dramaturgical perspective	*Blackwell dictionary of sociology: a user's guide to sociological language* (1995). Edited by Johnson, A.G. Oxford: Blackwell	87
	Matrix analysis	Bates, A.J. (2002) Matrix analysis as a complementary analytic strategy in qualitative inquiry. *Qualitative Health Research* 12 (6) 855–66	856
	Qualitative analysis	Polit, D.F. & Hungler, B.P. (1995) *Nursing research: principles and methods* (5th edition). Philadelphia, PA: Lippincott	650
	Qualitative meta-synthesis	Sandelowski, M., Docherty, S. & Emden, C. (1997) Focus on qualitative methods. Qualitative meta-synthesis: issues and techniques. *Research in Nursing and Health* 20 (4) 365–71	365–6

Sec-tion no.	Definition	Author(s)	Page in source text
2.87	Event history analysis	Allison, P.D. (1999) *Multiple regression: a primer*. Thousand Oaks, CA: Sage	185
	Exploratory data analysis	*Dictionary of nursing theory and research* (1995) 2nd edition. Edited by Powers, B.A. & Knapp, T.R. Thousand Oaks, CA: Sage	61
	Quantitative data analysis	Polit, D.F. & Hungler, B.P. (1995) *Nursing research: principles and methods* (5th edition). Philadelphia, PA: Lippincott	651
2.88	Content analysis	Polit, D.F. & Hungler, B.P. (1995) *Nursing research: principles and methods* (5th edition). Philadelphia, PA: Lippincott	638
2.89	Categorization analysis	www.sagepub.com/printerfriendly/aspx? pid=6572&ptype=B	
	Contextual analysis	Polit, D.F. & Hungler, B.P. (1995) *Nursing research: principles and methods* (5th edition). Philadelphia, PA: Lippincott	535
	Contextualization	DePoy, E. & Gitlin, L.N. (1994) *Introduction to research: multiple strategies for health and human services*. St Louis, MO: Mosby	296
	Conversation analysis	Heritage, J. (1997) Conversation analysis and institutional talk: analysing data. In Silverman, D. (ed.) *Qualitative research: theory, method and practice*. London: Sage Chapter 11	162
	Dialectical analysis	Harvey, L., MacDonald, M. & Hill, J. (2000) *Theories and methods*. London: Hodder & Stoughton	85
	Discourse analysis	Schwandt, T.A. (1997) *Qualitative inquiry: a dictionary of terms*. Thousand Oaks, CA: Sage	31
	Discourse theory	Schwandt, T.A. (1997) *Qualitative inquiry: a dictionary of terms*. Thousand Oaks, CA: Sage	31
	Network analysis	Miller, G. & Dingwall, R. (eds) (1997) *Context and method in qualitative research*. London: Sage	119
	Semiotics	Schwandt, T.A. (1997) *Qualitative inquiry: a dictionary of terms*. Thousand Oaks, CA: Sage	144
2.90	Primary data analysis	Woods, N.F. & Catanzaro, M. (1988) *Nursing research theory and practice*. St Louis, MO: Mosby	563
2.91	Meta-matrix construction	Wendler, M.C. (2001) Triangulation using a meta-matrix. *Journal of Advanced Nursing* 35 (4) 521–5	522
	Secondary data analysis	Polit, D.F. & Hungler, B.P. (1995) *Nursing research: principles and methods* (5th edition). Philadelphia, PA: Lippincott	653

Section no.	Definition	Author(s)	Page in source text
2.92	Cumulative meta-analysis	Clarke, M. & Oxman, A. (eds) (2002) *The Cochrane reviewers' handbook glossary.* Version 4.1.4 [Updated March 2001] In The Cochrane Library Issue 2. Oxford: Update Software. Updated Quarterly	9
	Meta-analysis	www.nlm.nih.gov/m/metaanal.htm	
	Meta-data analysis	Paterson, B.L., Thorne, S.E., Canam, C. & Jillings, C. (2001) *Meta-study of qualitative health research: a practical guide to meta-analysis and meta-synthesis.* Thousand Oaks, CA: Sage	10
	Meta-method	Paterson, B.L., Thorne, S.E., Canam, C. & Jillings, C. (2001) *Meta-study of qualitative health research: a practical guide to meta-analysis and meta-synthesis.* Thousand Oaks, CA: Sage	10
	Meta-study	Paterson, B.L., Thorne, S.E., Canam, C. & Jillings, C. (2001) *Meta-study of qualitative health research: a practical guide to meta-analysis and meta-synthesis.* Thousand Oaks, CA: Sage	1
	Meta-synthesis	Barroso, J. & Powell-Cope, G.M. (2000) Meta-synthesis of qualitative research on living with HIV infection. *Qualitative Health Research* 10 (3) 340–53	340
	Meta-theory	Paterson, B.L., Thorne, S.E., Canam, C. & Jillings, C. (2001) *Meta-study of qualitative health research: a practical guide to meta-analysis and meta-synthesis.* Thousand Oaks, CA: Sage	13
	QUOROM	Earl-Slater, A. (2002) *The handbook of clinical trials and other research.* Oxford: Radcliffe Medical Press	278
2.95	Evaluating research findings	Phillips, L.R.F. (1986) *A clinician's guide to the critique and utilization of nursing research.* Norwalk, CT: Appleton-Century-Crofts	462
2.96	Research proposal	Abdellah, F.G. & Levine, E. (1994) *Preparing nursing research for the 21st century: evolution, methodologies, challenges.* New York: Springer	392
2.97	Plagiarism	Baker, T.L. (1994) *Doing social research* (2nd edition). New York: McGraw-Hill	479
	Research report	Polit, D.F. & Hungler, B.P. (1995) *Nursing research: principles and methods* (5th edition). Philadelphia, PA: Lippincott	652
2.98	Diffusion	Lomas, J. (1994) Diffusion, dissemination and implementation: who should do what? *Annals of the New York Academy of Sciences* 703 (1)	226–35
	Diffusion of innovations	Jary, D. & Jary, J. (2000) *Collins dictionary of sociology* (3rd edition). Glasgow: Harper Collins	156
	Dissemination	Lomas, J. (1994) Diffusion, dissemination and implementation: who should do what? *Annals of the New York Academy of Sciences* 703 (1)	226–35

Section no.	Definition	Author(s)	Page in source text
2.99	Abstract	Polit, D.F. & Hungler, B.P. (1995) *Nursing research: principles and methods* (5th edition). Philadelphia, PA: Lippincott	635
	Galley proofs	Nieswiadomy, R.M. (2002) *Foundations of nursing research* (4th edition). Upper Saddle River, NJ: Prentice-Hall	360
	Peer review	Clarke, M. & Oxman, A. (eds) (2002) *The Cochrane reviewers' handbook glossary*. Version 4.1.4 [Updated March 2001] In The Cochrane Library Issue 2. Oxford: Update Software. Updated Quarterly	19
	Publication bias	Clarke, M. & Oxman, A. (eds) (2002) *The Cochrane reviewers' handbook glossary*. Version 4.1.4 [Updated March 2001] In The Cochrane Library Issue 2. Oxford: Update Software. Updated Quarterly	21
	Query letter	Nieswiadomy, R.M. (2002) *Foundations of nursing research* (4th edition). Upper Saddle River, NJ: Prentice-Hall	367
	Refereed journal	Polit, D.F. & Hungler, B.P. (1995) *Nursing research: principles and methods* (5th edition). Philadelphia, PA: Lippincott	651
2.101	Research utilization	Holm, K. & Llewellyn, J.G. (1986) *Nursing research for nursing practice*. Philadelphia, PA: W.B. Saunders	271
	Theory change	www.swif.uniba.it/lei/foldop/foldoc.cgi? theory+change	
2.102	Implementing research findings	Phillips, L.R.F. (1986) *A clinician's guide to the critique and utilization of nursing research*. Norwalk, CT: Appleton-Century-Crofts	465
3.7	Journal club	Polit, D.F. & Hungler, B.P. (1995) *Nursing research: principles and methods* (5th edition). Philadelphia, PA: Lippincott	644
3.8	Research/practice gap	Phillips, L.R.F. (1986) *A clinician's guide to the critique and utilization of nursing research*. Norwalk, CT: Appleton-Century-Crofts	463
3.9	Research governance	Earl-Slater, A. (2002) *The handbook of clinical trials and other research*. Oxford: Radcliffe Medical Press	301
3.11	Operational research	Rosenhead, J. (2001) Operational research. In Fulop, N., Allen, P., Clarke, A. & Black, N. (eds) *Studying the organization and delivery of health care services: research methods*. London: Routledge Chapter 10	154
3.16	Research assistant	Williamson, Y.M. (ed.) (1981) *Researchmethodology and its application to nursing*. New York: John Wiley	423
3.18	Research supervisor	Williamson, Y.M. (ed.) (1981) *Research methodology and its application to nursing*. New York: John Wiley	423–4

Appendix E: Buros Institute of Mental Measurements

For over 60 years the Buros Institute of Mental Measurements has worked to serve the public interest and advance the field of measurement. Founded in 1939 by Oscar K. Buros, the Institute is dedicated to monitoring the quality of commercially published tests. In addition to promoting appropriate test selection, use and practice, the Buros Institute works to encourage improved test development and research through thoughtful, critical analysis of individual instruments and the promotion of an open dialogue regarding contemporary measurement issues.

The titles published by the Buros Institute are focused on providing consumers and other test users with accurate evaluations of the usefulness and effectiveness of commercially available tests. Related volumes concerning issues and topics within the field of assessment are also published as part of the Buros Institute catalog.

MEASUREMENTS YEARBOOK AND SUPPLEMENT SERIES

The cornerstone of the Buros Institute's publishing activities is the *Mental Measurements Yearbook* (*MMY*). The *MMY* includes timely, consumer-oriented *test reviews*, providing evaluative information to promote and encourage informed test selection.

Typical *MMY* test entries include descriptive information, one or two professional reviews, and reviewer references. To be reviewed in the *MMY* a test must be commercially available, be published in the English language, and be new, revised, or widely used since it last appeared in the *MMY* series. Beginning in *The Fourteenth Mental Measurements Yearbook*, tests must also provide sufficient documentation supporting their technical quality to meet criteria for review.

Between the years 1988 and 1999, the Buros Institute produced Supplements to the *Ninth* through *Thirteenth Mental Measurements Yearbooks*. Beginning with the *Fourteenth Mental Measurements Yearbook*, volumes in the *MMY* series will be produced every 18 to 24 months and the Supplements will be discontinued.

ELECTRONIC ACCESS TO MENTAL MEASUREMENTS YEARBOOK SERIES

At the Buros Center for Testing's website (*www.unl.edu/buros*), search engines allow you to examine a large amount of information on tests and testing. 'Test Reviews Online' is a web-based service of the Buros Institute of Mental Measurements. Test reviews are available to individual users exactly as they appear in the *Ninth* through *Fifteenth Mental Measurements Yearbook* series. In addition, monthly updates are provided from our latest review database. For a small fee, users may download reviews for over 2,000 tests that include specifics on test purpose, population, publication date, administration time and descriptive test critiques.

The Mental Measurements Yearbook Database currently is available from OVID/SilverPlatter at many academic libraries. Containing the text of the *Ninth* through the *Fifteenth Mental Measurements Yearbooks*, the MMYD is updated every six months to ensure timely access to current information. The MMYD is available to libraries and organizations by subscription and may be provided as a stand-alone service for authorized users.

TESTS IN PRINT

Tests in Print (*TIP*) serves as a comprehensive bibliography to all known commercially available tests that are currently in print in the English language. Now in its sixth edition, *TIP* provides vital information to users, including test purpose, test publisher, in-print status, price, test acronym, intended test population, administration times, publication date(s), and test author(s). A score index permits users to identify what is being measured by each test. *Tests in Print* also guides readers to critical, candid test reviews published in the *Mental Measurements Yearbook* series. *Tests in Print* is an indispensable reference for professionals (including such areas as education, psychology, business) and anyone interested in the critical issues of tests and testing.

BUROS–NEBRASKA SERIES ON MEASUREMENT AND TESTING

Addressing contemporary issues in testing, the *Buros-Nebraska Series on Measurement and Testing* provides a valuable resource for professionals and students in a variety of disciplines. The series identifies movements and concerns affecting the future of measurement, and provides an overview of current thinking and past trends. Each volume in the series focuses on a topic within the assessment field. Individual chapters are authored by noted professionals and address issues relevant to that area. Together the volumes provide unique insight and perspective not found in any other publication or series. (Please note: All titles in this series only are distributed directly through the Buros Institute.)

MENTAL MEASUREMENTS YEARBOOK MONOGRAPHS

Mental Measurements Yearbook Monographs provide a unique historical perspective on the field of measurement. Each volume in the monograph series contains information and test reviews for instruments in a specialized area of testing. The reviews are drawn from the first seven editions in the *Mental Measurements Yearbook* series. A more recent collection of the monograph series is the *Buros Desk Reference* (BDR). These two books include test reviews compiled from the *Sixth* through the *Thirteenth* editions of the *Mental Measurement Yearbook* series in the specialist areas of school psychology and substance abuse.

(Permission has kindly been given by the Buros Institute of Mental Measurements to include the above material from the Publications Catalog on their website. For this we are most grateful. Further information about the publications themselves may be found on www.unl.edu/buros/catalog.html)

Key to Indexes

Author Index

Subject Index

Definitions and their page numbers are shown in **bold type**